Pharmaceutical Dictionary

English · Deutsch · Français · Español

Pharmaceutical Dictionary

English · Deutsch · Français · Español

Anita Maas / James Brawley

Fourth, revised and expanded edition

ECV Editio Cantor Verlag Aulendorf

Bibliografische Information der Deutschen Bibliothek
Die Deutsche Bibliothek verzeichnet diese Publikation in der Deutschen Nationalbibliografie; detaillierte bibliografische Daten sind im Internet über http://dnb.ddb.de abrufbar.

Bibliographic information published by Die Deutsche Bibliothek
Die Deutsche Bibliothek lists this publication in the Deutsche Nationalbibliografie; detailed bibliographic data is available in the Internet at http://dnb.ddb.de.

Printed and bound by: VEBU Druck GmbH, Bad Schussenried (Germany)

ISBN 3-87193-253-1 (Print); ISBN 3-87193-259-0 (Print + CD-ROM)

Content

Preface

The Pharmaceutical Dictionary has been something of a success story. In 1995, our idea was to produce a handy, pocket-sized reference booklet for those working in the pharmaceutical industry, principally in production, quality assurance, quality control and regulatory affairs and who regularly needed help with technical terminology that was becoming increasingly complex. We thus set ourselves the task of doing just this and the result was the first edition of the Pharmaceutical Dictionary of English and German technical terms published in 1995.

The dictionary was indeed a success and we soon had to produce a second edition. We took this opportunity to expand and in 1997 increased the number of terms to some 4000, still adhering to the original idea of the "pocket reference work".

In 1999, in the third edition, we took another important step by including French as the third language. At the same time we again expanded and increased the number of technical terms to some 5000.

This concept also proved successful and there was much demand so that, now, in 2002, we have decided again to expand and improve. We have added Spanish as the fourth language and have again expanded on the number of terms, bringing them up to 5,500. We have also changed the layout to cope more easily with the added language and to make it easier overall for the user.

We have, however, remained true to our initial idea: the Pharmaceutical Dictionary retains its pocket sized format so that it can be used as a "mobile work of reference" for those who need to look up something specific whilst e. g. working in production or in the lab. And we have kept the emphasis on production, quality assurance, quality control and regulatory affairs, simply expanding on the depth of treatment of these areas. We have also tried to be as consequent as possible in using the terminology used in the European Pharmacopoeias and e. g. GMP Guidelines and that recommended by the EU, EMEA and ICH.

We are most grateful for the help of our translators in fulfilling our idea: our thanks to **Dr. Alain Paillet**, Ingelheim (Germany), for the French translation and to **Dr. med. Juan-Francisco Sarti**, Germering (Germany), and his co-worker **Dr. Fernando Miragall**, Regensburg (Germany), for the Spanish translation. Our thanks too to our friends in the industry who helped us in expanding the range of terminology and providing us with what proved to be very constructive criticism.

Anita Maas James Brawley

Using the dictionary

The terms and their supplementary terms are arranged in alphabetical order. The principal terms are printed in bold type, the supplementary terms in grey half-tone.

The languages are designated with G (German), E (English), F (French) and S (Spanish).

Example: **density**
G Dichte
F densité
S densidad

absolute density
G absolute Dichte
F densité absolue
S densidad absoluta

There are some minor differences in spelling between British and American English. The British form has been used throughout the dictionary.

Examples:	**British English**	**American English**
	sterili***s***ation	sterili***z***ation
	licen***c***e	licen***s***e
	vap***ou***r	vap***o***r

Synonyms (sometimes several) are included in brackets after the principal term (i. e. they refer to the term immediately preceding).

Examples: source of error (failure) → source of error, source of failure
sonda de toma (de muestras) → sonda de toma, sonda de muestras

Some of the Spanish terms have two alternative methods of spelling. The letters involved are placed in brackets.

Example: lubri(fi)cante → lubricante, lubrificante

In order to emphasise how a particular term is used, an explanation is often indicated in brackets. No such indication is given if, in a particular language, this is not necessary.

Examples: anlaufen (Metall)
rugged (e. g. instrument, method)
élucider (une structure)
sellar (ampollas)

In the case of English infinitives, the "to" is entered after the term.

Examples: boil, to → to boil
collect, to; entrap, to → to collect, to entrap

For some terms, to enable a meaningful alphabetical sequence to be maintained, the order of words is reversed.

Examples: rest, at → at rest
Ruhezustand, im → im Ruhezustand
chaîne longue, à → à chaîne longue
paso seguro, de → de paso seguro

Benutzerhinweise

Haupt- und Untereinträge sind in alphabetischer Reihenfolge aufgelistet. Die Suchbegriffe der Haupteinträge erscheinen in fetter Schrift, die Suchbegriffe der Untereinträge in grauer Rasterschrift.

Die Begriffe der Referenzsprachen sind mit G (German – deutsch), E (English – englisch), F (French – französisch) und S (Spanish – spanisch) gekennzeichnet.

Beispiel: **Dichte**
E density
F densité
S densidad

absolute Dichte
E absolute density
F densité absolue
S densidad absoluta

Es gibt kleine Unterschiede in der Schreibweise zwischen dem britischen und dem amerikanischen Englisch. Für das Wörterbuch wurde die britisch-englische Schreibweise gewählt.

Beispiele:	**britisches Englisch**	**amerikanisches Englisch**
	sterili***s***ation	sterili***z***ation
	licen***c***e	licen***s***e
	vap***ou***r	vap***o***r

Das Synonym (ggf. auch mehrere) eines Begriffs ist in Klammern nach dem entsprechenden Begriff aufgeführt (d. h. es bezieht sich auf das unmittelbar davorstehende Wort).

Beispiele: source of error (failure) → source of error, source of failure
sonda de toma (de muestras) → sonda de toma, sonda de muestras

Bei einigen spanischen Begriffen bestehen zwei geringfügig unterschiedliche Schreibweisen. Die betreffenden Buchstaben sind in Klammern gesetzt.

Beispiel: lubri(fi)cante → lubricante, lubrificante

Um zu verdeutlichen, in welchem sachlichen Zusammenhang ein Begriff anzuwenden ist, steht in vielen Fällen ein entsprechender Hinweis in Klammern hinter dem Eintrag. Der Hinweis entfällt in der Sprache (den Sprachen), in der (denen) die Anwendung eindeutig ist.

Beispiele: anlaufen (Metall)
rugged (e. g. instrument, method)
élucider (une structure)
sellar (ampollas)

Das bei englischen Verben in der Infinitivform vorangestellte „to" ist im Wörterbuch nachgestellt.

Beispiele: boil, to → to boil
collect, to; entrap, to → to collect, to entrap

Bei einigen Einträgen sind die Wörter des Suchbegriffs umgestellt, um eine sinnvolle alphabetische Sortierung zu gewährleisten.

Beispiele: rest, at → at rest
Ruhezustand, im → im Ruhezustand
chaîne longue, à → à chaîne longue
paso seguro, de → de paso seguro

Indications pour l'emploi du dictionnaire

Les entrées principales et les entrées secondaires sont classées par ordre alphabétique. Dans les entrées principales, le terme-vedette est en caractères gras, dans les entrées secondaires, le terme-vedette est en caractères gris.
Les termes équivalents dans les langues de référence sont précédés respectivement de la lettre G (German – allemand), E (English – anglais), F (French – français) et S (Spanish – espagnol).

Exemple: densité
G Dichte
E density
S densidad

densité absolue
G absolute Dichte
E absolute density
S densidad absoluta

Il existe quelques différences orthographiques entre l'anglais britannique et l'anglais américain. Le présent dictionnaire est rédigé en anglais britannique.

Exemples:

	anglais britannique	**anglais américain**
	stérili***s***ation	sterili***z***ation
	licen***c***e	licen***s***e
	vap***ou***r	vap***o***r

Le, ou le cas échéant, les synonymes d'un terme figurent entre parenthèses à la suite du terme en question (c. a. d. qu'il/ils se rapporte/nt au terme précédent).

Exemples: margin of error (failure) → margin of error, margin of failure
sonda de toma (de muestras) → sonda de toma, sonda de muestras

Il existe pour certains termes espagnols des orthographies différentes. Les lettres concernées sont placées entre parenthèses.

Exemple: lubri(fi)cante → lubricante, lubrificante

Afin de préciser le domaine d'appartenance d'un terme, le terme-vedette de l'entrée principale est souvent suivi d'une indication correspondante placée entre parenthèses. Aucune indication n'est mentionnée dans la/les langue/s dans laquelle/lesquelles le domaine d'appartenance du terme est évident.

Exemples: anlaufen (Metall)
rugged (e. g. instrument, method)
élucider (une structure)
sellar (ampollas)

Dans le présent dictionnaire, le préfixe "to" accompagnant la forme infinitive des verbes anglais, est postposé.

Exemples: boil, to → to boil
collect, to; entrap, to → to collect, to entrap

Dans certaines entrées, des éléments appartenant au terme vedette sont postposés afin de permettre un classement alphabétique adéquat.

Exemples: rest, at → at rest
Ruhezustand, im → im Ruhezustand
chaîne longue, à → à chaîne longue
paso seguro, de → de paso seguro

Advertencias para el uso

Las voces principales y secundarias están ordenadas alfabéticamente. Los términos de búsqueda de las voces principales aparecen en negrilla, y los de las secundarias en fotograbado gris a media tinta.

Los términos de los idiomas de referencia están marcados con G (German – alemán), E (English – inglés), F (French – francés) y S (Spanish – español).

Ejemplo: **densidad**
G Dichte
E density
F densité

densidad absoluta
G absolute Dichte
E absolute density
F densité absolue

Existen pequeñas diferencias entre la forma de escribir inglés británica y la americana. En este diccionario se ha escogido el inglés británico.

Ejemplos:	**inglés británica**	**inglés americana**
	sterili***s***ation	sterili***z***ation
	licen***c***e	licen***s***e
	vap***ou***r	vap***o***r

El o los sinónimos de un término se encuentran entre paréntesis tras el término correspondiente (es decir que se refieren a la palabra inmediatamente anterior).

Ejemplos: margin of error (failure) → margin of error, margin of failure
sonda de toma (de muestras) → sonda de toma, sonda de muestras

Algunos términos españoles pueden escribirse de dos formas levemente distintas. Las diferentes letras correspondientes se encuentran entre paréntesis.

Ejemplo: lubri(fi)cante → lubricante, lubrificante

Para resaltar el contexto adecuado en el que se debe emplear un término, en muchos casos existe un aviso entre paréntesis detrás de la palabra correspondiente. Este aviso no existe en el idioma (los idiomas) en el (los) que el uso del término es inequívoco.

Ejemplos: anlaufen (Metall)
rugged (e. g. instrument, method)
élucider (une structure)
sellar (ampollas)

La preposición de infinitivo "to" de los verbos ingleses se encuentra en este diccionario detrás de una coma siguiendo al infinitivo.

Ejemplos: boil, to → to boil
collect, to; entrap, to → to collect, to entrap

En algunas voces se ha cambiado el orden de las palabras del término de búsqueda para garantizar un orden alfabético adecuado.

Ejemplos: rest, at → at rest
Ruhezustand, im → im Ruhezustand
chaîne longue, à → à chaîne longue
paso seguro, de → de paso seguro

Authors' profiles

Anita Maas studied pharmacy and qualified as a pharmacist in 1991. Since 1992, she has been involved in organising and carrying out training seminars for the pharmaceutical and supply industries. These seminars concentrate on GMP-relevant topics such as quality assurance, validation, documentation, pharmaceutical engineering and GMP guidelines and trends. One of these seminars is the one dealing with pharmaceutical English and is intended to train pharmaceutical executives in the use of the special vocabulary involved.
In 1999, Ms. Maas founded, in addition to her seminar activities, the Maas & Peither GMP-Verlag which edits among other books the GMP-BERATER, a reference book for the pharmaceutical and supply industries.

Anita Maas
PTS Pharma Training Service
Am Weißen Fels 4
66663 Merzig (Germany)

James Brawley, a qualified chemist, spent some 25 years in the chemical and pharmaceutical industries before setting up his own executive coaching business in 1992.
He carries out both public and in-house seminars, training executives within the pharmaceutical and chemical industries in the use of the specialised business English used in these fields. This comprises training executives – primarily from production, quality control and marketing – in how to meet and greet business partners, how to present their companies, how to describe their equipment and processes, how to discuss their plans and how to cope with e. g. an FDA inspection situation.

James Brawley
Executive Coaching
Scheffelweg 6
69251 Gaiberg (Germany)

English A – Z

English

German

French

Spanish

Using the dictionary:
p. 8–9

abrasion
G Abtrag, Abrieb
F abrasion
S abrasión

abridgement
G Abkürzung, Verkürzung
F raccourci
S abreviatura, abreviación, acortamiento

absence
G Abwesenheit
F absence
S ausencia

absolute
G absolut
F absolu
S absoluto, absolutamente

absorb, to
G absorbieren
F absorber
S absorber

absorbance
G Extinktion
F absorption
S extinción

absorbent
G Absorbens, Absorptionsmittel
F absorbant
S absorbente, medio de absorción

absorbing capacity
G Absorptionsvermögen
F capacité d'absorption
S capacidad de absorción

absorbing power
G Absorptionsvermögen
F capacité d'absorption
S capacidad de absorción

absorption
G Absorption
F absorption
S absorción

absorption base (for ointments)
G Absorptionsgrundlage (für Salben)
F base d'absorption (pour pommades)
S base de absorción (para pomadas)

absorption capacity
G Absorptionsfähigkeit
F capacité d'absorption
S capacidad de absorción

absorption coefficient
G Absorptionskoeffizient
F coefficient d'absorption
S coeficiente de absorción

absorption of medicinal substance
G Arzneistoffaufnahme
F adsorption d'un principe actif
S absorción del principio activo

absorption rate
G Absorptionsgeschwindigkeit
F vitesse d'absorption
S velocidad de absorción

absorptive capacity
G Saugfähigkeit
F capacité d'absorption
S capacidad de absorción

absorptivity
G Absorptionsfähigkeit
F capacité d'absorption
S capacidad de absorción

abuse
G Mißbrauch
F abus
S abuso

accelerate, to
G beschleunigen
F accélérer
S acelerar

accelerated stability test
G Streßtest
F test de stabilité accéléré
S estudio acelerado de estabilidad

accelerator
G Beschleuniger
F accélérateur
S acelerador

acceptable quality level (AQL)
G Annehmbare Qualitätsgrenzlage (AQL)
F niveau de qualité acceptable
S límite de calidad aceptable

class AQL
G Gesamt-AQL
F niveau absolu de qualité acceptable
S límite total de calidad aceptable

individual AQL
G Einzel-AQL
F niveau individuel de qualité acceptable
S límite individual de calidad aceptable

acceptance
G Annahme
F réception, acceptation, acceptance
S aceptación

acceptance criterion
G Akzeptanzkriterium
F critère d'acceptation
S criterio de aceptación

acceptance graph
G Annahmekennlinie
F courbe d'acceptance
S característica de aceptación

acceptance number
G Annahmezahl
F indice d'acceptance
S número de aceptación

acceptance test (e. g. for software)
G Akzeptanztest (z. B. für Software)
F test d'acceptance (par ex. pour logiciel)
S prueba de aceptación (p. ej. de software)

access
G Zugang, Zutritt
F accès
S acceso

authorised access
G autorisierter Zugang
F droit d'accès
S acceso autorizado

controlled access
G kontrollierter Zugang
F accès contrôlé
S acceso controlado

limited access, restricted access
G eingeschränkter Zugang
F accès limité
S acceso limitado

system access
G Zugang zum System
F accès au système
S acceso al sistema

access port
G Eintrittsstutzen
F tubulure d'accès
S tubuladura de acceso

accessibility
G Zugänglichkeit
F accessibilité
S accesibilidad

accessible
G begehbar
F accessible
S practicable, viable

poorly accessible points
G schwer zugängliche Stellen
F endroits difficilement accessibles
S lugares de difícil acceso

accessory
G Ausrüstungsteil, Zubehör
F accessoire
S accesorio

accident
G Unfall, Störfall
F accident, panne, incident
S accidente, avería, fallo, incidente

accident-proof
G unfallsicher
F protégé contre les accidents
S a prueba de accidentes

accredit, to
G akkreditieren
F accréditer
S acreditar

accredited calibration laboratory
G akkreditiertes Kalibrierlabor
F laboratoire d'étalonnage homologué
S laboratorio acreditado de calibración

accumulation
G Anhäufung
F accumulation
S acumulación

accumulation of particles
G Partikelansammlung
F accumulation de particules
S acumulación de partículas

accuracy
G Richtigkeit (einer Prüfmethode)
F exactitude
S corrección, exactitud (de un método de prueba)

acid
G Säure, sauer
F acide
S ácido

concentrated acid
G starke Säure
F acide concentré
S ácido concentrado

weak acid
G schwache Säure
F acide faible
S ácido débil

acid value
G Säurezahl
F indice d'acide
S índice de ácido

acidify, to
G ansäuern
F acidifier
S acidificar

acidity
G Azidität
F acidité
S acidez

acid-resistant
G säurebeständig
F résistant aux acides
S resistente a los ácidos

acoustic signal
G akustisches Signal
F signal acoustique
S señal acústica

acquire, to
G aufkaufen
F acquérir
S adquirir

acrylic glass
G Plexiglas
F plexiglas
S plexiglás

acrylic resin
G Acrylharz
F résine acrylique
S resina acrílica

action limit
G Aktionsgrenze, Stopgrenze
F limite d'action
S límite de acción

activated charcoal
G Aktivkohle
F charbon actif
S carbón activado

English German French Spanish

activation
G Aktivierung
F activation
S activación

activation energy
G Aktivierungsenergie
F énergie d'activation
S energía de activación

active ingredient
G wirksamer Bestandteil
F composant actif
S componente activo

active pharmaceutical ingredient (API)
G Wirkstoff (im Arzneimittel)
F principe actif (d'un médicament)
S principio activo (medicamento)

active substance
G wirksamer Bestandteil, Wirkstoff (im Arzneimittel)
F composant actif, principe actif (d'un médicament)
S componente activo, principio activo (medicamento)

active substance release
G Wirkstoff-Freigabe
F libération d'un principe actif
S liberación del principio activo

delayed release
G verzögerte Wirkstoff-Freigabe
F libération retardée d'un principe actif
S liberación retardada del principio activo

extended release
G verlängerte Wirkstoff-Freigabe
F libération prolongée d'un principe actif
S liberación prolongada del principio activo

active substance screening
G Wirkstoffscreening
F screening de principes actifs
S detección de sustancias activas

actual value
G Istwert
F valeur actuelle
S valor real

actual yield
G tatsächliche Ausbeute
F rendement réel
S rendimiento real

actuation
G Aktivierung
F activation
S activación

add, to
G zugeben
F ajouter
S añadir

addiction
G Sucht
F accoutumance
S adicción

addition
G Zugabe
F adjonction
S adición, suplemento

additive
G Zusatzstoff
F additif, adjuvant
S aditivo

adequate
G angemessen, geeignet
F approprié, adéquat
S adecuado, apropiado

adhere, to (tablets)
G kleben (bei Tabletten)
F adhérer
S adherir (comprimidos)

adherence
G Adhärenz
F adhérence
S adherencia

adhesion
G Haftung (physikalisch)
F adhésion
S adhesión (física)

adhesive
G Kleber
F colle
S sustancia adhesiva

adhesive film
G Klebefolie
F film adhésif
S película adhesiva

adhesive force
G Bindekraft
F force d'adhésion
S fuerza adhesiva

adhesive power
G Haftkraft
F force d'adhésion
S fuerza adhesiva

adhesive strength
G Klebekraft
F force d'adhérence
S fuerza adhesiva

adhesive tape
G Klebeband
F bande adhésive
S cinta adhesiva

adhesiveness
G Haftfähigkeit
F pouvoir d'adhésion
S adherencia, adhesividad

adiabatic reaction conditions
G adiabatische Reaktionsbedingungen
F conditions de réaction adiabatiques
S condiciones adiabáticas de reacción

adiabatic temperature
G adiabatische Temperatur
F température adiabatique
S temperatura adiabática

adjust, to
G einstellen, justieren
F ajuster, régler, étalonner
S ajustar, regular

adjustable
G einstellbar, regelbar, regulierbar
F ajustable
S ajustable, regulable

adjusting knob
G Einstellknopf
F bouton d'ajustement
S botón de ajuste

adjusting screw
G Justierschraube
F vis de mise au point
S tornillo de ajuste

adjustment
G Einstellung, Regulierung, Justierung
F ajustement, réglage, étalonnement
S ajuste, regulación

adjuvant
G Hilfsstoff
F excipient, adjuvant
S excipiente, sustancia auxiliar

administration (of a drug)
G Darreichung, Verabreichung (eines Medikaments), Verwaltung
F administration (d'un médicament)
S administración (de un medicamento)

administration form
G Darreichungsform
F forme du dosage, voie d'administration
S forma de administración

adsorbent
G Adsorptionsmittel
F adsorbant
S medio de adsorción

adsorption
G Adsorption
F adsorption
S adsorción

adsorption capacity
G Adsorptionsfähigkeit
F capacité d'adsorption
S capacidad de adsorción

adsorption chromatography
G Adsorptionschromatographie
F chromatographie d'adsorption
S cromatografía de adsorción

adsorptivity
G Adsorptionsfähigkeit
F capacité d'adsorption
S capacidad de adsorción

adverse reaction
G unerwünschte Reaktion
F réaction indésirable, effet adverse
S reacción indeseable

aerobic
G aerob
F aérobie
S aerobio

aerosol can
G Aerosoldose
F bidon d'aérosol, bombe aérosol
S tubo aerosol

aerosol measurement
G Aerosolmessung
F mesure (de la dose) d'un aérosol
S medida de aerosol

affinity
G Affinität
F affinité
S afinidad

affinity chromatography
G Affinitätschromatographie
F chromatographie d'affinité
S cromatografía de afinidad

affinity diagram
G Affinitätsdiagramm
F diagramme d'affinité
S diagrama de afinidad

after-taste
G Nachgeschmack
F arrière-goût
S regusto

agar
G Agar
F agar, agar-agar
S agar

age, to
G altern
F vieillir
S envejecer

ageing
G Alterung
F vieillissement
S envejecimiento

forced ageing
G beschleunigte Alterung (künstlich)
F vieillissement (forcé) prématuré
S envejecimiento acelerado (artificial)

age-resistant
G alterungsbeständig
F résistant au vieillissement
S resistente al envejecimiento

agglomerate
G Agglomerat
F agglomérat
S aglomerado

agglomerate, to
G agglomerieren
F agglomérer
S aglomerar

agglutination
G Agglutination
F agglutination
S aglutinación

aggregate
G Aggregat
F agrégat
S agregado

agitating speed
G Rührgeschwindigkeit
F vitesse d'agitation
S velocidad de agitación

agitator
G Rührwerk
F agitateur
S agitador

agreement
G Vereinbarung
F accord, convention
S acuerdo, convenio

air aspiration
G Luftabsaugung
F système d'évacuation d'air
S aspiración de aire

air attrition mill
G Luftstrahlmühle
F microniseur à jet d'air
S micronizador del chorro de aire

air bubble, entrapped
G eingeschlossene Luftblase
F bulle d'air piégée
S burbuja de aire capturada

air conditioner
G Klimaanlage
F appareil de climatisation
S aire acondicionado

air convection
G Luftkonvektion
F convection de l'air
S convección de aire

air current
G Luftstrom
F écoulement d'air
S corriente de aire

air duct
G Luftschacht
F canalisation d'air
S canalización de aire

air entrapment
G Lufteinschluß
F inclusion d'air
S inclusión de aire

air exchange
G Luftwechsel
F renouvellement d'air
S renovación del aire

air exchange rate
G Luftwechselrate
F taux de renouvellement d'air
S tasa de renovación de aire

air exhaust system
G Luftabsaugung
F système d'évacuation d'air
S aspiración de aire

air filter
G Luftfilter
F filtre à air
S filtro de aire

air flow
G Luftströmung
F circulation d'air
S flujo de aire

air flow controller
G Luftstromwächter
F régulateur d'écoulement d'air
S controlador de la corriente de aire

air flow direction
G Luftströmungsrichtung
F direction de l'écoulement d'air
S dirección del flujo aéreo

air flow pattern
G Luftführung
F modèle d'écoulement d'air
S patrón de conducción de aire

air impermeability
G Luftundurchlässigkeit
F imperméabilité à l'air
S impermeabilidad al aire

English German French Spanish

English German French Spanish

air inlet cover
G Zuluftklappe
F couvercle d'entrée d'air
S válvula de entrada de aire

air jet
G Luftstrahl
F jet d'air
S chorro de aire

air microbial count
G Luftkeimzahl
F nombre de micro-organismes de l'air
S número de gérmenes del aire

air outlet
G Luftaustrittsöffnung
F sortie d'air
S orificio de salida del aire

air permeability
G Luftdurchlässigkeit
F perméabilité à l'air
S permeabilidad al aire

air pressure
G Luftdruck
F pression d'air
S presión de aire

air pressure sensor
G Luftdruckfühler
F détecteur de pression atmosphérique
S sensor de presión atmosférica

air shaft
G Luftschacht
F canalisation d'air
S canalización de aire

air sieving
G Luftstrahlsiebung
F tamisage d'air
S tamizado del aire

air suction connection port
G Luftansaugstutzen
F tubulure d'aspiration d'air
S empalme para aspiración de aire

air supply
G Luftversorgung
F alimentation en air
S abastecimiento de aire

air throughput
G Luftdurchsatz
F débit d'écoulement d'air
S rendimiento de aire

air tightness
G Luftdichtheit
F imperméabilité à l'air
S hermeticidad para el aire

air turbulence
G Luftverwirbelung
F turbulence d'air
S turbulencia del aire

air velocity
G Luftgeschwindigkeit
F vitesse de l'air
S velocidad del aire

airborne
G aerogen
F aéroporté, transporté par l'air, en suspension dans l'air
S aerógeno

air-conditioned
G klimatisiert
F air conditionné
S climatizado

air-conditioning
G Klimatisierung
F climatisation
S climatizador

air-dried
G luftgetrocknet
F séché à l'air
S secado al aire

air-tight
G luftdicht
F étanche à l'air
S hermético, impermeable al aire

air-tight pack
G luftdichte Verpackung
F emballage étanche à l'air
S embalaje impermeable al aire

alarm
G Alarm, Warnsignal
F alarme, signal d'alarme
S alarma, señal de alarma

alarm limit
G Alarmlimit
F limite d'alarme
S límite de alarma

alarm signal
G Alarm
F signal d'alarme
S alarma

alarm system
G Alarmsystem
F système d'alarme
S sistema de alarma

alcoholate
G Alkoholauszug
F alcoolate
S extracto alcohólico

aldehyde
G Aldehyd
F aldéhyde
S aldehído

alert limit
G Warngrenze
F limite d'alerte
S límite de alerta

align, to
G ausrichten
F aligner, ajuster, centrer
S ajustar, alinear, orientar

alignment
G Justierung
F étalonnement
S ajuste

aliquot, to
G aliquotieren
F aliquoter
S alicuotar

alkaline
G alkalisch, basisch
F alcalin, basique
S alcalino, básico

alkaline solution
G Lauge
F soude
S lejía

alkaline treatment
G alkalische Behandlung
F traitement alcalin
S tratamiento alcalino

alkalinity
G Alkalinität
F alcalinité
S alcalinidad, basicidad

alkylation
G Alkylierung
F alkylation
S alquilación

Allen key
G Inbusschlüssel
F clé BTR
S llave hexagonal

Allen screw
G Inbusschraube
F vis à six pans creux femelle
S tornillo hexagonal

allergen
G Allergen
F allergène
S alergeno

allow to stand, to
G absetzen lassen
F laisser sédimenter, laisser se déposer
S dejar precipitar, dejar sedimentar

alloy
G Legierung
F alliage
S aleación

alpha helix (e. g. of protein)
G Alpha-Helix (z. B. eines Proteins)
F hélice alpha (structure des protéines)
S hélice alfa (p. ej. de proteína)

alternating current (AC)
G Wechselstrom
F courant alternatif
S corriente alterna

alternative medication
G Ausweichmedikation
F médication alternative
S medicación alternativa

alumina
G Aluminiumoxid
F oxyde d'aluminium
S óxido de aluminio

aluminium bottle
G Aluminiumflasche
F bouteille d'aluminium
S botella de aluminio

aluminium foil
G Aluminiumfolie
F feuille d'aluminium
S hoja de aluminio

aluminium oxide
G Aluminiumoxid
F oxyde d'aluminium
S óxido de aluminio

aluminium pallet
G Alupalette
F alupalette, palette en aluminium
S paleta de aluminio

ambient temperature
G Umgebungstemperatur, Raumtemperatur
F température ambiante
S temperatura ambiental, temperatura ambiente

amendment
G Änderungsanzeige
F amendement
S anuncio de enmienda

amines
G Amine
F amines
S aminas

aromatic amines
G aromatische Amine
F amines aromatiques
S aminas aromáticas

primary amines
G primäre Amine
F amines primaires
S aminas primarias

secondary amines
G sekundäre Amine
F amines secondaires
S aminas secundarias

tertiary amines
G tertiäre Amine
F amines tertiaires
S aminas terciarias

amino acid
G Aminosäure
F acide aminé
S aminoácido

essential amino acid
G essentielle Aminosäure
F acide aminé essentiel
S aminoácido esencial

amino acid derivative
G Aminosäurederivat
F dérivé d'acide aminé
S derivado de aminoácido

ammeter
G Amperemeter, Strommesser
F ampèremètre
S amperímetro

amorphous
G amorph
F amorphe
S amorfo

amount
G Menge
F quantité
S cantidad

amperage
G Stromstärke
F ampérage
S amperaje, intensidad de corriente

amperometric detection
G amperometrische Detektion
F détecteur ampérométrique
S detección amperométrica

amplification
G Verstärkung
F amplification
S amplificación, intensificación, refuerzo

amplifier
G Verstärker
F amplificateur
S amplificador

amplitude
G Amplitude
F amplitude
S amplitud

ampoule
G Ampulle
F ampoule
S ampolla

ampoule box
G Ampullenschachtel
F boîte d'ampoules
S caja de ampollas

ampoule cutter
G Ampullenfeile
F lime (pour ampoule)
S lima de ampolla

ampoule file
G Ampullenfeile
F lime (pour ampoule)
S lima de ampolla

ampoule filling
G Ampullenabfüllung
F remplissage d'une ampoule
S rellenado de una ampolla

ampoule neck
G Ampullenhals
F col d'une ampoule
S cuello de ampolla

anaerobic
G anaerob
F anaérobe
S anaerobio

analogue display
G Analoganzeige
F affichage numérique
S pantalla análoga

analysis
G Analyse, Prüfung
F analyse, test de contrôle
S análisis, examen, ensayo, prueba, test

analyte
G Analyt
F analyte, substance à analyser
S sustancia a analizar

analytical
G analytisch
F analytique
S analítico

analytical apparatus
G Analysengerät
F appareil d'analyses
S aparato de análisis

analytical balance
G Analysenwaage
F balance d'analyse
S báscula de análisis

English
German
French
Spanish

analytical chemistry
G analytische Chemie
F chimie analytique
S química analítica

analytical column
G analytische Säule
F colonne analytique
S columna analítica

analytical development
G Entwicklungsanalytik
F développement analytique
S analítica de desarrollo

analytical method
G Prüfmethode
F méthode analytique, méthode de contrôle
S método de prueba

analytical procedure
G Prüfverfahren
F procédure de test
S procedimiento de prueba

analytical result
G Testergebnis
F résultat d'analyse
S resultado de la prueba

analytical uncertainty
G analytische Unsicherheit
F incertitude analytique
S inseguridad analítica

anchor stirrer
G Ankerrührer
F agitateur à ancre
S agitador de ancla

angle
G Winkel
F angle
S ángulo

angle of gradient
G Neigungswinkel
F angle de pente
S ángulo de inclinación

angle of incidence
G Einfallswinkel
F angle d'incidence
S ángulo de incidencia

angle of reflection
G Reflektionswinkel
F angle de réflexion
S ángulo de reflexión

angle of refraction
G Brechungswinkel
F angle de réfraction
S ángulo de refracción

angle of slide
G Böschungswinkel
F angle de pente
S ángulo de la pendiente

angle of slope
G Neigungswinkel
F angle de pente
S ángulo de inclinación

angled
G abgewinkelt
F à angles, angulaire
S angulado, doblado, escuadrado

angular
G abgewinkelt
F à angles, angulaire
S angulado, doblado, escuadrado

anhydrous
G wasserfrei
F anhydre
S anhidro

animal experiment
G Tierversuch
F expériences réalisées sur animaux
S experimento con animales

animal sera
G tierische Seren
F sérums d'origine animale
S sueros de origen animal

anion exchanger
G Anionenaustauscher
F échangeur d'ions anioniques
S intercambiador de aniones

anneal, to
G glühen
F recuire
S incandescer

annual product report
G jährlicher Produktbericht
F rapport annuel de production
S informe anual de producción

anodised
G eloxiert
F oxydé (électrolytiquement)
S oxidado electrolíticamente

antibiotic
G Antibioticum
F antibiotique
S antibiótico

antibody
G Antikörper
F anticorps
S anticuerpo

anticlockwise
G gegen Uhrzeigersinn
F contre le sens des aiguilles d'une montre
S sentido antihorario

antidote
G Gegengift
F antidote
S antídoto

anti-foaming agent
G Antischaummittel, Entschäumer
F agent antimousse, antimousse
S agente antiespumante

anti-fungal
G pilzabtötend
F antifongique
S antifúngico, fungicida

anti-microbial agent
G Konservierungsmittel
F conservateur
S medio de conservación

anti-microbial effectiveness test
G Konservierungsmittelbelastungstest
F test d'efficacité anti-microbien
S prueba de eficacia antimicrobiana

anti-oxidant
G Antioxidans
F antioxydant
S antioxidante

anti-static agent
G Antistatikum
F agent antistatique
S antiestático

apathogenic
G apathogen
F apathogène
S apatógeno

aperture
G Lochblende
F diaphragme
S diafragma

apparatus
G Geräte
F appareillage expérimental
S aparatos

apparatus designation
G Gerätekennzeichnung
F marquage de l'appareil
S caracterización de aparatos

apparent density
G scheinbare Dichte
F densité apparente
S densidad aparente

appearance
G äußere Beschaffenheit
F aspect, apparence
S aspecto externo

appearance, general
G allgemeines Aussehen
F apparence (générale)
S aspecto general

appendix
G Anhang, Anlage (zur Dokumentation)
F annexe, appendice
S anexo, apéndice (de un documento)

applicability
G Anwendbarkeit
F applicabilité
S aplicabilidad

application
G Anwendung, Antrag
F application, utilisation, requête, demande
S aplicación, uso, solicitud, instancia

for external application
G zur äußerlichen Anwendung
F pour application externe
S para aplicación externa

application for marketing approval
G Antrag auf Vertriebsgenehmigung eines Arzneimittels bei der FDA (USA)
F demande d'autorisation de mise sur le marché (AMM)
S solicitud de permiso a la FDA (EE.UU.) para poner a la venta un medicamento

application for marketing authorisation
G Produktzulassungsantrag, Zulassungsantrag
F demande d'autorisation de mise sur le marché
S solicitud de autorización de un producto (para la venta)

application route
G Applikationsweg
F voie d'application
S vía de administración

application software
G Anwendungssoftware
F logiciel d'application
S sistema lógico de aplicación, software de aplicación

applicator
G Applikator
F applicateur
S aplicador

dropper applicator
G Verschluß mit Tropfer
F applicateur compte-gouttes
S cierre con cuentagotas

apply, to (sample)
G aufgeben (Probe), anbringen, aufbringen, auftragen
F appliquer (un échantillon), étendre, apposer, installer, poser
S aplicar (una muestra), extender, untar, instalar, montar

apprentice
G Auszubildender, Lehrling
F apprenti, stagiaire
S aprendiz

apprenticeship
G Lehre
F apprentissage
S aprendizaje, enseñanza

appropriate
G angemessen, geeignet
F approprié, adéquat
S adecuado, apropiado

approval
G Billigung, (behördliche) Genehmigung, Marktzulassung
F approbation, autorisation (d'une autorité réglementaire), autorisation de mise sur le marché (A.M.M.)
S aprobación, autorización (oficial), autorización para venta en el mercado

electronic approval
G elektronische Genehmigung
F autorisation électronique
S autorización electrónica

approval signature
G Unterschrift zur Genehmigung
F signature d'autorisation
S firma autorizante

approve, to
G billigen, genehmigen
F approuver, autoriser
S aprobar, autorizar

approved batch
G Verkaufscharge
F lot de production
S lote de venta

approved disinfectants
G zugelassene Desinfektionsmittel
F désinfectants autorisés
S desinfectantes autorizados

apron (of machine)
G Schürze, Abhängung
F tablier
S delantal

aqueous
G wäßrig
F aqueux
S acuoso

aqueous film coating
G wäßrige Filmbeschichtung
F film aqueux, couche aqueuse pelliculaire
S película acuosa de revestimiento

aqueous phase
G wäßrige Phase
F phase aqueuse
S fase acuosa

aqueous polymer
G wäßriges Polymer
F polymère aqueux
S polímero acuoso

aqueous waste
G Flüssigabfall
F effluent aqueux
S desecho fluido

archive
G Archiv
F archives
S archivo

archiving
G Archivierung, Aufbewahrung
F archivage, conservation, stockage
S archivado, conservación, almacenaje

archiving media
G Archivierungsmedien
F médium d'archivage
S medios de archivado

area
G Fläche
F surface, superficie
S superficie

segregated area
G abgetrennter Bereich
F zone séparée, zone isolée, zone de confinement
S área separada

area of application
G Anwendungsgebiet
F champ d'application, domaine d'application
S campo de aplicación

arithmetic mean
G arithmetisches Mittel
F moyenne arithmétique
S media aritmética

aromatic substance
G Aromastoff
F substance aromatique
S sustancia aromática

artificial fibre
G Kunstfaser
F fibre artificielle
S fibra artificial

English German French Spanish

as required
G bei Bedarf
F sur besoin, sur demande
S en caso necesario

asbestos
G Asbest
F amiante
S asbesto

asbestos filter
G Asbestfilter
F filtre en amiante
S filtro de asbesto

ascending curve
G Aufwärtskurve
F courbe ascendante
S curva ascendente

aseptic
G aseptisch
F aseptique
S aséptico

aseptic filling
G aseptische Abfüllung
F remplissage aseptique
S envasado aséptico

aseptic process
G aseptische Prozeßtechnik
F procédé aseptique, technique aseptique
S técnica de proceso aséptico

aseptic processing
G aseptische Herstellung
F fabrication aseptique
S fabricación aséptica

aseptic technology
G aseptische Prozeßtechnik
F procédé aseptique, technique aseptique
S técnica de proceso aséptico

ash
G Asche
F cendre
S ceniza

ashing
G Veraschung
F incinération
S incineración

aspirate, to
G absaugen, ansaugen
F aspirer
S aspirar, succionar

aspiration nipple
G Ansaugstutzen
F manchon d'aspiration
S empalme de aspiración

aspiration system
G Absaugvorrichtung
F système d'aspiration, système d'évacuation
S sistema de aspiración, sistema de evacuación

aspiration valve
G Ansaugventil
F vanne d'aspiration
S válvula de aspiración

aspirator bottle
G Saugflasche
F biberon
S biberón

assemble, to
G zusammensetzen
F assembler
S ensamblar, montar

assembly
G Montage, Zusammenbau
F assemblage, montage
S ensamblaje, montaje

assess, to
G bewerten
F évaluer
S evaluar

assessment (of data)
G Bewertung (von Daten)
F évaluation (de données)
S evaluación (de datos)

assessor
G Begutachter
F expert
S asesor, experto, perito

at rest
G im Ruhezustand
F à l'arrêt, immobilisé
S parado

in process
G im Betriebszustand
F à condition d'exploitation
S funcionando

atmospheric pressure
G Atmosphärendruck
F pression atmosphérique
S presión atmosférica

atomic emission spectroscopy
G Atomemissionsspektroskopie
F spectroscopie par émission atomique
S espectroscopia de emisión atómica

atomic layer epitaxy (ALE)
G Atomschichtepitaxie
F épitaxie d'une couche d'atomes
S epitaxia de un estrato atómico

atomise, to
G zerstäuben
F atomiser, pulvériser
S atomizar, pulverizar

atomiser
G Nebelgenerator, Zerstäuber
F atomiseur, pulvérisateur
S atomizador, pulverizador

atomising air
G Zerstäuberluft
F air d'atomiseur
S aire de atomizador

attach, to
G anbringen
F apposer, installer, poser
S instalar, montar

attachment
G Anbauteil, Befestigung
F accessoire, dispositif adaptable, module, fixation
S pieza de montaje, fijación

attenuated pathogen
G abgeschwächter Erreger
F agent pathogène atténué
S agente patógeno atenuado

attenuation (of a signal)
G Abschwächung (eines Signals)
F atténuation (d'un signal)
S atenuación (de una señal)

attenuator
G Schalldämpfer
F silencieux, amortisseur de son
S silenciador

audit
G Audit
F audit, inspection
S auditoría, inspección

audit function
G Auditfunktion
F fonction d'audit
S función de la auditoría

audit trail
G Auditweg
F trace-témoin de l'audit
S traza-testigo de la auditoría

auricular use
G Anwendung am Ohr
F pour usage auriculaire
S uso otológico

authorisation
G Genehmigung, behördliche Genehmigung
F autorisation, autorisation d'une autorité réglementaire
S autorización, autorización oficial

authorise, to
G genehmigen
F autoriser
S autorizar

English German French Spanish

authorised access
G autorisierter Zugang, Zugangsberechtigung
F droit d'accès, autorisation d'accès
S acceso autorizado, derecho de acceso

authorised individual
G autorisierte Person
F personne autorisée
S persona autorizada

authorised person
G befugte Person
F personne autorisée
S persona autorizada

authorities
G Behörde
F autorité réglementaire
S autoridades, organismos oficiales

authority
G Befugnis
F autorisation
S autorización, competencia

autoclavable
G autoklavierbar
F autoclavable
S esterilizable en autoclave

autoclave
G Autoklav, Sterilisator
F autoclave
S autoclave, esterilizador

autoclave (sterilisation) chamber
G Sterilisierkammer
F chambre d'autoclave
S cámara de esterilización

autoclave basket
G Korbeinsatz für Autoklaven
F corbeille d'autoclave
S cesto para autoclave

autoclave, to
G autoklavieren
F autoclaver
S esterilizar en autoclave

automate, to
G automatisieren
F automatiser
S automatizar

automatic operation
G automatischer Betrieb
F fonctionnement automatique
S funcionamiento automático

automation
G Automation
F automatisation
S automa(tiza)ción

auxilary area
G Nebenbereich
F zone auxiliaire
S área auxiliar

available
G verfügbar
F disponible
S disponible

average
G Durchschnitt
F moyenne
S media, promedio

average speed
G durchschnittliche Geschwindigkeit
F vitesse moyenne
S velocidad media

avoid, to
G vermeiden
F éviter
S eludir, evitar

axis of rotation
G Drehachse
F axe de rotation
S eje de rotación

back flow
G Rückfluß
F reflux
S reflujo

back flow flap
G Rückstauklappe
F clapet antirefouleur
S válvula de retención

back flow preventer
G Rückstauklappe
F clapet antirefouleur
S válvula de retención

back illumination
G Beleuchtung von hinten
F éclairage par l'arrière
S iluminación desde atrás

back pressure
G Gegendruck (in der Chromatographie)
F contre-pression
S contrapresión (en cromatografía)

back titration
G Rücktitration
F dosage en retour
S titulación retrógrada

back-up file
G Sicherheitskopie
F copie de sauvegarde
S copia de seguridad

back-up stack
G Nachlegestapel
F empilement de réserve
S montón de reserva

bacteria
G Bakterien
F bactérie
S bacterias

bacterial (microbial) content
G Keimgehalt
F teneur en micro-organismes
S contenido en gérmenes

bacterial endotoxin
G Bakterienendotoxin
F endotoxine bactérienne
S endotoxina bacteriana

bactericidal
G bakterizid
F bactéricide
S bactericida

baffle
G Ablenkplatte, Schikane, Umlenkblech, Leitblech, Zwischenwand
F plaque déflectrice, chicane, chicane de déviation, déflecteur, mur de séparation
S placa de desviación, vejación, chapa desviadora, deflector, disruptor, tabique

bag
G Beutel
F poche, sac, sachet
S sobre

package in bags, to
G in Beutel verpacken
F empaqueter (emballer) en sachets
S empaquetar en sobres

bag in bag
G Beutel in Außenbeutel
F sac à double paroi
S sobre de pared doble

bake off, to (column)
G verbacken (Säule)
F agglutiner (colonne)
S preparar (columna)

baking (e. g. of crystals)
G Zusammenbacken (z. B. von Kristallen)
F agglomération (par ex. de cristaux)
S cocción (p. ej. de cristales)

balance
G Waage
F balance
S balanza

top-loading balance
G oberschalige Waage
F balance à plat en haut
S balanza de carga superior

ball + socket joint
G Kugelgelenk
F rotule, joint à rotule
S articulación de rótula, unión esférica

ball bearing
G Kugellager
F roulement à billes
S rodamiento a bolas

ball hardness
G Kugeldruckhärte
F dureté à la bille
S dureza de la bola

ball mill
G Kugelmühle
F broyeur à boulets
S molinillo a bolas

ball nozzle
G Kugeldüse
F buse à billes
S aplicador de bola

ball valve
G Kugelventil
F clapet à billes, soupape à billes, vanne à billes
S válvula esférica

band
G Banderole
F banderole
S precinto

band balance
G Bandwaage
F balance de convoyeur
S báscula de cinta

band height (of tablets)
G Steghöhe (bei Tabletten)
F hauteur de bande
S altura de banda (de comprimidos)

bandage
G Verband
F pansement, bandage
S vendaje

banderole
G Banderole
F banderole
S precinto

barrel
G Faß
F tonneau
S tonel

barrier fluid
G Sperrflüssigkeit
F barrière fluidique
S barrera líquida

barrier layer
G Sperrschicht
F couche de barrage
S estrato barrera

base
G Base, Untergestell, Unterseite, Sockel
F base, socle, face inférieure
S base, pie, soporte, lado inferior, casquillo, zócalo

baseline
G Basislinie
F ligne de base
S línea de base

baseline drift
G Basisliniendrift
F dérive de la ligne de base
S desviación de la línea de base

baseline noise
G Basislinienrauschen
F bruit de fond de la ligne de base
S ruido de fondo de la línea de base

basic
G basisch
F basique, alcalin
S básico, alcalino

basic formulation
G Basisformulierung
F formulation de base
S formulación básica, formulación de base

basicity
G Basizität
F basicité
S basicidad, alcalinidad

basis
G Basis
F base
S base

basket apparatus
G Korbgerät
F appareil à corbeille
S aparato de cesto

basket stirring method
G Drehkörbchenmethode
F méthode d'agitation à corbeilles
S método de agitación con cesto rotatorio

batch
G Charge
F lot
S lote

sub-batch, partial batch
G Teilcharge
F sous-lot, lot partiel
S lote parcial

batch code
G Chargencode
F codage d'un lot
S código de un lote

batch consistency
G Chargenkonsistenz
F consistance d'un lot
S consistencia de un lote

batch control
G Chargenkontrolle
F contrôle des lots
S control de lotes

batch number
G Chargennummer
F numéro de lot
S número de lote

batch number coding
G Chargenbezeichnungsschlüssel
F système de codage pour les numéros de lot
S código de designación de lotes

batch packaging record
G Verpackungsprotokoll
F compte rendu de conditionnement
S protocolo de embalaje

batch processing record
G Herstellungsprotokoll
F protocole de fabrication
S protocolo de fabricación

batch record
G Chargenprotokoll
F relevé d'un lot, enregistrement d'un lot, compte rendu d'un lot
S protocolo de lotes

batch release
G Chargenfreigabe
F libération d'un lot
S liberación de un lote

batch size
G Chargengröße, Losgröße
F taille d'un lot
S tamaño de un lote

batch traceability
G Chargenrückverfolgbarkeit
F traçabilité d'un lot
S seguimiento de un lote

batch-related
G chargenspezifisch
F spécifique au lot
S específico del lote

bayonet connection
G Bajonettverschluß
F fermeture à baïonnette
S conexión de bayoneta

be in charge of, to
G beauftragt sein mit
F être chargé (d'une affaire)
S estar encargado de

English German French Spanish

bead
G Bördelrand
F bourrelet
S burlete rebordeado, canto rebordeado

bead, to
G umbördeln
F sertir
S bordear, rebordear, redondear

beaker
G Becherglas
F bécher, gobelet
S probeta

beam arrest (balance)
G Arretiervorrichtung (bei Waagen)
F relève-plateau
S dispositivo de fijación (en básculas)

bearing
G Peilung
F sondage, coussinet
S sondeo

bearing (mach.)
G Lager (Maschinenteil)
F assise, support
S asiento, cojinete, soporte

behaviour
G Verhalten
F comportement
S comportamiento

bellows
G Faltenbalg
F soufflet
S fuelle plegable

belt drive
G Keilriemenantrieb, Riemenantrieb
F entraînement par courroie, entraînement par courroie trapézoïdale
S propulsión por correa trapezoidal, propulsión por correa

belt speed
G Bandgeschwindigkeit
F vitesse du tapis
S velocidad de cinta

bench
G Labortisch, Arbeitstisch
F paillasse de laboratoire, table de travail, établi
S mesa de laboratorio, mesa de trabajo

bend
G Biegung
F courbure, pliage
S flexión, curvatura

bend, to
G knicken
F casser, couder
S doblar, quebrar

bevel
G Abschrägung, Facette
F biseau
S bisel, faceta

bill of materials
G Stückliste
F liste-inventaire, liste détaillée
S especificación, lista detallada, inventario

bimetal
G Bimetall
F bimétal
S bimetal

bin
G Behälter
F bac, container, cuve
S recipiente

binary nozzle
G Zweistoffdüse
F buse binaire
S aplicador binario

binding
G verbindlich
F obligatoire
S obligatorio

binding agent
G Bindemittel
F liant
S aglomerante, aglutinante

binding agent type
G Bindemitteltyp
F type de liant
S tipo de aglutinante

binding capacity
G Bindungsvermögen
F capacité de fixation
S capacidad de enlace, capacidad de fijación

bioavailability
G Bioverfügbarkeit
F biodisponibilité
S biodisponibilidad

bioburden
G Keimbelastung
F teneur en micro-organismes
S carga de gérmenes

biochemical oxygen demand (bod) analysis
G biochemischer Sauerstoffbedarf (BSB)
F analyse de la demande biologique d'oxygène (DBO)
S necesidades bioquímicas de oxígeno

biocompatible
G biokompatibel
F biocompatible
S biocompatible

biodegradable
G biologisch abbaubar
F biodégradable
S degradable biológicamente

biodegradation
G biologischer Abbau
F biodégradation
S degradación biológica

bioequivalence
G Bioäquivalenz
F bioéquivalence
S bioequivalencia

biogenerator
G Biogenerator
F biogénérateur
S biogenerador

biogenesis
G Biogenese
F biogenèse
S biogénesis

biogenic
G biogen
F biogène
S biógeno

biohazard
G Biogefahr, Gefahr durch biologische Agenzien
F danger biologique, risque biologique
S peligro biológico

biohazard cabinet
G Biosicherheitskabinett
F enceinte de risques biologiques
S gabinete de seguridad biológica

biohazard laboratory
G Biosicherheitslabor
F laboratoire de risques biologiques
S laboratorio de seguridad biológica

bioindicator
G Bioindikator
F indicateur biologique
S bioindicador

biological filter
G Biofilter
F filtre biologique
S filtro biológico

biological fluids
G biologische Flüssigkeiten
F liquides biologiques
S líquidos biológicos

English
German
French
Spanish

biological testing
G biologische Prüfung
F examens biologiques
S prueba biológica

biological treatment
G biologische Behandlung
F traitement biologique
S tratamiento biológico

bioluminescence
G Biolumineszenz
F bioluminescence
S bioluminiscencia

biomass
G Biomasse
F biomasse
S biomasa

biopharmaceutical
G biotechnologisch hergestelltes Arzneimittel
F produit biopharmaceutique
S medicamento producido biotecnológicamente

biosafety
G biologische Sicherheit
F bio-sécurité
S seguridad biológica

biosafety laboratory
G Biosicherheitslabor
F laboratoire de risques biologiques
S laboratorio de seguridad biológica

biosafety level
G biologische Sicherheitsstufe
F niveau de bio-sécurité
S grado de seguridad biológica

biosynthesis
G Biosynthese
F biosynthèse
S biosíntesis

biotechnology
G Biotechnologie
F biotechnologie
S biotecnología

biting capsule
G Zerbeißkapsel
F capsule à croquer
S cápsula mordible

bitter
G bitter
F amer
S amargo

bitter component
G Bitterstoff
F composant amer, substance amère
S sustancia amarga

blade
G Schaufel, Flügelrad
F pale, pelle, ailette
S pala, rueda de aletas, rueda de paletas

blade stirrer
G Flügelrührer
F agitateur à pales
S agitador de aletas

blank
G Blindprobe, Rohling
F valeur témoin, valeur à blanc, ébauche, pièce brute
S muestra en blanco, testigo, pieza bruta

blank value
G Blindwert, Leerwert
F valeur témoin, valeur à blanc
S valor en blanco, valor testigo

blend
G Mischung
F mixture, mélange
S mezcla, mixtura

blend, to
G mischen
F mélanger
S mezclar

blender
G Mischer
F mélangeur, malaxeur
S mezclador

forced-circulation mixer
G Zwangsmischer
F mélangeur excentrique
S mezclador de circulación forzada

high-shear mixer
G Mischer mit hohem Scherkraftanteil
F mélangeur avec forces de cisaillements importantes
S mezclador con gran fuerza de cizallamiento

tumble blender
G Taumelmischer
F mélangeur turbulent
S mezclador de turbulencia

blending apparatus
G Mischer
F mélangeur, malaxeur
S mezclador

blending cycle
G Mischzyklus
F cycle de mélange
S ciclo de mezcla

blending mixture
G Mischgut
F mélange homogénéisé
S mezcla homogeneizada

blending ratio
G Mischungsverhältnis
F titration, proportions de mélange
S proporción de mezcla

blinding
G Verblindung
F préparation pour essai en aveugle
S preparación para ensayo ciego

blister
G Blister, Blase
F blister, bulle
S blíster, ampolla, burbuja, vejiga

blister (forming) line
G Tiefziehmaschine
F machine pour conditionnements thermoformés
S máquina para troquelar en caliente

blister pack
G Blisterverpackung, Durchdrückpackung, Tiefziehverpackung
F conditionnement à bulles, conditionnement blister, plaquette, plaquette thermoformée, conditionnement thermoformé, conditionnement sous blister
S embalado en blísters, blíster, envase termoformado, envase blíster

blister tightness test
G Blisterdichtigkeitstest
F test d'étanchéité du blister
S prueba de estanqueidad del blíster

block, to
G blockieren
F bloquer
S bloquear

blockage
G Blockierung
F blocage
S bloqueo

blocked
G verstopft
F obstrué, bouché
S obstruido

blocking valve
G Sperrventil
F vanne de verrouillage
S válvula de bloqueo

blood bank
G Blutbank
F banque du sang
S banco de sangre

English German French Spanish

blood corpuscle
G Blutkörperchen
F globule sanguin
S eritrocito

blood donor service
G Blutspendewesen
F banque du sang
S servicio de donantes de sangre

blood plasma derivative
G Blutplasmaderivat
F produit d'origine plasmatique
S producto de plasma sanguíneo

blood plasma product
G Blutplasmaderivat
F produit d'origine plasmatique
S producto de plasma sanguíneo

blood product
G Blutprodukt
F produit sanguin
S producto sanguíneo

blossom
G Blüte
F fleur
S flor

blow moulding
G Blasverformung
F moulage par procédé pressé-soufflé
S moldeo por inyección

blow out, to
G ausblasen
F souffler, éteindre
S apagar soplando

blue dye bath test
G Blaubadtest
F test au bain bleu
S prueba de baño con colorante azul

blue silica gel
G Blaugel
F gel bleu
S gel azul de sílice

board of directors
G Vorstand
F comité de direction
S junta directiva

boil, to
G aufkochen, sieden
F bouillir
S hervir

boiler
G Kessel
F chaudière, bouilloire
S caldera, marmita

boiling capillary
G Siedekapillare
F capillaire d'ébullition
S capilar de ebullición

boiling chip
G Siedestein
F pierre facilitant l'ébullition
S piedra de ebullición

boiling point
G Siedepunkt
F point d'ébullition
S punto de ebullición

boiling retardation
G Siedeverzug
F retardement de l'ébullition
S retraso de la ebullición

bolt
G Bolzen
F boulon, cheville
S clavija, perno

bond
G Bindung
F liaison
S enlace

ion bonding
G ionische Bindung
F liaison ionique
S enlace iónico

trivalent bonding
G Dreifachbindung
F triple liaison
S enlace triple

bonding material
G Verbindungsmaterial
F substance de liaison
S material de unión

border, to
G umbördeln
F sertir
S bordear, rebordear, redondear

bore
G Bohrung
F forage, percement
S perforación

borosilicate glass
G Borosilikatglas
F verre de borosilicate
S vidrio de silicato bórico

bottle
G Flasche
F bouteille
S botella

bottle cap
G Flaschenverschluß
F capsule à bouteilles
S cierre de botella, tapa de botella

bottle neck
G Flaschenhals
F goulot, col de bouteille
S cuello de botella, gollete

bottle-closing machine
G Flaschenverschließmaschine
F machine d'encapsulage
S máquina de cierre de botellas

bottling line
G Abfüllinie, Abfüllstraße
F ligne de remplissage, rampe de remplissage, chaîne de remplissage
S cadena de envasado

bottling machine
G Flaschenabfüllmaschine
F machine de remplissage des bouteilles
S embotelladora

bottom plate
G Bodenplatte
F dalle (de sol)
S placa del suelo

bottom screen
G Bodensieb
F tamis bas, crible bas
S tamiz base

bovine prion
G Rinderprion
F prion bovin
S prión bovino

box
G Schachtel
F carton, boîte
S caja

branching
G Verzweigung
F ramification
S ramificación

brand name
G Markenname, Handelsmarke
F nom commercial, marque de commerce
S nombre comercial, marca comercial

break an ampoule, to
G Ampulle aufbrechen
F casser une ampoule
S romper una ampolla

break notch
G Bruchkerbe, Bruchrille
F encoche de rupture, entaille de rupture
S muesca de ruptura, ranura de ruptura, surco de ruptura

break point
G Bruchstelle
F point de rupture
S lugar de ruptura

break score
G Bruchrille
F encoche de rupture, entaille de rupture
S ranura de ruptura, surco de ruptura

breakage of glassware
G Glasbruch
F débris de verre
S ruptura de vidrio

breakdown
G Betriebsstörung, Ausfall, Panne
F perturbation de fonctionnement, panne, temps mort, défaillance
S interrupción del funcionamiento, avería, desperfecto, fallo

breaking current
G Ausschaltstrom
F courant de coupure
S corriente de desconexión

breaking notch
G Kreuzbruchkerbe
F encoche de rupture
S muesca de ruptura

breaking point
G Bruchstelle
F point de rupture
S lugar de ruptura

breaking resistance
G Bruchfestigkeit
F résistance à la rupture
S resistencia a la rotura

breaking strength
G Bruchfestigkeit
F résistance à la rupture
S resistencia a la rotura

brimful
G randvoll
F plein à ras-bord
S lleno a rebosar

brittle
G brüchig, spröde
F cassant, fragile
S frágil, quebradizo

brittleness
G Brüchigkeit
F fragilité
S fragilidad, friabilidad

bromination
G Bromierung
F bromage
S bromado

brush
G Bürste
F brosse
S cepillo

brush coat, to
G einstreichen (mit einer Bürste)
F enduire à la brosse
S untar con cepillo

bubble
G Blase
F bulle
S ampolla, burbuja, vejiga

bubble point test
G Blasendrucktest
F essai de point de bulle
S prueba de presión de vejiga, cistometría

Buchner funnel
G Nutsche
F entonnoir de Buchner
S embudo de Buchner

buckle, to
G knicken
F casser, couder
S doblar, quebrar

buffer
G Puffer
F tampon
S tampón

buffer solution
G Pufferlösung
F solution tampon
S solución de tamponamiento

buffering capacity
G Pufferkapazität
F capacité d'un tampon
S capacidad de tamponamiento

building
G Gebäude
F bâtiment, édifice
S edificio

building (facility) floor plan
G Gebäudeplan
F plan de l'édifice
S plan del edificio

bulb cooler
G Kugelkühler
F réfrigérant à boules
S refrigerador a bolas

bulk (material)
G Bulkware
F marchandise en vrac
S mercancía a granel

bulk density
G Schüttdichte
F densité apparente
S densidad de la masa comprimida

bulk material
G Schüttgut
F matériau en vrac
S carga a granel

bulk mixture
G Bulkmischung
F produits en vrac
S mezcla a granel

bulk pharmaceutical chemical (BPC)
G Wirkstoff (als Rohstoff)
F matière première en vrac
S sustancia activa (materia prima)

bulkhead connection
G Schottverschraubung
F connexion étanche
S atornillado hermético

bundle, to
G bündeln
F lier ensemble
S enfardar

bundling machine
G Bündelmaschine, Bündelpacker
F machine d'empaquetage, lieuse
S máquina de embalaje, enfardador

Bunsen burner
G Bunsenbrenner
F bec de gaz, bec de Bunsen
S mechero Bunsen

bur (of a tablet)
G Grat (einer Tablette)
F arête d'un comprimé
S borde (de un comprimido)

burette
G Bürette
F burette
S bureta

burst, to
G bersten
F éclater
S estallar, reventar

bursting disk
G Berstscheibe
F disque de rupture
S disco de ruptura

bursting pressure
G Berstdruck
F pression d'éclatement
S presión de rotura

bursting strength
G Berstdruckfestigkeit
F résistance à l'éclatement
S resistencia al estallido

English German French Spanish

bush
G Hülle
F douille, coussinet, manchon
S envoltura

bush (mach.)
G Muffe
F manchon, collet
S manguito

bushing (mach.)
G Muffe
F manchon, collet
S manguito

butterfly valve
G Drosselventil
F vanne papillon
S válvula de mariposa

butt-weld, to
G stumpfschweißen
F souder par rapprochement
S soldar a tope

butyl rubber stoppers
G Stopfen aus Butylgummi
F bouchon en caoutchouc butyle
S tapón de caucho butílico

by-product
G Nebenprodukt
F sous-produit, produit secondaire
S producto colateral, producto secundario

cable
G Kabel
F câble
S cable

cable clamp
G Kabelschelle
F serre-fils
S abrazadera de cable

cable duct
G Kabelkanal
F canal de câbles
S canal de cables

cable lug
G Kabelschuh
F cosse de câble
S terminal de cable

cable terminal
G Kabelklemme
F serre-fils
S terminal de cable

cachet
G Oblate, Oblatenkapsel
F capsule, cachet
S cápsula amilácea, oblea, gragea

cake formation
G Kuchenbildung
F prise en masse
S cuajamiento

caking
G Kuchenbildung
F prise en masse
S cuajamiento

calculate, to
G berechnen
F calculer
S calcular

calculation
G Berechnung, Rechnung
F calculation, calcul
S cálculo

calculation error
G Rechenfehler
F erreur de calcul
S error de cálculo

calibrate, to
G eichen, kalibrieren
F calibrer
S calibrar

calibrated pipette
G Vollpipette
F pipette calibrée
S pipeta calibrada

calibrating equipment
G Prüfmittel (zur Kalibrierung)
F équipement de calibration
S sistema de prueba (para calibrar)

calibration
G Kalibrierung, Eichung
F calibration
S calibración

multiple point calibration
G Kalibrierung anhand mehrerer Meßpunkte
F calibration par points de mesure multiples
S calibración por varios puntos

single point calibration
G Ein-Punkt-Kalibrierung
F calibration par un point de mesure
S calibración por punto único

calibration certificate
G Eichschein, Kalibrierschein
F certificat de calibration
S certificado de calibración

calibration curve
G Kalibrierkurve
F courbe de calibration
S curva de calibración

calibration interval
G Kalibrierintervall
F intervalle de calibration
S intervalo de calibración

calorimeter
G Kalorimeter
F calorimètre
S calorímetro

cam
G Nocke
F came
S leva

campaign
G Kampagne
F campagne
S campaña

camshaft
G Nockenwelle
F arbre à cames
S árbol de levas

can
G Dose
F canne
S bote, caja, lata

cane sugar
G Rohrzucker
F sucre de canne
S azúcar de caña

cannula
G Kanüle
F canule
S cánula

cant, to
G verkanten
F mettre sur l'arête
S ladear

canteen
G Kantine
F cantine
S cantina

cap
G Kopfhaube, Verschluß
F bonnet, bouchon, capuchon, couvercle
S capucha, cofia, cierre

cap, to (tablets)
G verbördeln, deckeln (bei Tabletten)
F capsuler (comprimés)
S rebordear cantos, cubrir, recubrir (comprimidos)

capable of flowing
G rieselfähig
F capable d'écoulement
S capaz de fluir

capacity
G Kapazität, Leistung, Fassungsvermögen
F capacité, contenance, performance
S capacidad, rendimiento

capillary
G Kapillare
F capillaire
S capilar

capillary electrophoresis
G Kapillarelektrophorese
F électrophorèse capillaire
S electroforesis capilar

capper
G Bördelmaschine
F boucheuse, capsuleuse
S máquina de rebordeo

capping machine
G Deckelverschließmaschine, Verschließmaschine
F encapsuleur, capsuleuse
S máquina para cerrar cápsulas, máquina de cierre

capsule
G Kapsel, Oblate
F capsule, cachet
S cápsula, oblea, gragea

capsule filling machine
G Kapselfüllmaschine
F encapsuleuse
S máquina de relleno de cápsulas

capsule shell
G Kapselhülse
F gousse d'une capsule
S cubierta de una cápsula

capsule size
G Kapselgröße
F taille d'une capsule
S tamaño de una cápsula

carbohydrates
G Kohlenhydrate
F hydrates de carbone, glucides
S hidratos de carbono

carbon
G Kohle
F carbone
S carbón

carbon chain
G Kohlenstoffkette
F chaîne carbonée
S cadena carbonada

carbon dioxide
G Kohlendioxyd
F dioxyde de carbone
S anhídrido carbónico

carbon filter
G Kohlefilter
F filtre au carbone
S filtro de carbón

carbon steel
G Karbonstahl
F acier au carbone
S acero al carbono

carboxylic acid
G Carbonsäure
F acide carboxylique
S ácido carbónico

carcinogenic
G cancerogen, karzinogen, krebserregend
F carcinogène, cancérogène
S cancerógeno, carcinógeno

cardboard
G Pappe
F carton
S cartón

carrier gas
G Trägergas
F gaz porteur
S gas portador

carry out, to
G durchführen
F réaliser, exécuter
S ejecutar, llevar a cabo, realizar

carryover
G Übertrag
F report, somme intermédiaire
S transporte

carton
G Karton, Schachtel, Pappschachtel
F carton, boîte
S cartón, caja, caja de cartón

carton, to
G kartonieren
F cartonner
S encartonar

cartoning machine
G Kartonierer
F machine à cartonner
S máquina encartonadora

cartoning section
G Kartonierteil
F aire d'encartonnage
S área de encartonamiento

cartoning technology
G Kartoniertechnik
F technique d'encartonnage
S técnica de encartonar

cartridge
G Kartusche, Patrone
F cartouche
S cartucho

cartridge gasket
G Patronendichtung
F joint de cartouche
S junta de cartucho

case report form
G Prüfbogen
F questionnaire
S cuestionario

casing
G Verkleidungsblech
F couvercle, capuchon
S chapa de revestimiento

casters
G Laufrollen, Lenkrollen
F rouleau porteur, galet de guidage, poulie de guidage
S polea, roldana

catalyst
G Katalysator
F catalyseur
S catalizador

catch basin
G Sinkkasten
F bassin de descente
S fuente (descendente) de recogida

catheter
G Katheter
F cathéter, sonde
S catéter

cathode
G Kathode
F cathode
S cátodo

cation
G Kation
F cation
S catión

cation chromatography
G Kationenchromatographie
F chromatographie sur résine échangeuse de cations
S cromatografía de cationes

cation exchanger
G Kationentauscher
F échangeur de cations
S intercambiador de cationes

cause of failure
G Fehlerursache
F cause du défaut
S causa de error

cause, to
G verursachen
F provoquer
S causar, provocar

caustic
G ätzend
F caustique
S cáustico

English German French Spanish

cavity
G Hohlraum, Vertiefung
F cavité, espace creux, puits
S cavidad, espacio hueco, depresión

CE symbol
G CE-Zeichen
F symbole CE
S símbolo CE

ceiling
G Decke
F plafond
S techo

false ceiling
G eingezogene Decke
F faux plafond
S techo falso

suspended ceiling
G abgehängte Decke
F faux plafond
S techo suspendido

ceiling lighting
G Deckenbeleuchtung
F éclairage plafonnier
S alumbrado de techo

cell
G Zelle, Küvette
F cellule, cuvette
S célula, cubeta

cell changer
G Küvettenwechsler
F échangeur de cuvette
S intercambiador de cubetas

cell counter
G Zellzähler
F compteur de cellules
S contador de células

cell culture
G Zellkultur
F culture de cellules
S cultivo celular

cell density
G Zelldichte
F densité de cellules
S densidad de células

cell growth
G Zellwachstum
F croissance de cellules
S crecimiento celular

cell harvesting
G Zellernte
F récolte de cellules
S recolección de células

cell holder
G Küvettenhalter
F support de cuvette
S portacubetas

cell mount
G Küvettenhalter
F support de cuvette
S portacubetas

cell population
G Zellpopulation
F population de cellules
S población celular

cell proliferation
G Zellvermehrung
F prolifération de cellules
S proliferación celular

cell wall
G Zellwand
F membrane cellulaire
S pared celular

cellular anomaly
G zelluläre Anomalie
F anomalie cellulaire
S anomalía celular

cellular prion (prpc)
G zelluläres Prion
F prion cellulaire (prpc)
S prión celular (prpc)

cellulose
G Zellstoff
F cellulose
S celulosa

cement flooring
G Zementestrich
F chape de ciment
S suelo de cemento

censored
G zensiert
F censuré
S censado

central receiving
G zentrale Warenannahme
F réception de marchandises
S recepción central de mercancías

central weighing area
G zentrale Einwaage
F aire centrale de pesage
S área central de pesado

centre of gravity
G Schwerpunkt
F centre de gravité
S baricentro, centro de gravedad

centre, to
G zentrieren
F centrer
S centrar

centrifugal fan
G Zentrifugalventilator
F ventilateur centrifuge
S ventilador centrífugo

centrifugal force
G Fliehkraft, Zentrifugalkraft
F force de centrifugation
S fuerza centrífuga

centrifugation
G Zentrifugation
F centrifugation
S centrifugación

centrifuge
G Zentrifuge
F centrifugeuse
S centrífuga

centrifuge, to
G zentrifugieren
F centrifuger
S centrifugar

certificate
G Urkunde, Zertifikat
F certificat
S certificado, documento

certificate of analysis
G Analysenzertifikat
F certificat d'analyse
S certificado de análisis

certificate of conformity
G Konformitätszertifikat
F certificat de conformité
S certificado de conformidad

certificate, to
G zertifizieren
F certifier
S certificar

certification
G Zertifizierung
F certification
S certificación

cessation (of a reaction)
G Unterbrechung (einer Reaktion)
F interruption d'une réaction
S interrupción (de una reacción)

chain drive
G Kettenantrieb
F entraînement par chaînes
S propulsión por cadena

chairman
G Vorsitzender, Obmann
F porte-parole
S portavoz, presidente

challenge test
G Belastungstest
F test de stimulation
S prueba de carga

chamber
G Kammer
F chambre
S cámara

change
G Änderung, Wechsel
F changement
S cambio, modificación, variación

change control
G Änderungskontrolle
F contrôle des changements, contrôle des modifications
S control de modificaciones

change management
G Änderungskontrolle
F contrôle des changements, contrôle des modifications
S control de modificaciones

change of location
G Standortwechsel
F déménagement
S cambio de emplazamiento

change of site
G Standortwechsel
F déménagement
S cambio de emplazamiento

change request
G Änderungsantrag
F demande de modification
S solicitud de cambio

changing room
G Umkleide
F vestiaire
S vestuario

channel
G Kanal
F canal, canalisation, voie
S canal, tubo, conducto

characterisation (of a compound)
G Charakterisierung (einer Verbindung)
F caractérisation (d'un composé organique)
S caracterización (de un compuesto)

charge
G Füllgut
F matière de remplissage
S material de relleno

charge (electricity)
G Ladung (Elektrizität)
F charge (électricité)
S carga (electricidad)

charge chute
G Befüllrutsche
F toboggan de charge, toboggan d'alimentation, glissoir de charge
S tobogán de carga

charge port
G Befüllstutzen
F orifice de charge, orifice d'alimentation
S tubuladura de carga, tubuladura de alimentación

charge tube
G Befüllrohr
F conduite de charge, conduite d'alimentation
S conducto de carga, conducto de alimentación

charge, to
G einfüllen, beladen
F charger, alimenter
S envasar, llenar

charged ion
G geladenes Ion
F ion chargé
S ion cargado

charging device
G Einfüllvorrichtung
F dispositif d'alimentation, appareillage d'alimentation
S dispositivo de relleno

charging funnel
G Einfülltrichter
F trémie de charge
S embudo de relleno

charging tube
G Einfüllrohr
F conduite d'alimentation
S tubo de relleno

charging valve
G Einfüllklappe
F vanne d'alimentation
S válvula de relleno

chart recorder
G Diagrammschreiber, Schreiber
F enregistreur graphique, enregistreur
S registrador gráfico, registradora

check
G Kontrolle, Überprüfung
F contrôle, vérification
S control, comprobación

check valve
G Rückschlagventil
F vanne anti-retour
S válvula de retención

check, to
G überprüfen
F contrôler, vérifier
S comprobar

checked
G geprüft
F contrôlé, inspecté, vérifié
S comprobado

chelate
G Chelatkomplex
F chélate, complexe de chélation
S complejo de quelatos

chelate complex
G Chelatkomplex
F chélate, complexe de chélation
S complejo de quelatos

chelate formation
G Chelatbildung
F formation de chélate
S formación de quelatos

chelated compound
G Chelatverbindung
F composé organique chélaté
S compuesto quelado

chelating agent
G Komplexiermittel
F agent chélatant
S agente quelante

chemical agents
G chemische Agenzien, chemische Mittel
F agents chimiques
S agentes químicos

chemical compound
G chemische Verbindung
F combinaison chimique
S compuesto químico

chemical modification
G chemische Modifikation
F modification chimique
S modificación química

chemical plant
G Chemiebetrieb
F usine chimique
S planta química

chemical profile
G chemisches Profil
F profil chimique
S perfil químico

chemical purity
G chemische Reinheit
F pureté chimique
S pureza química

chemically pure
G chemisch rein
F chimiquement pur
S químicamente puro

chemicals
G Chemikalien
F produits chimiques
S productos químicos

chemiluminescence
G Chemilumineszenz
F chimiluminescence, chimioluminescence
S quimioluminiscencia

chewing tablet
G Kautablette
F comprimé à mâcher
S comprimidos masticables

child-proof
G kindersicher
F inaccessible aux enfants
S inaccesible para niños

child-proof packaging
G kindersichere Verpackung
F emballage de sécurité pour enfants
S embalaje a prueba de niños

child-resistant closure
G kindersicherer Verschluß
F fermeture de sécurité pour enfants
S cierre a prueba de niños

chiral ligand exchange chromatography
G chirale Ligandenaustauschchromatographie
F chromatographie d'échange de ligands optiquement actifs
S cromatografía de intercambio de ligandos ópticamente activos

chiral medicinal substance
G chiraler Arzneistoff
F médicament optiquement actif
S sustancia medicamentosa ópticamente activa

chiral purity
G chirale Reinheit
F pureté chirale
S pureza quiral

chirality
G Chiralität
F chiralité
S quiralidad

chlorinate, to
G chlorieren
F chlorurer
S clorar

chlorinated water
G Chlorwasser
F eau chlorée
S agua clorada

chlorine
G Chlor
F chlor
S cloro

chocolate agar
G Schokoladenagar
F gélose chocolat
S agar chocolate

chopper
G Zerhacker
F hachoir, couperet
S troceadora

chopper speed
G Zerhackergeschwindigkeit
F vitesse de hachoir
S velocidad de troceo

chromatogram
G Chromatogramm
F chromatogramme
S cromatograma

chromatographic assay
G chromatographische Methode
F méthode chromatographique
S método cromatográfico

chromatography
G Chromatographie
F chromatographie
S cromatografía

ascending chromatography
G aufsteigende Chromatographie
F chromatographie ascendante
S cromatografía ascendente

descending chromatography
G absteigende Chromatographie
F chromatographie descendante
S cromatografía descendente

chrome steel
G Chromstahl
F acier chromé
S acero cromado

chromium plated
G verchromt
F chromé
S cromado

chromosulphuric acid
G Chromschwefelsäure
F acide sulfurique chromique
S ácido sulfúrico crómico

chute
G Rutsche
F toboggan
S tobogán

circuit
G Stromkreis
F circuit
S circuito eléctrico

circuit (electrical)
G Schaltung (elektrisch)
F circuit, connexion (électrique)
S conexión (eléctrica)

circuit board
G Platine
F platine
S platino

circuit diagram
G Schaltbild
F schéma de montage, schéma des connexions
S diagrama de circuito

circulatory dryer
G Umlufttrockner
F séchoir à circulation d'air
S secador de circulación de aire

circulatory pump
G Umwälzpumpe
F pompe de circulation
S bomba de circulación

circumference
G Umfang
F circonférence, périmètre, étendue
S circunferencia, perímetro, extensión

cladding (of piping)
G Verkleidung (von Rohrleitungen)
F revêtement (de tuyauteries)
S recubrimiento (de conducciones)

clamp
G Klammer
F pinces
S pinzas

clarity
G Klarheit
F clareté
S claridad

classify, to
G sichten, klassieren
F classifier
S clasificar, ordenar

clean air
G Reinluft
F air filtré
S aire limpio

clean area
G Reinraum, reiner Bereich
F zone aseptique, zone d'atmosphère contrôlée
S área estéril, área limpia

clean bench
G reine Werkbank
F paillasse sous flux laminaire
S banco de trabajo estéril

English
German
French
Spanish

clean room
G Reinraum
F zone d'atmosphère contrôlée
S área estéril

clean room class
G Reinraumklasse
F niveau de stérilité
S nivel de esterilidad

clean room clothing
G Reinraumkleidung
F vêtement protecteur pour zone d'atmosphère contrôlée
S ropa para área estéril

clean room engineering
G Reinraumtechnik
F ingénierie des zones d'atmosphère contrôlée
S técnica para el área estéril

clean room grade
G Reinraumklasse
F niveau de stérilité
S nivel de esterilidad

clean room operations
G Arbeitsvorgänge im Reinraum
F opérations en zone d'atmosphère contrôlée
S procesos de trabajo en área estéril

clean steam
G Reinstdampf
F vapeur pure
S vapor puro

cleaning
G Reinigung
F nettoyage
S limpieza

cleaning cloth
G Reinigungstuch
F chiffon, serpillière
S paño de limpieza

cleaning equipment
G Reinigungsgerät
F équipement de nettoyage
S aparato de limpieza

cleaning in-place (CIP)
G Reinigung (von Anlagen) im geschlossenen System
F nettoyage en place (CIP)
S limpieza (de instalaciones) en sistema cerrado

cleaning nozzle
G Waschdüse
F buse de nettoyage
S aplicador de lavado

cleaning procedure
G Reinigungsvorschrift
F procédure de nettoyage
S instrucción de limpieza

cleaning schedule
G Reinigungsplan
F programme de nettoyage
S plan de limpieza

cleaning tissue
G Reinigungstuch
F chiffon, serpillière
S paño de limpieza

cleaning validation
G Reinigungsvalidierung
F validation du nettoyage
S validación de la limpieza

cleanliness
G Sauberkeit
F propreté
S limpieza

cleanliness class
G Reinheitsklasse
F classe d'environnement
S nivel de pureza

cleanliness grade (e. g. room)
G Reinheitsgrad, Reinigungsgrad, Reinheitsklasse
F niveau de propreté, niveau de pureté, classe d'environnement
S grado de pureza, grado de limpieza, nivel de pureza

cleansing agent
G Reinigungsmittel
F agent de nettoyage
S detergente, producto de limpieza

clear
G klar, deutlich, eindeutig
F transparent, clair, distinct, précis
S claro, transparente, distinto, inequívoco, unívoco

clearance
G Freiraum
F espace libre
S espacio libre

cleft
G Spalte
F fissure, fente, crevasse
S fisura

clerk
G Sachbearbeiter
F responsable
S encargado, ponente

client
G Auftraggeber
F client, commettant, donneur d'ordre
S cliente, comitente, comisionista

climate-controlled area
G Bereich mit kontrolliertem Klima
F zone d'atmosphère contrôlée
S zona de atmósfera controlada

climatic chamber
G Klimaprüfkammer
F chambre de climatisation
S cámara de aclimat(iz)ación

clinical research
G klinische Forschung
F recherche clinique
S investigación clínica

clinical study
G klinische Studie
F essai clinique
S estudio clínico

clinical trial
G klinische Prüfung, klinische Studie
F essai clinique
S ensayo clínico, estudio clínico

for clinical trial use
G zur klinischen Prüfung bestimmt
F réservé aux essais cliniques
S reservado para ensayos clínicos

clinical trial location
G klinische Prüfeinrichtung
F emplacement des essais cliniques
S centro de investigación clínica

clinical trial sample
G klinisches Prüfmuster
F échantillon clinique
S muestra para ensayos clínicos

clip
G Schelle
F collier
S abrazadera, collar

clockwise
G im Uhrzeigersinn
F dans le sens des aiguilles d'une montre
S sentido horario

clogged
G verstopft
F obstrué, bouché
S obstruido

cloning
G Klonierung
F clonage
S clonación

close off, to
G absperren
F fermer
S cerrar, cortar

closed loop
G geschlossener Kreislauf
F circulation fermée
S circulación cerrada

English German French Spanish

closure
G Verschluß
F bouchon, capuchon, couvercle
S cierre

tube closure
G Tubenverschluß
F bouchon de tube
S cierre de un tubo

closure material
G Verschlußmaterial
F matériau de fermeture
S material de cierre

clothing receptacle
G Kleidungsaufnahmebehälter
F corbeille pour vêtements de travail
S cesto para ropa de trabajo

cloudy
G trüb
F turbide, trouble
S turbio

coagulate, to
G gerinnen
F coaguler
S coagular

coagulation
G Gerinnung, Koagulation
F coagulation
S coagulación

coalescing filter
G Koaleszenzfilter
F filtre coalescent
S filtro de coalescencia

coarse
G grob
F brut, grossier
S grosero, grueso

coarse granules
G Grobgranulat
F granulés grossiers
S granulado grueso

coarse particle
G Grobkorn
F particule grossière
S grano grueso

coarse sieve
G Grobsieb
F tamis grossier
S tamiz de malla gruesa

coat
G Überzug
F couche, pellicule
S cubierta, revestimiento

coat, to (tablets)
G beschichten, überziehen (Tabletten)
F enduire, enrober (comprimés)
S laminar, recubrir (comprimidos)

coated (tablets)
G überzogen (Tabletten)
F enduit (comprimés)
S recubierto (comprimidos)

coated film
G beschichtete Folie
F feuille enduite
S lámina recubierta

coated foil
G beschichtete Folie
F feuille enduite
S lámina recubierta

coated tablet
G Filmtablette
F comprimé pelliculé
S gragea

coating
G Belag, Beschichtung, Filmüberzug
F revêtement, film de revêtement, couche, enduction
S recubrimiento, revestimiento, película de revestimiento

coating lacquer
G Überzugslack
F vernis de couverture
S barniz de cobertura

coating pan
G Dragierkessel
F dragéification (à la turbine)
S caldera para gragear

coating quantity
G Auftragsmenge (beim Coating)
F quantité (d'enduit) appliquée
S cantidad a aplicar (al recubrir)

coating thickness
G Auftragsdicke
F épaisseur de l'enduit, épaisseur de la couche
S espesor de la capa

code bars
G Codestriche
F code à barres
S barras de código

code reader, electronic
G elektronisches Codelesegerät
F déchiffreur électronique de codage
S lector electrónico de códigos

code reading
G Codelesung
F lecture du codage
S lectura de códigos

coding station
G Prägestation
F station d'estampage
S estación de troquelado

coefficient of absorbance
G Extinktionskoeffizient
F coefficient d'absorption
S coeficiente de extinción

coefficient of expansion
G Dehnungskoeffizient
F coefficient d'expansion
S coeficiente de dilatación

coefficient of friction
G Reibungskoeffizient
F coefficient de friction, coefficient de frottement
S coeficiente de fricción

coefficient of variation
G Variationskoeffizient
F coefficient de variation
S coeficiente de validación

coenzyme
G Koenzym
F coenzyme
S coenzima

coherent
G kohärent
F cohérent
S coherente

cohesion
G Kohäsion
F cohésion
S cohesión

cohesive power
G Kohäsionskraft
F force de cohésion
S fuerza de cohesión

cold room
G Kühlraum
F chambre froide
S cámara frigorífica

cold storage
G Kühllager
F stockage à froid
S almacén frigorífico

cold store
G Kühllager
F stockage à froid
S almacén frigorífico

coldest spot (autoclave)
G kältester Punkt (beim Autoklav)
F point le plus froid
S punto más frío (en autoclave)

collar
G Manschette
F collier, bague, anneau
S manguito

collation of data
G Datenüberprüfung
F collation de données
S comprobación de datos

collect, to
G auffangen
F capter, recueillir
S captar, colectar, recoger

collection system
G Sammelsystem
F système de collecte
S sistema colector

collection vessel
G Auffanggefäß
F cuve de collecte, récipient de collecte
S recipiente colector

collector
G Sammelbehälter
F réservoir, collecteur
S depósito (colector)

collodion
G filmbildende Flüssigkeit
F collodion
S colodión

colloidal dispersion
G Kolloiddispersion
F dispersion colloïdale
S dispersión coloidal

colony-forming unit (CFU)
G koloniebildende Einheit (KBE)
F unité formant colonie
S unidad formadora de colonias

colorimetric solution
G Farbvergleichslösung
F solution colorimétrique
S solución colorimétrica

colour capacity
G Färbevermögen
F capacité de coloration
S capacidad colorante

colour change
G Farbumschlag
F changement de couleur
S cambio de color

colour coating
G Farbüberzug
F revêtement de couleur
S revestimiento coloreado

colour code
G Farbcodierung
F codage de couleurs
S codificación de colores

colour code specification
G Farbcodierungsspezifikation
F spécification du codage de couleurs
S especificación de la codificación de colores

colour dispersion
G Farbdispersion
F dispersion de la couleur
S dispersión cromática

colour ring code reader
G Farbringleser
F lecteur de codage de couleurs
S lector de anillo cromático

colour scale
G Farbabstufung, Farbskala
F gradation de couleurs, gamme de couleurs
S gradación de colores, escala cromática

colour shade
G Farbton
F teinte, nuance d'une couleur
S matiz del color

colour uniformity
G Farbuniformität
F uniformité de couleur
S uniformidad cromática

colouration
G Färbung
F coloration, teinture
S coloración

colouring agent
G Färbemittel, Farbstoff
F colorant, pigment
S colorante

colourless
G farblos
F incolore
S incoloro

column conditioning
G Säulenkonditionierung
F conditionnement d'une colonne
S acondicionamiento de la columna

column coupling
G Säulenverbindung
F couplage de colonnes
S acople de columna

column diameter
G Säulendurchmesser
F diamètre de colonne
S diámetro de la columna

column filler
G Säulenfüllmaterial
F matériel de remplissage d'une colonne
S material de relleno de la columna

column length
G Säulenlänge
F longueur de colonne
S longitud de la columna

column outlet
G Auslaßöffnung einer Säule
F sortie d'une colonne
S orificio de salida de una columna

column oven
G Säulenofen
F four pour colonne
S horno de columna

column overloading
G Säulenüberladung
F surcharge de la colonne
S sobrecarga de columna

column packing
G Säulenfüllung
F package de colonne
S llenado de la columna

column performance
G Trennleistung der Säule
F performance d'une colonne
S rendimiento separador de la columna

combustible
G brennbar
F combustible
S combustible, inflamable

combustion
G Verbrennung
F combustion, incinération
S combustión, incineración

command
G Befehlseingabe
F entrée d'une commande
S entrada de un comando

commercial name
G Handelsname
F nom de commerce
S nombre comercial

commercial product
G Handelsware
F produit commercial
S producto comercial

compact line
G Kompaktanlage
F appareillage compact
S instalación compacta

compactible mixture
G preßfertige Mischung
F mélange comprimable
S mezcla comprimible

compaction
G Tablettierung
F fabrication de comprimés
S fabricación de comprimidos

English German French Spanish

compaction device
G Tablettierwerkzeug, Preßwerkzeug
F instrument de fabrication de comprimés, outil de compression
S instrumentos para fabricar comprimidos, instrumental de compresión

compaction force
G Preßkraft
F force de compression
S fuerza de compresión

compaction roll (tablet press)
G Druckrolle (an der Tablettenpresse)
F cylindre de compression
S cilindro compresor (en la prensa de comprimidos)

compactor
G Kompaktierer
F compacteur
S compactador

company
G Gesellschaft, Konzern
F société, compagnie, consortium
S sociedad, consorcio

company management
G Geschäftsleitung
F direction d'une société
S gerencia

company secret
G Betriebsgeheimnis
F secret d'entreprise
S secreto empresarial

compatibility
G Verträglichkeit, Kompatibilität
F compatibilité
S compatibilidad

compatible
G kompatibel
F compatible
S compatible

competitor
G Mitbewerber
F compétiteur
S competidor

compilation (of documents)
G Erstellung (von Dokumenten)
F compilation (de documents)
S redacción (de documentos)

compile, to
G erstellen
F compiler, produire
S elaborar, producir, redactar

complaint
G Beanstandung, Reklamation
F réclamation
S reclamación

complaint report
G Beanstandungsbericht
F compte-rendu de réclamation
S informe de reclamaciones

completion
G Beendigung
F achèvement
S conclusión, terminación

complex formation
G Komplexbildung
F formation de complexes
S secuestración

complex former
G Komplexbildner
F substance complexante
S agente secuestrante

compliance
G Einhaltung
F conformité
S cumplimiento, observancia

component (of a tablet press)
G Bestandteil, Formatteil (bei einer Tablettenpresse)
F composant, constituant, ingrédient (d'une presse à comprimés)
S componente, ingrediente, componente formador (de una prensa de comprimidos)

components
G Einzelteile
F composants
S componentes

composite foil
G Verbundfolie
F feuille stratifiée
S hoja laminada, lámina estratificada

composite sample
G Mischmuster
F échantillon mixte
S muestra mixta

composition
G Zusammensetzung
F composition
S composición

comprehensible
G verständlich
F compréhensible
S comprensible

compress
G Kompresse
F compresse
S compresa

compress, to
G verdichten
F comprimer, concentrer
S concentrar, comprimir

compressed air
G Druckluft, Preßluft
F air comprimé
S aire comprimido

compressed air cylinder
G Druckluftzylinder
F cylindre de compression
S cilindro de aire comprimido

compressed air plant
G Druckluftanlage
F installation servant à la production d'air comprimé
S instalación de aire comprimido

compressed core
G Preßling
F implant, pastille, boulette
S masa comprimida

compressed gases
G komprimierte Gase
F gaz comprimés
S gases comprimidos

compressed tablets
G Preßtabletten
F comprimés
S comprimidos

compression
G Tablettierung, Verdichtung
F fabrication de comprimés, compression, concentration
S fabricación de comprimidos, concentración, compresión

compression chamber
G Preßkammer
F chambre de compression
S cámara de compresión

compression characteristics
G Preßeigenschaften
F caractéristiques de compression
S características de compresión

compression format
G Preßformat
F format de compression
S formato de compresión

compression material
G Preßmasse
F composé comprimable, matière moulée
S masa comprimible

compression mould
G Preßwerkzeug
F outil de compression
S instrumental de compresión

English German French Spanish

compression roll (tablet press)
G Druckrolle (an der Tablettenpresse)
F cylindre de compression
S cilindro compresor (en la prensa de comprimidos)

compression speed
G Preßgeschwindigkeit
F vitesse de compression
S velocidad de compresión

compression station
G Druckstation
F station de compression
S estación de compresión

compulsory
G obligatorisch, verpflichtend
F obligatoire
S obligatorio

computer security
G Computersicherheit
F sécurité informatique
S seguridad informática

computer validation
G Computervalidierung
F validation d'ordinateur, validation informatique
S validación informática

computer-assisted
G computergestützt
F assisté par ordinateur
S asistido por ordenador

computer-controlled
G computergesteuert
F contrôlé par ordinateur
S controlado por ordenador

computerised
G computergestützt
F assisté par ordinateur
S asistido por ordenador

concave
G nach innen gewölbt, konkav
F concave
S cóncavo

concentrate
G Dickextrakt
F concentré
S extracto concentrado

dried concentrate
G Trockenextrakt
F concentré sec
S concentrado seco

concentrate, to
G verdichten, einengen (Konzentration), anreichern, eindicken, verdicken
F comprimer, concentrer, épaissir
S concentrar, comprimir, espesar, enriquecer, condensar

concentration
G Verdichtung, Konzentration, Anreicherung
F compression, concentration
S concentración, compresión, enriquecimiento

concentration medium
G Anreicherungsmedium
F médium de concentration
S medio de concentración, medio de enriquecimiento

concern
G Konzern
F compagnie, consortium
S consorcio

concrete ceiling
G Betondecke
F plafond en béton
S techo de hormigón

concurrent validation
G produktionsbegleitende Validierung
F validation concurrente
S validación concomitante a la producción

condensate
G Kondensat
F condensat
S condensado

condensation
G Kondensation
F condensation
S condensación

condense water
G Kondenswasser
F eau condensée
S agua condensada

condenser
G Kondensator, Kühler
F condenseur, réfrigérant
S condensador, refrigerador

conditions
G Bedingungen
F conditions
S condiciones

conductive
G leitfähig
F conducteur
S conductor

conductive heat
G Wärmeleitung
F conduction thermique
S conducción térmica

conductivity
G elektrische Leitfähigkeit, Leitfähigkeit
F conductivité électrique, conductivité
S conductividad eléctrica, conductibilidad

conductivity cell
G Leitfähigkeitsmeßzelle
F cellule de mesure de conductivité
S célula de medida de la conductividad

conductivity detector
G Wärmeleitfähigkeitsdetektor
F conductimètre
S detector de conductividad térmica

conductivity meter
G Leitfähigkeitsmesser
F conductimètre
S conductímetro

conductivity sensor
G Leitfähigkeitsmesser
F capteur de conductivité
S sensor de conductividad

cone
G Kegel, Konus
F cône
S cono

confidence area
G Vertrauensbereich
F plage de confiance
S área de confianza, intervalo de confianza

confidence interval
G Vertrauensintervall
F intervalle de confiance
S intervalo de confianza

confidence level
G Vertrauensniveau
F niveau de confiance
S nivel de confianza

confidence limits
G Vertrauensgrenzen
F limites de confiance
S límites de confianza

confidentiality
G Vertraulichkeit
F confidentialité
S confidencialidad

configurable software
G konfigurierbare Software
F logiciel configurable
S software configurable

conform with, to
G übereinstimmen mit
F être en conformité avec
S coincidir con

conformation isomers
G Konformationsisomere
F isomères de conformation
S isómeros de conformación

English German French Spanish

conformity
G Konformität, Übereinstimmung
F conformité
S conformidad, concordancia, coincidencia

conformity assurance
G Konformitätssicherung
F assurance de conformité
S aseguramiento de conformidad

confusion
G Verwechslung
F méprise, erreur
S confusión

conical
G kegelförmig, verjüngt, konisch
F conique
S disminuido, estrechado, cónico

conical flask
G Spitzkolben
F ballon conique
S matraz cónico

conical screener
G konischer Abschirmer
F protection cônique
S protector cónico

conicalness
G Verjüngung, Konizität
F amincissement
S conicidad, disminución

conicity
G Verjüngung, Konizität
F amincissement
S conicidad, disminución

connect, to
G anschließen
F connecter
S conectar

connected
G angeschlossen
F connecté
S conectado

wrongly connected
G falsch angeschlossen
F faussement connecté
S mal conectado

connection
G Anschluß, Verbindung
F connexion
S conexión

connection nipple
G Anschlußstutzen
F douille de connexion, manchon de connexion
S empalme de conexión

connection port
G Anschlußstutzen
F douille de connexion, manchon de connexion
S empalme de conexión

connector
G Verbindungsstück
F raccord
S pieza de unión

consistency
G Konsistenz, Gleichförmigkeit
F uniformité, consistance
S consistencia, homogeneidad, uniformidad

constant weight
G Gewichtskonstanz
F constance d'un poids
S constancia del peso

constituent
G Bestandteil
F composant, constituant, ingrédient
S componente, ingrediente

constriction
G Verengung
F constriction
S constricción, estrechamiento

construction joints
G Arbeitsfugen
F joints de construction
S juntas de construcción

consumables
G Verbrauchsmaterial
F consommables
S material consumible

consumer
G Verbraucher
F consommateur
S consumidor

consumption
G Verbrauch
F consommation
S consumo

contact person
G Ansprechpartner
F interlocuteur
S interlocutor

contact plate
G Abklatschplatte
F plaque de contact
S placa de contacto

contact time
G Kontaktzeit
F temps de contact
S tiempo de contacto

container
G Ansatzbehälter, Behälter, Behältnis, Gebinde
F bac, container, cuve, récipient, conditionnement
S contenedor, recipiente

final container
G Endbehältnis
F récipient final
S recipiente final

mobile container
G fahrbarer Ansatzbehälter, fahrbarer Behälter
F cuve sur roues, cuve mobile
S contenedor portátil, recipiente portátil

contaminants
G kontaminierende Stoffe
F contaminants
S sustancias contaminantes

contaminate, to
G kontaminieren, verschmutzen
F contaminer
S contaminar, ensuciar

contaminated
G kontaminiert
F contaminé
S contaminado

contamination
G Verunreinigung
F impureté, contamination
S contaminación, impureza

contamination level
G Kontaminationsgrad
F niveau de contamination
S grado de contaminación

contamination profile (of a product)
G Kontaminationsprofil (eines Produktes)
F profil de contamination (d'un produit)
S perfil de contaminación (de un producto)

contamination, airborne
G aus der Luft stammende Kontamination
F contamination transportée par l'air, contamination aéroportée
S contaminación procedente del aire

content
G Gehalt, Inhalt
F contenu
S contenido

content control
G Füllgutkontrolle
F contrôle du contenu
S control del contenido

content uniformity (CU)
G Einheitlichkeit des Gehaltes, Gehaltseinheitlichkeit
F uniformité du contenu
S uniformidad del contenido

contents
G Füllgut, Verzeichnis
F matière de remplissage, répertoire, registre
S material de relleno, índice

continuous
G stufenlos
F continu
S continuo

continuous band
G Endlosbahn
F bande continue
S cinta sin fin

continuous culture
G kontinuierliche Kultur
F culture en continu
S cultivo continuo

continuous film
G endlose Folie
F feuille continue
S lámina continua

continuous foil
G endlose Folie
F feuille continue
S lámina continua

continuous monitoring
G ständige Überwachung
F contrôle continu
S vigilancia continua

continuous operation
G kontinuierlicher Betrieb, Dauerbetrieb
F fabrication en continu, opération continue
S funcionamiento continuo

contract
G Vertrag
F contrat
S contrato

contract acceptor
G Auftragnehmer
F client
S comisionista

contract cleaner
G Reinigungsfirma
F entreprise de nettoyage
S empresa de limpieza

contract laboratory
G Auftragslabor
F laboratoire sous-traitant
S laboratorio comisionado

contract manufacture
G Herstellung im Lohnauftrag, Lohnherstellung
F fabrication en sous-traitance, fabrication par sous-traitance
S fabricación por comisión

contract manufacturer
G Auftragshersteller
F producteur sous-traintant
S fabricante por comisión

contract manufacturer order
G Lohnherstellungsauftrag
F commande de fabrication par sous-traitance
S encargo de fabricación por comisión

contract manufacturing
G Auftragsherstellung, Auftragsproduktion
F production par un sous-traitant
S producción por contrata, producción por encargo

contract packager
G Lohnabpacker
F empaqueteur
S empaquetador comisionado

contract packaging
G Lohnverpackung
F empaquetage par sous-traitance
S embalaje por comisión

contract provider
G Auftraggeber
F donneur d'ordre, commettant, client
S cliente, comitente

English German French Spanish

contraindicated
G kontraindiziert
F contre-indiqué
S contraindicado

contraindication
G Gegenanzeige, Kontraindikation
F contre-indication
S contraindicación

contrast medium
G Kontrastmittel
F substance de contraste
S medio de contraste

control
G Steuerung, Kontrolle
F contrôle
S control

control accuracy
G Regelgenauigkeit
F exactitude de réglage, exactitude de contrôle
S exactitud de la regulación

control balance
G Kontrollwaage
F balance de contrôle
S báscula de control

control box
G Schaltkasten
F armoire électrique
S caja de distribución

control flap
G Regelklappe
F clapet de réglage
S válvula reguladora

control instrumentation
G Kontrollinstrumentierung
F instruments de contrôle
S instrumentos de control

control knob
G Bedienungselement
F bouton de contrôle
S elemento de manejo

control lamp
G Signallampe
F lampe de contrôle
S lámpara de señales

control loop
G Regelkreis
F boucle d'asservissement
S circuito regulador

control panel
G Bedienterminal, Schalttafel
F terminal de contrôle, pupitre de commande, tableau de commande
S terminal de control, cuadro de distribución, cuadro de mando

control system
G Leitsystem
F système de contrôle
S sistema de control

control test
G Prüfung
F analyse, test de contrôle
S examen, ensayo, prueba, test

control valve
G Regelklappe, Regler
F clapet de réglage, régulateur
S válvula reguladora, regulador

control, to
G überprüfen
F contrôler, vérifier
S comprobar

controllable
G regulierbar
F ajustable
S regulable

controlled access
G kontrollierter Zugang
F accès contrôlé
S acceso controlado

controlled access area
G kontrollierter Zugangsbereich
F zone d'accès contrôlé
S zona de acceso controlado

English German French Spanish

controlled release
G kontrollierte Freisetzung
F libération contrôlée
S liberación controlada

controller
G Regler
F régulateur
S regulador

controller set point
G Reglereinstellung
F réglage d'un régulateur
S ajuste de un regulador

convective heat
G Wärmestrahlung
F rayonnement thermique
S radiación térmica

conversion
G Umrechnung
F conversion
S conversión

converter
G Umwandler
F convertisseur
S transformador

convertibility (of a substance in a reaction)
G Umwandlungsfähigkeit (einer Substanz in einer Reaktion)
F convertibilité (d'une substance en une réaction)
S convertibilidad (de una sustancia en una reacción)

convex
G nach außen gewölbt, konvex
F convexe
S convexo

convey, to
G fördern
F transporter
S fomentar, promover

conveyor
G Bandzufuhr, Förder-
F convoyeur
S suministro por cinta, transportador

conveyor balance
G Bandwaage
F balance de convoyeur
S báscula de cinta

conveyor belt
G Bandförderer, Fließband, Förderband, Transportband
F convoyeur, convoyeur à bande, tapis roulant,
S transportador de cinta, cinta transportadora

coolant
G Kühlflüssigkeit, Kühlmittel
F réfrigérant, liquide de refroidissement
S líquido refrigerante, medio refrigerante

cool-down time
G Abkühlzeit
F temps de refroidissement
S tiempo de enfriamiento

cooler
G Kühler
F réfrigérant
S refrigerador

cooling
G Abkühlung
F refroidissement, réfrigération
S enfriamiento

cooling coil
G Schlangenkühler
F serpentin de refroidissement
S serpentín refrigerador

cooling device
G Abkühlvorrichtung
F dispositif de refroidissement
S dispositivo de enfriamiento

cooling jacket
G Kühlmantel, Mantelkühlung
F manteau de refroidissement, chemise de refroidissement
S camisa refrigerante, camisa de refrigeración

cooling phase
G Abkühlphase
F phase de refroidissement
S fase de enfriamento

cooling rate
G Abkühlungsgeschwindigkeit
F vitesse de refroidissement
S velocidad de enfriamiento

cooling tower
G Kühlturm
F tour de refroidissement
S torre de refrigeración

cooling water
G Kühlwasser
F eau de refroidissement
S agua de refrigeración

cooling water loop
G Kühlwasserschleife
F boucle d'eau de refroidissement
S serpentín para el agua de refrigeración

copper
G Kupfer
F cuivre
S cobre

corn starch
G Maisstärke
F amidon du maïs
S almidón de maíz

corner
G Ecke
F coin
S esquina

correction
G Berichtigung, Korrektur
F correction
S corrección, enmienda, rectificación

corrective action
G Korrekturmaßnahme
F action corrective
S acción correctora

correspond, to
G entsprechen
F correspondre (à)
S corresponder

not corresponding to
G nicht entsprechen
F différent de
S no corresponder

corridor
G Flur
F corridor
S corredor

corrode, to
G korrodieren
F corroder
S corroer

corrodible
G korrosionsempfindlich
F sensible à la corrosion
S sensible a la corrosión

corrosion
G Korrosion
F corrosion
S corrosión

corrosive
G korrodierend
F corrosif
S corroyente

corrugate, to
G riffeln
F canneler, strier
S acanalar, estriar

corrugated
G geriffelt
F cannelé, strié
S acanalado, estriado

corrugated cardboard (carton)
G Wellpappe
F carton ondulé
S cartón ondulado

English German French Spanish

corrugation
G Riffelung
F cannelure, striage
S acanaladura, estría, ranura

cosmetics
G Kosmetika
F cosmétiques
S cosméticos

cost-efficient
G kosteneffizient
F économique
S económico

cotton
G Baumwolle
F coton
S algodón

cotton plug
G Wattebausch
F tampon d'ouate
S torunda de algodón

cotton wool
G Verbandwatte, Watte
F ouate à pansement, ouate
S algodón de vendaje, algodón

cough drops
G Hustentropfen
F gouttes antitussives
S gotas antitusivas

cough syrup
G Hustensaft
F sirop contre la toux
S jarabe antitusígeno

coulometric analysis
G coulometrische Analyse
F analyse coulométrique
S análisis coulométrico

counter
G Zähler
F compteur
S contador

counter-flange
G Gegenflansch
F contre-bride
S contrabrida

counter-ion
G Gegenion
F contre-ion, ion complémentaire
S contraión, ion complementario

counter-spring
G Rückzugfeder
F ressort de rappel
S muelle de retorno

countersunk rivet
G Senkniete
F rivet conique
S remache avellanado

countersunk screw
G Senkschraube
F vis conique
S tornillo avellanado

counter-weight
G Gegengewicht
F contrepoids
S contrapeso

couple, to
G ankuppeln
F accoupler, accrocher
S acoplar

coupling
G Kupplung
F couplage
S acoplamiento, embrague

course of a reaction
G Reaktionsverlauf
F déroulement d'une réaction
S transcurso de la reacción

course-grained
G grobkristallin
F grossièrement cristallin
S groseramente cristalino

covalent
G kovalent
F covalent
S covalente

cover
G Abdeckhaube, Verkleidung, Verkleidungsblech, Haube, Abdeckung, Deckel
F couvercle, capuchon, revêtement
S chapa de revestimiento, casquete, cubierta, revestimiento, sombrerete, tapa, tapadera

cover fitting
G Haubenhalterung
F garniture de couvercle
S soporte del casquete

cover foil
G Deckfolie
F feuille de protection
S hoja de recubrimiento

cover glass (microscopy)
G Abdeckplatte, Deckglas (Mikroskopie)
F verre de protection, lame, lame de protection (microscopie)
S cubreobjetos (microscopio)

cover slip (microscopy)
G Deckglas (Mikroskopie)
F plaquette en verre (microscopie)
S cubreobjetos (microscopio)

covered
G verkleidet
F revêtu, recouvert
S recubierto, revestido

covering power
G Deckkraft
F propriété couvrante
S capacidad de cubrir

crack
G Riß
F déchirure, fissure
S desgarro, fisura

cracked (glass)
G gesprungen (Glas)
F fêlé
S quebrado (vidrio)

crack-filling
G rißüberbrückend
F colmatant (une fissure)
S rellenante de una fisura

cream
G Creme
F crème
S crema

creaming (of emulsions)
G Aufrahmung (bei Emulsionen)
F crémage (d'une émulsion)
S cremado (de emulsiones)

crimp (of a tube)
G Falz (einer Tube), Tubenfalz
F joint (d'un tube)
S encaje, juntura (de un tubo)

crimp, to
G verbördeln, falzen
F capsuler, plier
S rebordear cantos, plegar

crimping cap
G Bördelkappe
F bouchon, couvercle, calotte
S calota de rebordeo

crimping machine
G Bördelmaschine
F boucheuse, capsuleuse
S máquina de rebordeo

crimping tongs
G Falzzange
F pincettes, pinces, tenailles
S tenazas para cerrar tubos

criterion
G Kriterium
F critère
S criterio

according to stringent criteria (e. g. testing)
G gemäß strengen Kriterien (z. B. Test)
F selon des critères sévères (par ex. un test)
S siguiendo criterios estrictos (p. ej. test)

critical micelle concentration
G kritische Micellkonzentration, kritische Mizellkonzentration
F concentration critique de micelles
S concentración crítica de micelas, concentración micelar crítica

critical parameter
G kritischer Parameter
F paramètre critique
S parámetro crítico

critical processing step
G kritischer Prozeßschritt
F étape critique d'un procédé
S etapa crítica de un proceso

cross bar
G Querstange
F tige transversale
S barra transversal

cross reference
G Querverweis
F référence
S referencia

cross-bellows controller
G Kreuzbalgregler
F régleur pneumatique
S regulador de fuelle cruzado

cross-contamination
G Untermischung, Kreuzkontamination
F contamination croisée
S contaminación cruzada, mezcla cruzada

cross-functional guideline
G abteilungsübergreifende Richtlinie
F lignes directrices générales
S línea directriz general

cross-linking
G Quervernetzung
F connexion latérale
S conexión lateral

cross-mix
G Untermischung, Kreuzkontamination
F contamination croisée
S contaminación cruzada, mezcla cruzada

cross-section
G Querschnitt
F section transversale, coupe transversale
S sección transversal

crosswires
G Fadenkreuz
F réticule
S retículo

crucible
G Tiegel
F creuset
S crisol

crude product
G Rohprodukt
F produit brut
S producto bruto

crush, to
G zerstoßen, mahlen
F broyer, concasser, piler
S machacar, moler, pulverizar, triturar

cryotube
G Gefrierröhrchen
F tube de congélation
S tubo de congelación

crystal structure
G Kristallaufbau
F structure cristalline
S estructura cristalina

crystalline
G kristallin
F cristallin
S cristalino

crystallisation
G Auskristallisierung, Kristallisierung
F cristallisation
S cristalización

crystallise out, to
G auskristallisieren
F se cristalliser complètement
S cristalizar completamente

crystallise, to
G kristallisieren
F cristalliser
S cristalizar

cube mixer
G Kubusmischer
F mélangeur en cube
S mezclador cúbico

culture broth
G Kulturbouillon, Nährbouillon, Nährlösung
F bouillon de culture
S caldo de cultivo, solución de cultivo, solución nutritiva

culture media preparation
G Nährmedienherstellung
F préparation des milieux de culture
S preparación de medio de cultivo

culture media preparation room
G Nährmedienküche
F salle de préparation des milieux de culture
S sala de preparación de medios de cultivo

culture medium
G Nährboden, Nährmedium
F milieu de culture
S medio de cultivo

dehydrated medium
G Trockennährmedium
F milieu de culture déhydraté
S medio de cultivo deshidratado

culture medium filling
G Nährmedienabfüllung
F remplissage des milieux de culture
S relleno con medio de cultivo

culture surface
G Kulturrasen
F surface de culture
S superficie de cultivo

cup (of blister)
G Napf (beim Blister)
F blister, coupe, emballage à bulles, gobelet
S pocillo del blíster

cure, to
G aushärten
F tremper
S curar

curing
G Aushärtung
F trempe
S curado

current
G laufend, Strom
F courant, électricité
S corriente, corriente eléctrica

current cost
G laufende Kosten
F coûts d'exploitation
S costes de explotación

cursor
G Schieber
F curseur
S compuerta, corredera, cursor

curve
G Kennlinie
F caractéristique
S característica

customer
G Abnehmer, Kunde
F client
S cliente

English German French Spanish

cutaneous foam
G Schaum zur Anwendung auf der Haut
F mousse pour utilisation cutanée
S espuma cutánea

cutaneous paste
G Paste zur Anwendung auf der Haut
F pâte pour utilisation cutanée
S pasta cutánea

cutaneous use
G Anwendung auf der Haut
F pour usage cutané
S uso cutáneo

cutting point (of an ampoule)
G Brechpunkt (einer Ampulle)
F point de rupture (d'une ampoule)
S punto de ruptura (de una ampolla)

cuvette
G Küvette
F cuvette
S cubeta

cycle
G Zyklus
F cycle
S ciclo

cycle number
G Taktzahl
F cadence
S número de ciclos

cycle sequence
G Zyklussequenz
F séquence de cycles
S secuencia de ciclos

cyclone separation
G Zyklonabscheidung
F séparateur à cyclone
S separación por centrifugación

cylindrical
G zylindrisch
F cylindrique
S cilíndrico

cytostatics
G Zytostatica
F cytostatiques
S citostáticos, agentes citostáticos

daily
G täglich
F journalier
S diario

daily dosage
G Tagesdosis
F dose journalière
S dosis diaria

damage
G Beschädigung, Beeinträchtigung
F dommage, dégâts, préjudice
S daño, merma, perjuicio

damage to health
G Gesundheitsschaden
F préjudice à la santé
S perjuicio para la salud

damaged
G beschädigt
F défectueux, endommagé
S dañado, estropeado, perjudicado

dangerous
G gefährlich
F dangereux
S peligroso

dangerous material
G Gefahrstoff
F matériel dangereux
S sustancia peligrosa

darken
G Verdunkelung
F obscurcissement
S oscurecimiento

data
G Daten, Angaben
F données, spécifications
S datos, especificaciones

data base backup
G Datenbanksicherheitskopie
F backup d'une base de données
S copia de seguridad de un banco de datos

data entry
G Dateneingabe
F saisie de données
S entrada de datos

data processing, electronic
G elektronische Datenverarbeitung
F système de traitement électronique de données
S proceso electrónico de datos

data recording
G Datenaufnahme
F enregistrement de données
S registro de datos

data security
G Datensicherheit
F sécurité des données
S seguridad de datos

data transcription
G Datentranskription
F transcription de données
S transcripción de datos

database screening
G Datenbankscreening
F screening d'une banque de données
S búsqueda en banco de datos

deacidify, to
G entsäuern
F alcaliniser
S alcalinizar, desacidificar

deactivation
G Inaktivierung
F inactivation
S inactivación

dead space
G Totraum
F espace mort
S espacio muerto

dead spots
G tote Enden
F extrémités
S extremos de desecho

dead time
G Totzeit
F temps mort
S tiempo muerto

dead volume
G Totvolumen
F volume mort
S volumen muerto

dead volume-free
G totraumfrei
F dépourvu de volume mort
S sin espacios muertos

dead weight
G Leergewicht
F poids à vide
S peso en vacío, tara

deadline
G Frist
F délai, terme
S plazo

deadline extension
G Fristverlängerung
F prolongation d'un délai
S prolongación de un plazo

deaerate, to
G entgasen, entlüften
F dégazer, désaérer, ventiler
S airear, desgasificar, ventilar

deaeration (of liquids)
G Entgasung (von Flüssigkeiten)
F dégazage
S desgasificación (de líquidos)

debris
G Bruch, Trümmer
F débris
S despojos, escombros, restos

deburr, to
G entgraten
F ébarber
S desbarbar

deburrer
G Entgrater
F ébarbeur
S desbarbador, desbastador

deburring
G Entgratung
F ébarbage
S desbarbado

decalcifier
G Entkalker
F détartrant
S agente descalcificante

decalcify, to
G entkalken
F détartrer
S descalcificar

decant, to
G abgießen, dekantieren
F décanter, transvaser
S decantar, verter

decoction
G Abkochung, Decoct
F décoction
S decocción

decoder
G Entschlüssler
F décodeur
S descodificador

decomposition
G Zersetzung
F décomposition
S degradación, descomposición

decomposition product
G Zersetzungsprodukt
F produit de décomposition
S producto de degradación

deconcentration
G Abreicherung
F élimination
S eliminación, reducción

decontamination
G Dekontamination
F décontamination
S descontaminar

dedicated equipment
G Mono-Anlage
F équipement dédié
S instalación para uso único

deduster
G Entstauber
F dépoussiéreur
S desempolvante

dedusting
G Entstaubung
F action de dépoussiérer, dépoussiérage
S desempolvamiento

deep draw, to
G tiefziehen
F emboutir
S embutir a profundidad

deep freezing
G Tiefkühlung
F surgélation
S congelación

deep-freeze, to
G tieffrieren
F congeler
S congelar

deep-frozen
G tiefgefroren
F congelé
S congelado

defect
G Fehler, Qualitätsmangel
F défaut, défaut de qualité, erreur
S error, defecto de calidad

human error
G menschlicher Fehler
F erreur d'origine humaine
S error humano

random error
G zufälliger Fehler
F erreur aléatoire
S error casual

defect (error, failure) evaluation list
G Fehlerbewertungsliste
F registre d'évaluation d'erreurs
S lista de evaluación de errores

defect characteristic
G Fehlermerkmal
F caractéristique du défaut
S característica de defecto

defective
G beschädigt, fehlerhaft
F défectueux, endommagé
S dañado, defectuoso, estropeado, perjudicado

defective batch
G Fehlcharge
F lot défectueux
S lote defectuoso

defective units
G fehlerhafte Einheiten
F unités défectueuses
S unidades defectuosas

deficiency
G Mangel
F déficience, carence, insuffisance
S carencia, defecto, deficiencia, insuficiencia

deficiency protocol
G Mängelprotokoll
F procès-verbal des défauts
S protocolo de deficiencias

deficiency report
G Mängelrüge
F compte-rendu des insuffisances
S reclamación por vicios

deflect, to
G ablenken
F dévier
S desviar

deflection (of pointer)
G Ausschlag (eines Zeigers)
F déviation (d'une aiguille)
S desviación (de una aguja indicadora)

deflector
G Leitblech
F déflecteur
S deflector, disruptor

defoamer
G Entschäumer
F antimousse
S agente antiespumante

deformation
G Verformung
F déformation
S deformación

defrost, to
G auftauen
F dégeler
S descongelar

degas, to
G entgasen
F dégazer, désaérer
S desgasificar

degassing (of liquids)
G Entgasung (von Flüssigkeiten)
F dégazage
S desgasificación (de líquidos)

degradable
G abbaubar
F dégradable
S degradable

degradation
G Abbau
F dégradation
S degradación

English German French Spanish

degradation granulation
G Abbaugranulierung
F granulation de dégradation
S granulación de degradación

degradation path
G Abbauweg
F chemin de dégradation
S vía de degradación

degradation product
G Abbauprodukt, Zerfallsprodukt
F produit de dégradation
S producto de degradación, producto de desintegración

degrease, to
G entfetten
F dégraisser
S desengrasar

degree of freedom
G Freiheitsgrad
F degré de liberté
S grado de libertad

dehydrated culture medium
G Trockennährmedium
F milieu déhydraté
S medio de cultivo deshidratado

dehydration
G Dehydratisierung
F déhydratation
S deshidratación

deionise, to
G entmineralisieren
F déminéraliser
S desmineralizar

deionised water
G entionisiertes Wasser
F eau déionisée
S agua desionizada

delay
G Verzögerung
F retard
S retardo, retraso

delay time
G Verzögerungszeit
F retard
S tiempo de retraso

delayed
G verzögert
F retardé
S retardado, retrasado

delayed action tablet
G Retardtablette
F comprimé à libération retardée
S comprimido retard

delivery
G Ausgabe, Auslieferung, Lieferung
F livraison
S distribución, entrega

delivery date
G Liefertermin, Lieferdatum
F date de livraison
S fecha de entrega

delivery note
G Lieferschein
F bordereau de livraison
S talón de entrega

demand, to
G fordern
F exiger
S exigir

demineralised
G vollentsalzt
F complètement désalinisé
S completamente desmineralizado

demineralised water
G demineralisiertes Wasser, entmineralisiertes Wasser, VE-Wasser
F eau déminéralisée
S agua completamente desmineralizada, agua desmineralizada

demixing
G Entmischung
F démixtion
S separación

denatured
G denaturiert, vergällt
F dénaturé
S desnaturalizado

denaturing
G Denaturierung
F dénaturation
S desnaturalización

denaturing agent
G Denaturierungsmittel, Vergällungsmittel
F agent dénaturant
S agente desnaturalizante

density
G Dichte
F densité
S densidad

absolute density
G absolute Dichte
F densité absolue
S densidad absoluta

bulk density
G Schüttdichte
F densité apparente
S densidad aparente

relative density
G relative Dichte
F densité relative
S densidad relativa

tapped density, packed density
G Stampfdichte
F densité de package, densité de damage
S densidad de compresión

dental use
G dentale Anwendung
F usage dental
S uso dental

department
G Abteilung
F département, service
S departamento

deplete, to (e. g. viruses)
G abreichern (z. B. Viren)
F éliminer (par exemple des virus)
S eliminar (p. ej. virus)

deposit
G Wandbelag
F dépôt
S recubrimiento de la pared, depósito

depot drug
G Depotpräparat
F médicament retard
S preparado retard

depression of freezing point
G Gefrierpunktserniedrigung
F abaissement du point de congélation
S reducción del punto de congelación

deprotonation
G Deprotonierung
F déprotonation
S desprotonización

depth filter
G Tiefenfilter
F filtre profondeur
S filtro de profundidad

deputisation
G Stellvertretung
F suppléance
S suplencia, sustitución

deputy
G Stellvertreter
F suppléant, remplaçant
S suplente, sustituto

depyrogenate, to
G entpyrogenisieren
F dépyrogéner
S despirogenar, eliminar pirógenos

depyrogenation
G Entpyrogenisierung
F dépyrogénation
S despirogenación, eliminación de pirógenos

derivative
G Abkömmling, Derivat
F dérivé
S derivado

desalt, to
G entsalzen
F dessaler
S desalinizar

description
G Beschreibung
F description
S descripción

desiccant
G Trocknungsmittel
F déshydratant, desséchant
S desecante, deshidratante

desiccate, to
G austrocknen, trocknen
F dessiquer, sécher
S desecar, secar

desiccator
G Exsiccator
F dessicateur
S desecante, exicante

design
G Bauart
F design
S tipo de construcción

designate, to
G bezeichnen
F étiqueter
S denominar, marcar, rotular

designated (for)
G bestimmt (für)
F désigné (pour)
S designado (para)

designation
G Bezeichnung
F désignation, appellation
S denominación, marcado, rotulación

designed for
G ausgelegt für
F prévu pour, construit pour
S construido para, diseñado para

destroy, to
G abtöten, vernichten
F tuer, détruire
S destruir, matar

destruction
G Vernichtung
F destruction
S destrucción

detachable
G entfernbar, abnehmbar
F amovible, démontable, détachable
S desmontable

detectable
G detektierbar, nachweisbar
F détectable
S detectable

undetectable
G nicht nachweisbar
F indétectable
S no detectable

detection
G Nachweis
F détection, preuve
S demostración, prueba

detection precision
G Detektionsgenauigkeit
F précision de détection
S exactitud de detección

detection range
G Detektionsbereich
F zone de détection
S zona de detección

detection sensitivity
G Detektionsempfindlichkeit
F sensibilité de détection
S sensibilidad de detección

detector cell
G Detektorzelle
F cellule de détection
S célula de detección

detector inlet
G Detektoreinlaß
F entrée de détecteur
S entrada al detector

detector outlet
G Detektorauslaß
F sortie de détecteur
S salida del detector

detergent
G Reinigungsmittel
F agent de nettoyage
S detergente, producto de limpieza

deteriorate, to
G verderben
F se détériorer, s'abîmer
S deteriorar, deteriorarse

deterioration
G Verderb
F détérioration, altération
S deterioro

determination
G Bestimmung
F détermination, évaluation
S análisis, determinación

determination of content
G Gehaltsbestimmung
F détermination du contenu
S determinación del contenido

determine, to
G bestimmen, ermitteln
F déterminer, évaluer
S averiguar, determinar

developing chamber (chromatography)
G Chromatographiekammer
F chambre de développement (chromatographie)
S cámara cromatográfica

development
G Entwicklung
F développement
S desarrollo, evolución

development of resistance
G Resistenzentwicklung
F développement d'une résistance
S desarrollo de resistencia

development report
G Entwicklungsbericht
F rapport de développement
S informe de desarrollo

development route
G Entwicklungsweg
F route de développement
S vía de desarrollo, vía evolutiva

development stage
G Entwicklungsstufe
F phase de développement
S etapa de desarrollo, nivel de desarrollo

development status
G Entwicklungsstatus
F état de développement
S status de desarrollo

deviation
G Abweichung
F déviation, écart
S desviación

device
G Vorrichtung
F appareillage, dispositif
S dispositivo

dewpoint
G Taupunkt
F point de rosée
S punto de descongelación

dextro-rotatory
G rechtsdrehend
F dextrogyre
S dextrógiro

English German French Spanish

diagnosis
G Befund
F diagnose
S diagnóstico

diagnostics
G Diagnostica
F diagnostiques
S agentes diagnósticos

diagram
G Diagramm
F diagramme
S diagrama

diameter
G Durchmesser
F diamètre
S diámetro

diaphragm
G Lochblende, Membran
F diaphragme, membrane
S diafragma, membrana

diaphragm valve
G Membranventil
F vanne à membrane
S válvula de membrana

die (of tabletting machine)
G Matrize (an der Tablettenpresse)
F matrice (d'une presse à comprimés)
S matriz (de una prensa de comprimidos)

die alignment
G Matrizenausrichtung
F ajustage de la matrice
S disposición de matrices

die block
G Formblock
F bloc de moulage
S bloque de moldeo

die bore
G Matrizenöffnung
F cavité de matrice
S abertura de matriz

die opening
G Matrizenöffnung
F ouverture d'une matrice
S abertura de matriz

die plate
G Matrizenscheibe
F plateau d'une matrice
S disco matriz

die plate diameter
G Matrizenscheibendurchmesser
F diamètre du plateau d'une matrice
S diámetro del disco matriz

die plate height
G Matrizentischhöhe
F hauteur du plateau d'une matrice
S altura de la mesa para matriz

die plate speed
G Matrizentischgeschwindigkeit
F vitesse de la table d'une matrice
S velocidad de la mesa para matriz

die table
G Matrizentisch
F table d'une matrice
S mesa para matriz

die wall
G Matrizenwand
F paroi d'une matrice
S pared de matriz

die-cut, to
G ausstanzen
F découper à l'emporte-pièce, poinçonner
S estampar, perforar, punzonar

die-cutting station
G Stanzstation
F station de poinçonnage
S estación de troquelado

differential manometer
G Differenzdruckmesser
F manomètre différentiel
S manómetro diferencial

diffraction
G Lichtbeugung
F diffraction de la lumière
S difracción luminosa

diffusion
G Diffusion
F diffusion
S difusión

diffusion flow
G Diffusionsfluß
F débit de diffusion
S flujo de difusión

diffusion speed
G Diffusionsgeschwindigkeit
F vitesse de diffusion
S velocidad de difusión

digital read out
G digitale Ausgabe
F édition numérique
S edición digital

diluent
G Verdünnungsmittel
F diluant
S diluyente

dilute
G verdünnt
F dilué
S diluido

dilute, to
G verdünnen
F diluer
S diluir

dilution
G Verdünnung
F dilution
S dilución

dilution series
G Verdünnungsreihe
F séries de dilution
S serie de dilución

dimensions
G Abmessungen, Ausmaß
F dimensions
S cuantía, dimensiones, medidas

diminish, to
G vermindern
F diminuer
S disminuir, reducir

dip tube
G Eintauchrohr, Steigrohr, Tauchrohr
F tube plongeur, colonne d'ascension, colonne d'immersion
S tubo ascensional, tubo montante, tubo de inmersión

dip, to
G eintauchen
F immerger
S sumergir

diploid cell culture
G diploide Zellkultur
F culture de cellules diploides
S cultivo de células diploides

dipole-dipole interaction
G Dipol-Dipol-Wechselwirkung
F interaction dipolaire
S interacción entre dipolos

direct contact test
G Abklatschtest
F test de contact direct
S prueba de contacto directo

direct current
G Gleichstrom
F courant continu
S corriente continua

direct current source
G Gleichstromquelle
F source de courant continu
S fuente de corriente continua

English German French Spanish

direct inoculation (for microbial count determination)
G Direktbeschickung (zur Keimzahlbestimmung)
F inoculation directe
S inoculación directa (para recuento microbiano)

direct tablet compression
G Direkttablettierung
F compression directe
S compresión directa

direction of rotation
G Drehrichtung
F direction de rotation
S sentido de la rotación

directive
G Richtlinie
F directive
S directriz

director
G Direktor, Vorstand, Vorstandsmitglied
F comité de direction, directeur
S director, junta directiva, miembro de la junta directiva

disassembly
G Ausbau, Demontage, Zerlegung
F démontage
S desmontaje

discharge cock
G Ablaßhahn
F robinet de purge
S grifo de salida

discharge nipple
G Ablaßstutzen
F manchon d'écoulement, manchon de drainage
S empalme de salida

discharge outlet
G Auslauf
F sortie de vidange, sortie de purge
S desagüe, salida

discharge port
G Ablaufstutzen
F manchon d'écoulement
S empalme de salida

discharge, to (liquids)
G entladen, ablassen (Flüssigkeiten)
F décharger, faire couler, laisser s'écouler
S descargar, dar salida, dejar escapar

discharge, to (ointment from container)
G austragen (Salbe aus Container)
F décharger (la pommade du conteneur)
S descargar (pomada del contenedor)

discoloration
G Verfärbung
F décoloration
S decoloración

discrepancy
G Diskrepanz
F disparité, écart
S discrepancia

disinfect, to
G desinfizieren, entkeimen
F désinfecter
S desinfectar

disinfectable
G desinfizierbar
F désinfectable
S desinfectable

disinfectant
G Desinfektionsmittel
F désinfectant
S agente desinfectante

disinfecting effectiveness
G desinfizierende Wirksamkeit
F efficacité de la désinfection
S eficacia desinfectante

disinfecting procedure
G Desinfektionsverfahren
F procédé de désinfection
S procedimiento de desinfección

disinfection
G Desinfektion
F désinfection
S desinfección

disintegrant
G Sprengmittel
F agent délitant, désintégrant
S desintegrante

disintegrate, to
G zerfallen
F se désintégrer, se désagréger
S desintegrar(se)

disintegration
G Zerfall
F désintégration
S desintegración

disintegration test
G Zerfallsprüfung
F essai de désintégration
S ensayo de desintegración

disintegration time
G Zerfallszeit
F temps de désintégration
S tiempo de desintegración

disk drive (computer)
G Laufwerk (Computer)
F minuterie, lecteur (d'un ordinateur)
S unidad (de un ordenador)

dismantling
G Zerlegung
F démontage
S desmontaje

dispatch
G Versand
F expédition, envoi
S envío, expedición

dispatch unit
G Versandeinheit
F unité d'expédition
S unidad de envío

dispatch, to
G versenden
F expédier
S enviar, expedir

dispense, to
G ausgeben
F dépenser, distribuer
S distribuir, gastar

dispenser
G Spender, Verteiler
F distributeur
S distribuidor

dispensing (of a liquid)
G Verteilung (einer Flüssigkeit)
F délivrance (d'un liquide)
S distribución (de un líquido)

dispensing volume
G Verteilungsvolumen
F volume de délivrance
S volumen de distribución

disperse, to
G dispergieren
F disperser
S dispersar

dispersion
G Dispersion, Streubreite
F dispersion
S dispersión

dispersion agent
G Dispersionsmittel
F agent de dispersion
S agente dispersor

display
G Anzeige, optische Anzeige
F indicateur, indication visuelle
S indicación, pantalla, señal óptica

integrated display
G integrierte Anzeige
F indicateur intégré
S pantalla integrada

visual display
G optische Anzeige
F indicateur optique
S pantalla óptica

display, to
G anzeigen
F indiquer, afficher
S indicar, mostrar

disposable
G Einweg-
F jetable, à usage unique
S de uso único

disposable cover
G Einmalabdeckung
F couvercle à usage unique, capuchon à usage unique
S cubierta de uso único

disposable gloves
G Einmalhandschuhe
F gants à usage unique
S guantes de uso único

disposable jump-suit
G Einmalanzug
F combinaison à usage unique
S ropa de uso único

disposable packaging
G Einwegverpackung, Wegwerfpackung
F conditionnement à usage unique
S embalaje de uso único

disposable syringe
G Einmalspritze
F seringue à usage unique
S jeringa de uso único

disposable towels
G Einmalhandtücher
F serviette à usage unique
S toallas de uso único

disposal
G Beseitigung, Entsorgung
F élimination, rejet
S desecho, eliminación

waste disposal
G Abfallbeseitigung
F élimination de déchets
S eliminación de desechos

disposal regulations
G Entsorgungsvorschriften
F régulations concernant les rejets
S prescripciones de eliminación

disposal system
G Entsorgungssystem
F système d'élimination
S sistema de eliminación

dissemination of (dust)
G Verbreitung von (Staub)
F dissémination de (poussière)
S diseminación de (polvo)

dissociation
G Dissoziation
F dissociation
S disociación

dissolution
G Auflösung
F dissolution
S dilución, disolución

dissolution behaviour
G Auflösungsverhalten
F comportement de dissolution
S comportamiento en disolución

dissolution medium
G Auflösemedium, Lösemedium
F milieu de dissolution
S diluyente, disolvente, medio de disolución

dissolution rate
G Auflösungsrate, Auflösegeschwindigkeit
F vitesse de dissolution
S tasa de disolución, velocidad de disolución

dissolution speed
G Auflösegeschwindigkeit
F vitesse de dissolution
S velocidad de disolución

dissolution study
G Auflösungsstudie
F essai de dissolution
S estudio de dilución

dissolve, to
G auflösen, lösen
F dissoudre
S diluir, disolver

dissolved oxygen (DO)
G gelöster Sauerstoff
F oxygène dissous
S oxígeno disuelto

distil off, to
G abdestillieren
F distiller
S destilar

distil, to
G destillieren
F distiller
S destilar

distillate
G Destillat
F distillat
S destilado

distillation bottom
G Destillationsboden
F bas de la colonne de distillation
S fondo de destilación

distillation process
G Destillationsprozeß
F processus de distillation
S proceso de destilación

distillation range
G Destillationsbereich
F intervalle de distillation
S intervalo de destilación

distillation residue
G Destillationsrückstand
F résidu de distillation
S residuo de destilación

distilled water
G Aqua dest., destilliertes Wasser
F eau distillée
S agua destilada

distinct
G deutlich
F distinct, clair
S claro, distinto

distribution (of values)
G Streuung (von Werten), Verteilung
F diffusion, dispersion (de valeurs), distribution
S dispersión (de valores), distribución

division
G Sparte
F département, section
S especialidad, rama, sector

docking system
G Andocksystem
F système d'amarrage, système de fixation
S sistema de fijación, sistema de acoplamiento

doctor of veterinary medicine
G Tierarzt
F vétérinaire
S veterinario

document, to
G dokumentieren, protokollieren
F enregistrer, documenter
S documentar, levantar acta, protocolar

documentation
G Dokumentation
F documentation
S documentación

English German French Spanish

donor (person)
G Spender (als Person)
F donneur (personne)
S donante

door handle
G Klinke, Türklinke
F loquet, poignée de porte
S picaporte, gatillo, trinquete

door seal
G Türdichtung
F joint de porte
S junta de una puerta

dosage
G Dosierung
F posologie
S dosificación, posología

dosage form
G Arzneiform, Darreichungsform
F forme du dosage, forme pharmaceutique, voie d'administration
S forma de administración, forma farmacéutica

dosage security
G Dosierungssicherheit
F sécurité de dosage
S seguridad de dosificación

dosage unit
G Dosiereinheit, Dosierungseinheit
F dose unitaire, unité de dosage
S unidad de dosificación

dose
G Dosis
F dose
S dosis

multi-dose container
G Mehrdosenbehältnis
F récipient multi-doses
S recipiente de dosis múltiple

single dose
G Einzeldosis
F dose unique
S dosis única

single unit dose container
G Einzeldosisbehältnis
F récipient à dose unique
S recipiente de dosis única

dose criterion
G Dosiskriterium
F critère de dosage
S criterio de dosificación

dose reliability
G Zuverlässigkeit der Dosierung
F fiabilité d'une dose
S fiabilidad de la dosificación

dose uniformity
G Einheitlichkeit der Dosierung
F uniformité d'une dose
S uniformidad de la dosificación

dose, to
G abmessen, dosieren
F doser
S dosificar, calibrar, medir

dosing aid
G Dosierhilfe
F dispositif d'aide au dosage
S dispositivo para dosificar

dosing chamber
G Dosierkammer
F chambre de dosage
S cámara de dosificación

dosing device
G Dosiereinrichtung
F appareil doseur
S dispositivo dosificante

dosing loop
G Dosierschleife
F boucle de dosage
S bucle de dosificación

dosing pattern
G Dosierungsschema
F schéma de dosage
S muestra de dosificación

dosing piston
G Dosierkolben
F piston doseur
S matraz de dosificación

dosing screw
G Dosierschnecke
F vis de dosage
S tornillo dosificante

dosing screw conveyor
G Schneckendosiermaschine
F convoyeur à vis doseuse
S máquina dosificadora de tornillo sin fin

dosing wheel
G Dosierrad, Dosierstern
F roue de dosage
S rueda de dosificación

dotted-line recorder
G Punktschreiber
F enregistreur par ligne pointillée
S registradora de línea de puntos

double beam
G Doppelstrahl
F double faisceau
S haz doble, rayo doble

double jacket
G Doppelmantel
F double manchon, double manteau
S cubierta doble

double peak
G Doppelpeak
F pic double
S pico doble

double rotary press
G Doppelrundläuferpresse
F presse rotative double
S prensa rotatoria doble

double-blind
G doppelblind
F en double aveugle
S doble ciego

double-blind study
G Doppelblindversuch
F essai en double aveugle
S ensayo de doble ciego

double-distilled water
G Aqua bidest.
F eau pour préparation injectable (PPI)
S agua bidestilada

double-layer compression
G Zweischichtverpressung
F compression à double couche
S compresión de doble capa

doubling time
G Generationszeit
F temps de doublement
S tiempo de generación

doughy
G teigartig
F pâteux
S pastoso

downtime (machine)
G Ausfall
F panne, temps mort, défaillance
S avería, desperfecto, fallo

draft
G Entwurf
F ébauche
S bosquejo, diseño, esbozo, proyecto

draft bill
G Gesetzesentwurf
F projet de loi
S proyecto de ley

drain
G Abfluß, Abguß, Ablauf, Sinkkasten
F bassin de descente, conduit d'écoulement, drain, sortie, tuyau d'écoulement
S decantación, desagüe, escape, fuente (descendente) de recogida, salida, vaciado

drain cock
G Ablaßhahn
F robinet de purge
S grifo de salida

drain duct
G Abflußrinne
F rigole d'écoulement
S desaguadero

drain nipple
G Ablaßstutzen
F manchon d'écoulement, manchon de drainage
S empalme de salida

drain valve
G Ablaßventil
F vanne de purge, vanne de sortie
S válvula de salida

drain, to (liquids)
G ablassen (Flüssigkeiten)
F faire couler, laisser s'écouler
S dar salida, dejar escapar

drawing
G Zeichnung
F dessin, figure, schéma
S dibujo

drinking water
G Trinkwasser
F eau potable
S agua potable

drip, to
G träufeln
F verser au goutte à goutte
S gotear

drive
G Antrieb, Getriebe
F engrenage, entraînement, transmission
S engranaje, impulso, propulsión, tracción, transmisión

drive motor
G Antriebsmotor
F moteur de transmission, moteur propulsif
S motor de propulsión

drive shaft
G Antriebswelle
F arbre de transmission
S árbol motor

drive speed
G Antriebsgeschwindigkeit, Laufradgeschwindigkeit
F vitesse de roulement, vitesse de transmission
S velocidad de propulsión, velocidad de revolución, velocidad de rodamiento

drive unit
G Antriebseinheit
F unité de transmission
S unidad propulsora

drop closure
G Tropfverschluß
F obturateur doseur
S tapón cuentagotas

drop counter
G Tropfenzähler
F compte-gouttes
S cuentagotas

drop height
G Fallhöhe
F hauteur de chute
S altura de caída

drop protection
G Tropfschutz
F protection anti-gouttes
S protección frente al goteo

drop, to
G tropfen
F fuire
S gotear

drop-collection
G Tröpfchenabscheidung
F collecte de gouttelettes
S separación de gotitas

droplet
G Tröpfchen
F gouttelettes
S gotita

dropper applicator
G Verschluß mit Tropfer
F applicateur compte-gouttes
S cierre con cuentagotas

dropper insert
G Tropfeinsatz
F bouchon à compte-gouttes
S tapón cuentagotas

dropping bottle
G Tropfflasche
F flacon compte-gouttes, flacon doseur
S frasco cuentagotas

dropping point
G Tropfpunkt
F point de goutte, température de liquéfaction
S punto de goteo

drug
G Arzneimittel, Arzneistoff
F médicament, principe actif, produit pharmaceutique
S medicamento, sustancia medicamentosa

drug mechanism
G Wirkungsmechanismus
F mécanisme d'action
S mecanismo de acción

drug premix
G Arzneimittelvormischung
F préparation pharmaceutique
S elaboración previa del medicamento

drug safety manager
G Stufenplanbeauftragter
F personne responsable de la pharmaco-vigilance
S responsable de farmacovigilancia

drugs for animal feed
G Fütterungsarzneimittel
F médicament pour nourriture animale
S medicamento para el pienso

drum
G Trommel, Walze
F rouleau, cylindre, tambour
S cilindro, rodillo, tambor

drum dryer
G Walzentrockner
F séchoir à cylindres
S secador de cilindros

drum mixer
G Trommelmischer
F mélangeur à tambour
S mezclador de tambor

dry extract
G Trockenextrakt
F extrait sec
S extracto seco

dry granulation
G Trockengranulierung
F granulation par séchage
S granulación en seco

dry heat oven
G Trockenofen
F étuve
S estufa de secado, horno de secado

dry heat sterilisation
G Heißluftsterilisation
F stérilisation à l'air chaud
S esterilización por aire caliente

dry heat steriliser
G Trockenhitzesterilisator
F stérilisateur à chaleur sèche
S esterilizador de calor seco

dry out, to
G austrocknen
F dessiquer
S desecar

dry weight
G Trockengewicht
F poids sec, extrait sec
S peso seco

dry weight analysis
G Trockengewichtanalyse
F analyse à poids sec
S análisis de peso seco

dry, to
G eintrocknen, trocknen
F sécher, dessiquer
S desecar, secar

drying agent
G Trockenmittel
F agent de dessication
S agente desecante

drying cycle
G Trocknungszyklus
F cycle de séchage
S ciclo de desecación

drying oven
G Trockenschrank
F séchoir
S secador

drying time
G Trocknungszeit
F temps de séchage
S tiempo de desecación

dual-component reagent
G Zweikomponenten-Reagenz
F réactifs à deux composants
S reactivo de doble componente

duct
G Kanal, Schacht
F bouche, canal, canalisation, conduite, voie
S canal, conducto, pozo, tubo

duct network
G Kanalnetz
F système de canalisation
S red de canales

ducting
G Kanalnetz
F système de canalisation
S red de canales

ducting system
G Schachtsystem
F système de canalisation
S sistema de conducciones

due date
G Lieferdatum
F date de livraison
S fecha de entrega

duplicate
G Duplikat
F duplicata
S duplicado

durability
G Beständigkeit
F stabilité à long terme, résistance
S estabilidad, inalterabilidad

durable
G dauerhaft
F durable, stable
S duradero

duration
G Dauer
F durée
S duración

duration of exposure to radiation
G Bestrahlungsdauer
F durée d'exposition à l'irradiation
S duración de la irradiación

duration of sterilisation
G Sterilisationszeit
F durée de stérilisation
S tiempo de esterilización

duration of trial
G Studiendauer
F durée d'un essai
S duración de prueba

dust concentration
G Staubanteil
F concentration en poussière
S proporción de polvo

dust control
G Staubkontrolle
F contrôle de la poussière
S control de polvo

dust exhausting device
G Staubabsauganlage
F système d'aspiration de la poussière
S sistema de aspiración de polvo

dust extraction
G Staubabsauganlage
F système d'aspiration de la poussière
S sistema de aspiración de polvo

dust guard
G Staubschutz
F protection contre les poussières
S protección contra el polvo

dust mask
G Staubmaske
F masque contre la poussière
S máscara contra el polvo

dust particles
G Staubpartikel
F particules de poussière
S partícula de polvo

dust production
G Staubentwicklung
F production de poussière
S producción de polvo

dusting powder
G Streupulver
F poudrage
S polvo vulnerario

dustproof
G staubgeschützt
F imperméable à la poussière
S protegido frente al polvo

dust-tight
G staubdicht
F étanche à la poussière
S hermético para el polvo

dwell time
G Aufenthaltsdauer
F temps de résidence
S duración de la permanencia

dye
G Färbemittel, Farbe, Farbstoff
F colorant, pigment, teinture
S color, colorante, pigmento, tintura

dye concentration
G Farbstoffkonzentration
F concentration d'un colorant
S concentración de colorante

dyeing power
G Färbkraft
F pouvoir colorant
S poder colorante

ear cream
G Ohrencreme
F crème auriculaire
S crema auricular

ear defender
G Gehörschutz
F protection auriculaire
S protección auricular

ear drops
G Ohrentropfen
F gouttes auriculaires
S gotas auriculares

ear gel
G Ohrengel
F gel auriculaire
S gel auricular

ear ointment
G Ohrensalbe
F pommade auriculaire
S pomada auricular

ear protector
G Gehörschutz
F protection auriculaire
S protección auricular

English German French Spanish

ear wash
G Ohrenspüllösung
F solution de lavage auriculaire
S solución de lavado auricular

earth
G Ableitung, Erdung
F mise à la terre, prise de terre
S derivación, toma de tierra

earth, to
G erden
F mettre à la terre
S conectar a tierra

earthing
G Erdung
F mise la terre, prise de terre
S toma de tierra

easy punch sliding
G Stempelleichtgängigkeit
F facilité de glissement d'un poinçon
S facilidad de deslizamiento del troquel

eccentric band
G Exzenterband
F courroie excentrique
S cinta excéntrica

eccentric machine
G Exzentermaschine
F machine excentrique
S máquina excéntrica

eccentric tablet press
G Exzenterpresse
F presse excentrique à comprimés
S prensa excéntrica

EC-GMP Guideline
G EG-GMP-Leitfaden
F directives GMP de la CE
S Líneas directrices de la EC sobre GMP

ecologist
G Umweltschützer
F écologiste
S ecologista

edge
G Rand
F arête, bord
S arista, borde

edition
G Ausgabe, Version
F édition, version
S edición, versión

EDP (Electronic Data Processing)
G EDV (Elektronische Datenverarbeitung)
F traitement électronique des données, informatique
S proceso electrónico de datos

education
G Ausbildung
F éducation
S educación, formación

effect
G Einwirkung
F effet
S efecto

effective
G wirksam
F efficace
S activo, eficaz

effective volume
G Nutzungsvolumen
F volume effectif
S volumen efectivo

effervescent
G schäumend
F effervescent
S espumante

effervescent tablet
G Brausetablette
F comprimé effervescent
S comprimido efervescente

efficacy
G Wirksamkeit
F efficacité
S eficacia

efficiency
G Effizienz
F efficacité
S eficiencia

effluvium
G Ausdünstung
F effluent, efflux
S evaporación, transpiración

eject, to
G ausstoßen
F éjecter, expulser, rejeter
S emitir, expeler, expulsar

ejection
G Ausstoß, Auswurf
F éjection, rejet
S eyección

automatic ejection
G automatischer Auswurf
F éjection automatique
S eyección automática

ejection control
G Auswurfgegenkontrolle
F contrôle de l'éjection
S control de la expulsión

ejection force
G Ausstoßkraft
F force d'éjection
S fuerza de eyección

ejection time
G Ausstoßzeit
F temps d'éjection
S tiempo de eyección

ejector cam
G Auswurfkurve (bei der Tablettenpresse)
F came d'éjection
S curva de expulsión (de prensa de comprimidos)

elastic
G elastisch
F élastique
S elástico

elasticity
G Elastizität
F élasticité
S elasticidad

electrical cables
G elektrische Zuleitungen
F câbles électriques
S cables de conducción eléctrica

electrical charge
G elektrische Ladung
F charge électrique
S carga eléctrica

electrical power source
G elektrische Stromquelle
F source d'un courant électrique
S fuente de corriente eléctrica

electricity
G Strom
F courant, électricité
S corriente eléctrica

electrode
G Elektrode
F électrode
S electrodo

electrolysis
G Elektrolyse
F électrolyse
S electrólisis

electrolyte
G Elektrolyt
F électrolyte
S electrólito

electromagnetic interference
G elektromagnetische Interferenz
F interférence électromagnétique
S interferencia electromagnética

electron beam accelerator
G Elektronenstrahlbeschleuniger
F accélérateur de faisceau d'électrons
S acelerador de haz de electrones

English German French Spanish

English German French Spanish

electron capture detector (ECD)
G Elektroneneinfangdetektor
F détecteur à capture électronique
S detector de captura electrónica

electronic batch recording
G elektronische Chargendokumentation
F documentation électronique
S documentación electrónica de lotes

electronic batch recording system
G elektronische Chargendokumentation
F système de documentation électronique de lots
S documentación electrónica de lotes

electronic data processing
G elektronische Datenverarbeitung
F traitement électronique des données
S proceso electrónico de datos

electronic data storage
G Datenspeicherung
F sauvegarde électronique de données
S almacenamiento de datos

electronic identification (EID)
G elektronische Identifikation (EID)
F identification électronique
S identificación electrónica

electronic signature
G elektronische Unterschrift
F signature électronique
S firma electrónica

electro-pneumatic operation
G elektro-pneumatischer Betrieb
F opération électro-pneumatique
S funcionamiento electroneumático

electro-polished
G elektropoliert
F électro-poli
S pulido eléctricamente

electrostatic charge
G elektrostatische Aufladung
F charge électrostatique
S carga electrostática

elementary analysis
G Elementaranalyse
F analyse élémentaire
S análisis elemental

elevator
G Aufzug
F ascenseur
S ascensor

eliminate a failure (fault), to
G Fehler beseitigen
F éliminer une erreur
S eliminar errores

eluant
G Elutionsmittel
F éluant
S agente levigante

eluate
G Eluat
F éluat
S levigado, eluado

elucidate, to (a structure)
G aufklären (Struktur)
F élucider (une structure)
S aclarar, esclarecer (una estructura)

embed, to
G einbetten
F inclure
S incluir

emboss, to
G aufprägen, einprägen, einstanzen, prägen, stanzen
F empreindre, estamper, imprimer, poinçonner
S acuñar, estampar, imprimir, punzonar, troquelar

embossed
G geprägt
F estampé
S acuñado, estampado

embossed film
G Prägefolie
F feuille estampée
S lámina de estampado

embossing station
G Prägestation
F station d'estampage
S estación de troquelado

embossment
G Prägung
F estampage
S acuñado, estampado, troquelado

embrocation
G Einreibung, Einreibemittel
F beaume, embrocation, liniment, onguent
S bálsamo, fricción, frotamiento, linimento

emergency
G Notfall
F urgence
S caso de urgencia

emergency off
G Not-Aus
F arrêt d'urgence
S interruptor de emergencia

emergency power supply
G Notstromaggregat
F générateur de courant d'urgence
S generador eléctrico de emergencia

emission
G Emission
F émission
S emisión

empirical
G empirisch
F empirique
S empírico

empirical formula
G empirische Formel
F formule empirique
S fórmula empírica

employee
G Angestellter
F employé
S empleado

employee suggestion scheme
G betriebliches Vorschlagswesen
F schéma interne de suggestions pour employés
S sistema empresarial de propuestas

employment
G Arbeitsstelle
F emploi
S puesto de trabajo

empty, to
G entleeren
F vider, évacuer
S vaciar

emptying valve
G Entleerventil
F valve de vidange
S válvula de vaciamiento

emulsifier
G Emulgator, Emulgiergerät
F émulseur, émulsifiant
S emulsivo, emulsor

emulsify, to
G emulgieren
F émulsionner
S emulsionar

emulsifying agent
G Emulgator
F émulsifiant
S emulsivo

emulsion
G Emulsion
F émulsion
S emulsión

oil/water emulsion
G Öl-in-Wasser Emulsion
F émulsion d'huile dans l'eau
S emulsión de aceite en agua

water/oil emulsion
G Wasser-in-Öl Emulsion
F émulsion d'eau dans l'huile
S emulsión de agua en aceite

enamel
G Email
F émail
S esmalte

enamelled
G emailliert
F émaillé
S esmaltado

enantiomer
G Enantiomere
F énantiomère
S enantiómero

enantiomeric purity
G enantiomere Reinheit
F pureté énantiomère
S pureza enantiómera

encapsulate, to
G verkapseln
F encapsuler
S capsular

encapsulator
G Kapselmaschine
F encapsuleuse
S máquina encapsuladora

encased
G eingeschlossen, umgeben von
F enchâssé
S rodeado de

enclosure
G Anlage (zur Dokumentation)
F annexe, appendice
S anexo, apéndice (de un documento)

end of study
G Studienende
F fin d'un essai clinique
S fin del estudio

end of trial
G Studienende
F fin d'un essai clinique
S fin del estudio

endanger, to (quality)
G gefährden (Qualität)
F mettre en danger, compromettre (la qualité)
S arriesgar, poner en peligro (la calidad)

endocervical gel
G Gel zur endozervikalen Anwendung
F gel pour utilisation endo-cervicale
S gel de uso endocervical

endocervical use
G endozervikale Anwendung
F usage endo-cervical
S uso endocervical

endosinusial use
G Anwendung in den Nebenhöhlen
F pour usage sinusien
S uso endosinusal

endothermic reaction
G endothermische Reaktion
F réaction endothermique
S reacción endotérmica

endothermic split-off
G endothermische Abspaltung
F scission endothermique
S escisión endotérmica

endotoxin
G Endotoxin
F endotoxine
S endotoxina

enema
G Darmspülung, Klistier
F lavement, lavement intestinal
S enema, lavativa

energy consumption
G Energieverbrauch
F consommation d'énergie
S consumo energético

engineer
G Ingenieur
F ingénieur
S ingeniero

engineering
G Ingenieurwesen, Technik (als Abteilung)
F ingénieurie, ingénierie
S ingeniería, departamento técnico

engineering drawing
G technische Zeichnung
F dessin technique
S dibujo técnico

engrave, to
G eingravieren
F graver
S grabar

engraving roll
G Gravurrolle
F rouleau de gravure
S rollo de grabado

enlargement
G Vergrößerung
F agrandissement
S agrandamiento

enrich, to
G anreichern
F concentrer
S concentrar, enriquecer

enrichment
G Anreicherung
F concentration
S concentración, enriquecimiento

enrichment medium
G Anreicherungsmedium
F médium de concentration
S medio de concentración, medio de enriquecimiento

ensure, to
G sicherstellen
F assurer, garantir
S asegurar, garantizar

enter, to
G eintragen
F inscrire, enregistrer
S inscribir, registrar

enteric-coated
G magensaftresistent überzogen
F à enrobage entérique
S con cubierta resistente al jugo gástrico

entero-soluble
G dünndarmlöslich
F entéro-soluble
S soluble en el intestino delgado

entrap, to
G auffangen
F capter, recueillir
S captar, colectar, recoger

entry
G Befehlseingabe
F entrée d'une commande
S entrada de un comando

environment
G Umgebung, Umwelt
F environnement
S entorno, medio ambiente

non-aqueous environment
G nicht-wäßrige Umgebung
F milieu non aquatique
S entorno no acuoso

uncontrolled environment
G nicht kontrollierte Umgebung
F environnement non controlé
S entorno no controlado

environmental analysis
G Umweltanalyse
F analyse de l'environnement
S análisis del medio ambiente

environmental awareness
G Umweltbewußtsein
F conscience de l'environnement
S conciencia del medio ambiente

English
German
French
Spanish

environmental conditions
G Umgebungsbedingungen
F conditions de l'environnement
S condiciones ambientales

environmental control
G Umweltkontrolle
F contrôle de l'environnement
S control ecológico

environmental damage
G Umweltschaden
F atteinte à l'environnement
S daño ecológico

environmental influence
G Umwelteinfluß
F influence de l'environnement
S influencia del medio ambiente

environmental management
G Umweltschutzmanagement
F gestion de l'environnement
S gestión ecológica

environmental monitoring
G Umgebungskontrolle
F contrôle de l'environnement
S control del entorno

environmental protection agency (EPA)
G Umweltschutzbehörde
F agence pour la protection de l'environnement
S autoridades de protección del medio ambiente

environmental report
G Umweltschutzbericht
F rapport sur l'écologie
S informe ecológico

environmental waste
G Umweltverschmutzung
F pollution de l'environnement
S desgaste ecológico, degradación ecológica

environmentalist
G Umweltschützer
F écologiste
S ecologista

environmentally friendly
G umweltfreundlich
F écologique
S ecológico

enzyme
G Enzym
F enzyme
S enzima

DNA-modifying enzyme
G DNA-modifizierendes Enzym
F enzyme de modification de l'ADN
S enzima modificador del ADN

eperimisation
G Epimerisierung
F épimérisation
S epimerización

epidural use
G epidurale Anwendung
F usage épidural
S uso epidural

epoxy resin
G Epoxidharz
F résine époxy
S epoxirresina

Eppendorf reaction vessel
G Eppendorf-Reaktionsgefäß
F fiole Eppendorf
S tubo de ensayo Eppendorf

equation
G Gleichung (mathematisch)
F équation
S ecuación (matemática)

equilibrium
G Gleichgewicht
F équilibre
S equilibrio

re-equilibrium
G erneutes Gleichgewicht
F rééquilibre
S reequilibrio

equip, to
G ausrüsten
F équiper, outiller
S equipar

equipment
G Ausrüstung, Geräte
F équipement, appareillage expérimental
S equipamiento, aparatos

dedicated equipment
G Ausrüstung nur für ein Produkt
F équipement dédié
S equipamiento sólo para un producto

multipurpose equipment
G Ausrüstung für verschiedene Produkte
F équipement multi-usage
S equipamiento para diferentes productos

equipment maintenance
G Wartung der Ausrüstung
F entretien de l'équipement
S mantenimiento del equipo

equipment manufacturer
G Gerätehersteller
F fabricant d'équipement
S fabricante de aparatos

equipment qualification
G Qualifizierung der Ausrüstung
F qualification de l'équipement
S cualificación del equipamiento

equipment test
G Gerätetest
F test d'appareils
S comprobación de aparatos

equivalency
G Äquivalenz
F équivalence
S equivalencia

equivalent
G äquivalent
F équivalent
S equivalente

Erlenmeyer flask
G Erlenmeyerkolben
F Erlenmeyer, flacon à fond plat
S matraz de Erlenmeyer

error
G Fehler
F défaut, erreur
S error

human error
G menschlicher Fehler
F erreur humaine
S error humano

random error
G zufälliger Fehler
F erreur aléatoire
S error casual

error (failure) investigation
G Fehleruntersuchung
F investigation des sources d'une erreur
S investigación de errores

essential oil
G ätherisches Öl
F huile essentielle
S aceite etérico

ester number
G Esterzahl
F nombre d'ester
S número de éster

esterification
G Veresterung
F estérification
S esterificación

etch, to
G einätzen
F corroder, décaper
S grabar (al aguafuerte)

ethical
G ethisch
F éthique
S ético

ethical products
G ethische Produkte
F produits éthiques
S productos éticos

ethics committee
G Ethikkomission
F commission d'éthique
S comisión ética

European Pharmacopoeia (PhEur)
G Europäisches Arzneibuch (PhEur)
F pharmacopée européenne (PhEur)
S Farmacopea Europea

eutectic
G eutektisch
F eutectique
S eutéctico

eutectic point
G Eutektikum
F point d'eutexie
S punto eutéctico

evacuate, to
G entleeren
F vider, évacuer
S vaciar

evacuation system
G Absaugvorrichtung
F système d'aspiration, système d'évacuation
S sistema de aspiración, sistema de evacuación

evaluate, to
G bewerten
F évaluer
S evaluar

evaluation (of data)
G Auswertung, Bewertung (von Daten)
F interprétation, évaluation (de données)
S evaluación, interpretación (de datos)

evaluation range
G Auswertebereich
F plage d'évaluation
S área de evaluación

evaporate, to
G abdampfen, ausdampfen, eindampfen, verdampfen, verdunsten
F évaporer, faire s'évaporer, faire évaporer, passer à la vapeur
S evaporar, evaporarse, volatilizar

evaporating dish
G Abdampfschale
F capsule d'évaporation
S cápsula de evaporación

evaporation
G Verdunstung
F évaporation
S evaporación, vaporización

evaporative loss
G Verdunstungsverlust
F perte due à l'évaporisation
S pérdida de evaporación

evaporator
G Verdampfer
F évaporateur
S evaporador

evidence
G Nachweis
F détection, preuve
S demostración, prueba

exact
G genau
F exact
S exacto

examination on receipt
G Eingangsprüfung
F examen d'entrée
S examen inicial

exceed, to
G überschreiten
F excéder
S exceder

excess
G Überschuß
F excès
S excedente, sobrante

excess atmospheric pressure
G Atmosphärenüberdruck
F surpression atmosphérique
S sobrepresión atmosférica

excess pressure
G Überdruck
F surpression
S sobrepresión

excess weight
G Mehrgewicht
F excédent de poids
S excedente de peso

exchangeable
G austauschbar, auswechselbar
F interchangeable
S intercambiable

excipient
G Hilfsstoff
F excipient, adjuvant
S excipiente, sustancia auxiliar

exclusion limit
G Ausschlußgrenze
F limite d'exclusion
S límite de exclusión

excretion
G Exkretion
F excrétion
S excreción

excretion of medicinal substance
G Arzneistoffausscheidung
F élimination d'un principe actif
S eliminación del principio activo

ex-duct
G Ex-Kanal
F canal de purge anti-déflagrant, orifice de purge anti-déflagrant
S orificio (válvula) de seguridad (antideflagrante)

execute, to
G durchführen
F réaliser, exécuter
S ejecutar, llevar a cabo, realizar

executive
G Führungskraft
F directeur, cadre dirigeant
S directivo, ejecutivo

executive with power of procuration
G Prokurist
F fondé de pouvoirs
S apoderado general

exhaust air
G Abluft, Prozeßabluft, Raumabluft
F air d'évacuation, air d'échappement
S aire de escape de un proceso, aire de escape

exhaust air duct
G Abluftkanal
F canal d'évacuation de l'air
S canal del aire de escape

exhaust air filter
G Abluftfilter
F filtre à air d'évacuation
S filtro del aire de escape

exhaust air flue
G Abluftschacht
F puits d'évacuation d'air
S pozo de evacuación de aire

exhaust air shaft
G Abluftschacht
F puits d'évacuation d'air
S pozo de evacuación de aire

exhaust gas
G Abgas
F gaz d'échappement, gaz d'évacuation
S gas de escape

exhaust line
G Abluftleitung
F conduite d'évacuation
S conducto de evacuación de aire

English German French Spanish

exhaust pipe
G Abluftrohr
F conduite d'évacuation d'air
S tubo de evacuación de aire

exhaust valve
G Abluftregelklappe
F clapet d'évacuation d'air
S válvula de evacuación de aire

exothermic reaction
G exothermische Reaktion
F réaction exothermique
S reacción exotérmica

expanded polystyrene (EPS)
G expandiertes Polystyrol (EPS)
F polystyrène expansé
S poliesterol expandido

expansion
G Ausdehnung
F expansion
S ampliación, dilatación, expansión, extensión

expansion joint
G Dehnungsfuge
F joint dilatable
S junta de dilatación

experiment
G Versuch
F essai, expérience
S ensayo, experimento, prueba

experimental conditions
G Versuchsbedingungen
F conditions expérimentales
S condiciones experimentales

expert
G Begutachter, Sachverständiger
F expert
S asesor, experto, perito

expert opinion
G Begutachtung
F opinion d'expert
S dictamen, peritaje

expert system
G Expertensystem
F système expert
S sistema de expertos

expertise
G Gutachten
F expertise, avis d'expert
S dictamen

expiration coding
G Codierung des Verfalldatums
F codage de la date d'expiration
S codificación de la fecha de caducidad

expiration date
G Verfallsdatum
F date d'expiration
S fecha de caducidad, fecha de expiración

expire, to
G verfallen
F expirer
S caducar, expirar

expiry date
G Verfallsdatum
F date d'expiration
S fecha de caducidad, fecha de expiración

explosion hazard
G Explosionsgefahr
F danger d'explosion
S peligro de explosión

explosion panel
G Ex-Klappen
F clapet anti-déflagrant
S válvula antideflagrante

explosion relief
G Explosionsentlastung
F décharge d'explosion
S descarga de explosión

explosion relief duct cover
G Ex-Kanalabdeckung
F couvercle de canalisation anti-déflagrant
S cubierta del orificio de seguridad

explosion vent
G Ex-Kanal
F canal de purge anti-déflagrant, orifice de purge anti-déflagrant
S orificio o válvula de seguridad (antideflagrante)

explosion-proof
G explosionssicher
F anti-déflagrant
S a prueba de explosión

explosion-protected
G explosionsgeschützt, Ex-geschützt
F protégé contre une explosion
S protegido contra explosión, protegido frente a explosión

explosiveness
G Explosivität
F explosivité
S explosividad

export package
G Exportverpackung
F emballage à l'export
S embalaje de exportación

express, to
G auspressen
F presser
S exprimir, prensar

extend, to
G verlängern
F prolonger, rallonger
S alargar, prolongar

extended release
G verlängerte Wirkstoff-Freigabe
F libération prolongée
S liberación prolongada de sustancia activa

extension
G Ansatzstück
F rallonge
S pieza de empalme, pieza insertable

extension cable
G Verlängerungskabel
F câble de rallonge
S alargadera, cable de prolongación

extension pipe
G Ansatzrohr
F tuyau de rallonge
S tubo de empalme

external
G äußerlich
F externe
S externo

external air
G Außenluft
F air frais, air libre
S aire fresco, aire libre

external dimensions
G Außenmaße
F dimensions externes
S dimensiones externas

external steam
G externe Dampfzufuhr
F vapeur externe
S suministro de vapor externo

external steam heating
G Beheizung mit externer Dampfzufuhr
F chauffage avec apport de vapeur externe
S calefacción con suministro de vapor externo

extract
G Auszug, Extrakt
F extrait
S extracto

liquid extract
G Flüssigextrakt
F extrait liquide
S extracto líquido

extract, to
G extrahieren
F extraire
S extraer

English
German
French
Spanish

extractable substance
G extrahierbare Substanz
F substance extractible
S sustancia extraíble

extraction
G Extraktion, Gewinnung
F extraction, production
S extracción, obtención, producción

extrude, to
G extrudieren
F extruder
S extrudir

extruder
G Extruder, Strangpresse
F extrudeuse
S extrusor, prensa extrusora

extrusion
G Extrusion
F extrusion
S extrusión

eye
G Öse
F œillet
S ojal

eye cream
G Augencreme
F crème ophtalmique
S crema oftálmica

eye drops
G Augentropfen
F gouttes ophtalmiques
S gotas oftálmicas

eye gel
G Augengel
F gel pour œil
S gel oftálmico

eye lid
G Augenlid
F paupière
S párpado

eye lotion
G Augenbad
F lotion pour œil
S loción oftálmica

eye ointment
G Augensalbe
F pommade pour les yeux
S pomada oftálmica

eye protection
G Augenschutz
F protection oculaire
S protección ocular

eye wash equipment
G Augendusche
F douche de rinçage pour les yeux
S equipo de lavado oftálmico

eyelet
G Öse
F œillet
S ojal

face mask
G Mundschutz
F masque de protection facial
S protección bucal

face protection
G Gesichtsschutz
F protection faciale
S protección facial

facility (machines)
G Anlage (Maschine), Betriebsstätte, Einrichtung (in Gebäuden)
F usine, établissement industriel, site de fabrication, installation industrielle
S equipo, instalación (máquina), plantas empresariales, instalación (en edificios)

factory
G Betriebsstätte
F usine, installations, site de fabrication
S plantas empresariales

factory acceptance test (FAT)
G Vorabnahme (beim Hersteller), Werksabnahme
F contrôle avant livraison, réception en usine
S control antes de entrega, test de aceptación en fábrica

fade, to
G verblassen
F perdre sa couleur, se défraîchir
S empalidecer

faeces test
G Stuhluntersuchung
F analyse des selles
S examen de heces

fail, to
G versagen
F faillir à sa tâche
S fracasar

failed batch
G Fehlcharge
F lot défectueux
S lote defectuoso

fail-safe mode
G fehlersicherer Modus
F mode indéréglable
S modo a prueba de errores

failure
G Ausfall, Panne, Störfall, Versagen, Fehler
F défaillance, incident, panne, temps mort, défaut, erreur
S avería, desperfecto, incidente, fallo, error

failure alarm
G Störungsmeldung
F alarme de mauvais fonctionnement
S aviso de avería

failure message
G Fehlermeldung
F message d'erreur
S aviso de errores

failure mode and effect analysis (FMEA)
G Fehlermöglichkeits- und Einflußanalyse (FMEA)
F analyse de modes et effets des pannes (FMEA)
S análisis de influencia y posibilidad de defectos

failure rate
G Fehlerrate
F taux d'erreur
S tasa de errores

failure rectification
G Fehlerbehebung
F dépannage, action de corriger
S corrección de errores

falling sphere viscosimeter
G Kugelfallviskosimeter
F viscosimètre à sphère descendante
S viscosímetro de esfera descendiente

falsification
G Fälschung, Verfälschung
F falsification
S falsificación

falsify, to
G verfälschen
F falsifier
S falsificar

fan
G Gebläse, Ventilator
F ventilateur
S ventilador

fan belt
G Keilriemen
F courroie trapézoïdale
S correa trapezoidal

fan wheel
G Flügelrad, Gebläserad
F ailette, roue de ventilateur
S rueda de aletas, rueda de paletas, rueda de ventilador

fan wheel anemometer
G Flügelradanemometer
F anémomètre à moulinet, anémomètre à ailettes
S anemómetro de rueda de aletas

fast fuse
G flinke Sicherung
F fusible à action instantanée
S fusible rápido

fast-clamping device
G Schnellspannvorrichtung
F dispositif de serrage rapide
S dispositivo tensor rápido

fatal dose
G tödliche Dosis
F dose mortelle
S dosis mortal

fatty acid
G Fettsäure
F acide gras
S ácido graso

fatty ointment
G Fettsalbe
F pommade
S pomada con elevado contenido en grasa

fault
G Fehler, Störfall
F défaut, erreur, incident, panne
S avería, error, fallo, incidente

fault (failure) display
G Störanzeige
F affichage d'une erreur
S pantalla de aviso de avería

faultless
G einwandfrei
F irréprochable
S intacto

faulty
G fehlerhaft
F défectueux
S defectuoso

feature
G Merkmal
F caractéristique, particularité
S característica

feed
G Beschickung, Zufuhr, Zuleitung
F alimentation, charge, tuyauterie d'alimentation
S alimentación, carga, suministro, tubería de alimentación

feed chute
G Zufuhrrinne
F rigole d'alimentation, conduit d'alimentation
S canal de alimentación

feed hopper
G Beschickungstrichter, Fülleinrichtung
F trémie de charge, trémie de remplissage
S embudo de carga, dispositivo de relleno

feed screw
G Dosierschnecke
F vis de dosage
S tornillo dosificante

feed shoe
G Füllschuh
F sabot distributeur
S zueco distribuidor

feed silo
G Beschickungssilo
F trémie de charge
S depósito de carga

feed system
G Eintragsvorrichtung
F système d'alimentation
S sistema de alimentación

feed table
G Zuführtisch
F table de chargement, table d'alimentation
S mesa de abastecimiento

feed tube
G Füllrohr
F tube de remplissage
S tubo de llenado

feed water
G Speisewasser
F eau d'alimentation
S agua de alimentación

ferment, to
G fermentieren
F faire fermenter
S fermentar

fermentation
G Fermentation, Gärung
F fermentation
S fermentación

fermentation laboratory
G Fermentationslabor
F laboratoire de fermentation
S laboratorio de fermentación

fermentation room
G Fermentationsraum
F aire de fermentation
S área de fermentación

fermentation vessel
G Fermentationskessel
F cuve de fermentation
S caldera de fermentación

fermenter
G Fermenter
F fermenteur
S fermentador

fertiliser
G Düngemittel
F engrais
S abono, fertilizante

fibre
G Faser
F fibre
S fibra

fibre cardboard
G Fiberkarton
F carton à fibres
S cartón de fibra

fibre catcher
G Faserfänger
F capteur de fibres
S captador de fibras

fibre drum
G Fibertrommel
F tambour à fibres
S tambor de fibras

fibreglass
G Glasfaser
F fibre de verre
S fibra de vidrio

fibreglass-reinforced filter
G glasfaserverstärkter Filter
F filtre renforcé à la fibre de verre
S filtro reforzado con fibra de vidrio

field force
G Außendienst
F force de vente
S servicio externo de ventas

fill, to
G einfüllen, beladen
F charger, alimenter
S envasar, llenar

filler
G Füllmittel
F moyen de remplissage
S medio de relleno

filling
G Abfüllung
F remplissage
S envasado, embotellamiento

filling cam (tablet press)
G Füllkurve (bei der Tablettenpresse)
F came de remplissage
S curva de relleno (prensa de comprimidos)

English German French Spanish

English German French Spanish

filling depth
G Fülltiefe
F hauteur de remplissage
S altura del relleno

filling device
G Einfüllvorrichtung
F dispositif d'alimentation, appareillage d'alimentation
S dispositivo de relleno

filling funnel
G Einfülltrichter
F trémie de charge
S embudo de relleno

filling hose
G Abfüllrohr
F conduite de remplissage
S conducto de envasado

filling level
G Füllhöhe
F niveau de remplissage
S nivel de llenado

filling line
G Abfüllinie, Abfüllstraße
F ligne de remplissage, rampe de remplissage, chaîne de remplissage
S cadena de envasado

filling machine
G Abfüllmaschine
F remplisseuse
S máquina de envasado

filling needle
G Abfüllnadel
F aiguille de remplissage
S aguja de envasado

filling nozzle
G Düsennadel, Füllventil
F aiguille d'injection, buse de remplissage, injecteur à aiguille
S aguja de inyección, válvula de relleno

filling pipe
G Abfüllrohr
F conduite de remplissage
S conducto de envasado

filling port
G Einfüllöffnung
F ouverture de chargement
S abertura de relleno

filling quantity
G Abfüllmenge, Füllmenge
F quantité de remplissage, volume de remplissage
S cantidad envasada, cantidad de relleno

filling section
G Abfüllstrecke, Füllbereich
F chemin de remplissage, zone de remplissage
S sección de llenado, zona de relleno

filling station
G Abfüllort, Abfüllstation, Füllstation
F station de remplissage, station de mise en bouteilles, station en bidons
S estación de envasado, estación de llenado

filling tube
G Abfüllschlauch, Einfüllrohr
F conduite d'alimentation, tuyau de remplissage
S tubo de envasado, tubo de relleno

filling valve
G Einfüllklappe
F vanne d'alimentation
S válvula de relleno

filling volume
G Füllvolumen
F volume de charge
S volumen de relleno

filling weight
G Füllgewicht
F poids de remplissage
S peso al envasar

film
G Folie, Überzug
F couche, feuille, pellicule
S cubierta, hoja, lámina, revestimiento

film forming
G Folienverformung
F façonnage de feuilles
S deformación de láminas

film laminating adhesive
G Folienverbundkleber
F adhésif pour feuilles
S adhesivo para láminas

film printing
G Folienbedruckung
F impression de feuilles
S impresión de láminas

film slippage
G Folienschlupf
F glissement d'une feuille
S deslizamiento de una lámina

film supply
G Folienbeschickung
F alimentation en feuilles
S abastecimiento de láminas

film tear sensor
G Folienrißkontrolle
F contrôle des déchirures de feuilles
S control de desgarro de láminas

film thickness
G Foliendicke
F épaisseur de feuille
S espesor de lámina

film tube
G Schlauchfolie
F feuille en gaine
S película tubular

film-forming agent
G Filmbildner
F agent filmogène
S agente formador de películas

film-forming liquid
G filmbildende Flüssigkeit
F collodion
S colodión

filter
G Filter
F filtre
S filtro

terminal filter
G endständiger Filter
F filtre terminal
S filtro terminal

filter bag
G Filterbeutel, Filtersack
F filtre à poches, sac de filtration
S bolsa filtro

filter bed
G Filterbett
F lit de filtre
S lecho filtrante

filter cartridge
G Filterkerze, Filterpatrone
F chandelle filtrante, cartouche de filtre
S candela filtrante, cartucho de filtro

filter cleaning device
G Filterabreinigungsvorrichtung
F dispositif de nettoyage de filtre
S dispositivo de limpieza de filtros

filter housing
G Filtergehäuse
F boîtier de filtre
S armazón del filtro

filter insert
G Filtereinsatz
F support de filtre
S inserción del filtro

filter installation
G Filtereinbau
F installation d'un filtre
S instalación de un filtro

filter integrity
G Filterintegrität
F intégrité d'un filtre
S integridad del filtro

filter integrity test
G Filterintegritätstest
F test d'intégrité de filtre
S prueba de integridad del filtro

filter materials
G Filtermaterialien
F matériaux de filtre
S materiales de filtración

filter paper
G Filtrierpapier
F papier filtre
S papel de filtro

filter removal
G Filterausbau
F démontage de filtre
S desmontaje de un filtro

filter residue
G Filterrückstand
F résidu de filtration
S residuo de filtración

filter resistance
G Filterwiderstand
F résistance du filtre
S resistencia del filtro

filter seal
G Filterabdichtung
F étanchement d'un filtre
S cierre hermético de un filtro

filter stand
G Filtergestell
F support de filtre
S soporte del filtro

filter surface
G Filterfläche, Filteroberfläche
F surface d'un filtre, superficie d'un filtre
S superficie del filtro

filter suspension rack
G Filteraufhängevorrichtung
F crémaillère pour filtre
S dispositivo de suspensión de filtros

filter, to
G abnutschen, filtrieren, kolieren
F filtrer
S filtrar

filtrate
G Filtrat
F filtrat
S filtrado

filtrate waste
G Filtrationsabfall
F effluent de filtration
S desecho de filtración

filtration
G Filtration
F filtration
S filtración

filtration method
G Filtrationsmethode
F méthode de filtration
S método de filtración

filtration resistance
G Filtrationswiderstand
F résistance au filtrage
S resistencia a la filtración

final acceptance (of a machine)
G Abnahme (einer Maschine)
F réception technique (d'une machine)
S recepción técnica (de una máquina)

final container
G Endbehältnis
F conditionnement final, conteneur final, récipient final
S recipiente final

final drying
G Nachtrocknen
F séchage final
S secado final

final sterilisation
G Endsterilisation
F stérilisation finale
S esterilización final

final yield
G Endausbeute
F rendement final
S rendimiento final

finding
G Befund
F diagnose
S diagnóstico

fine adjusting screw
G Mikrometerschraube
F micromètre, vis micromètre
S tornillo micrométrico

fine adjustment
G Feineinstellung, Feinregulierung
F réglage fin, mise au point précise
S ajuste fino, regulación fina

fine dust filter
G Feinstaubfilter
F filtre à poussières fines
S filtro de polvo fino

fine particle
G Feinkorn
F particule fine
S partícula fina

fine sieve
G Feinsieb
F tamis fin
S tamiz fino

fine tissue
G Feingewebe
F tissu fragile
S tejido fino

fine-grained
G feinkörnig
F à grain fin
S de grano fino

fines (sieve)
G Siebdurchgang
F passant (tamisage)
S paso de tamiz, tamizado

finished goods
G Fertigwaren
F produits manufacturés
S productos manufacturados

finished medicinal product
G Fertigarzneimittel
F médicament fini, produit pharmaceutique fini
S medicamento manufacturado, especialidad farmacéutica manufacturada

finished pack
G Fertigpackung
F emballage fini
S envase terminado

finished product
G Fertigprodukt
F produit fini
S producto acabado

fire alarm
G Feuermelder
F alarme d'incendie
S alarma de incendio

fire extinguisher
G Feuerlöscher
F extincteur
S extintor (de incendios)

fire hazard
G Feuergefahr
F risque d'incendie
S peligro de incendio

fire protection door
G Brandschutzklappe
F porte de protection anti-incendie
S puerta de protección contra incendios

fire-proof
G feuergeschützt
F ignifugé, à l'épreuve du feu
S protegido frente al fuego

fire-resistant
G feuerfest
F in-inflammable
S ignífugo, resistente al fuego

firmness
G Festigkeit
F solidité
S firmeza, solidez

first aid
G Erste Hilfe
F secours d'urgence, premiers secours
S primeros auxilios

first-order reaction
G Reaktion 1. Ordnung
F réaction de premier ordre
S reacción de primer orden

fit, to
G einbauen
F installer
S instalar, montar

fitted
G eingebaut
F encastré
S incorporado, instalado, montado

fitting
G Armatur
F garniture
S armadura, accesorios

fixing
G Befestigung
F fixation
S fijación

fixing solution
G Fixierlösung
F solution de fixation
S solución fijadora

flake, to
G ausflocken
F floculer
S flocular

flaky
G flockig
F floconneux
S flocular

flame emission spectroscopy
G Flammenemissionsspektroskopie
F spectroscopie à émission de flamme
S espectroscopia de emisión de llama

flame gun
G Flammpistole
F pistolet chalumeau
S pistola de llama

flame ionisation detector (FID)
G Flammenionisationsdetektor (FID)
F détecteur à ionisation de flamme
S detector de ionización de llama

flame photometer
G Flammenphotometer
F photomètre de flamme
S fotómetro de llama

flame photometry
G Flammenphotometrie
F photométrie de flamme
S fotometría de llama

flame protector (of instrument)
G Brandschutz (eines Gerätes)
F ignifugation, ignifugeage (d'un instrument)
S protección frente al fuego (de un aparato)

flame steriliser
G Flammensterilisator
F stérilisateur à flammes
S esterilizador a la llama

flame-seal, to (ampoules)
G zuschmelzen (Ampullen)
F obturer par vitrification (ampoules)
S obturar por vitrificación, cerrar ampollas a la llama

flammability
G Brennbarkeit
F combustibilité
S combustibilidad, inflamabilidad

flammable
G brennbar, entflammbar, feuergefährlich
F combustible, inflammable
S combustible, inflamable

highly flammable
G leicht entflammbar
F facilement inflammable
S fácilmente inflamable

non-flammable
G nicht brennbar
F in-inflammable
S no combustible, no inflamable

flange
G Flansch
F bride, collerette
S brida, collar

flange, to
G flanschen, umbördeln
F brider, sertir
S bridar, bordear, rebordear, redondear

flap
G Klappe
F clapet, volet
S tapa, válvula

flap control
G Klappensteuerung
F guidage de clapet
S control de las válvulas

flap positioner
G Klappensteller
F positionneur de clapet
S posicionador de válvulas

flap trap
G Rückschlagklappe
F clapet anti-retour
S válvula de retención

flash light
G Blinklicht
F feux clignotant
S luz intermitente

flash point
G Flammpunkt
F point d'inflammation
S punto de ignición

flask
G Kolben
F ballon, flacon
S alambique, matraz, retorta

flat bag
G Flachbeutel
F sachet plat, sachet plan
S bolsa plana

flat surface
G ebene Fläche
F surface plane
S superficie plana

flattened
G abgeflacht
F aplati
S aplanado

flattening
G Abflachung
F aplatissement
S aplanamiento

flavour
G Geschmackstoff, Geschmack
F agent aromatique, goût
S agente saporífero, gusto

flavouring agent
G Geschmackstoff
F agent aromatique
S agente saporífero

flavourless
G geschmacklos
F insipide, fade
S insípido

fleece
G Vlies
F toison
S vellocino

flexible
G biegsam
F flexible, pliable
S flexible, maleable, plegable

flexing resistance
G Falzechtheit
F résistance au pliage
S resistencia al plegado

flexional strain
G Biegebeanspruchung
F sollicitation à la flexion
S tensión de flexión

flexional strength
G Beugungsfestigkeit
F résistance à la flexion
S resistencia a la flexión

flexural strength
G Biegefestigkeit
F résistance au pliage, résistance au fléchissement
S resistencia a la flexión

flexural stress
G Biegespannung
F tension de pliage, tension de fléchissement
S tensión de flexión

flexure
G Biegung
F courbure, pliage
S flexión, curvatura

floc
G Flocke
F bourre
S copo, flóculo

flocculate, to
G ausflocken
F floculer
S flocular

flocculation
G Flockung
F floculation
S floculación

floor
G Boden
F sol, plancher
S suelo

floor covering
G Fußbodenbelag, Bodenbelag
F revêtement de sol
S pavimento, revestimiento del suelo

floor drain
G Bodenabfluß, Fußbodenabfluß, Gulli
F égoût, bouche d'égout
S sumidero

floor finishing
G Fußbodenbelag, Bodenbelag
F revêtement de sol
S pavimento, revestimiento del suelo

floor leveller
G Ausgleichsestrich
F chape de compensation
S pavimento compensador

floor plan
G Stockwerksplan
F plan d'étage
S plano de los pisos

flooring
G Fußbodenbelag, Bodenbelag
F revêtement de sol
S pavimento, revestimiento del suelo

flow
G Durchfluß
F débit
S paso (de un líquido), flujo

flow cell
G Durchflußzelle
F cellule de mesure du débit
S célula de fluxometría

flow chart
G Ablaufschema, Flußdiagramm, Fließdiagramm
F schéma opérationnel, schéma de marche, schéma de principe, schéma de fabrication, schéma fonctionnel
S esquema operacional, diagrama de flujo, diagrama operacional

flow cytometry
G Durchflußzytometrie
F cytométrie à débit liquide
S citometría de flujo

flow gradient
G Fließgradient
F gradient d'écoulement
S gradiente de flujo

flow meter
G Strömungswächter
F débitmètre
S fluxómetro

flow promoter (in tabletting)
G Fließmittel (in der Tablettierung)
F fluidifiant
S fluidificante (fabricación de comprimidos)

flow property
G Fließeigenschaft
F propriété d'écoulement
S propiedad fluida

flow rate
G Durchflußgeschwindigkeit, Fließgeschwindigkeit, Strömungsgeschwindigkeit
F débit
S velocidad de flujo

flow regulation
G Durchflußregulierung
F régulation du débit
S regulación del flujo

flowability
G Fließfähigkeit
F fluidité
S fluidez

flowable
G rieselfähig
F capable d'écoulement
S capaz de fluir

flowing property
G Rieselfähigkeit
F propriété d'écoulement
S capacidad de fluir

flowmeter
G Durchflußmesser
F débimètre
S fluxómetro

flowmeter, variable
G variabler Volumenstromregler
F débitmètre
S regulador variable de flujo

flow-through cell
G Durchflußzelle
F cellule de mesure du débit
S célula de fluxometría

fluctuate, to
G schwanken
F fluctuer
S fluctuar, variar

fluid bed
G Wirbelschicht
F lit fluidisé
S lecho fluidificado

fluid bed dryer
G Wirbelschichttrockner
F sécheur en lit fluidisé
S secador de lecho fluidificado

fluid bed spray granulator
G Wirbelschichtgranulator
F granulateur en lit fluidisé
S granulador de lecho fluidificado

fluid energy mill
G Luftstrahlmühle
F microniseur à jet d'air
S micronizador del chorro de aire

English German French Spanish

fluidisation
G Wirbelschichtverfahren
F fluidisation
S procedimiento de lecho fluidificado

fluidise, to
G verflüssigen
F liquéfier
S licuar, licuefacer

fluidity
G Rieselfähigkeit
F propriété d'écoulement
S capacidad de fluir

fluorescence
G Fluoreszenz
F fluorescence
S fluorescencia

fluorescent
G fluoreszierend
F fluorescent
S fluorescente

fluorination
G Fluorierung
F fluoruration
S fluoración

fluorometry
G Fluorometrie
F fluorométrie
S fluorometría

flush
G bündig
F lié
S enrasado

flush, to (with)
G durchströmen (mit)
F rincer (avec), purger
S inundar (con), purgar (con)

flushing
G Begasung
F fumigation
S fumigación

fluted filter
G Faltenfilter
F filtre nervuré, filtre cannelé
S filtro acanalado

fluted skirting
G Hohlkehlsockel
F plinthe à gorge arrondie
S rodapié en forma de garganta

foam
G Schaum
F mousse
S espuma

foam formation
G Schaumbildung
F formation de mousse, moussage, production de mousse
S formación de espuma

foam plastic
G Schaumstoff
F mousse en plastique
S espuma

foam spray
G Schaumspray
F aérosol pour mousse
S aerosol de espuma

foam, to
G schäumen
F mousser
S espumar

foaming
G Schaumbildung
F formation de mousse, moussage, production de mousse
S formación de espuma

foetal calf serum (FCS)
G fötales Kälberserum
F sérum de veau fœtal
S suero bovino fetal

fog
G Nebel
F brouillard
S niebla

foil
G Folie
F feuille
S hoja, lámina

fold
G Falte
F pli
S arruga, pliegue

fold, to
G falzen
F plier
S plegar

foldable
G abklappbar
F pouvant être rabattu, rabattable
S plegable

folding carton
G Faltschachtel
F boîte pliante
S caja plegable

folding carton sealing machine
G Faltschachtelverschließmaschine
F machine à sceller les boîtes pliantes
S máquina de cierre de cajas plegables

folding carton set-up machine
G Faltschachtelaufrichtmaschine
F plieuse pour boîtes pliantes
S máquina plegadora de cajas

folding machine
G Falzmaschine
F plieuse
S plegadora

folding station
G Falzstation
F station de pliage
S estación de plegado

food
G Lebensmittel
F aliment, nourriture
S alimento

food additive
G Nahrungsergänzungsmittel
F additif alimentaire
S aditivo alimentario

food grade
G lebensmittelecht
F qualité alimentaire
S calidad alimenticia

force
G Kraft
F force
S fuerza

force of attraction
G Anziehungskraft
F force d'attraction
S fuerza de atracción

forced-circulation mixer
G Zwangsmischer
F mélangeur à circulation forcée
S mezclador de circulación forzada

foreign body
G Fremdkörper
F corps étranger
S cuerpo extraño

foreman
G Vorarbeiter, Meister
F contremaître, maître
S capataz, maestro

fork-lift truck
G Gabelstapler
F chariot élévateur
S carretilla elevadora de horquilla

form
G Formular
F formulaire
S formulario

format
G Format
F taille, format
S formato, tamaño

forming foil
G Verformfolie
F feuille thermoformée
S lámina termoformada

formula
G Formel
F formule
S fórmula

formulation
G Formgebung, Formulierung, Galenik, Rezeptur, Zubereitung
F préparation, formulation
S fórmula galénica, formulación (galénica), preparación

controlled release formulation
G Formulierung mit kontrollierter Freisetzung
F formulation avec libération contrôlée
S formulación con liberación controlada

fraction
G Bruchstück, Fraktion
F fraction, fragment, morceau
S fracción, fragmento

fraction collector
G Fraktionssammler
F collecteur de fractions
S colector de fracciones

fractional sterilisation
G Tyndallisation
F tyndallisation
S tindalización

fractionate, to
G fraktionieren
F fractionner
S fraccionar

fracture line
G Bruchlinie
F ligne de rupture, ligne de fracture
S línea de ruptura, línea de fractura

fragile
G zerbrechlich
F fragile
S frágil

fragment
G Bruchstück
F morceau, fragment
S fragmento

fragment control
G Bruchstückkontrolle
F contrôle des fragments
S control de fragmentos

fragrance
G Duft
F odeur
S aroma, olor

frame
G Gestell
F support, cadre
S armazón, bastidor, soporte

free flowing
G freifließend
F fluide, s'écoulant librement
S fluyendo libremente

freeze dryer
G Gefriertrockner
F lyophilisateur
S liofilizador

freeze drying
G Gefriertrocknung, Lyophilisation
F lyophilisation
S liofilización

freeze-dried
G gefriergetrocknet
F lyophilisé
S liofilizado

freezer
G Gefrierschrank
F congélateur
S congelador

freezing point
G Eispunkt, Gefrierpunkt
F point de congélation
S punto de congelación

frequency
G Häufigkeit
F fréquence
S frecuencia

frequency distribution
G Häufigkeitsverteilung
F distribution de fréquences
S distribución de frecuencias

fresh air inlet
G Frischluftzufuhr
F arrivée d'air frais
S entrada de aire fresco

friability
G Abrieb
F abrasion
S abrasión

friction
G Reibung
F friction
S fricción, frotamiento

frictional force
G Reibungskraft
F force de friction, force de frottement
S fuerza de fricción

frictional resistance
G Abriebfestigkeit, Reibungswiderstand
F résistance à la friction, résistance au frottement
S resistencia a la abrasión, resistencia a la fricción

fronting (in HPLC)
G Frontbildung (HPLC)
F formation d'un front (HPLC)
S formación de frente (HPLC)

frozen storage
G Tiefkühllager
F stockage à très basse température
S almacén congelador

FTIR spectroscopy
G FTIR-Spektroskopie
F spectroscopie IR par transformation de Fourier
S espectroscopia infrarroja en transformación de Fourier

fulfilment
G Erfüllung
F réalisation
S cumplimiento, realización

fully automatic
G vollautomatisch
F entièrement automatique
S completamente automático

fume cupboard
G Abzug
F hotte à flux laminaire, hotte chimique
S escape, campana de extracción de gases

fumigant
G Begasungsmittel
F fumigant
S fumigante

fumigation
G Begasung, Raumbegasung
F fumigation
S fumigación

fuming acid
G rauchende Säure
F acide fumant
S ácido fumante

function keys
G Funktionstasten
F touche de fonctionnement
S botones de operación

function specification
G Funktionsspezifizierung
F spécification de fonctionnement
S especificación funcional

functionality
G Funktionsfähigkeit
F fonctionnalité
S capacidad funcional

fungi
G Pilze
F champignons
S hongos

fungicidal
G fungizid
F fongicide
S fungicida

fungicide
G Fungizid
F fongicide
S fungicida

fungus
G Schimmelpilz
F champignon
S moho

funnel
G Trichter, Schütt-Trichter
F entonnoir, trémie (d'alimentation)
S embudo, tolva

funnel opening
G Trichteröffnung
F ouverture d'un entonnoir, ouverture d'un trémie
S abertura del embudo

funnel, to
G eintrichtern
F remplir à l'aide d'un entonnoir
S llenar con embudo

furnace
G Schmelzofen
F four
S horno fundidor

fuse (electrical)
G Sicherung, Schütz (elektrisch)
F fusible, protection (électrique)
S cortacircuito, fusible, protección (eléctrica)

fuse box
G Sicherungskasten
F boîte de fusibles
S caja de fusibles

fuse, to
G einschmelzen
F fondre, faire fondre
S fundir

fused glass
G Sinterglas
F verre fritté
S vidrio sinterizado

fused glass particles
G Sinterglasteilchen
F particules de verre fritté
S partículas de vidrio sinterizado

fusion
G Zusammenschluß von Firmen
F fusion (d'entreprises)
S fusión de empresas

fusion point (of ampoules)
G Abschmelzhöhe (von Ampullen)
F point de fusion (d'ampoules)
S punto de fusión (de ampollas)

galenical development department
G Galenikabteilung
F département de développement galénique
S departamento de farmacia galénica

galvanised
G verzinkt
F galvanisé au zinc
S galvanizado con zinc

gamma rays
G Gammastrahlen
F rayons gamma
S rayos gamma

gargle
G Gurgellösung
F solution pour gargarisme
S solución para gargarismos

gas
G Gas
F gaz
S gas

pressure-dissolved gases
G unter Druck gelöste Gase
F gaz dissous sous pression
S gas diluido a presión

gas bubble
G Gasblase
F bulle de gaz
S burbuja de gas

gas chromatography
G Gaschromatographie
F chromatographie en phase gazeuse
S cromatografía de gases

gas cylinder
G Druckgasflasche, Gasflasche
F bouteille de gaz
S botella de gas a presión, botella de gas

gas flow
G Gasstrom
F débit de gaz
S corriente gaseosa

gas flow-through process
G Gasdurchströmungsverfahren
F procédé de circulation des gaz
S procedimiento de purga gaseosa

gas sterilisation
G Gassterilisation
F stérilisation au gaz
S esterilización por gas

gas supply
G Gaszufuhr
F alimentation en gaz
S alimentación de gas

gaseous
G gasförmig
F gazeux
S gaseoso

gaseous phase
G Gasphase
F phase gazeuse
S fase gaseosa

gasket
G Dichtung, Dichtungsscheibe
F joint (rondelle)
S junta, disco para cierre hermético

inflatable gasket
G aufblasbare Dichtung
F joint gonflable
S junta hinchable

gasket channel
G Dichtungsführung
F cannelure pour joint
S guía para la junta

gasket ring
G Dichtungsring
F joint torique en forme de rondelle
S arandela para junta hermética

gas-tight
G gasdicht
F étanche au gaz
S impermeable al gas

gastric duration
G Aufenthalt im Magen
F durée de résidence gastrique
S permanencia en el estómago

gastric fluid
G Magensaft
F suc gastrique
S jugo gástrico

English German French Spanish

gastric juice
G Magensaft
F suc gastrique
S jugo gástrico

gastric residence
G Aufenthalt im Magen
F durée de résidence gastrique
S permanencia en el estómago

gastro-enteral use
G gastrointestinale Anwendung
F utilisation gastro-intestinale
S aplicación gastrointestinal

gastro-resistant
G magensaftresistent
F résistant au suc gastrique
S resistente al jugo gástrico

gastro-resistant granules
G magensaftresistentes Granulat
F granules gastro-résistantes
S granulado resistente al jugo gástrico

gauge
G Meßlehre
F jauge
S galga, gálibo, calibre

gauze
G Mull, Tupfer
F gaze, tampon d'ouate
S gasa, torunda

gauze bandage
G Mullbinde
F bande de gaze
S venda de gasa

gear ratio
G Übersetzung (im Getriebe)
F transmission
S transmisión

gel
G Gel
F gel
S gel

gel chromatography
G Gelchromatographie
F chromatographie sur gel
S cromatografía sobre gel

gel filtration
G Gelfiltration
F filtration sur gel
S filtración por gel

gel formation
G Gelbildung
F formation de gel
S gelación

gel seal
G Gelverschluß
F fermeture pour gel
S cierre por gel

gel, to
G gelieren
F geler
S gelar

gelatine capsule
G Gelatinekapsel
F capsule de gélatine
S cápsula de gelatina

hard gelatine capsule
G Hartgelatinekapsel
F gélule
S cápsula de gelatina dura

soft gelatine capsule
G Weichgelatinekapsel
F gélule molle
S cápsula de gelatina blanda

gel-forming agent
G Gelbildner
F gélifiant
S gelificante

gellant
G Geliermittel
F gélifiant
S gelificante

gelling agent
G Geliermittel
F gélifiant
S gelificante

gene technology
G Gentechnologie
F génie génétique
S tecnología genética

general manager
G Geschäftsführer
F président directeur général (PDG)
S gerente

generation (of)
G Erzeugung
F engendrement, production
S generación, producción

generator
G Generator
F générateur
S generador

generic
G Genericum
F générique
S genérico

generic marketing authorisation
G Zulassung als Generikum
F autorisation de mise sur le marché comme médicament générique
S autorización como genérico

genetic engineering
G Genmanipulation
F manipulation génétique
S manipulación genética

genetically modified organisms (GMO)
G genetisch veränderte Organismen
F organismes génétiquement modifiés (OGM)
S organismos modificados genéticamente

genomic data
G Genomdaten
F données génomiques
S datos genómicos

genomics
G Genomlehre
F génomique
S teoría del genoma

German Hazardous Substance Act
G Deutsches Gefahrstoffgesetz
F législation allemande sur les substances dangereuses
S Ley Alemana de Sustancias Peligrosas

germination
G Auskeimung (von Sporen)
F germination
S germinación (de esporas)

ghost peak
G Geisterpeak
F pic fantôme
S pico fantasma

gingival use
G Anwendung am Zahnfleisch
F pour usage gingival
S uso gingival

glass ampoule
G Spießampulle
F ampoule de verre
S ampolla de vidrio

glass balloon
G Glasballon
F ballon de verre
S balón de vidrio

glass cuvette
G Glasküvette
F cuvette en verre
S cubeta de vidrio

glass electrode
G Glaselektrode
F électrode de verre
S electrodo de vidrio

English German French Spanish

glass particle
G Glaspartikel
F particule de verre
S partícula de vidrio

glass rod
G Glasstab
F baguette de verre
S barra de vidrio, bastón de vidrio

glass sinter
G Glassinter
F fritte de verre
S sínter de vidrio

glass splinters
G Glassplitter
F éclats de verre
S añicos de vidrio

glass tube
G Glasröhrchen
F tube de verre
S tubo (de ensayo) de vidrio

glass type
G Glasart
F type de verre
S tipo de vidrio

glass vial
G Glasfläschchen
F flacon en verre, fiole en verre
S vial de vidrio

glassware
G Glasgeräte
F verrerie
S instrumental de vidrio

gloss
G Glanz
F lustre, brillance
S brillo, lustre

glossy
G glänzend
F brillant, lustré
S brillante, lustrado

glove box
G Isolator
F isolateur
S aislante

gloves
G Handschuhe
F gants
S guante

glue
G Kleber, Leim
F colle
S cola, sustancia adhesiva

glue, to
G leimen, kleben
F coller
S encolar, pegar

GMP compliance
G GMP-Entsprechung
F conformité aux bonnes pratiques de fabrication
S conformidad con GMP

GMP guidelines
G GMP-Richtlinien
F règles GMP
S directrices de GMP

implementation of GMP guidelines
G Umsetzung von GMP-Richtlinien
F mise en pratique des règles GMP
S puesta en práctica de directices de GMP

observance of GMP guidelines
G Befolgung von GMP-Richtlinien
F respect des règles GMP
S observancia de directrices de GMP

GMP-conform
G GMP-gerecht
F conforme aux bonnes pratiques de fabrication
S conforme a GMP

GMP-controlled laboratory
G GMP-Labor
F laboratoire conforme aux GMP
S laboratorio controlado para GMP

Good Clinical Practice (GCP)
G Gute Klinische Praxis
F bonnes pratiques cliniques (GCP)
S Prácticas Clínicas Correctas (GCP)

Good Laboratory Practice (GLP)
G Gute Laborpraxis (GLP)
F bonnes pratiques de laboratoire (GLP)
S Prácticas Correctas de Laboratorio (GLP)

Good Manufacturing Practice (GMP)
G Gute Herstellungspraxis (GMP)
F bonnes pratiques de fabrication (GMP)
S Prácticas Correctas de Fabricación (GMP)

gown
G Kittel, Laborkittel
F blouse de laboratoire
S bata, bata de laboratorio

gowning procedure
G Bekleidungsvorschrift
F règles vestimentaires, instructions vestimentaires
S prescripción de vestuario

gowning room
G Ankleideraum
F vestiaire
S vestuario

grade
G Einstufung
F classification
S clasificación

grade of gloss
G Glanzgrad
F degré de lustre
S grado de brillantez

grade of lustre
G Glanzgrad
F degré de lustre
S grado de brillantez

grade, to
G einstufen
F classifier
S clasificar

gradient
G Gefälle, Gradient, Neigung
F gradient, inclinaison, pente
S declive, gradiente, inclinación, pendiente

gradient pump
G Gradientenpumpe
F pompe à gradient
S bomba de gradiente

graduate (with doctorate), PhD
G promoviert
F titulaire d'un doctorat
S doctorado

graduated
G graduiert
F gradué
S graduado

graduated measuring cylinder
G graduierter Meßzylinder
F éprouvette graduée
S probeta graduada

graduated plan
G Stufenplan
F plan échelonné
S plan escalonado, plan graduado

graduation
G Skaleneinteilung
F graduation
S graduación de una escala

graduation mark
G Strichmarkierung, Teilstrich
F marque de graduation
S marca de graduación

grain
G Körnung
F granulation
S granulación

fine grain
G feine Körnung
F granulation fine
S granulación fina

Gram staining
G Gramfärbung
F méthode de coloration de Gram
S tinción de Gram

Gram-negative
G Gram-negativ
F Gram-négatif
S Gram negativo

Gram-positive
G Gram-positiv
F Gram-positif
S Gram positivo

granular
G körnig
F granulaire
S granular

granulate
G Granulat
F granulé
S granulado

granulate, to
G granulieren
F granuler
S granular

granulating fluid
G Granulierflüssigkeit
F liquide de granulation
S líquido de granulación

granulating process
G Granulierverfahren
F procédé de granulation
S procedimiento de granulación

granulation performance
G Granulationsleistung
F rendement de transformation en granulé
S rendimiento de granulación

granule
G Granulatkorn
F granule
S gránulo

granuloma formation
G Bildung eines Granuloms
F formation d'un granulome
S formación de un granuloma

graph
G grafische Darstellung
F graphe
S representación gráfica

grating
G Gitter, Gitterrost
F grille
S retícula

gravel filter
G Kiesbettfilter
F filtre de graviers
S filtro de grava

gravimetric analysis
G Gewichtsanalyse
F analyse du poids
S análisis del peso

gravity
G Schwerkraft
F force de gravité
S fuerza de gravedad

gravity feed
G Zufuhr durch Gefälle
F alimentation par gravité
S alimentación por gravedad

grease
G Schmierfett
F graisse
S grasa lubri(fi)cante

grease, to
G einfetten, schmieren
F graisser, lubrifier
S engrasar, lubri(fi)car

grid
G Netz
F grille
S red

grind, to
G mahlen, pulverisieren, zerstoßen
F broyer, concasser, piler, pulvériser
S machacar, moler, pulverizar, triturar

grinding
G Vermahlung
F moulage
S molienda, molturado

grip
G Bügel, Griff
F prise, poignée
S asa, estribo, empuñadura, mango

groove
G Nut, Rille
F cannelure, rainure, sillon
S acanaladura, estría, muesca, ranura

gross margin
G Bruttomarge
F marge brute
S margen bruto

ground
G Ableitung, Erdung, geschliffen
F mise à la terre, prise de terre, moulu, poli
S derivación, toma de tierra, bruñido, pulido, tallado

ground glass
G Glasschliff
F polissage de verre
S pulido del vidrio

ground stopper
G Schliffstopfen
F bouchon rodé
S tapón esmerilado

ground, to
G erden
F mettre à la terre
S conectar a tierra

grounding
G Erdung
F mise la terre, prise de terre
S toma de tierra

ground-joint flask
G Schliffkolben
F ballon rodé
S matraz esmerilado

group manager
G Gruppenleiter
F chef de département
S director de grupo

growth defect
G Wachstumsdefekt
F défaut de croissance
S defecto de crecimiento

growth factors
G Wachstumsfaktoren
F facteurs de croissance
S factores de crecimiento

growth promotion
G Wachstumsförderung
F promotion de la croissance
S estimulación del crecimiento

guarantee
G Garantie
F garantie
S garantía

guarantee, to
G sicherstellen
F assurer, garantir
S asegurar, garantizar

guide
G Führungsvorrichtung
F guide, dispositif de guidage, mécanisme de guidage
S dispositivo de guía, guía

guide rollers
G Führungsrollen
F rouleaux de guidage
S poleas de guía

guide, to
G leiten
F diriger
S conducir, dirigir

guideline
G Leitlinie, Richtlinie
F directive
S directiva, directriz

cross-functional guideline
G abteilungsübergreifende Richtlinie
F lignes directrices générales
S directriz general

guiding device
G Führungsvorrichtung
F guide, dispositif de guidage, mécanisme de guidage
S dispositivo de guía, guía

guiding mechanism
G Führungsvorrichtung
F guide, dispositif de guidage, mécanisme de guidage
S dispositivo de guía, guía

gum, to
G gummieren
F gommer
S engomar, impermeabilizar

gutter
G Rinne
F gouttière
S canal, reguera, surco

hair hygrometer
G Haarhygrometer
F hygromètre à cheveux
S higrómetro capilar

hairline crack
G Haarriß
F fissure capillaire
S fisura capilar

half-life
G Halbwertszeit
F demi-vie
S tiempo de vida media

halogen exchange
G Halogenaustausch
F échange d'halogène
S intercambio de halógenos

halogenated compounds
G halogenierte Verbindungen
F substances halogènes
S compuestos halogenados

halogenation
G Halogenierung
F halogénation
S halogenación

halogen-containing organic solvents
G halogenhaltige organische Lösungsmittel
F solvants organiques halogènes
S diluyentes orgánicos halogenados

halogen-free organic solvents
G halogenfreie organische Lösungsmittel
F solvants organiques non halogènes
S diluyentes orgánicos no halogenados

hammer mill
G Hammermühle
F broyeur à marteau
S molino triturador

hand disinfection
G Händedesinfektion
F désinfection des mains
S desinfección de manos

hand press
G Handpresse
F presse manuelle
S prensa manual

hand wash facility
G Handwaschgelegenheit
F possibilité de lavage des mains
S posibilidad de lavar las manos

handle
G Bügel, Griff
F prise, poignée
S asa, estribo, empuñadura, mango

handling (of)
G Handhabung, Umgang (mit)
F maniement, traitement
S manejo, tratamiento, trato (con)

hand-operated
G von Hand
F manuel
S manual

hard capsule
G Steckkapsel
F gélule
S cápsula gelatinosa dura

hard copy
G Papierausdruck
F imprimé sur papier
S impreso (en papel, sobre papel)

hard gelatine capsule
G Hartgelatinekapsel
F gélule
S cápsula de gelatina dura

hard hat
G Schutzhelm
F casque de protection
S casco protector

hard rubber
G Hartgummi
F caoutchouc durci, ébonite
S ebonita

hardening
G Härten
F durcissage
S endurecimiento

hardness
G Härte
F dureté
S dureza

hardness tester
G Härtetester
F machine à tester la dureté
S máquina de comprobación de dureza

hard-wearing
G trittsicher
F sûr à la marche
S de paso seguro

harmful
G gesundheitsschädlich, schädlich, umweltverschmutzend
F dangereux, nocif, polluant
S dañino, nocivo, perjudicial, polucionante

harmful by inhalation
G gesundheitsschädlich bei Inhalation
F dangereux pour la santé si inhalé
S perjudicial para la salud si se inhala

harmful if swallowed
G gesundheitsschädlich beim Verschlucken
F dangereux pour la santé si ingéré
S perjudicial para la salud si se ingiere

harmful in contact with skin
G gesundheitsschädlich bei Hautkontakt
F dangereux pour la santé lors d'un contact cutané
S perjudicial para la salud si entra en contacto con la piel

harmful agent
G schädliches Mittel
F agent nocif
S agente nocivo

harmless products
G unschädliche Mittel
F produits inoffensifs
S productos inocuos

harvest, to
G ernten
F récolter
S cosechar

hatch
G Durchreiche
F porte coupée
S postigo

hazard class
G Gefahrenklasse
F classe de dangers
S clase de peligro

hazard indication
G Gefahrenhinweis
F mise en garde
S aviso de peligro

causes (severe) burns
G verursacht (schwere) Verbrennungen
F peut provoquer de (sévères) brûlures
S causa (graves) quemaduras

irritating to eyes
G reizt die Augen
F peut provoquer des irritations aux yeux
S irrita los ojos

irritating to respiratory system
G reizt die Atemwege
F peut irriter le système respiratoire
S irrita las vías respiratorias

may cause cancer
G kann Krebs erzeugen
F peut provoquer un cancer
S puede causar cáncer

may cause cancer by inhalation
G kann beim Einatmen Krebs erzeugen
F cancéreux si inhalé
S cancerógeno si se inhala

may cause harm to unborn child
G gefährdet ungeborene Kinder
F dangereux pour les enfants pendant une grossesse
S peligroso para el feto

may cause heritable genetic damage
G kann vererbliche Genschäden verursachen
F peut être la cause de dommages génétiques héréditaires
S puede originar daños genéticos hereditarios

may impair fertility
G kann die Fruchtbarkeit beeinträchtigen
F peut altérer la fertilité
S puede dañar la fertilidad

toxic by inhalation
G giftig beim Einatmen
F toxique si inhalé
S tóxico si se inhala

toxic if swallowed
G giftig beim Verschlucken
F toxique si ingéré
S tóxico si se ingiere

toxic in contact with skin
G giftig bei Hautkontakt
F toxique au contact de la peau
S tóxico para la piel

hazard potential
G Gefahrenpotential
F potentiel de danger
S potencial de riesgos

hazard symbol
G Gefahrensymbol
F symbole de danger
S símbolo de peligro

hazardous
G gefährlich, schädlich
F dangereux, nocif
S dañino, nocivo, peligroso

hazardous material
G Gefahrstoff
F matériel dangereux
S sustancia peligrosa

head (person)
G Leiter
F directeur
S director

head covering
G Kopfbedeckung, Kopfhaube
F bonnet
S capucha, cofia, sombrero

head of department
G Abteilungsleiter
F chef de département, chef de service
S director de departamento

head of engineering department
G Technischer Leiter
F directeur du département d'ingénierie
S director del departamento técnico

head of production
G Herstellungsleiter
F directeur de production
S director de producción

head of quality control
G Kontrolleiter
F responsable du contrôle-qualité
S director de control

head space
G Kopfraum, Gasraum
F espace de tête
S espacio para la cabeza

headgear
G Kopfbedeckung
F bonnet
S sombrero

health care
G Gesundheitswesen
F système de santé
S sistema sanitario

health care products
G Gesundheitsprodukte
F produits d'hygiène grand public
S productos para la salud

health check, periodic
G regelmäßige Gesundheitsuntersuchung
F visite médicale périodique
S inspección médica periódica

health risk
G Gesundheitsrisiko
F risque pour la santé
S riesgo para la salud

healthy volunteer
G gesunder Freiwilliger
F volontaire sain
S voluntario sano

heat
G Wärme
F chaleur
S calor

heat distribution
G Hitzeverteilung, Temperaturverteilung, Wärmeverteilung
F distribution de chaleur, répartition de la température
S distribución de calor, distribución de temperatura

heat exchanger
G Wärmetauscher
F échangeur de chaleur
S intercambiador de calor

heat flow calorimeter
G Wärmeflußkalorimeter
F calorimètre à flux de chaleur
S calorímetro de flujo de calor

heat insulation
G Wärmeisolierung
F isolation thermique
S aislamiento térmico

heat loss
G Wärmeverlust
F déperdition de chaleur
S pérdida calórica

heat of evaporation
G Verdampfungswärme
F chaleur d'évaporation
S calor de evaporación

heat of reaction
G Reaktionswärme
F chaleur due à la réaction
S calor de reacción

heat penetration test
G Hitzedurchdringungstest
F essai de pénétration thermique
S prueba de penetración térmica

English German French Spanish

heat recovery
G Wärmerückgewinnung
F récupération de la chaleur
S recuperación de calor

heat seal, to
G heißsiegeln
F thermosceller
S sellar al calor

heat sensor
G Thermofühler
F sonde thermique
S sonda térmica

heat sterilisation
G Hitzesterilisation
F stérilisation à la chaleur
S esterilización al calor

heat transfer
G Wärmeübertragung
F transfert de chaleur
S transferencia térmica

heat treatment
G Wärmebehandlung
F traitement thermique
S tratamiento térmico

heat, to
G beheizen
F chauffer
S caldear

heated storage
G Heißlagerung
F stockage thermique
S almacenamiento caliente

heating
G Erwärmung
F réchauffement
S calentamiento

heating aggregate
G Heizaggregat
F appareil de chauffage
S aparato de calefacción

heating coil
G Aufheizspirale, Heizschlange
F serpentin chauffant
S serpentín de calentamiento, serpentín de calefacción

heating element
G Heizelement
F élément chauffant
S elemento calefactor

heating jaw
G Heizbacke
F mâchoire chauffante
S mordaza de calefacción

heating mantle
G Heizpilz
F manteau chauffant
S manguito de caldeo

heating source
G Heizquelle
F source de chauffage, source de chaleur
S fuente de calor

heat-labile
G hitzelabil
F sensible à la chaleur
S lábil al calor

heat-resistant
G hitzebeständig
F résistant à la chaleur
S resistente al calor

heat-sealing adhesive
G Heißsiegelkleber
F adhésif thermofusible
S adhesivo termofusible

heat-sealing lacquer
G Heißsiegellack
F laque thermofusible
S laca termofusible

heat-sensitive
G hitzeempfindlich
F sensible à la chaleur
S sensible al calor

heat-stable
G hitzestabil
F stable à la chaleur
S estable al calor

heat-transmitting oil
G wärmeübertragendes Öl
F huile conductrice de chaleur
S aceite transmisor de calor

heat-up time
G Aufheizzeit
F temps de réchauffement
S tiempo de calentamiento

heavy metal
G Schwermetall
F métal lourd
S metal pesado

height
G Höhe
F hauteur
S altura

height-adjustable
G höhenverstellbar
F à hauteur ajustable
S de altura regulable

HEPA filters (high efficiency particulate air)
G HEPA-Filter
F filtres HEPA
S filtro HEPA

herbal medicines
G Phytopharmaka, pflanzliche Arzneimittel
F phytopharmaceutiques
S fitofármacos

herbicide
G Unkrautvernichtungsmittel
F herbicide
S herbicida

hermetic seal
G hermetischer Verschluß
F fermeture hermétique
S cierre hermético

heterocyclic
G heterozyklisch
F hétérocyclique
S heterocíclico

heteroploid cell culture
G heteroploide Zellkultur
F culture de cellules hétéroploïde
S cultivo celular heteroploide

hiding power
G Deckkraft
F propriété couvrante
S capacidad de cubrir

high efficiency particulate air (HEPA) filter
G Hochleistungsschwebstoffilter
F filtre antipoussières à haute performance
S filtro antipolvo de gran rendimiento

high performance
G Hochleistungs-
F haute performance
S gran rendimiento

high pressure liquid chromatography (HPLC)
G Hochdruckflüssigkeitschromatographie
F chromatographie liquide sous haute pression
S cromatografía líquida a alta presión

high purity water
G Reinstwasser
F eau de haute pureté
S agua ultrapurificada

high shear mixer
G Pflugscharmischer
F mélangeur à forces de cisaillement
S mezclador de cizallamiento intenso

English
German
French
Spanish

high speed blender
G Pflugscharmischer
F mélangeur à forces de cisaillement
S mezclador de cizallamiento

high-bay storage
G Hochregallager
F étagère de stockage
S almacén de estanterías altas

highly dosed
G hoch dosiert
F à haute dose
S altamente dosificado

highly effective
G hochwirksam
F très efficace
S muy eficaz

highly infectious material
G hochinfektiöses Material
F matière hautement infectieuse
S material muy infeccioso

highly polished
G hochglanzpoliert
F poli-miroir
S muy pulido

highly potent
G hochwirksam
F très efficace
S muy eficaz

high-resolution
G hochauflösend
F haute-résolution
S de alta resolución

high-speed press
G Hochleistungspresse
F presse rapide
S prensa rápida

high-speed tabletting press
G Hochgeschwindigkeitstablettenpresse
F presse à comprimés haute vitesse
S prensa de alta velocidad

hinged
G schwenkbar
F pivotable
S giratorio

hob
G Prägestempel
F poinçon
S cuño, troquel

holding tank
G Lagertank
F récipient de stockage, cuve de stockage
S tanque depósito

hollow
G hohl
F creux
S hueco

hollow article
G Hohlkörper
F corps creux
S cuerpo hueco

hollow body
G Hohlkörper
F corps creux
S cuerpo hueco

hollow space
G Hohlraum
F cavité, espace creux
S cavidad, espacio hueco

homeopathic products
G homöopathische Erzeugnisse
F produits homéopathiques
S productos homeopáticos

homogeneity
G Homogenität
F homogénéité
S homogeneidad

homogeneous
G homogen
F homogène
S homogéneo

homogenise, to
G homogenisieren, zerkleinern
F homogénéiser, hacher
S homogenizar, triturar

homogeniser
G Homogenisator, Zerkleinerer
F homogénéiseur, hachoir
S homogenizador, trituradora

homologous
G homolog
F homologue
S homólogo

hood
G Haube, Abdeckung
F couvercle, capuchon
S casquete, cubierta, sombrerete

hopper
G Trichter, Fülltrichter, Schütt-Trichter
F entonnoir, trémie, entonnoir d'alimentation, trémie d'alimentation
S embudo, embudo de llenado, tolva

horizontal
G waagerecht
F horizontal
S horizontal

horizontal electrophoresis
G Horizontalelektrophorese
F électrophorèse horizontale
S electroforesis horizontal

hospital pack
G Anstaltspackung, Klinikpackung
F emballage pour hôpitaux, conditionnement pour hôpitaux
S envase clínico, embalaje para clínica

hot air oven
G Heißluftofen
F four à air chaud
S horno de aire caliente

hot air steriliser
G Heißluftsterilisator
F stérilisateur à air chaud
S esterilizador de aire caliente

hot water spraying
G Heißwasserberieselung
F aspersion d'eau chaude
S rociado con agua caliente

hot-wire anemometer
G Hitzedrahtanemometer
F anémomètre à résistance électrique
S anemómetro de resistencia eléctrica

housing
G Gehäuse
F boîtier
S caja, estuche

HPLC pump
G HPLC-Pumpe
F pompe HPLC
S bomba de HPLC

hue
G Farbton
F teinte, nuance d'une couleur
S matiz del color

humidification
G Befeuchtung
F humidification
S humectación, humidificación

humidifier
G Befeuchter, Luftbefeuchter
F humidificateur
S humidificador de aire

humidify, to
G befeuchten
F humidifier
S humectar, humedecer

humidise, to
G anfeuchten
F humidifier
S humectar, humedecer

English German French Spanish

humidity
G Feuchtigkeit, Luftfeuchtigkeit
F humidité
S humedad, humedad del aire

bound moisture
G gebundene Feuchtigkeit
F humidité adhérente
S humedad adherente

unbound moisture
G nicht gebundene Feuchtigkeit
F humidité non liée
S humedad no adherente

humidity detector
G Feuchtesensor
F détecteur d'humidité
S detector de humedad

hydrate
G Hydrat
F hydrate
S hidrato

hydrocarbon
G Kohlenwasserstoff
F composé hydrocarboné
S hidrocarburo

hydrochloric acid
G Salzsäure
F acide chlorhydrique
S ácido clorhídrico

hydrogen
G Wasserstoff
F hydrogène
S hidrógeno

hydrogen bond
G Wasserstoffbrückenbindung
F liaison hydrogène
S puente de hidrógeno

hydrogen peroxide
G Wasserstoffperoxid
F eau oxygénée, peroxide d'hydrogène
S peróxido de hidrógeno

hydrogenation
G Hydrogenierung
F hydrogénation
S hidrogenación

hydrolysis
G Hydrolyse
F hydrolyse
S hidrólisis

hydrolytic grade
G hydrolytischer Grad
F degré hydrolytique
S grado hidrolítico

hydrophilic
G hydrophil
F hydrophile
S hidrófilo

hydrophobic
G hydrophob, wasserabweisend
F hydrophobe
S hidrófobo, hidrófugo

hydroxyl number
G Hydroxylzahl
F indice d'hydroxyle
S índice hidroxílico

hygienic area
G Hygienezone
F zone d'hygiène
S área higiénica

hygrometer
G Feuchtemesser, Feuchtigkeitsmesser, Hygrometer
F hygromètre
S higrómetro

hygroscopic
G hygroskopisch, wasseranziehend
F hygroscopique
S higroscópico, hidrófilo

hygroscopicity
G Hygroskopizität
F hygroscopie
S higroscopicidad

hypertonic
G hypertonisch
F hypertonique
S hipertónico

hypotonic
G hypotonisch
F hypotonique
S hipotónico

ice water
G Eiswasser
F eau glacée
S agua helada

identification
G Identifikation
F identification
S identificación

identity
G Identität
F identité
S identidad

identity test
G Identitätsprüfung
F test d'identité
S prueba de identidad

ignitable
G entzündbar
F inflammable
S inflamable

ignite, to
G ausglühen
F faire rougir, se calciner
S calcinar

ignition
G Zündung
F inflammation
S encendido, ignición

ignition source
G Zündquelle
F source d'inflammation
S fuente de ignición

illumination
G Beleuchtung
F éclairage
S iluminación

immerse, to
G eintauchen, untertauchen
F immerger
S sumergir, sumergirse

immersed heating coil
G untergetauchte Heizschlange
F serpentin chauffant immergé
S serpentín de calefacción sumergido

immersion bath
G Tauchbad
F bain d'immersion
S baño de sumersión

immersion depth
G Eintauchtiefe
F profondeur d'immersion
S profundidad de inmersión

immersion heater
G Tauchsieder
F chauffe-liquide
S calentador de inmersión

immersion lacquer
G Tauchlack
F laque par immersion
S barniz de inmersión

immersion period
G Eintauchzeit
F période d'immersion
S tiempo de inmersión

immersion sword
G Tauchschwert
F lame d'immersion
S lámina de inmersión

immersion, by
G im Tauchverfahren
F procédé par immersion
S en procedimiento de inmersión

English German French Spanish

immiscible
G nicht mischbar
F non miscible
S no miscible

immune electrophoresis
G Immunelektrophorese
F immunoélectrophorèse
S inmunoelectroforesis

immunological
G immunologisch
F immunologique
S inmunológico

impact
G Schlag, Stoß
F impact, coup, choc
S choque, golpe, impacto

impact force
G Schlagkraft
F force de frappe, force d'impact
S fuerza impactante, fuerza de percusión

impact protection
G Stoßschutz
F protection anti-chocs
S protección frente a la colisión

impact resistance
G Schlagfestigkeit
F résistance au choc
S resistencia a los choques

impact-resistant
G stoßfest
F résistant aux chocs
S resistente a los golpes

impairment
G Beeinträchtigung
F préjudice, dommage
S merma, perjuicio

impeller
G Laufrad, Flügelrad
F ailette
S rueda portante, rueda de aletas

impeller speed
G Antriebsgeschwindigkeit, Laufradgeschwindigkeit
F vitesse de roulement, vitesse de transmission
S velocidad de propulsión, velocidad de rodamiento, velocidad de revolución

impermeability
G Undurchlässigkeit
F imperméabilité
S impermeabilidad

impermeable
G undurchlässig
F imperméable
S impermeable

impermeable to air
G luftundurchlässig
F imperméable à l'air
S impermeable al aire

impervious
G undurchlässig
F imperméable
S impermeable

impervious to moisture
G feuchtigkeitsundurchlässig
F étanche
S impermeable a la humedad

imperviousness
G Undurchlässigkeit
F imperméabilité
S impermeabilidad

implant
G Implantat
F implant
S implantado

implanter
G Implantatinjektor
F injecteur d'implant
S inyector de implantados

implement, to
G implementieren
F implémenter, établir
S establecer, realizar

import licence
G Einfuhrerlaubnis
F license d'importation
S licencia de importación

impregnate, to
G imprägnieren, tränken
F imprégner
S impregnar, empapar, embeber

imprint
G Aufdruck
F impression
S impresión

imprint, to
G aufdrucken, aufprägen, einprägen
F imprimer, empreindre
S estampar, imprimir

improve, to
G verbessern
F améliorer
S mejorar

impurity
G Verunreinigung
F impureté, contamination
S contaminación, impureza

reducing impurity
G reduzierende Verunreinigung
F pollution réductrice
S impureza reductora

trace impurity
G Verunreinigung in Spuren
F impureté à l'état de traces
S impureza vestigial

impurity profile
G Verunreinigungsprofil
F profil d'impuretés
S perfil de impurezas

inaccessible
G unzugänglich
F inaccessible
S inaccesible

inaccessible points
G unzugängliche Stellen
F endroits inaccessibles
S lugares inaccesibles

inactivated
G inaktiviert
F inactivées
S inactivado

inactivating substance (for disinfectant)
G Enthemmer (zur Inaktivierung von Desinfektionsmitteln)
F substance neutralisante
S sustancia neutralizante (para inactivar desinfectantes)

inactivation
G Inaktivierung
F inactivation
S inactivación

inactivation agent
G Inaktivierungsmittel
F agent d'inactivation
S agente inactivador

inactivation vessel
G Inaktivierungsgefäß
F récipient servant à l'inactivation
S recipiente de inactivación

inactive raw material
G inaktiver Rohstoff
F matière première inactive
S materia prima inactiva

inadvertent use
G versehentlicher Gebrauch
F utilisation par inadvertance
S uso por inadvertencia

incident
G Vorfall, Zwischenfall
F incident
S incidente

incineration
G Verbrennung
F combustion, incinération
S combustión, incineración

incinerator
G Verbrennungsanlage
F incinérateur
S crematorio

inclined plane
G schiefe Ebene
F plan incliné
S plano inclinado

inclusion
G Einschluß
F inclusion
S inclusión

inclusion crystallisation
G Einschlußkristallisation
F cristallisation occlusive
S cristalización de inclusión

incoming goods
G angelieferte Materialien
F marchandises receptionnées
S materiales suministrados

incompatibility
G Inkompatibilität, Unverträglichkeit
F incompatibilité
S incompatibilidad, intolerancia

incompatible
G inkompatibel
F incompatible
S incompatible

incomplete
G unvollständig
F incomplet
S incompleto

incubate, to
G bebrüten, inkubieren
F incuber
S incubar

incubation room
G Inkubationsraum
F chambre d'incubation
S cámara de incubación

incubation time
G Bebrütungszeit
F temps d'incubation
S tiempo de incubación

incubator
G Brutschrank, Wärmeschrank
F incubateur
S incubadora

indelible
G unauslöschbar
F indélébile
S indeleble

index
G Verzeichnis
F répertoire, registre
S índice

indicate, to
G anzeigen
F indiquer, afficher
S indicar, mostrar

indicator
G Indikator
F indicateur
S indicador

indicator organism
G Indikatorkeim
F organisme indicateur
S germen indicador

individual characteristic
G Einzelmerkmal
F caractéristique individuelle
S característica individual

individual weight
G Einzelgewicht
F poids individuel
S peso individual

industrial scale manufacture
G Herstellung im industriellen Maßstab
F fabrication à l'échelle industrielle
S fabricación a escala industrial

inert
G inert
F inerte
S inerte

inert gas
G Edelgas, Schutzgas
F gaz inerte, gaz rare
S gas inerte, gas noble

inert gas packaging
G Schutzgasverpackung
F emballage avec gaz inerte
S embalaje con gas inerte

inert gas purging
G Inertbegasung
F purge au gaz rare
S purga con gases inertes

infectious
G infektiös
F infectieux
S infeccioso

infectious disease
G ansteckende Krankheit
F maladie infectieuse
S enfermedad contagiosa

inferior
G minderwertig
F de mauvaise qualité
S de menor calidad

inflammability class
G Brandklasse
F classe d'inflammables
S clase inflamable

inflammable
G entzündbar
F inflammable
S inflamable

inflammatory reaction
G Entzündungsreaktion
F réaction inflammatoire
S reacción inflamatoria

inflatable
G aufblasbar
F gonflable
S hinchable

inflatable silicone seal
G aufblasbare Silikondichtung
F joint de silicone gonflable
S cierre inflable de silicona

infrared radiation
G Infrarotstrahlung
F rayonnement infrarouge
S radiación infrarroja

infringement
G Verletzung
F contrefaire un brevet
S lesión (herida), infracción

infusion
G Aufguß, Infus
F infusion
S infusión

infusion assembly
G Infusionsbesteck
F nécessaire pour infusion
S instrumental de infusión

infusion solution
G Infusionslösung
F solution de perfusion
S solución de infusión

ingredient
G Bestandteil
F composant, constituant, ingrédient
S componente, ingrediente

inhalation
G Inhalation
F inhalation
S inhalación

inherent uncertainty (e. g. of a technique)
G inhärente Ungenauigkeit (z. B. einer Technik)
F imprécision inhérente (par ex. d'une technologie)
S inexactitud inherente (p. ej. de una técnica)

English German French Spanish

inhibition
G Hemmung
F inhibition
S inhibición

inhibitor
G Hemmstoff
F inhibiteur
S inhibidor

initial speed
G Anfangsgeschwindigkeit
F vitesse initiale
S velocidad inicial

initial weight
G Einwaage
F poids initial
S peso inicial

initials
G Namenszeichen
F initiales
S iniciales

initiation (of a reaction)
G Initiierung (einer Reaktion)
F initiation (d'une réaction)
S iniciación (de una reacción)

inject, to
G injizieren
F injecter
S inyectar

injectible
G injizierbar
F injectable
S inyectable

injection
G Einspritzung
F injection
S inyección

injection block
G Einspritzblock
F bloc d'injection
S bloque de inyección

injection needle
G Injektionsnadel, Kanüle
F aiguille pour injection, canule
S aguja de inyección, cánula

injection port
G Einspritzdüse
F buse d'injection
S inyector

injection solution
G Injektionslösung
F solution injectable
S solución inyectable

injection syringe
G Injektionsspritze
F seringue d'injection
S jeringuilla

injection tip
G Injektionsspitze
F pointe d'injection
S punta de jeringa

injection valve
G Einspritzventil
F vanne d'injection
S válvula de inyección

injection vial
G Injektionsflasche
F flacon d'injection
S vial de inyección

injection volume
G Einspritzvolumen
F volume d'injection
S volumen de inyección

injection-moulded component
G Spritzgußteil
F composant moulé par injection
S componente moldeado por inyección

injector, automatic
G automatischer Injektor
F injecteur automatique
S inyector automático

ink
G Tinte
F encre
S tinta

ink jet printer
G Tintenstrahldrucker
F imprimante à jet d'encre
S impresora de chorro de tinta

inlet
G Einfluß
F orifice d'entrée de liquide
S orificio de entrada de líquido

inlet air
G Zuluft
F entrée d'air
S entrada de aire

inlet filter
G Eingangsfilter, Einlaßfilter
F filtre d'entrée, filtre d'admission
S filtro de entrada

inlet temperature
G Eingangstemperatur, Einlaßtemperatur
F température d'entrée, température d'admission
S temperatura de entrada

inlet valve
G Einlaßventil
F vanne d'entrée
S válvula de entrada

innovative
G innovativ
F innovant
S innovador

inoculate, to
G beimpfen (mit Keimen)
F ensemencer, inoculer
S inocular, sembrar

inoculating loop
G Impföse
F œillet d'inoculation
S ojal de inoculación

inoculation
G Inokulation, Beimpfung
F inoculation
S inoculación, siembra

inorganic
G anorganisch
F anorganique
S anorgánico

in-process control (IPC)
G In-Prozeß-Kontrolle
F contrôle lors de la fabrication
S control durante el proceso

insect infestation
G Insektenbefall
F invasion d'insectes
S infestación con insectos

insect trap
G Insektenfalle
F piège à insectes
S trampa de insectos

insecticide
G Insektizid, insektizid
F insecticide
S insecticida

insert
G Beilage
F annexe
S anexo

in-situ
G in-situ
F in situ
S in situ

in-situ sterilisation
G In-situ-Dämpfen
F stérilisation in situ
S esterilización in situ

insoluble
G unlöslich
F insoluble
S insoluble

English German French Spanish

inspected
G geprüft
F contrôlé, inspecté, vérifié
S comprobado

inspection
G Inspektion
F inspection
S inspección

inspection of incoming goods
G Wareneingangsprüfung
F contrôle des livraisons de marchandises
S control de entrada de mercancías

inspectorate
G Inspektorat
F inspection (entité admin.)
S inspectoría

install, to
G einbauen
F installer
S instalar, montar

installation
G Einbau, Installation
F installation, montage
S instalación, montaje

installation costs
G Installationskosten
F coûts d'une installation
S costes de instalación

installation location
G Aufstellungsort
F lieu d'installation
S lugar de instalación

installation qualification
G Installationsqualifizierung
F qualification de l'installation
S cualificación de una instalación

installation scheme
G R+I-Schema
F schéma de l'installation, des canalisations et diagrammes des instruments
S esquema de instalación, de canalización y diagramas de instrumentos

instant coupling
G Schnellkupplung
F connexion instantanée
S conexión rápida

instant melting point
G Sofortschmelzpunkt
F point de fusion instantané
S punto de fusión instantánea

instruction
G Anweisung, Arbeitsvorschrift, Vorschrift
F instruction, mode d'emploi, procédure opératoire, spécification
S instrucción, norma de trabajo, prescripción

instruction manual
G Handbuch
F manuel (d'utilisation)
S manual de instrucciones

instructions for use
G Gebrauchsanweisung
F instructions pour l'utilisation
S instrucción de uso

instrument accessories
G Gerätezubehör
F accessoires d'un équipement
S accesorios del aparato

instrument calibration
G Gerätekalibrierung
F calibration de l'équipement
S calibración de aparatos

instrument configuration
G Gerätekonfiguration
F configuration de l'instrument
S configuración de aparatos

instrument disinfection
G Gerätedesinfektion
F désinfection des instruments
S desinfección de instrumentos

instrument lubrication
G Geräteschmierung
F lubrification d'un instrument
S lubricación del aparato

instrument manual
G Gerätehandbuch
F manuel d'instructions
S manual de instrucciones

instrument memory
G Gerätespeicher
F mémoire d'un instrument
S memoria de un instrumento

instrument options
G Geräteoptionen
F options d'un équipement
S opciones del aparato

instrument panel
G Instrumententafel
F tableau d'instruments
S tablero de instrumentos

instrument set-up
G instrumenteller Aufbau
F montage des instruments
S montaje de instrumentos

instrument specification
G Gerätespezifikation
F spécification de l'instrument
S especificación de aparatos

insulating layer
G Isolierschicht
F couche d'isolation
S capa aislante

insulation
G Isolierung
F isolation
S aislamiento

intact
G intakt
F intact
S intacto

integrity
G Integrität, Unversehrtheit
F intégrité
S integridad

integrity test
G Integritätstest
F test d'intégrité
S prueba (test) de integridad

integrity testing
G Integritätsprüfung
F test d'intégrité
S prueba de integridad

intellectual property
G intellektuelles Eigentum
F propriété intellectuelle
S propiedad intelectual

interaction
G Wechselwirkung
F interaction, action réciproque
S acción recíproca, interacción

interchangeable
G austauschbar
F interchangeable
S intercambiable

interface
G Grenzfläche
F surface de séparation, interface
S interfase, superficie limitante

interference
G Interferenz, Störung
F interférence, dérangement, perturbation
S interferencia, avería, fallo

electrical interference
G elektrische Störung
F interférence électrique
S avería eléctrica

English German French Spanish

English German French Spanish

interfering bands
G Störbanden, interferierende Banden
F bandes d'interférence
S bandas de interferencia

interim storage
G Zwischenlagerung
F stockage intermédiaire
S almacenaje intermediario

intermediate ceiling
G Zwischendecke
F faux plafond
S techo intermedio

intermediate control
G Zwischenkontrolle
F contrôle intermédiaire
S control intermediario

intermediate product
G Zwischenprodukt
F produit intermédiaire
S producto intermediario

intermediate stage
G Zwischenstufe
F état intermédiaire
S nivel intermediario

internal audit
G internes Audit
F audit interne
S auditoría interna

internal bag
G Innenbeutel
F poche intérieure
S bolsa interior

internal diameter
G lichter Durchmesser
F diamètre interne
S diámetro interno

internal dimension
G Innenmaß
F dimension interne
S dimensión interna

internal lacquer
G Innenlack, Innenlackierung
F laque interne, vernissage interne
S barniz interno, barnizado interno

internal pressure
G Innendruck
F pression interne
S presión interna

internal protective lacquer
G Innenschutzlack
F laque interne de protection
S barniz protector interno

internal standard
G Hausstandard, interner Standard
F étalon interne, standard interne
S estándar interno

interpretation
G Auswertung
F interprétation, évaluation
S evaluación, interpretación

interruption
G Unterbrechung
F interruption
S interrupción

intervention
G Eingriff
F intervention
S intervención

invalid
G ungültig
F non valable
S inválido

inventory
G Lagerbestand
F inventaire, stock
S existencias en almacén, stocks

investigate, to
G untersuchen
F inspecter
S examinar, explorar, investigar

investigation
G Untersuchung
F inspection
S examen, exploración, investigación

Investigational New Drug Application (IND)
G Antrag an die FDA (USA) zur klinischen Prüfung eines Arzneimittels
F demande d'autorisation d'étude clinique d'un nouveau médicament (IND) auprès de la FDA
S solicitud a la FDA (EE.UU.) para investigar clínicamente un nuevo medicamento

investigator
G Prüfarzt
F médecin responsable d'essais cliniques
S médico investigador

investment costs
G Investitionskosten
F coûts d'investissements
S costes de inversión

in-vitro diagnosis
G In-vitro-Diagnose
F diagnostic in-vitro
S diagnóstico in vitro

in-vitro release
G In-vitro-Freisetzung
F libération in-vitro
S liberación in vitro

in-vitro release rate
G In-vitro-Freisetzungsrate
F vitesse de libération in-vitro
S tasa de liberación in vitro

involvement
G Beteiligung
F participation
S participación

iodine flask
G Iodzahlkolben
F flacon d'iode
S matraz de índice de iodo

iodine number
G Iodzahl
F indice d'iode, nombre d'iode
S índice de iodo

ion exchange
G Ionenaustausch
F échange d'ions
S intercambio de iones

ion exchange chromatography
G Ionenaustauschchromatographie
F chromatographie par échange d'ions
S cromatografía de intercambio iónico

ion exchange resin
G Austauscherharz
F résine échangeuse d'ions
S resina de intercambio iónico

ion exchanger
G Ionenaustauscher
F échangeur d'ions
S intercambiador de iones

ion exclusion chromatography
G Ionenausschlußchromatographie
F chromatographie d'exclusion ionique
S cromatografía de exclusión iónica

ion pair chromatography
G Ionenpaarchromatographie
F chromatographie par paires d'ions
S cromatografía de pares de iones

ionisation
G Ionisierung
F ionisation
S ionización

IR fingerprint
G IR-Fingerabdruck
F empreinte digitale IR
S huella dactilar IR

IR spectroscopy
G IR-Spektroskopie
F spectroscopie IR
S espectroscopia IR

IR spectrum
G IR-Spektrum
F spectre infrarouge
S espectro infrarrojo

irradiate, to (with)
G bestrahlen mit
F irradier avec
S irradiar con

irradiation
G Bestrahlung
F irradiation
S irradiación

irritating substance
G reizende Substanz
F substance irritante
S sustancia irritante

irritating to eyes
G reizt die Augen
F irritant pour les yeux
S irrita los ojos

irritating to respiratory system
G reizt die Atemwege
F irritant pour le système respiratoire
S irrita las vías respiratorias

irritating to skin
G hautreizend
F irritant pour la peau
S irritante cutáneo

irritation (chem.)
G Reizung (chemisch)
F irritation (chimique)
S irritación (química)

ISO-certificated
G ISO-zertifiziert
F certifié ISO
S ISO-certificado

isocratic
G isokratisch
F isocratique
S isocrático

isolator
G Isolator
F isolateur
S aislante

isotonic
G isoton
F isotonique
S isotónico

issue
G Ausgabe, Version
F édition, version
S edición, versión

itemised goods
G Stückgut
F colis
S bultos sueltos

jacket
G Ummantelung
F gaine, enveloppe
S revestimiento

jam, to
G blockieren
F bloquer
S bloquear

jar
G Weithalsgefäß
F fiole, jarre
S recipiente de cuello ancho

jaw (tech.)
G Backe (techn.)
F mâchoire
S mandíbula, mordaza

job
G Arbeitsstelle
F emploi
S puesto de trabajo

job description
G Stellenbeschreibung
F description d'un emploi
S descripción de un puesto de trabajo

joint
G Fuge, Naht, Trennfuge
F joint
S junta, soldadura, sutura

construction joint
G Arbeitsfuge
F joint de construction
S junta de construcción

expansion joint
G Dehnungsfuge
F joint de compensation
S junta de dilatación

settling joint
G Bewegungsfuge
F joint de dilatation
S junta de movimiento

jointing material
G Fugenmaterial
F matériau pour joint
S material de junta

juice
G Saft
F jus
S jugo (animal), zumo (vegetal)

junction box
G Verteilerkasten
F boîte de distribution
S caja de distribución

Karl Fischer reagent
G Karl-Fischer-Lösung
F réactif de Karl Fischer
S reactivo de Karl Fischer

key (of punch)
G Paßfeder, Schlüssel (des Stempels), Taste
F clavette, ressort d'ajustage (de poinçon), touche
S llave (de troquel), tecla

key board
G Tastatur(feld)
F clavier
S teclado

key component
G Schlüsselkomponente
F composant clé
S componente clave

key personnel
G Personal in Schlüsselstellung
F personnel occupant un poste à responsabilités
S personal en posición clave

kill, to
G abtöten
F tuer, détruire
S destruir, matar

killing
G Abtötung
F action de tuer
S destrucción

kinetic reaction
G kinetische Reaktion
F réaction cinétique
S reacción cinética

kinetics
G Kinetik
F cinétique
S cinética

kit
G Bausatz
F kit, prêt-à-monter
S kit

knead, to
G kneten
F pétrir, malaxer
S amasar

knurled nut
G Rändelmutter
F écrou moleté
S tuerca moleteada

knurled screw
G Rändelschraube
F vis moletée
S tornillo moleteado

English German French Spanish

lab
G Labor
F laboratoire
S laboratorio

lab coat
G Kittel, Laborkittel
F blouse de laboratoire
S bata, bata de laboratorio

lab ware
G Laborartikel
F matériel de laboratoire
S artículo de laboratorio

label
G Etikett
F étiquette
S etiqueta

loose labels, cut labels
G lose Etiketten
F étiquettes prédécoupées
S etiquetas sueltas

roll-fed labels
G Etiketten auf Rollen
F étiquettes en rouleaux
S etiquetas en rollo

self-adhesive labels
G selbstklebende Etiketten
F étiquettes autoadhésives
S etiquetas autoadhesivas

label count
G Etikettenzählung
F comptage d'étiquettes
S recuento de etiquetas

label counter
G Etikettenzähler
F compteur d'étiquettes
S contador de etiquetas

label reconciliation
G Etikettenbilanzierung
F bilan d'étiquettes
S balance de etiquetas

label, to
G bezeichnen, kennzeichnen
F étiqueter, marquer
S denominar, etiquetar, marcar, rotular

labelling
G Beschriftung, Etikettierung, Kennzeichnung
F étiquetage, marquage
S etiquetado, marcado, rotulado

labelling rules
G Etikettierungsregeln
F règles d'étiquetage
S reglas de etiquetado

laboratory
G Labor
F laboratoire
S laboratorio

laboratory assistant
G Laborant
F assistant de laboratoire, laborantin
S asistente de laboratorio

laboratory information management system (LIMS)
G Laborinformations- und -management-System (LIMS)
F système de gestion des données de laboratoire (LIMS)
S sistema de gestión de datos de laboratorio (LIMS)

laboratory notebook
G Laborjournal
F cahier de laboratoire
S diario de laboratorio

laboratory scale
G Labormaßstab
F échelle de laboratoire
S escala de laboratorio

laboratory shoes
G Laborschuhe
F chaussures de laboratoire
S calzado de laboratorio

lacquer
G Lack
F laque
S barniz, laca

lacquer, to
G lackieren
F laquer
S barnizar, lacar

lacquering fluid
G Lackiersuspension
F suspension de laquage
S suspensión de lacado

lacrimal fluid
G Tränenflüssigkeit
F liquide lacrymal
S líquido lacrimal

lactone
G Lacton
F lactone
S lactona

lactose
G Lactose
F lactose
S lactosa

ladle
G Schöpfkelle
F louche
S cazo, vasija

laevo-rotary
G linksdrehend
F lévogyre
S levógiro

lamella
G Lamelle
F lamelle
S arandela, disco, laminilla

laminar air flow
G Laminarströmung
F flux d'air laminaire
S corriente laminar

laminar flow
G Laminarfluß, laminare Strömung
F flux laminaire
S flujo laminar

laminate, to
G beschichten
F enduire
S laminar, recubrir

laminated foil
G Verbundfolie
F feuille stratifiée
S hoja laminada, lámina estratificada

laminated glass
G laminiertes Glas
F verre stratifié
S vidrio laminado

laminated tablet
G Manteltablette
F comprimé multicouche
S comprimido de cubierta estratificada

large volume parenterals (LVP)
G großvolumige Parenteralia
F produits injectables de grand volume
S productos inyectables de gran volumen

laser printer
G Laserdrucker
F imprimante à laser
S impresora de láser

latch
G Klinke
F loquet, poignée de porte
S picaporte, gatillo, trinquete

lattice
G Kristallgitter
F réseau cristallin
S retículo cristalino

launch
G Markteinführung
F introduction sur le marché, lancement d'un produit
S introducción en el mercado

law
G Gesetz
F loi
S ley

layer
G Lage, Schicht
F couche, phase
S estrato

layout
G Lageplan
F schéma, plans du site
S plano del lugar

leaflet feed
G Prospektzuführung
F approvisionnement en dépliants
S suministro de prospectos

leak
G Leck, Undichtigkeit
F fuite
S escape, permeabilidad

leak test
G Lecktest, Dichtigkeitsprüfung
F essai d'étanchéité, essai de fuite, essai de perte
S prueba de escape, prueba de estanqueidad

leakage
G Leck, Undichtigkeit
F fuite
S escape, permeabilidad

leakage current
G Kriechstrom
F courant de cheminement
S corriente de fuga

leak-tight
G dicht
F étanche
S hermético

leak-tight connection
G dichte Verbindung
F raccordement étanche
S conexión hermética

leaky
G undicht
F non étanche
S permeable

LED readout
G LED-Anzeige
F affichage électroluminescent
S pantalla electroluminiscente

leech
G Blutegel
F sangsue
S sanguijuela

left-hand
G linksgängig
F à pas gauche
S de paso izquierdo

legend
G Zeichenerklärung
F légende
S leyenda

legible
G lesbar
F lisible
S legible

legislation
G Gesetzgebung
F législation
S legislación

length
G Länge
F longueur
S longitud

lens
G Linse
F lentille
S lente

lettering
G Beschriftung
F étiquetage, marquage
S etiquetado, marcado, rotulado

level
G Füllstand, Pegel, Pegelstand, eben
F niveau, plat
S nivel de relleno, nivel, liso, llano, plano

level detector
G Füllstandsmelder
F détecteur de niveau
S detector de nivel de relleno

level sensor
G Pegelmesser
F détecteur de niveau
S sensor de nivel

levelling
G Nivellierung
F nivellement
S nivelación

level-measuring device
G Füllstandsmesser
F dispositif de mesure d'un niveau
S sistema de medida del nivel de relleno

lever
G Hebel
F levier
S palanca

lever press
G Hebelpresse
F presse à bascule
S prensa de palanca

lever switch controls
G Kippschalter-Kontrollen
F interrupteurs à bascule
S controles de interruptor unipolar

liability (financial)
G Verbindlichkeit (finanz.)
F passif (finance)
S obligación, pasivo (contabilidad)

liability (legal)
G Haftung (rechtlich)
F responsabilité (juridique)
S responsabilidad (jurídica)

licence
G Lizenz, behördliche Genehmigung
F licence, autorisation d'une autorité réglementaire
S licencia, autorización oficial

licensing agreement
G Lizenzabkommen
F contrat de licence
S acuerdo de licencia

lid
G Deckel
F couvercle
S tapa, tapadera

lid flap
G Verschlußklappe
F clapet de fermeture
S válvula de cierre

life cycle
G Lebenszyklus
F cycle de vie
S ciclo vital

lift
G Aufzug
F ascenseur
S ascensor

lifting cam (of upper punch)
G Aufzugsschiene (des Oberstempels)
F came (de poinçon) ascendante
S carril de ascenso (del troquel superior)

lifting device
G Hebevorrichtung, Hubvorrichtung
F dispositif de levage, appareillage élévateur
S dispositivo elevador

lifting platform
G Hebebühne
F plate-forme de levage
S plataforma elevadora

English German French Spanish

lifting truck
G Hubwagen
F chariot élévateur
S carro elevador

light
G Beleuchtungskörper
F appareil d'éclairage
S aparato de iluminación

light barrier
G Lichtschranke
F barrière optique
S barrera luminosa, barrera óptica

light fittings
G Beleuchtungskörper
F appareil d'éclairage
S aparato de iluminación

light scattering
G Lichtstreuung
F dispersion de la lumière
S dispersión luminosa

light source
G Lichtquelle
F source de lumière
S fuente luminosa

light transmittance
G Lichtdurchlässigkeit
F transparence
S transparencia para la luz

light-fast
G lichtbeständig
F résistant à la lumière
S resistente a la luz

light-fastness
G Lichtbeständigkeit
F résistance à la lumière
S resistencia a la luz

lighting
G Beleuchtung
F éclairage
S iluminación

light-scattering detector
G Streulicht-Detektor
F détecteur de lumière diffuse
S detector de luz dispersa

light-sensitive
G lichtempfindlich
F photo-sensible, sensible à la lumière
S fotosensible

limit
G Grenzwert
F limite
S valor límite

limit of detection (LOD)
G Nachweisgrenze
F limite de détection
S límite de detección

limit of quantitation (LOQ)
G Bestimmungsgrenze
F limite de quantitation
S límite de análisis, límite de determinación

lower limit of quantitation
G untere Bestimmungsgrenze
F limite inférieure de quantitation
S límite inferior de determinación

upper limit of quantitation
G obere Bestimmungsgrenze
F limite supérieure de quantitation
S límite superior de determinación

limit test
G Grenzprüfung
F test de limites
S prueba de límites

limitation
G Einschränkung
F limitation
S limitación, restricción

limited access
G beschränkter Zugang, eingeschränkter Zugang
F accès limité, accès restrictif
S acceso limitado

limited access area
G Bereich mit eingeschränktem Zugang
F zone d'accès limité
S zona de acceso limitado

line clearance (at a packaging line)
G Linienabnahme (an der Verpackungslinie)
F ligne de dégagement (d'une chaîne de conditionnement)
S punto de descarga (de la cadena de envasado)

line voltage
G Netzspannung
F tension du secteur
S tensión de la red

linear extension
G Längenausdehnung
F extension longitudinale
S expansión longitudinal

linear range
G Linearbereich
F intervalle linéaire
S área lineal

linearity
G Linearität
F linéarité
S linealidad

liniment
G Einreibemittel, Liniment
F beaume, onguent, liniment
S bálsamo, linimento

lining (of containers)
G Auskleidung (von Behältern)
F garnissage (de récipients)
S revestimiento (de recipientes)

lint-free clothes
G fusselfreie Kleidung
F vêtement qui ne peluche pas
S ropa sin pelusa

lipid
G Lipid
F lipide
S lípido

lipophilic
G lipophil
F lipophile
S lipófilo

lipophobic
G lipophob
F lipophobe
S lipófobo

liquid
G Flüssigkeit, flüssig
F liquide
S líquido

thin
G dünnflüssig
F (très) fluide
S (muy) fluido

viscous
G dickflüssig
F visqueux
S viscoso

liquid crystal display (LCD)
G Flüssigkristallanzeige
F affichage à cristaux liquides
S pantalla de cristal líquido

liquid extract
G Flüssigextrakt
F extrait liquide
S extracto fluido

liquid form
G flüssige Form
F forme liquide (spécialités pharmaceutiques)
S forma líquida de administración

liquid gas
G Flüssiggas
F gaz liquide
S gas líquido

liquid level
G Flüssigkeitsstand
F niveau du liquide
S nivel de líquido

English German French Spanish

liquid level indicator
G Flüssigkeitsstandsanzeige
F indicateur du niveau de liquide
S indicador de nivel de líquido

liquid media
G Flüssigmedien
F milieux liquides
S medios líquidos

liquid phase
G flüssige Phase
F phase liquide
S fase líquida

liquid-liquid extraction
G flüssig-flüssig-Extraktion
F extraction liquide-liquide
S extracción líquido-líquido

liquified gases
G verflüssigte Gase
F gaz liquéfiés
S gases licuados

liquify, to
G verflüssigen
F liquéfier
S licuar, licuefacer

list
G Verzeichnis
F répertoire, registre
S índice

list of items
G Stückliste
F liste-inventaire, liste détaillée
S especificación, lista detallada, inventario

litmus
G Lackmus
F tournesol
S litmus, tornasol

litmus paper
G Lackmuspapier
F papier de tournesol
S papel de tornasol

live vaccine
G Lebendimpfstoff
F vaccin vivant
S vacuna viva

load
G Ladung, Beschickung
F charge
S alimentación, carga

dynamic load
G dynamische Belastung
F charge dynamique
S carga dinámica

microbial load
G mikrobielle Belastung
F présence microbienne
S carga microbiana

load capacity
G Belastbarkeit
F capacité de chargement
S capacidad de carga

load pattern (for autoclaves)
G Beschickungsmuster (für Autoklaven)
F schéma de charge (pour autoclave)
S esquema de carga (para autoclave)

loading
G Beladung, Belastung
F chargement, charge
S carga

loading capacity
G Tragfähigkeit
F limite de charge, force portante
S capacidad de carga

loading configuration
G Beladungsschema
F schéma de chargement
S esquema de carga

loading height (e. g. of autoclave)
G Beladungshöhe
(z. B. eines Autoklaven)
F hauteur de chargement
(p. ex. d'un autoclave)
S altura de carga
(p. ej. de autoclave)

loading limit
G Belastungsgrenze
F limite de charge
S límite de carga

load-resisting
G belastungsstabil
F stable au chargement
S estable a la carga

local code
G regionales Regelwerk
F code régional
S código regional

locate a failure (fault), to
G Fehler finden
F identifier une erreur
S encontrar errores

location
G Lage, Ort, Standort
F emplacement, endroit, lieu
S emplazamiento, lugar, posición, situación, ubicación

lock
G Schleuse
F sas
S esclusa

material lock
G Materialschleuse
F sas réservé aux fournitures
S esclusa de material

personnel lock
G Personenschleuse
F sas réservé au personnel
S esclusa de personal

lock seam
G Falznaht
F couture de pliage
S soldadura del encaje

lock, to
G arretieren
F fermer à clef
S fijar, parar, retener

locked location
G unter Verschluß
F enfermé
S cerrado

locker
G Spind
F placard de vestiaire
S armario estrecho

locker room
G Spindraum
F vestiaire
S vestuario

log
G Aufzeichnung
F enregistrement
S registro

log book
G Logbuch, Laborjournal
F cahier de route,
cahier de laboratoire
S cuaderno de bitácora,
diario de laboratorio

log data, to
G Daten erfassen
F enregistrer des données
S registrar datos

log, to (data)
G aufzeichnen (Daten)
F enregistrer (des données)
S registrar (datos)

logistic systems
G logistische Systeme
F systèmes logistiques
S sistemas logísticos

logistics
G Logistik
F logistique
S logística

logo
G Firmenzeichen, Logo
F logo
S logotipo

long-chained
G langkettig
F à chaîne longue
S de cadena larga

longitudinal axis
G Längsachse
F axe longitudinal
S eje longitudinal

long-term stability
G Langzeitstabilität
F stabilité à long terme
S estabilidad a largo plazo

long-term therapy
G Langzeittherapie
F thérapie à long terme
S terapia a largo plazo

loop
G Stromkreis
F circuit
S circuito eléctrico

loop volume
G Schleifenvolumen
F volume de la boucle
S volumen de bucle

loose powder
G loses Pulver
F poudre en vrac
S polvo suelto

loss
G Verlust
F perte
S pérdida

loss of quality
G Güteminderung
F perte de qualité, baisse de qualité
S pérdida de calidad

loss on drying
G Trocknungsverlust
F pertes dues au séchage
S pérdidas por desecación

lot
G Charge
F lot
S lote

lotion
G Lotion
F lotion
S loción

low dosage
G niedrige Dosis
F dose faible
S dosis baja

low-dosed
G niedrig dosiert
F à dose faible
S a dosis baja

lower punch
G Unterstempel
F poinçon inférieur
S troquel inferior

lower, to
G senken
F abaisser, baisser
S bajar, reducir

lozenge
G Lutschtablette
F pastille, tablette à sucer
S comprimido para chupar

lubricant
G Gleitmittel, Schmiermittel
F lubrifiant
S lubri(fi)cante

lubricate, to
G schmieren
F graisser, lubrifier
S engrasar, lubri(fi)car

lubricating nipple
G Schmiernippel
F bouchon graisseur
S boquilla lubri(fi)cante

lubrication pump
G Schmierstoffpumpe
F pompe lubrifiante
S bomba de lubri(fi)cante

luminescence scanner
G Lumineszenztaster
F scanner à luminescence
S sensor de luminiscencia

lye
G Lauge
F soude
S lejía

lyophilisate
G Lyophilisat
F lyophilisat
S liofilizado

lyophilisation
G Gefriertrocknung, Lyophilisation
F lyophilisation
S liofilización

lyophilised
G gefriergetrocknet
F lyophilisé
S liofilizado

lyophiliser
G Gefriertrockner
F lyophilisateur
S liofilizador

lysate
G Lysat
F lysat
S lisado

MAC value
G MAK-Wert
F taux de concentration maximal de travail
S valor de concentración máxima de trabajo

maceration
G Mazeration
F macération
S maceración

machine breakdown
G Maschinenausfall
F défaillance de machine
S avería de una máquina

machine cover
G Maschinenabdeckung
F couvercle de machine
S cubierta de la máquina

machine room
G Maschinenraum
F salle des machines
S sala de máquinas

machine speed
G Maschinengeschwindigkeit
F vitesse de machine
S velocidad de una máquina

machine stoppage
G Maschinenstillstand
F arrêt de machine
S detención de la máquina

macromolecule
G Makromolekül
F macro-molécule
S macromolécula

macropores
G Makroporen
F macropores
S macroporos

magnetic cell separation
G magnetische Zelltrennung
F clivage cellulaire magnétique
S separación magnética de células

magnetic clutch
G Magnetkupplung
F embrayage magnétique
S acoplamiento magnético

magnetic stirrer
G Magnetrührer
F agitateur magnétique
S agitador magnético

magnetic stirring bar
G Rührfisch
F agitateur magnétique, barreau aimanté
S agitador magnético

magnetic tape
G Magnetband
F bande magnétique
S cinta magnética

magnification
G Vergrößerung
F agrandissement
S aumento

magnifying glass
G Lupe
F loupe
S lupa

main circuit
G Hauptstromkreis
F circuit principal
S circuito eléctrico principal

main compression roll
G Hauptdruckrolle
F rouleau presseur principal
S rollo principal de prensa

main ring
G Ringleitung
F boucle de recirculation
S cañería en anillo, red anular

main switch
G Hauptschalter, Netzschalter
F interrupteur principal, interrupteur de courant
S interruptor principal, interruptor a la red

maintenance
G Instandhaltung, Wartung
F entretien, maintenance
S entretenimiento, mantenimiento

maintenance dosage
G Erhaltungsdosis
F dose de maintien
S dosis de mantenimiento

make redundant, to
G entlassen
F renvoyer, licencier, congédier
S despedir

malfunction
G Funktionsstörung, Störung
F dérangement, dysfonctionnement, perturbation
S avería, disfunción, fallo

malfunction alarm
G Störungsmeldung
F alarme de mauvais fonctionnement
S aviso de avería

malfunction indication
G Störungsmeldung
F alarme de mauvais fonctionnement
S aviso de avería

mammalian cell culture
G Säugetierzellkultur
F culture de cellules de mammifère
S cultivo de células de mamífero

mammalian cell line
G Säugetierzellinie
F lignée de cellule de mammifère
S línea de células de mamífero

managing director
G Geschäftsführer
F président directeur général (PDG)
S gerente

manhole
G Mannloch
F trou d'homme
S registro

manometer
G Manometer, Druckmeßgerät
F manomètre, manomètre de pression
S manómetro

mantle
G Ummantelung
F gaine, enveloppe
S revestimiento

manual
G manuell, von Hand
F manuel
S manual

manual packaging
G Handverpackung
F emballage manuel
S empaquetado manual

manufacture
G Herstellung, Produktion
F fabrication, production
S fabricación, producción

computer-integrated manufacturing (CIM)
G computerintegrierte Herstellung
F fabrication informatisée
S fabricación informatizada

manufactured biotechnologically
G biotechnologisch hergestellt
F manufacturé par biotechnologie
S fabricado biotecnológicamente

manufactured goods
G Fertigwaren
F produits manufacturés
S productos manufacturados

manufacturer
G Hersteller
F fabricant
S fabricante

manufacturer audit
G Herstelleraudit
F audit d'un fabricant
S inspección de un fabricante

manufacturer's specification
G Herstellerangaben
F spécifications du fabricant
S especificaciones del fabricante

manufacturing authorisation
G Herstellerlaubnis
F autorisation de fabrication
S permiso de fabricación

manufacturing conditions
G Herstellungsbedingungen
F conditions de production
S condiciones de producción

manufacturing contract
G Lohnauftrag
F contrat de fabrication
S negocio de comisión

manufacturing environment
G Herstellungsumgebung
F zone de fabrication
S entorno de producción

manufacturing instructions
G Herstellungsanweisung, Herstellungsvorschrift
F instructions de fabrication
S instrucción de fabricación, prescripciones de fabricación

manufacturing location/site
G Produktionsort
F lieu de production
S lugar de producción

manufacturing order
G Herstellungsauftrag
F commande de fabrication
S encargo de producción

manufacturing procedure
G Herstellungsverfahren
F procédure de fabrication
S procedimiento de fabricación

manufacturing site
G Produktionsstätte
F site de production
S lugar de producción

manufacturing step
G Herstellungsstufe
F étape de fabrication
S etapa de producción

margin of error
G Fehlergrenze
F marge d'erreur
S límite de error, margen de error

marinate, to
G beizen
F mariner
S adobar, cauterizar, desinfectar

mark, to
G kennzeichnen, stempeln
F étiqueter, marquer, poinçonner
S etiquetar, marcar, troquelar

marker (on leaflet)
G Flattermarke, Leitsubstanz
F marque inconstante, marqueur, traceur
S marca inconstante, marcador

marketing authorisation
G Marktzulassung, Zulassung
F autorisation de mise sur le marché (A.M.M.)
S autorización de (para) venta en el mercado

mask
G Maske
F masque
S máscara

mask, to
G maskieren
F masquer
S enmascarar

masking
G Maskierung
F masque
S enmascaramiento

master formula
G Herstellungsvorschrift
F instructions de fabrication
S prescripciones de fabricación

mat
G matt
F mat
S mate

material
G Werkstoff
F matériau
S material

material compatibility
G Materialverträglichkeit
F compatibilité des matériaux
S compatibilidad de materiales

material fatigue
G Materialermüdung
F fatigue du matériel
S fatiga del material

material flow
G Materialfluß
F flux des matériaux
S flujo de material

material lock
G Materialschleuse
F sas réservé au matériel
S esclusa de material

material movement
G Materialbewegung
F mouvement des matériaux
S movimiento de material

material safety data sheet (MSDS)
G Sicherheitsdatenblatt
F feuille de données de sécurité
S hoja de datos de seguridad, pliego de datos de seguridad

material specifications
G Materialspezifikationen
F spécifications des matériaux
S especificaciones del material

material stress
G Materialbeanspruchung
F sollicitation du matériel
S tensión sobre el material

material wastage
G Materialverschwendung
F gaspillage
S derroche de material

materials handling
G Materialwirtschaft
F manipulation des matériaux
S administración del material

materials management
G Materialwirtschaft
F manipulation des matériaux
S administración del material

matrix data analysis
G Matrixdatenanalyse
F analyse de données matricielles
S análisis de datos en matriz

matrix diagram
G Matrixdiagramm
F diagramme matriciel
S diagrama en matriz

maturing
G Alterung
F vieillissement
S envejecimiento

maximum allowable concentration (MAC)
G maximale Arbeitsplatzkonzentration (MAK)
F concentration maximale de postes de travail
S concentración máxima de puestos de trabajo

maximum dosage
G Höchstdosis
F dose maximale
S dosis máxima

maximum load
G Höchstlast
F charge maximale
S carga máxima

maximum speed
G Höchstgeschwindigkeit
F vitesse maximale
S velocidad máxima

maximum valid dilution (MVD)
G maximal zulässige Verdünnung (MZV)
F dilution maximale autorisée
S dilución máxima permitida

maximum weight
G Höchstgewicht
F poids maximum
S peso máximo

mean
G Durchschnitt
F moyenne
S media, promedio

measurable
G meßbar
F mesurable
S medible, mensurable

measure
G Maßnahme
F mesure
S medida

measure, to
G messen
F mesurer
S medir

measurement
G Messung
F mesure
S medición, medida

measurement converter
G Meßumformer
F convertisseur
S convertidor de mediciones

measuring and control technology
G Elektro-, Meß- und Regeltechnik (EMR), Meß-Steuer-Regel (MSR)-Technik
F électrotechnique et techniques de mesure et de réglage; techniques de mesure, de réglage et de contrôle
S electrotécnica y técnicas de medida y regulación; técnica de medición, regulación y control

English
German
French
Spanish

English German French Spanish

measuring device
G Meßmittel
F instrument de mesure
S dispositivo de medición

measuring error
G Meßfehler
F erreur de mesure
S error de medición

measuring instrument
G Meßgerät
F instrument de mesure
S aparato de medición

measuring point
G Meßpunkt
F point de mesure
S punto de medida

measuring range
G Meßbereich
F gamme de mesure
S zona de medición

measuring spoon
G Meßlöffel
F cuillère-mesure
S cuchara de medida

mechanical
G maschinell
F mécanique
S mecánico

mechanical seal
G mechanischer Verschluß
F fermeture mécanique
S cierre mecánico

media fill
G Nährmedienabfüllung
F remplissage des milieux de culture
S relleno con medio de cultivo

media steriliser
G Mediensterilisator
F stérilisateur de milieu
S esterilizador de medios

medical device
G Medizinprodukt
F produit à usage médical
S producto médico

medical examination
G ärztliche Untersuchung
F examen médical
S exploración médica

medical examination on starting a new job
G Einstellungsuntersuchung
F examen médical suite à une embauche
S exploración médica al ser empleado

medical prescription
G ärztliche Verordnung
F ordonnance, prescription
S prescripción médica

medical science
G Medizinische Wissenschaft
F science médicale
S ciencia médica

medicated chewing gum
G medizinisches Kaugummi
F chewing-gum médicamenté
S goma de mascar medicamentosa

medicated hair tonic
G medizinisches Haarwasser
F lotion capillaire
S loción capilar

medicated vaginal tampon
G Vaginaltampon
F tampon vaginal
S tampón vaginal

medication
G Medikation
F médication
S medicación

medicinal product
G Arzneimittel
F médicament, produit pharmaceutique
S medicamento

genetically manufactured medicinal product
G gentechnologisch hergestelltes Arzneimittel
F médicament produit par génie génétique
S medicamento producido mediante tecnología genética

medicinal product premix
G Arzneimittelvormischung
F préparation pharmaceutique
S elaboración previa del medicamento

medicinal substance
G Arzneistoff
F principe actif
S sustancia medicamentosa

medicinal water
G Heilwasser
F eau médicinale
S agua medicinal

Medicines Marketing Authorisation Application (MAA)
G Antrag auf Zulassung zum Inverkehrbringen von Arzneimitteln in der EU
F demande d'autorisation de mise sur le marché (AMM)
S solicitud de autorización de venta de medicamentos en la UE

medium
G Medium
F milieu
S medio

dehydrated medium
G Trockennährmedium
F milieu de culture déhydraté
S medio de cultivo deshidratado

melt
G Schmelze
F fusion
S fundición, fusión

melt, to
G einschmelzen, schmelzen
F fondre, faire fondre
S fundir

melting index
G Schmelzindex
F indice de fusion
S índice de fusión

melting point
G Schmelzpunkt
F point de fusion
S punto de fusión

instant melting point
G Sofortschmelzpunkt
F point de fusion instantané
S punto de fusión inmediata

melting range
G Schmelzbereich
F plage de fusion
S márgenes de fusión

member state
G Mitgliedstaat
F état membre
S estado miembro

membrane
G Membran
F membrane
S membrana

membrane area
G Membranfläche
F surface de membrane
S superficie de la membrana

membrane filter
G Membranfilter
F filtre à membrane, filtre microporeux
S filtro de membrana

membrane filtration
G Membranfiltration
F filtration par membrane
S filtración por membrana

membrane key pad
G Folientastatur
F clavier à effleurement
S teclado de membrana plástica

membrane type
G Membrantyp
F type de membrane
S tipo de membrana

membrane vacuum
G Membranvakuum
F vide à diaphragme
S vacío de membrana

menu-controlled
G menügesteuert
F commandé par menu
S dirigido por minuta

merger
G Zusammenschluß von Firmen
F fusion (d'entreprises)
S fusión de empresas

mesh size
G Maschenweite
F ouverture de maille
S tamaño del orificio de la malla

mesh wire
G Drahtnetz
F tamis métallique
S red de alambre

mesopores
G Mesoporen
F mésopores
S mesoporos

metabolic path
G Abbauweg
F chemin de dégradation
S vía de degradación

metal
G Metall
F métal
S metal

metal detector
G Metallsuchgerät
F détecteur de métaux
S detector de metales

metal fracture
G Metallbruch
F fracture du métal
S fractura de un metal

meter, to
G abmessen, dosieren
F doser
S dosificar, calibrar, medir

metered dose inhaler
G Dosieraerosol
F inhalateur doseur
S aerosol dosificante

metering accuracy
G Dosiergenauigkeit
F exactitude de dosage
S exactitud de la dosificación

metering aid
G Dosierhilfe
F dispositif d'aide au dosage
S dispositivo para dosificar

metering chamber
G Dosierkammer
F chambre de dosage
S cámara de dosificación

metering device
G Dosiereinrichtung
F appareil doseur
S dispositivo dosificante

method
G Technik, Methode
F technique, méthode
S técnica, método

method of administration
G Verwaltungsverfahren
F méthode d'administration
S procedimiento administrativo

mezzanine
G Zwischengeschoß
F étage intermédiaire
S piso intermedio

microbial
G mikrobiell
F microbien
S microbiano

microbial by-products
G mikrobielle Nebenprodukte
F produits secondaires microbiens
S productos colaterales microbianos

microbial challenge test
G Bakterienbelastungstest
F test de stimulation microbien
S prueba de estimulación con bacterias

microbial collector
G Luftkeimsammler
F échantillonneur d'air
S colector de gérmenes del aire

microbial contaminants
G mikrobielle Kontaminanten
F contaminants microbiens
S contaminantes microbianos

microbial control
G mikrobielle Kontrolle
F contrôle microbien
S control microbiano

microbial count
G Keimzahl
F nombre de micro-organismes
S número de gérmenes

microbial count determination
G Keimzahlbestimmung
F détermination du nombre de micro-organismes
S recuento de gérmenes

microbial differentiation
G Keimdifferenzierung
F différentiation microbienne
S diferenciación de gérmenes

microbial growth
G mikrobielles Wachstum
F croissance microbienne
S crecimiento microbiano

microbial reduction
G Keimreduktion
F réduction microbienne
S reducción de gérmenes

microbiological
G mikrobiologisch
F microbiologique
S microbiológico

microbiology
G Mikrobiologie
F microbiologie
S microbiología

microcrystalline
G mikrokristallin
F microcristallin
S microcristalino

micro-encapsulated
G mikroverkapselt
F micro-encapsulé
S microencapsulado

micro-filtration
G Mikrofiltration
F micro-filtration
S microfiltración

micro-filtration membrane
G Mikrofiltrationsmembran
F membrane de micro-filtration
S membrana de microfiltración

micrometer screw
G Mikrometerschraube
F micromètre, vis micromètre
S tornillo micrométrico

micronisation
G Mikronisierung
F micronisation
S micronización

English German French Spanish

microorganisms
G Mikroorganismen
F micro-organismes
S microorganismos

non-pathogenic microorganisms
G apathogene Mikroorganismen
F micro-organismes non-pathogènes
S microorganismos no patógenos

pathogenic microorganisms
G pathogene Mikroorganismen
F micro-organismes pathogènes
S microorganismos patógenos

viable microorganisms
G lebensfähige Mikroorganismen
F micro-organismes viables
S microorganismos viables

micro-pipetting
G Mikropipettierung
F micro-pipettage
S micropipetado

micro-plasma
G Mikroplasma
F micro-plasma
S microplasma

microscope
G Mikroskop
F microcospe
S microscopio

microwave
G Mikrowelle
F micro-onde
S microonda

microwave drying
G Mikrowellentrocknung
F séchage à micro-ondes
S desecación por microondas

migration
G Migration, Wanderung
F migration
S migración

mildewed
G schimmelig
F moisi
S enmohecido, mohoso

mill
G Mühle
F broyeur
S molino

mill, to
G mahlen, zerstoßen
F broyer, concasser, piler
S machacar, moler, pulverizar, triturar

minimum contents
G Mindestinhalt
F contenu minimal
S contenido mínimo

miscible
G mischbar
F miscible
S miscible

immiscible
G nicht mischbar
F non miscible
S no miscible

misidentification
G Verwechslung
F méprise, erreur
S confusión

mistake
G Fehler
F défaut, erreur
S error

mix
G Untermischung, Vermischung
F mélange
S entremezcla

mix in
G Untermischung, Vermischung
F mélange
S entremezcla

mix, to
G mischen
F mélanger
S mezclar

mixed bed
G Mischbett
F lit mixe
S lecho mixto

mixed bed ion exchanger
G Mischbettionentauscher, Gemischtbett-Ionenaustauscher
F échangeur d'ions à lit mixte
S intercambiador de iones de lecho mixto

mixture
G Gemisch, Mischung
F mixture, mélange
S mezcla, mixtura

mixture to be shaken
G Schüttelmixtur
F mixture devant être agitée
S mezcla a agitar

mm water
G mm Wassersäule
F mm de pression d'eau
S mm de presión de agua

mobile
G fahrbar
F mobile
S móvil, portátil

mobile phase (in chromotography)
G Fließmittel (in der Chromatographie)
F phase mobile
S fase móvil (en cromatografía)

modified
G modifiziert
F modifié
S modificado

modified release granules
G Granulat mit veränderter Wirkstoff-Freisetzung
F libération modifiée de granules
S granulado con liberación modificada de la sustancia activa

modular design
G Baukastenprinzip, Modularbauweise
F design modulaire
S diseño modular, principio de unidades de montaje

module
G Anbauteil, Baustein
F accessoire, dispositif adaptable, module
S módulo, piedra de construcción, pieza de montaje

moiety
G Teil
F partie, portion
S parte

moist
G feucht
F humide
S húmedo

moisten, to
G anfeuchten, befeuchten, benetzen
F humidifier, mouiller
S humectar, humedecer, mojar, rociar

moisture
G Feuchtigkeit
F humidité
S humedad

bound moisture
G gebundene Feuchtigkeit
F humidité adhérente
S humedad adherente

unbound moisture
G nicht gebundene Feuchtigkeit
F humidité non liée
S humedad no adherente

moisture content
G Feuchtigkeitsgehalt
F teneur en humidité
S contenido en humedad

moisture uptake
G Feuchtigkeitsaufnahme
F absorption d'humidité
S absorción de humedad

moisture-repelling
G feuchtigkeitsabweisend
F qui répulse l'humidité
S repelente de la humedad

moisture-resistant
G feuchtigkeitsbeständig
F résistant à l'humidité
S resistente a la humedad

moisture-sensitive
G feuchtigkeitsempfindlich
F sensible à l'humidité
S sensible a la humedad

molar
G molar
F molaire
S molar

molarity
G Molarität
F molarité
S molaridad

mole
G Mol
F mole
S mol

molecular
G molekular
F moléculaire
S molecular

molecular biology
G Molekularbiologie
F biologie moléculaire
S biología molecular

molecular formula
G Molekularformel
F formule brute
S fórmula molecular

molecular modelling
G Molekularmodellierung
F modelage moléculaire
S modelado molecular

molecular size
G Molekülgröße
F taille moléculaire
S tamaño molecular

molecular weight
G Molekulargewicht
F poids moléculaire
S peso molecular

monitor, to
G überwachen
F contrôler, surveiller
S supervisar, vigilar

monitoring
G Überwachung
F contrôle, surveillance
S supervisión, vigilancia

monitoring by the authorities
G behördliche Überwachung
F surveillance par les autorités
S control oficial

monitoring device
G Überwachungseinrichtung
F appareil de contrôle,
appareil de surveillance
S dispositivo de vigilancia

monitoring system
G Überwachungssystem
F système de contrôle,
système de surveillance
S sistema de vigilancia

monochromatic
G monochrom
F monochromatique
S monocromo

monochromator
G Monochromator
F monochromateur
S monocromador

monoclonal antibody
G monoklonaler Antikörper
F anticorps monoclonal
S anticuerpo monoclonal

monolithic material
G monolithisches Material
F matériau monolithique
S material monolítico

monomer
G Monomer
F monomère
S monómero

monovalent
G einwertig
F monovalent
S monovalente

mortality rate
G Absterberate
F taux de mortalité
S tasa de extinción, tasa de mortalidad

mortar
G Mörser, Reibschale
F mortier
S mortero

mortar bed
G Mörtelbett
F lit de mortier
S lecho de mortero

mother liquor
G Mutterlauge
F eau mère, lessive-mère
S lejía madre

motor housing
G Motorgehäuse
F carter d'un moteur
S cárter del motor

motor performance
G Motorleistung
F performance d'un moteur
S rendimiento de un motor

motor revolutions
G Motordrehzahl
F vitesse de rotation d'un moteur
S número de revoluciones del motor

mottled
G gesprenkelt
F madré
S moteado, salpicado

mould
G Schimmel, Schimmelpilz
F champignon, moisissure
S moho

mould growth
G Schimmelbefall
F formation de moisissure
S crecimiento de moho

mould, to (suppositories)
G Zäpfchen gießen
F mouler des suppositoires
S moldear supositorios

moulded
G geformt, gepreßt
F moulu
S comprimido, moldeado

moulding compound
G Preßmasse
F composé comprimable, matière moulée
S masa comprimible

moulding granulate
G Preßgranulat
F granule moulée
S granulado de compresión

moulding pressure
G Preßdruck
F pression de pressage, pression de moulage
S presión de prensado

English German French Spanish

English German French Spanish

moulding trial
G Preßversuch
F essai de compression
S ensayo de compresión

moulds
G Pilze
F champignons
S hongos

mouldy
G schimmelig
F moisi
S enmohecido, mohoso

mount
G Halterung
F support
S soporte

mounting
G Montage, Einbau
F assemblage, installation, montage
S instalación, montaje

mounting trolley
G Montagewagen
F chariot de montage
S carro de montaje

mouthpiece
G Mundstück
F embout
S boquilla, embocadura

mouthwash
G Mundwasser, Mundspüllösung
F bain de bouche, solution pour bain de bouche
S enjuague bucal, solución de enjuague bucal

movable parts
G bewegliche Teile
F pièces mobiles
S piezas móviles

mucilage
G Schleim
F mucilage, mucus
S mucosidad

mucosal tissue
G Schleimhautgewebe
F tissu d'une muqueuse
S tejido mucoso

mucous
G schleimig
F muqueux
S mucoso, mucilaginoso

mucous membrane
G Schleimhaut
F muqueuse
S mucosa

mud pack preparation
G Moorzubereitung
F préparation de tourbe
S preparación de turba

muffle furnace
G Muffelofen
F four à moufle
S horno de manguito

multi-bore die
G Matrize für Mehrfachwerkzeug
F matrice pour outil multiple
S matrices para herramientas de uso múltiple

multicentric
G multizentrisch
F multicentrique
S multicéntrico

multi-channel pipetting system
G Vielfachkanalpipettiersystem
F système de pipettage à canaux multiples
S sistema de pipeteo con canales múltiples

multi-channel recorder
G Mehrkanalschreiber
F enregistreur à canaux multiples
S registradora de canales múltiples

multiple disk brake
G Lamellenbremse
F frein à disques multiples
S freno de discos múltiples

multiple-dose container
G Mehrdosenbehältnis
F conditionnement multi-doses
S recipiente de dosis múltiple

multi-purpose equipment
G Mehrzweckanlage
F installation technique multi-usages
S instalación de uso múltiple

multi-stage distillation unit
G Mehrstufendestillationsanlage
F unité de distillation à plusieurs étages
S unidad de destilación a etapas múltiples

multivalent
G mehrwertig
F polyvalent
S polivalente

mutagenic
G mutagen
F mutagène
S mutágeno

Mutual Recognition Agreement (MRA)
G Abkommen zur gegenseitigen Anerkennung
F procédure de reconnaissance mutuelle
S Acuerdo de Reconocimiento Mutuo de Procedimientos Administrativos en la UE

Mutual Recognition Procedure (MRP)
G Gegenseitiges Anerkennungsverfahren bei der Zulassung von Arzneimitteln in der EU
F procédure de reconnaissance mutuelle
S Procedimiento de Reconocimiento Mutuo en la UE

naked flame
G offene Flamme
F flamme ouverte
S llama abierta

narcotic
G Rauschmittel
F narcotique
S narcótico

narcotic substance
G Betäubungsmittel
F substance narcotique
S sustancia narcótica

narcotics regulation
G Betäubungsmittelgesetz
F décret concernant les narcotiques
S decreto sobre narcóticos

nasal applicator
G Nasenolive
F applicateur nasal
S aplicador nasal

nasal cream
G Nasencreme
F crème nasale
S crema nasal

nasal gel
G Nasengel
F gel nasal
S gel nasal

nasal ointment
G Nasensalbe
F pommade nasale
S pomada nasal

nasal use
G nasale Anwendung
F utilisation nasale
S aplicación nasal

natural active substances
G natürlich vorkommende Wirkstoffe
F principes actifs naturels
S sustancias activas naturales

English German French Spanish

natural product
G Naturprodukt
F produit naturel
S producto natural

nature (of a substance)
G Beschaffenheit (einer Substanz)
F nature (d'une substance)
S naturaleza (de una sustancia)

nebulise, to
G vernebeln
F nébuliser
S nebulizar

nebuliser
G Vernebler
F nébuliseur
S nebulizador

negative pressure
G Unterdruck
F sous-pression, depression
S depresión, hipotensión

net
G Netz
F grille
S red

net weight
G Leergewicht
F poids à vide
S peso en vacío, tara

net-like
G netzförmig
F réticulaire
S reticular

network
G Netzwerk
F réseau
S obra de malla, retículo

neutralising substance (for disinfectant)
G Enthemmer (zur Inaktivierung von Desinfektionsmitteln)
F substance neutralisante
S sustancia neutralizante (para inactivar desinfectantes)

neutron activation analysis
G Neutronenaktivierungsanalyse
F analyse par activation neutronique
S análisis de activación de neutrones

New Drug Application (NDA)
G Antrag auf Produktbewilligung bei der FDA
F demande d'autorisation d'un médicament auprès de la FDA
S solicitud de aprobación de un producto por la FDA

new product development
G Entwicklung eines neuen Produktes
F développement d'un nouveau produit
S desarrollo de un producto nuevo

niche
G Nische
F niche
S nicho

nichrome steel
G Chromnickelstahl
F acier chromé et nickelé
S acero cromado y niquelado

nipple
G Befüllstutzen
F orifice de charge, orifice d'alimentation
S tubuladura de carga, tubuladura de alimentación

nitric acid
G Salpetersäure
F acide nitrique
S ácido nítrico

nitrogen
G Stickstoff
F azote
S nitrógeno

nitrogen-phosphorous detector (NPD)
G Stickstoff-Phosphor-Detektor
F détecteur d'azote phosphorisé
S detector de nitrógeno fosforado

noise
G Lärmbelastung, Rauschen
F bruit, pollution par le bruit
S ruido (de fondo)

baseline noise
G Basislinienrauschen
F bruit de fond d'une ligne de base
S ruido (de fondo) en la línea de base

noise development
G Geräuschentwicklung
F émissions sonores
S producción de ruido

noise insulation
G Geräuschisolierung
F insonorisation du bruit
S aislamiento sonoro

noise level
G Geräuschpegel
F niveau du bruit
S nivel sonoro

noise-proof
G geräuschdämmend
F insonorisé
S insonorizado

nominal size
G Nenngröße
F taille nominale
S tamaño nominal

nominal value
G Nennwert
F valeur nominale
S valor nominal

nominal volume
G Nennvolumen
F volume nominal
S volumen nominal

nominal width
G Nennweite
F largeur nominale
S anchura nominal

non-abrasive
G abriebfest
F résistant à l'abrasion
S resistente a la abrasión

non-aqueous
G nicht-wäßrig
F non aqueux
S no acuoso

non-compliance
G Nichteinhaltung
F non conformité
S no observancia

non-crushing
G trittsicher
F sûr à la marche
S de paso seguro

non-linear
G nichtlinear
F non linéaire
S no lineal

non-polar
G unpolar
F non polaire
S no polar

non-polluting
G umweltfreundlich
F écologique
S ecológico

non-return valve
G Rückschlagventil
F vanne anti-retour
S válvula de retención

non-slip
G rutschsicher
F anti-dérapant
S antideslizante

non-sterility
G Unsterilität
F fécondité
S fertilidad, fecundidad

English German French Spanish

non-viscous
G dünnflüssig
F fluide, très fluide
S fluido

non-volatile
G nichtflüchtig
F non volatile
S no volátil

normality (of a solution)
G Normalität (einer Lösung)
F normalité (d'une solution)
S normalidad (de una disolución)

nose drops
G Nasentropfen
F gouttes nasales
S gotas nasales

notch
G Kerbe
F fente, gorge
S muesca

Notified Body
G Benannte Stelle
F organisme cité
S departamento citado

novelty (e. g. of a product)
G Neuheitsgrad (z. B. eines Produktes)
F degré d'innovation (par ex. d'un produit)
S grado de novedad (p. ej. de un producto)

nozzle
G Düse
F buse, gicleur, tuyère
S aplicador, inyector, tobera

nozzle head
G Sprühkopf
F gicleur, buse
S cabeza del inyector

nozzle insert
G Düseneinsatz
F garniture d'un gicleur
S inserción de la tobera

nuclear magnetic resonance (NMR) spectroscopy
G Kernresonanzspektroskopie
F spectroscopie nucléaire à résonance magnétique
S espectroscopia de resonancia nuclear

nuclease-free water
G nukleasefreies Wasser
F eau dénuée de nucléase
S agua sin nucleasas

nucleic acid
G Nukleinsäure
F acide nucléique
S ácido nucleico

nucleophilic substitution
G nukleophile Substitution
F substitution nucléophilique
S sustitución nucleófila

nucleus
G Kern
F noyau
S núcleo

number of items
G Stückzahl
F nombre de pièces
S número de piezas

number of theoretical plates
G Zahl der theoretischen Böden
F nombre de plateaux théoriques
S número de placas teóricas

nut
G Mutter, Schraubenmutter
F écrou
S tuerca

nutrient
G Nährstoff
F aliment, produit nutritif, nutriment
S alimento, nutriente, sustancia nutricia

nutrient medium
G Nährmedium
F milieu de culture
S medio de cultivo

object lens
G Objektlinse
F lentille-objet
S lente del objetivo

obligatory
G verbindlich
F obligatoire
S obligatorio

without obligation
G unverbindlich
F ne comportant aucune obligation
S no obligatorio

oblong tablet
G längliche Tablette, Oblongtablette
F comprimé allongé, comprimé oblong
S comprimido elongado, comprimido oblongo

observation port
G Schauglas
F fenêtre d'observation
S ventana de observación

observation window
G Beobachtungsfenster, Schauglas, Sichtfenster
F fenêtre d'observation, fenêtre de visée
S ventana de observación, ventana visual

observation, special
G besondere Beobachtung
F observation particulière
S observación especial

obsolete
G veraltet, überholt
F obsolète, périmé, suranné, vieillot
S envejecido, obsoleto

occlusive dressing
G Okklusivverband
F bandage d'occlusion
S vendaje oclusivo

ocular
G Okular
F occulaire
S ocular

ocular use
G Anwendung am Auge
F pour usage ophtalmique
S uso oftálmico

odour
G Duft, Geruch
F odeur
S aroma, olor

odourless
G geruchlos
F sans odeur
S inodoro

oil bath
G Ölbad
F bain d'huile
S baño de aceite

oil separator
G Ölabscheider
F siphon de dépôt d'huile, séparateur d'huile, déshuileur
S separador de aceite

oil trap
G Ölabscheider
F siphon de dépôt d'huile, séparateur d'huile, déshuileur
S separador de aceite

oil/water emulsion
G Öl-in-Wasser-Emulsion
F émulsion d'huile dans l'eau
S emulsión de aceite en agua

oil-separating filter
G Ölabscheidefilter
F filtre de retenue d'huile
S filtro de separación de aceite

oily
G ölig
F huileux
S oleaginoso, oleoso

ointment
G Salbe
F pommade
S pomada, ungüento

ointment base
G Salbengrundlage
F ingrédient de base d'une pommade
S excipiente de una pomada

ointment mill
G Salbenmühle
F broyeur à pommade
S molino de pomada

oligomers
G Oligomere
F oligomères
S oligómero

omission
G Auslassung
F omission
S omisión

on/off switch
G Abschalter, Ausschalter
F interrupteur, bouton marche/arrêt
S interruptor (de desconexión)

on/off valve
G Absperrventil
F valve d'arrêt
S válvula de cierre

one-point cut (OPC) ampoule
G Brechampulle
F ampoule autocassable
S ampolla de apertura manual

on-site
G vor Ort
F sur site
S en el lugar

on-site installation
G Installation vor Ort
F installation sur site
S instalación in situ

on-site visit
G Ortsbesichtigung
F visite sur site
S visita del lugar

opalescence
G Opaleszenz
F opalescence
S opalescencia

opaque
G lichtundurchlässig, undurchsichtig
F opaque
S opaco

open case
G Anbruch
F emballage ouvert, emballage entamé
S envase abierto

open package
G Anbruch
F emballage ouvert, emballage entamé
S envase abierto

opening
G Öffnung
F ouverture
S abertura

operability
G Funktionsfähigkeit
F fonctionnalité
S capacidad funcional

operating conditions
G Betriebsbedingungen
F conditions de service
S condiciones de funcionamiento

operating instructions
G Bedienungsanleitung, Betriebsanleitung, Gebrauchsanweisung
F mode d'emploi, instructions opératoires, instructions de service, instructions pour l'utilisation
S instrucción de uso, instrucción de manejo, instrucción de servicio, instrucciones de funcionamiento

operating limit
G Betriebsgrenze
F limite de service, limite d'utilisation
S límite de funcionamiento

operating manual
G Betriebsanleitung
F mode d'emploi, instructions de service
S instrucciones de funcionamiento

operating mode
G Bedienungsmodus
F mode d'utilisation
S modo de servicio

operating panel
G Bedienungsfeld
F tableau d'utilisation
S panel de mandos

operating personnel
G Bedienungspersonal
F personnel de service
S personal de servicio

operating platform
G Bedienungsbühne
F plate-forme de commande
S plataforma de control

operating procedure
G Arbeitsanweisung, Arbeitsvorschrift
F procédure opératoire, instruction
S instrucción de trabajo, norma de trabajo

operating system
G Bedienungssystem
F système d'exploitation
S sistema de servicio

operating voltage
G Betriebsspannung
F voltage, tension de régime
S voltaje de funcionamiento

operation
G Arbeitsgang, Vorgang
F opération, processus
S proceso, turno de trabajo

unattended operation
G nicht unter Beobachtung stehender Vorgang
F processus non soumis à un contrôle
S proceso no observado

operational adjustment
G betriebliche Anpassung, Prozeßanpassung
F ajustement de fonctionnement, ajustement d'un procédé
S ajuste del funcionamiento, ajuste de un proceso

operational costs
G Betriebskosten
F coûts de fonctionnement
S costes de funcionamiento

operational cycle
G Arbeitsablauf
F cycle de fonctionnement
S ciclo de funcionamiento

operational parameter
G Betriebsparameter
F paramètre de service
S parámetro de servicio

operational qualification (OQ)
G Funktionsqualifizierung
F qualification opérationnelle
S cualificación funcional

operative aids
G Bedienhilfen
F aides au fonctionnement
S ayudas de funcionamiento

operator
G Durchführender
F exécutant, opérateur
S ejecutante, operador

operator console
G Bedienpult
F pupitre de commande, tableau de commande
S pupitre de mando, tablero de control

English German French Spanish

ophthalmic products
G Ophthalmica
F produits ophtalmiques
S productos oftálmicos

ophthalmic use
G Anwendung am Auge
F pour usage ophtalmique
S uso oftálmico

opinion leader
G Meinungsbildner
F leader d'opinion
S líder de opinión

optical antipodes
G optische Antipoden
F antipodes optiques
S antípodas ópticos

optical barrier
G Lichtschranke
F barrière optique
S barrera luminosa, barrera óptica

optical purity
G optische Reinheit
F pureté optique
S pureza óptica

optical rotation
G optische Drehung
F rotation optique
S rotación óptica

optimisation
G Optimierung
F optimisation
S optim(iz)ación

oral
G oral
F oral
S oral

oral administration
G perorale Darreichung
F administration orale
S administración peroral

oral ampoule
G Trinkampulle
F ampoule buvable
S ampolla bebible

oral drops
G Tropfen zum Einnehmen
F gouttes pour voie orale
S gotas orales

oral gel
G Gel zum Einnehmen
F gel pour administration orale
S gel oral

oral paste
G Paste zum Einnehmen
F pâte pour utilisation orale
S pasta oral

oral powder
G Pulver zum Einnehmen
F poudre à utilisation orale
S polvo oral

oral use, for
G zum Einnehmen
F pour administration orale
S para uso oral

orbital fusion welding
G Orbitalschweißen
F soudure orbitale
S soldadura orbital

orbitally welded
G orbital geschweißt
F soudé par soudure orbitale
S soldado orbitalmente

order
G Bestellung
F commande
S pedido

order number
G Auftragsnummer, Bestellnummer
F numéro de commande
S número del encargo,
número de pedido

order of magnitude
G Größenordnung
F ordre de magnitude
S orden de magnitud

organic base
G organische Base
F base organique
S base orgánica

organic phase
G organische Phase
F phase organique
S fase orgánica

organic solvent
G organisches Lösungsmittel
F solvant organique
S diluyente orgánico

organisation chart
G Organigramm
F organigramme
S organigrama

organism
G Keim
F germe, organisme microbien
S germen

organogram
G Organigramm
F organigramme
S organigrama

organoleptic testing
G Sinnesprüfung
F test organoleptique
S prueba organoléptica

organo-metallic compound
G metallorganische Verbindung
F composé organo-métallique
S compuesto organometálico

orifice
G Auslaß, Austritt, Mündung
F sortie, orifice
S descarga, desembocadura, escape, orificio, salida

origin of species
G Ursprungsart
F espèce d'origine
S especie de origen

original package
G Orginalpackung
F conditionnement d'origine
S envase original

O-ring
G O-Ring
F joint torique
S anillo tórico

oromucosal use
G Anwendung in der Mundhöhle
F usage bucco-mucosal
S uso bucal

oscillation
G Oszillation
F oscillation
S oscilación

osmolality
G Osmolalität
F osmolalité
S osmolalidad

osmometer
G Osmometer
F osmomètre
S osmómetro

osmosis
G Osmose
F osmose
S ósmosis

osmotic pressure
G osmotischer Druck
F pression osmotique
S presión osmótica

out-dated
G überholt
F périmé, suranné, vieillot
S obsoleto, envejecido

English
German
French
Spanish

outer carton
G Umkarton
F boîte, carton, carton d'expédition
S caja, cartón, cartón externo

outer lacquer
G Außenlack
F laque extérieure
S barniz externo

outer packaging
G Umverpackung
F emballage externe
S embalaje externo

outlet
G Ablauf, Auslaß, Auslauf, Austritt
F sortie de vidange, sortie de purge, orifice
S desagüe, descarga, escape, salida

outlet air
G Abluft
F air d'évacuation, air d'échappement
S aire de escape

outlet filter
G Auslaßfilter
F filtre de sortie
S filtro de descarga, filtro de salida

outlet nipple
G Ablaßstutzen, Auslaufstutzen
F manchon d'écoulement, manchon de drainage, manchon de purge
S empalme de salida

outlet port
G Ablaufstutzen
F manchon d'écoulement
S empalme de salida

outlet temperature
G Auslaßtemperatur
F température de sortie
S temperatura de salida

outlet valve
G Ablaßventil, Auslaßventil
F valve de sortie, vanne de purge, vanne de sortie
S válvula de salida

outlier
G Ausreißer
F valeur aberrante, anormale
S elemento fuera de los márgenes habituales

output
G Ausstoß (Menge)
F niveau de production, niveau de rendement
S volumen de producción

output per hour
G Stundenleistung
F rendement horaire, débit horaire
S rendimiento horario

outside air
G Außenluft
F air frais, air libre
S aire fresco, aire libre

ovality
G Ovalität
F forme ovale
S ovalidad

oven
G Wärmeschrank
F incubateur
S incubadora

overage
G Aufschlag
F supplément, majoration
S aumento, suplemento

overall dimensions
G Gesamtabmessungen
F dimensions totales
S dimensiones totales

overall height
G Gesamthöhe
F hauteur totale
S altura total

overall length
G Gesamtlänge
F longueur totale
S longitud total

overall width
G Gesamtbreite
F largeur totale
S anchura total

overdose
G Überdosierung
F surdosage, surdose
S sobredosificación

overdosed
G überdosiert
F surdosé, surdosage
S sobredosificado

overfill(ing)
G Überfüllung
F quantité en excès
S repleción

overflow
G Überlauf
F débordement
S desbordamiento, rebosadero

overflow vessel
G Überlaufgefäß
F récipient de débordement
S recipiente de desbordamiento

overlap
G Überschneidung
F chevauchement, recouvrement
S entrecruzamiento, interferencia

overload
G Überlastung
F surcharge
S sobrecarga

overloading
G Überlastung
F surcharge
S sobrecarga

overs
G Siebrückstand
F résidu de tamisage
S residuo de tamizado

overshoe
G Überschuhe
F couvre-chaussure
S chanclos

over-the-counter (OTC) product
G frei verkäufliches Produkt, OTC-Produkt, Selbstmedikationsprodukt
F produit sans ordonnance, produit en vente libre
S producto de venta libre, producto para automedicación

overwrite function
G Überschreibfunktion
F fonction d'écrasement
S función sobreescribir

oxidation
G Oxydierung
F oxydation
S oxidación

oxidisable
G oxydierbar
F oxydable
S oxidable

oxidising agent
G Oxydationsmittel
F oxydant
S oxidante

oximation
G Oximierung, Oximbildung
F oximation
S oximación

oxygen
G Sauerstoff
F oxygène
S oxígeno

oxygen content
G Sauerstoffgehalt
F teneur en oxygène
S contenido en oxígeno

oxygen release
G Sauerstoffentwicklung
F évolution de la teneur en oxygène
S liberación de oxígeno

English German French Spanish

English German French Spanish

oxygenation
G Oxigenierung
F oxygénation
S oxigenación

ozone
G Ozon
F ozone
S ozono

ozonisation
G Ozonisierung
F ozonisation, ozonation
S ozon(iz)ación

pack
G Gebinde, Packung
F emballage, conditionnement
S embalaje, envase, envoltura, haz

child-resistant pack
G kindergesicherte Verpackung
F conditionnement de sécurité pour enfants
S envase a prueba de niños

shrink-pack
G eingeschrumpftes Gebinde
F emballage sous film rétractable
S haz contraído, haz comprimido

pack, to
G einpacken
F emballer
S embalar, empaquetar, envasar

package
G Packung
F emballage, conditionnement
S embalaje, envase, envoltura

package design
G Verpackungsdesign
F design du conditionnement
S diseño de un envase

package insert
G Beipackzettel, Packungsbeilage
F notice (d'un emballage), notice explicative
S prospecto acompañante (del medicamento), prospecto informativo del medicamento

package integrity
G Unversehrtheit der Verpackung
F intégrité d'un conditionnement
S integridad de un embalaje

package leaflet
G Beipackzettel, Packungsbeilage
F notice (d'un emballage), notice explicative
S prospecto acompañante (del medicamento), prospecto informativo del medicamento

package loading
G Packguteinschub
F passage intercalé de conditionnements
S inserción de embalajes

package size
G Packungsgröße
F taille de l'emballage
S tamaño del envase

package stacking
G Packungsstapelung
F empilage de conditionnement
S apilamiento de envases

package, to
G konfektionieren, verpacken
F emballer
S embalar, empaquetar, envasar

packaging
G Konfektionierung, Verpackung (als Vorgang)
F conditionnement, emballage
S embalaje, empaquetado, envasado

packaging aids
G Packhilfsmittel
F auxiliaires de conditionnement
S materiales auxilares para envasado

packaging components
G Bestandteile der Packung
F constituants d'un emballage
S componentes del envase

packaging defect
G Verpackungsfehler
F défaut de conditionnement
S defecto de embalaje

packaging instruction
G Verpackungsanweisung
F instruction d'emballage
S instrucción de embalaje

packaging line
G Verpackungslinie
F chaîne de conditionnement, rampe de conditionnement
S cadena de empaquetado

packaging machine
G Verpackungsmaschine
F conditionneuse
S empaquetadora

packaging material
G Packmaterial, Packmittel, Verpackungsmaterial
F matériel d'emballage
S material de embalaje

printed packaging material
G bedrucktes Packmaterial
F matériel d'emballage imprimé
S material impreso de embalaje

packaging material dispensary
G Packmittelausgabe
F distribution du matériel d'emballage
S distribución de material de embalaje

packaging material manufacturer
G Packmittelhersteller
F fabricant de matériel d'emballage
S fabricante de material de embalaje

packaging material, primary
G primäres Packmittel
F conditionnement primaire
S medio de envasado primario

packaging material, secondary
G sekundäres Packmittel
F conditionnement secondaire
S medio de envasado secundario

packaging material, unprinted
G unbedrucktes Packmittel
F conditionnement non-imprimé
S medio de envasado no impreso

packaging order
G Verpackungsauftrag
F commande de conditionnement
S encargo de embalaje

packaging warehouse
G Packmittel-Lager
F magasin d'articles de conditionnement
S almacén de medios de envasado

packed density
G Stampfdichte
F densité de tassement
S densidad de apisonamiento

pad
G Tupfer
F tampon d'ouate, gaze
S torunda

paddle stirrer
G Blattrührerapparatur
F pale d'agitation
S pala de agitación

pallet
G Palette
F palette
S paleta

aluminium pallet
G Alupalette
F alupalette, palette en aluminium
S paleta de aluminio

plastic pallet
G Kunststoffpalette
F palette en plastique
S paleta de plástico

wooden pallet
G Holzpalette
F palette en bois
S paleta de madera

pallet store
G Palettenstellplatz
F dépôt de palettes
S almacén para paletas

palletise, to
G palettieren
F palettiser
S cargar con paleta

palletiser
G Palettiermaschine
F palettiseur
S máquina de carga con paleta

pan coater
G Trommelcoater
F machine d'enrobage à tambour
S máquina de tambor para gragear

pan-coat, to
G dragieren
F dragéifier
S preparar grageas (con cubierta de azúcar), gragear

panel
G Armaturentafel, Bedienpult
F pupitre de commande, tableau de bord, tableau de commande
S cuadro de mandos, pupitre de mando, tablero de control, tablero de instrumentos

paper printout
G Papierausdruck
F imprimé sur papier
S impreso (en papel, sobre papel)

parallel connection
G Parallelschaltung
F connection parallèle
S conexión paralela

parameter, critical
G kritischer Parameter
F paramètre critique
S parámetro crítico

parent company
G Mutterfirma
F société mère
S sociedad matriz

parenterals
G Parenteralia
F préparations injectables
S inyectables

large volume parenterals (LVP)
G großvolumige Parenteralia
F préparations injectables de grand volume
S inyectables voluminosos

small volume parenterals (SVP)
G kleinvolumige Parenteralia
F préparations injectables de petit volume
S inyectables de escaso volumen

part
G Teil
F partie, portion
S parte

part subject to wear
G Verschleißteil
F pièce sujette à l'usure
S pieza desgastable

partial batch
G Teilcharge
F sous-lot
S lote parcial, sublote

partial hydrolysis
G partielle Hydrolyse
F hydrolyse partielle
S hidrólisis parcial

partial pressure
G Partialdruck
F pression partielle
S presión parcial

participation
G Beteiligung
F participation
S participación

particle
G Partikel, Teilchen
F particule
S partícula

airborne particles
G aus der Luft stammende Partikel
F particules aéroportées
S partículas procedentes del aire

fine particles
G feine Körnung
F granulation fine
S granulación fina

viable particles
G lebensfähige Partikel
F particules viables
S partículas viables

particle count
G Partikelzahlen
F nombre de particules
S número de partículas

particle counter
G Partikelzähler
F compteur de particules
S contador de partículas

particle distribution
G Partikelverteilung
F distribution des particules
S distribución de partículas

particle filter
G Partikelfilter
F filtre à particules
S filtro de partículas

particle form
G Partikelform, Teilchenform
F forme d'une particule
S forma de la partícula

particle generation
G Partikelerzeugung
F génération de particules
S producción de partículas

particle measuring instrument
G Partikelmeßgerät
F appareil de mesure des particules
S aparato de medición de partículas

particle monitoring
G Partikelmonitoring
F contrôle des particules
S control de partículas

particle separation rate
G Partikelabscheiderate
F taux de retenue des particules
S tasa de separación de partículas

particle shape
G Teilchenform
F forme d'une particule
S forma de la partícula

particle size
G Korngröße, Partikelgröße, Teilchengröße
F taille des particules
S tamaño del grano, tamaño de la partícula

particle size distribution
G Korngrößenverteilung
F distribution de la taille des particules
S distribución del tamaño de los granos

particle spectrometer
G Teilchenspektrometer
F spectomètre de particules
S espectrometría de partículas

particle-free
G partikelfrei
F libre de particules
S sin partículas

particle-releasing material
G partikelabgebendes Material
F matériau libérant des particules
S material que desprende partículas

particulate matter
G Partikel
F particules
S partículas

parting agent
G Formentrennmittel
F séparateur de formes
S separador de formas

partition (wall)
G Stellwand, Trennwand, Zwischenwand
F mur de partage, mur de séparation
S pantalla protectora, tabique (de separación)

part-time employee
G Teilzeitkraft
F employé à mi-temps
S empleado a tiempo parcial

passage
G Durchlauf
F passage
S paso

passivated
G passiviert
F passivé
S pasivado

passivation (e. g. of steel)
G Passivierung (z. B. von Stahl)
F passivation (par ex. de l'acier inoxydable)
S pasivación (p. ej. de acero)

password
G Paßwort
F mot de passe
S consigna

paste
G Paste
F pâte
S pasta

pasteboard
G Pappe
F carton
S cartón

paste-like
G pastenartig
F pâteux
S pastoso

pasteurisation
G Pasteurisierung
F pasteurisation
S paste(u)rización

pastille
G Lutschtablette, Pastille
F pastille, tablette à sucer
S comprimido para chupar, pastilla

pasty
G teigartig, pastös, pastenartig
F pâteux
S pastoso

patent
G Patent
F brevet
S patente

infringement of a patent
G Verletzung eines Patentes
F violation de brevet
S violación de patente

patent application
G Patentbeantragung
F demande de brevet
S solicitud de patente

patent approval
G Erteilung eines Patentes
F approbation de brevet
S aprobación de patente

patent claim
G Patentanspruch
F droits liés à un brevet
S reclamación de patente

patent duration
G Patentgültigkeitsdauer
F durée de validité d'un brevet
S duración de la validez de una patente

patent expiry
G Auslaufen des Patentes
F expiration d'un brevet
S expiración de una patente

patent filing
G Patentanmeldung, Patenteinreichung
F dépôt de demande de brevet
S solicitud de patente

patent life
G Patentgültigkeitsdauer
F durée de validité d'un brevet
S duración de la validez de una patente

patent office
G Patentamt
F office des brevets
S oficina de patentes

patent prolongation
G Patentfristerneuerung
F prorogation d'un brevet
S prolongación del plazo de patente

patent protection
G Patentschutz
F protection d'un brevet
S protección de patentes

patent scope
G Patentumfang
F étendue d'un brevet
S extensión de una patente

patented
G patentiert
F breveté
S patentado

pathogen
G Erreger (Mikroorganismus), Krankheitserreger
F pathogène
S agente patógeno (microorganismo), patógeno

pathogenic
G pathogen
F pathogénique
S patógeno

pathological
G pathologisch
F pathologique
S patológico

patient
G Patient
F patient
S paciente

patient identification number
G Patientennummer
F numéro d'identification d'un patient
S número de identificación del paciente

patient information leaflet
G Patientenbroschüre
F brochure d'information pour patient
S folleto de información del paciente

peak
G Peak
F pic
S pico

extraneous peak
G nicht zugehöriger Peak
F pic étranger
S pico extraño

peak area
G Peakfläche
F surface de pic
S superficie del pico

peak height
G Peakhöhe
F hauteur de pic
S altura del pico

peak purity
G Peakreinheit
F pureté de pic
S pureza del pico

peak shoulder
G Peakschulter
F épaulement de pic
S hombro del pico

English German French Spanish

peak spreading
G Peakverbreiterung
F étalement de pic
S ensanchamiento del pico

peak width
G Peakbreite
F largeur de pic
S anchura del pico

pebble mill
G Kugelmühle
F broyeur à boulets
S molinillo a bolas

pellet
G Pellet, Preßling
F pellet, implant, pastille, boulette
S pellet, masa comprimida

pelletise, to
G pelletieren
F pastiller, transformer en pastilles
S transformar en pellets

penetrate, to
G eindringen
F pénétrer
S penetrar

penetration
G Durchdringung, Penetration
F pénétration
S penetración

penetration depth
G Eindringtiefe
F profondeur de pénétration
S profundidad de penetración

peptone
G Pepton
F peptone
S peptona

percolate, to
G perkolieren
F extrahir par percolation
S percolar

percolation
G Perkolation
F percolation
S percolación

perforable bottle
G Durchstechflasche
F bouteille perforable
S botella perforable

perforate, to
G perforieren
F perforer
S perforar

perforated
G gelocht
F perforé
S perforado

perforated base
G Lochboden
F base perforée
S suelo perforado

perforation
G Perforierung
F perforation
S perforación

perforation tool
G Perforierwerkzeug
F outil de perforation
S instrumentos de perforación

performance
G Leistung
F performance
S rendimiento

performance qualification
G Leistungsqualifizierung, Verfahrensqualifizierung
F qualification des performances (d'un procédé)
S cualificación del rendimiento, cualificación de un procedimiento

period of incubation
G Inkubationsdauer
F période d'incubation
S período de incubación

period of use (of filters)
G Standzeit (von Filtern)
F période d'utilisation (de filtres)
S período de uso (de filtros)

period of validity
G Gültigkeitsdauer
F durée de validité
S período de validez

peripheral instrumentation
G periphere Geräte
F appareils périphériques
S aparatos periféricos

peristaltic pump
G Dosierpumpe, Schlauchpumpe
F pompe doseuse, pompe péristaltique
S bomba de dosificación, bomba peristáltica

permanent hardness (of water)
G permanente Härte (von Wasser)
F dureté permamente (de l'eau)
S dureza permanente (del agua)

permanently installed
G fest installiert
F installé de manière permanente
S instalado fijamente

permeability
G Durchlässigkeit, Permeabilität
F perméabilité
S permeabilidad

permeable
G durchlässig, permeabel
F perméable
S permeable

permeable membrane
G permeable Membran
F membrane perméable
S membrana permeable

permeable to air
G luftdurchlässig
F perméable à l'air
S permeable al aire

permeation
G Durchdringung
F pénétration
S penetración

permissible
G zulässig
F permis
S permitido

peroxide index
G Peroxydzahl
F index de peroxyde
S índice de peróxido

peroxide number
G Peroxydzahl
F index de peroxyde
S índice de peróxido

person responsible
G Sachbearbeiter
F responsable
S encargado, ponente

personnel cost
G Personalkosten
F coûts du personnel
S costes del personal

personnel department
G Personalabteilung
F service de personnel
S departamento de personal

personnel file
G Personalakte
F acte du personnel
S acta personal

personnel flow
G Personalfluß
F flux du personnel
S flujo de personal

personnel hygiene
G Personalhygiene
F hygiène du personnel
S higiene personal

personnel lock
G Personalschleuse
F sas réservé au personnel
S entrada para el personal

personnel protection
G Personenschutz
F sécurité du personnel
S seguridad del personal

personnel safety
G Personenschutz
F sécurité du personnel
S seguridad del personal

personnel training
G Personalschulung
F formation du personnel
S formación del personal

pertinent
G relevant
F pertinent, approprié
S relevante

pessary
G Vaginalzäpfchen
F suppositoire vaginal
S supositorio vaginal

pest control
G Schädlingsbekämpfung
F lutte antiparasitaire
S control de plagas, lucha antiparasitaria

pesticide
G Pestizid, Schädlingsvertilgungsmittel
F pesticide
S pesticida

pestle
G Pistill
F pilon
S pistilo

Petri dish
G Petrischale
F boîte de Petri
S placa de Petri

petrochemicals
G petrochemische Substanzen
F substances pétrochimiques
S sustancias petroquímicas

pH
G pH-Wert
F pH
S pH

pH adjustment
G pH-Wert-Einstellung
F ajustement du pH
S ajuste del pH

pH meter
G pH-Meter
F pH-mètre
S pH metro

pharmaceutical division
G Pharma-Sparte
F division pharmaceutique
S sector farmacéutico

pharmaceutical grade
G entspricht Arzneibuchqualität
F qualité pharmaceutique
S calidad farmacéutica

pharmaceutical manufacturer
G pharmazeutischer Unternehmer
F industriel de la pharmacie
S fabricante farmacéutico

pharmaceutical sample
G Ärztemuster
F échantillon pharmaceutique
S muestra farmacéutica

pharmaceutical water
G Pharma-Wasser
F eau pharmaceutique
S agua farmacéutica

pharmacist
G Apotheker
F pharmacien
S farmacéutico

pharmacokinetics
G Pharmakokinetik
F pharmacocinétique
S farmacocinética

pharmacological activity
G pharmakologische Aktivität
F activité pharmacologique
S actividad farmacológica

pharmacology
G Pharmakologie
F pharmacologie
S farmacología

pharmacopoeia
G Arzneibuch, Pharmakopöe
F pharmacopée
S farmacopea

pharmacopoeial monograph
G Arzneibuchmonographie
F monographie de la pharmacopée
S monografía de farmacopea

pharmaco-vigilance manager
G Stufenplanbeauftragter
F personne responsable de la pharmaco-vigilance
S responsable de farmacovigilancia

phase diagram
G Phasendiagramm
F diagramme de phases
S diagrama de fases

phase distribution
G Phasenverteilung
F distribution de phases
S distribución de fases

phase transition
G Phasenübergang
F transition de phase
S transición de fase

phosphorescence
G Phosphoreszenz
F phosphorescence
S fosforescencia

photo cell
G Photozelle
F cellule photoélectrique
S célula fotoeléctrica

photochemical
G photochemisch
F photochimique
S fotoquímico

photoelectric cell
G Photozelle
F cellule photoélectrique
S célula fotoeléctrica

photolysis
G Photolyse
F photolyse
S fotólisis

photometer
G Photometer
F photomètre
S fotómetro

photometry
G Photometrie
F photométrie
S fotometría

physical characteristics
G physikalische Eigenschaften
F caractéristiques physiques
S propiedades físicas

physical examination
G körperliche Untersuchung
F inspection physique
S exploración física

physical inspection
G körperliche Untersuchung
F inspection physique
S exploración física

physical segregation
G räumliche Trennung
F ségrégation physique
S separación espacial

physical-chemical characteristics
G physikalisch-chemische Eigenschaften
F caractéristiques physico-chimiques
S propiedades fisicoquímicas

physiological saline
G physiologische Kochsalzlösung
F solution saline physiologique
S solución salina fisiológica

physiological testing
G physiologische Prüfung
F examen physiologique
S prueba fisiológica

phyto-
G pflanzlich
F végétal
S vegetal

phytochemistry
G Phytochemie
F phytochimie
S fitoquímica

phytopharmaceuticals
G Phytopharmaka, pflanzliche Arzneimittel
F phytopharmaceutiques
S fitofármacos

pickle, to
G beizen
F mariner
S adobar, cauterizar, desinfectar

pickled
G gebeizt
F décapé
S decapado, macerado

pickled and blasted
G gebeizt und gestrahlt
F poncé et décapé
S decapado y pulido

pie chart
G Kreisdiagramm
F diagramme à secteurs
S diagrama circular

piece
G Bruchstück
F morceau, fragment
S fragmento

pierce, to
G durchstechen
F transpercer
S perforar

piezo ignition
G piezoelektrische Zündung
F allumage piezoélectrique
S encendido piezoeléctrico

pigment
G Farbe, Pigment
F colorant, teinture, pigment
S color, pigmento, tintura

pile
G Stapel
F pile
S montón, pila

pill
G Pille
F pilule
S píldora

pilot batch
G Versuchscharge
F lot pilote
S lote piloto

pilot plant
G Versuchsanlage
F usine pilote
S instalación piloto

pilot scale
G Versuchsmaßstab
F échelle pilote
S escala piloto

pilot scale production
G Produktion im Versuchsmaßstab
F production à l'échelle pilote
S producción a escala piloto

pin
G Stift
F broche, pointeau, goupille
S clavija, perno, pivote

pin holes
G Nadellöcher
F perforations d'aiguille
S perforaciones de aguja

pin mill
G Stiftmühle
F broyeur à broches
S molino de clavija

pinch, to
G quetschen
F écraser
S aplastar

pinion
G Ritzel
F pignon
S piñón

pipe bend
G Knierohr
F tuyau coudé
S tubo acodado

pipe(work)
G Rohrleitung
F canalisation
S canalización

pipeline
G Rohrleitung
F canalisation
S canalización

pipette
G Pipette
F pipette
S pipeta

pipette bottle
G Pipettenflasche
F flacon de pipette
S frasco de pipeteo

pipette off, to
G abpipettieren
F pipetter
S pipetear

pipette tip
G Pipettenspitze
F pointe de pipette
S punta de pipeta

pipetting aid
G Pipettierhilfe
F système d'aide au pipettage
S sistema de ayuda para pipetear

pipetting system
G Pipettiersystem
F système de pipettage
S sistema de pipeteo

pipettor
G Pipettiersystem
F système de pipettage
S sistema de pipeteo

piping (gas, water)
G Leitung (Gas, Wasser)
F conduite (de gaz, d'eau)
S conducción, tubería (gas, agua)

piping and instrument diagram (P&ID)
G R+I-Schema
F schéma fonctionnel et instrumental; schéma de l'installation, des canalisations et diagrammes des instruments
S esquema de procesos e instrumentos; esquema de instalación, de canalización y diagramas de instrumentos

piping designation
G Rohrleitungskennzeichnung
F marquage des tuyaux
S caracterización de cañerías

piping system
G Rohrleitungssystem
F système de canalisation
S sistema de canalización

English German French Spanish

piston
G Kolben
F piston
S émbolo, pistón

piston drive
G Kolbenantrieb
F entraînement par piston
S propulsión por émbolo

piston rod
G Kolbenstange
F tige de piston
S barra del émbolo

pitch die
G Matrizenbohrung
F forure d'une matrice
S orificio de matriz

pivotable
G schwenkbar
F pivotable
S giratorio

pivotted
G ausgeschwenkt
F pivoté
S girado hacia fuera

pixel
G Pixel
F pixel
S píxel

place of work
G Arbeitsplatz
F poste de travail
S puesto de trabajo, empleo

placebo
G Placebo
F placebo
S placebo

placebo-controlled
G placebokontrolliert
F contrôlé par placebo
S controlado por placebo

placement
G Plazierung
F placement
S colocación

placing on the market
G Inverkehrbringen
F introduction sur le marché
S introducción en el mercado

plan
G Grundriß
F plan (horizontal)
S plano (horizontal)

plane
G eben
F plat
S liso, llano, plano

planetary mixer
G Planetenmischer
F mélangeur planétaire
S mezclador planetario

plant (machines)
G Anlage (Maschine), Betriebsstätte, Einrichtung (in Gebäuden), pflanzlich
F usine, établissement industriel, installation, installation industrielle, site de fabrication, végétal
S equipo, instalación (máquina), instalación (en edificios), plantas empresariales, vegetal

dedicated plant
G Einrichtung für einen bestimmten Zweck
F installation industrielle dédiée
S instalación para un fin determinado

plant area
G Betriebsfläche
F surface d'une installation
S área de las instalaciones empresariales

plant audit
G Betriebsprüfung
F audit d'une installation
S auditoría de empresa

plant control
G Anlagensteuerung
F système de contrôle d'une installation
S control de plantas e instalaciones

plant expansion
G Betriebserweiterung
F agrandissement d'une installation
S ampliación de la empresa

plant hygiene
G Betriebshygiene
F hygiène des installations
S higiene de la empresa

plant maintenance
G Anlagenwartung
F maintenance d'une installation
S mantenimiento de equipo e instalaciones

plant management
G Betriebsführung
F management d'une installation
S gestión empresarial

plant manager
G Betriebsleiter, Werksleiter
F directeur d'usine, directeur technique
S director de taller, director técnico de la empresa

plant sanitation
G Betriebshygiene
F hygiène des installations
S higiene de la empresa

plant steam
G Betriebsdampf
F vapeur d'une installation
S vapor de una planta

plant-based
G pflanzlich
F végétal
S vegetal

plastered
G verputzt
F crépi
S enlucido, revocado

plastered wall
G verputzte Wand
F mur revêtu d'un crépi
S pared revocada

plastic
G Kunststoff, plastisch
F plastique
S plástico

plastic ampoule
G Kunststoffampulle
F ampoule en plastique
S ampolla de plástico

plastic barrel
G Kunststoffaß
F tonneau en plastique
S tonel de plástico

plastic bottle
G Kunststoff-Flasche
F bouteille en plastique
S botella de plástico

plastic coating
G Kunststoffbeschichtung
F revêtement plastique
S revestimiento plástico

plastic film
G Plastikfolie
F film plastique
S lámina de plástico

plastic material
G Kunststoff
F plastique
S plástico

plastic packaging
G Kunststoffverpackung
F emballage plastique
S embalaje de plástico

plastic pallet
G Kunststoffpalette
F palette en plastique
S paleta de plástico

plastic-coated
G kunststoffbeschichtet
F revêtu de plastique
S revestido de plástico

plasticiser
G Weichmacher
F plastifiant
S plastificante

plasticity
G Plastizität
F plasticité
S plasticidad

plate
G Blech
F tôle
S chapa, lámina, plancha

plate method (in microbiology)
G Plattengußverfahren (Mikrobiologie)
F coulage de plaques (microbiologie)
S método de placas (microbiología)

plate number
G Bodenzahl
F nombre de plateaux
S número de placa

plate spacing
G Plattenabstand
F distance entre plateaux
S distancia entre placas

Plexiglas
G Plexiglas
F plexiglas
S plexiglás

pliable
G biegsam
F flexible, pliable
S flexible, maleable, plegable

plug
G Stopfen
F bouchon, tampon
S tapón

plug connection
G Steckkupplung
F connexion à fiche(s)
S conexión de enchufe

plumbing
G Verrohrung
F plomberie
S instalación de conducciones

pneumatic
G pneumatisch
F pneumatique
S neumático

point of withdrawal
G Entnahmestelle
F point de retrait
S lugar de extracción

pointer
G Zeiger
F aiguille, indicateur
S indicador

poison
G Gift, Giftstoff, Toxin
F poison, toxine
S sustancia venenosa, tóxico, toxina, veneno

poisonous
G giftig, toxisch
F toxique
S tóxico, venenoso

polar
G polar
F polaire
S polar

polarimeter
G Polarimeter
F polarimètre
S polarímetro

polariser
G Polarisator
F polariseur
S polarizador

polarity
G Polarität
F polarité
S polaridad

policy
G Leitlinie
F directive
S directiva

polish
G Poliermittel
F produit de polissage
S producto para pulir

polish, to
G polieren
F polir
S bruñir, pulir

polluting
G umweltverschmutzend
F polluant
S polucionante

polyaromatic hydrocarbons (PAH)
G polyaromatische Kohlenwasserstoffe (PAK)
F hydrocarbures polyaromatiques
S hidrocarburos poliaromáticos

polycyclic
G polycyclisch
F polycyclique
S policíclico

polyethylene coating
G Polyethylenbeschichtung
F couverture en polyéthylène
S cubierta de polietileno

polymer
G polymer
F polymère
S polímero

polystyrene insert
G Polystyrol-Einsatz
F insert en polystyrène
S inserción de poliestirol

polyvinyl chloride (PVC)
G Polyvinylchlorid (PVC)
F chlorure de polyvinyl (PVC)
S cloruro de polivinilo

polyvinylidene fluoride (PVDF)
G Polyvinylidenfluorid
F fluorure de polyvinylidène (PVDF)
S fluoruro de polivinilideno

poorly reactive
G reaktionsträge
F inerte
S inerte

pore diameter
G Porendurchmesser
F diamètre d'un pore
S diámetro de poro

pore size
G Porengröße
F taille d'un pore
S tamaño del poro

pore volume
G Porenvolumen
F volume d'un pore
S volumen del poro

pore-free
G porenfrei
F dépourvu de pores
S sin poros

porosity
G Porosität
F porosité
S porosidad

porous
G porös
F poreux
S poroso

portioned packaging
G portionierte Abpackung
F conditionnement en plusieurs phases
S envase porcionado

positive pressure
G Überdruck
F surpression
S sobrepresión

potable water
G Trinkwasser
F eau potable
S agua corriente potable

potent
G wirksam
F efficace
S activo, eficaz

potentation
G Potenzierung
F potentialisation
S potenciación

potential applications
G potentielle Anwendungen
F applications potentielles
S aplicaciones potenciales

potentiometer
G Potentiometer
F potentiomètre
S potenciómetro

poultice
G Umschlagpaste
F cataplasme
S cataplasma

powder
G Puder, Pulver
F poudre
S polvo

loose powder
G loses Pulver
F poudre en vrac
S polvo suelto

powder bed
G Pulverbett
F lit de poudre
S lecho de polvo

powder density
G Pulverdichte
F densité d'une poudre
S densidad del polvo

powder feeder
G Pulverdosierschnecke
F vis doseuse pour poudre
S tornillo sin fin dosificador de polvo

powder fraction
G Pulverfraktion
F fraction de poudre
S fracción de polvo

powder sampler
G Stechheber
F dispositif d'échantillonnage, pipette de prélèvement
S pipeta (de toma de muestras)

powder, to
G pulverisieren
F pulvériser
S pulverizar

powdered mixture
G Pulvermischung
F mélange de poudre
S mezcla de polvo

powdery
G pudrig
F poudreux
S pulverulento

power absorber
G Kraftaufnehmer
F absorbeur d'énergie
S absorbedor de fuerza

power consumption
G Leistungsverbrauch, Stromaufnahme
F consommation d'énergie, consommation d'électricité
S consumo de energía, consumo de electricidad

power failure
G Stromausfall
F coupure de courant
S corte de corriente

intermittent power interruption
G zeitweiser Stromausfall
F coupure de courant intermittente
S corte intermitente de corriente, corte transitorio de corriente

power input
G Leistungsaufnahme
F puissance absorbée
S absorción de potencia

power source
G Stromquelle
F source d'électricité
S fuente de electricidad

power station
G Kraftwerk
F centrale énergétique
S central energética

power supply
G Netzgerät, Stromversorgung, Versorgungsstrom
F alimentation en courant électrique, courant d'alimentation
S alimentador a la red, corriente de alimentación, suministro eléctrico

power supply fluctuation
G Netzschwankungen, Stromversorgungsschwankungen
F variations de l'intensité du courant
S fluctuaciones de la intensidad de corriente eléctrica, fluctuaciones del suministro eléctrico

power switch
G Hauptschalter, Netzschalter
F interrupteur principal, interrupteur de courant
S interruptor principal, interruptor a la red

pre-amplification
G Vorverstärkung
F préamplification
S preamplificación

pre-assembly
G Vormontage
F pré-assemblé
S montaje previo

pre-blend, to
G vormischen
F mélanger à l'avance
S mezclar previamente

precaution
G Vorsichtsmaßnahme
F précaution
S medida precautoria

precious metal
G Edelmetall
F métal précieux
S metal noble

precipitate
G Fällung, Niederschlag
F précipitation, précipité
S precipitación, precipitado

precipitate, to
G ausfällen
F précipiter
S precipitar

precipitating agent
G Fällungsmittel
F agent de précipitation
S agente de precipitación

precipitation
G Ausfällung, Fällung
F précipitation, précipité
S precipitación, precipitado

precipitation agent
G Ausfällungsmittel
F agent de précipitation
S agente precipitador

precipitation titration
G Fällungstitration
F titrage de précipitation, dosage de précipitation
S volumetría de precipitación

precise
G präzise
F précis
S preciso

precision
G Genauigkeit (einer Prüfmethode), Präzision
F précision
S exactitud (de un método de prueba), precisión

precision balance
G Feinwaage, Präzisionswaage
F balance de précision
S balanza de precisión

precision repeatability
G Wiederholbarkeit der Präzision
F répétitivité de la précision
S repetitividad de la precisión

precoat, to (tablets)
G andecken (beim Dragieren)
F pré-enrober
S prerrecubrir (grageas)

pre-column
G Vorsäule
F colonne préalable
S columna previa

pre-compression force
G Vorpreßkraft
F force de compression préalable
S fuerza de compresión previa

predecessor
G Vorgänger
F prédécesseur
S predecesor

pre-delivery check
G Vorabnahme (beim Hersteller)
F contrôle avant livraison
S control antes de entrega

prefilled syringe
G Fertigspritze
F seringue prête à l'usage
S jeringa dispuesta para el uso

pre-filter
G Vorfilter
F filtre préalable
S filtro previo

pre-folded package insert
G vorgefaltete Packungsbeilage
F notice explicative dépliante
S prospecto informativo del medicamento previamente plegado

pre-formulation
G Präformulierung
F préformulation
S preformulación

pre-insertion
G Voreinschub
F pré-insertion
S preinserción

preliminary batch
G Vorcharge
F lot préliminaire
S carga previa

premises
G Räumlichkeiten
F locaux
S locales

pre-mix
G Vormischung
F pré-mélange
S mezcla previa

pre-mix, to
G vormischen
F mélanger à l'avance
S mezclar previamente

pre-mixed
G vorgemischt
F mélangé à l'avance
S mezclado previamente

preparation
G Zubereitung
F préparation, formulation
S formulación, preparación

preparation of solution
G Lösungsherstellung
F préparation d'une solution
S preparación de una solución

pre-pressing roller
G Vordruckrolle (Tablettenpresse)
F rouleau presseur
S rollo de prensado previo (comprimidos)

pre-printed
G vorbedruckt
F imprimé à l'avance
S preimpreso

pre-printed form
G Vordruck
F formulaire
S formulario

prescription
G Rezept, Verschreibung, verschreibungspflichtig
F ordonnance, vendu sur ordonnance
S prescripción, receta, de receta obligatoria

non-prescription
G nicht verschreibungspflichtig
F vendu sans ordonnance
S de venta libre

prescription only
G rezeptpflichtig
F disponible seulement sur ordonnance
S con receta médica

pre-selection
G Vorauswahl
F pré-sélection
S preselección

presence
G Anwesenheit
F présence
S presencia

preservation
G Konservierung
F conservation
S conservación

preservative
G Konservierungsmittel
F conservateur
S medio de conservación

preserve, to
G konservieren
F conserver
S conservar

preserved
G konserviert
F conservé
S conservado

pre-setting
G Voreinstellung
F pré-réglage
S prerreglaje

pressing material
G Preßmaterial
F matériel de moulage, matériel de pressage
S material de prensado

pressure
G Druck
F pression
S presión

negative pressure
G Unterdruck
F souspression
S presión baja

positive pressure
G Überdruck
F surpression
S sobrepresión

pressure column
G Druckkolonne
F colonne sous pression
S columna a presión

English German French Spanish

English German French Spanish

pressure column distillation plant
G Druckkolonnendestillationsanlage
F appareil de distillation à colonnes multiples
S aparato de destilación a columna de presión

pressure control (excess pressure)
G Druckkontrolle (bei Überdruck)
F contrôle de la pression
S control de presión (en caso de sobrepresión)

pressure differential
G Differenzdruck, Druckdifferenz
F différence de pression, pression différentielle
S diferencia de presión, presión diferencial

pressure differential indicator
G Differenzdruckanzeiger
F indicateur de pression différentielle
S indicador de presión diferencial

pressure drop
G Druckabfall
F chute de pression, dépressurisation
S descenso de presión

pressure equilibrium
G Druckausgleich
F compensation de pression
S equilibrio de presión

pressure fluctuation
G Druckschwankung
F fluctuation de pression
S fluctuación de presión

pressure gauge
G Druckmeßgerät
F manomètre
S manómetro

pressure increase
G Druckanstieg
F augmentation de pression
S aumento de presión

pressure loading
G Druckbelastung
F charge de pression
S carga de presión

pressure reading
G Druckablesung
F relevé de la pression
S lectura de la presión

pressure regulator
G Druckregler
F régulateur de pression
S regulador de presión

pressure release outlet
G Druckablaß
F sortie de régulation de pression
S salida de presión

pressure relief duct
G Druckentlastungskanal
F canalisation de décompression
S canal de descompresión

pressure relief opening
G Druckentlastungsöffnung
F ouverture de décompression
S orificio de descompresión

pressure relief valve
G Druckentlastungsklappe
F soupape de sûreté (pour la pression)
S válvula de descompresión

pressure resistance
G Druckfestigkeit
F résistance à la pression
S resistencia a la presión

pressure test
G Druckhaltetest
F test de pression de retenue
S prueba de retención de la presión

pressure transmitter
G Druckaufnehmer
F transmetteur de pression
S transmisor de presión

pressure tubing
G Druckschlauch
F tuyauterie apte à la pression
S tubo de presión

pressure vessel
G Druckgefäß
F récipient sous pression
S recipiente a presión

pressure-measuring point
G Druckmeßdose
F point de mesure de la pression
S punto de medida de presión

pressure-resistant
G druckfest
F résistant à la pression
S resistente a la presión

pressurisation level
G Druckhöhe
F niveau de pressurisation
S altura de presión

pressurisation system
G Drucksystem
F système de pressurisation
S sistema de presurización

pressurised container
G Druckbehälter
F récipient pressurisé, récipient soumis à la pression
S recipiente presurizado

pressurised reaction vessel
G Druckreaktionskessel
F cuve à réaction sous pression
S caldera presurizada de reacción

pre-treatment
G Vorbehandlung
F traitement préalable
S pretratamiento

prevent, to
G verhindern
F empêcher, éviter
S evitar, impedir

prevention
G Vermeidung
F prévention
S evitación

preventive maintenance
G vorbeugende Wartung
F entretien préventif
S mantenimiento preventivo

primary contamination
G Primärkontamination
F contamination primaire
S contaminación primaria

primary formulation
G Primärformulierung
F formulation primaire
S formulación primaria

primary packaging material
G Primärpackmittel
F matériel d'emballage primaire
S material primario de envase

primary steam
G Primärdampf
F vapeur primaire
S vapor primario

prime, to
G grundieren
F amorcer
S enderezar, dar la primera capa

principal
G Auftraggeber
F donneur d'ordre, commettant, client
S cliente, comitente

print control (printed matter)
G Druckkontrolle (von Aufdruckdaten)
F contrôle de l'impression
S control de impresos

print recognition
G Druckerkennung
F identification de l'impression
S identificación del impreso

English German French Spanish

print release
G Druckfreigabe
F autorisation d'imprimer
S autorización para imprimir

print, to
G bedrucken
F imprimer
S imprimir, estampar

printer
G Drucker
F imprimante
S impresora

ink jet printer
G Tintenstrahldrucker
F imprimante à jet d'encre
S impresora de chorro de tinta

laser printer
G Laserdrucker
F imprimante à laser
S impresora de láser

printer ink
G Druckerfarbe
F couleur d'imprimante
S impresora a color

printing block
G Klischee
F cliché
S cliché

printing roller
G Druckwalze
F cylindre à imprimer
S rodillo de imprenta

print-out, printout
G Ausdruck, Schreiberausdruck
F imprimé
S impreso

paper printout, hard copy
G Papierausdruck
F imprimé sur papier
S impreso sobre papel

prion proteins (prp)
G Prionproteine
F protéines-prions (prp)
S proteína priónica (prp)

probe
G Sonde
F sonde
S sonda

problem decision plan
G Problementscheidungsplan
F plan de solutionnement d'un problème
S plan para decidir problemas

procedural change
G Verfahrensänderung
F modification d'un procédé
S modificación del procedimiento

procedure
G Verfahren
F procédé
S procedimiento

process adjustment
G betriebliche Anpassung, Prozeßanpassung
F ajustement de fonctionnement, ajustement d'un procédé
S ajuste del funcionamiento, ajuste de un proceso

process automation
G Prozeßautomatisierung
F automatisation d'un procédé
S automa(tiza)ción de un proceso

process control
G Prozeßsteuerung
F contrôle d'un procédé
S control de un proceso

process control system
G Prozeßleitsystem
F système de gestion d'un procédé
S sistema de gestión de un proceso

process development
G Verfahrensentwicklung
F développement d'un procédé
S desarrollo de un procedimiento

process documentation
G Prozeßdokumentation
F documentation d'un procédé
S documentación de un proceso

process environment
G Prozeßumgebung
F environnement d'un procédé
S entorno de un proceso

process equipment
G Produktionsanlagen
F équipement d'un procédé de fabrication
S equipo de instrumentos para el proceso de producción

process flow diagram (PFD)
G Prozeßflußdiagramm
F schéma fonctionnel
S diagrama de flujo de procesos

process robustness
G Robustheit des Prozesses
F robustesse d'un procédé
S robustez del proceso

process technology
G Verfahrenstechnik
F technique des procédés
S técnica del procedimiento

process temperature
G Prozeßtemperatur
F température d'un procédé
S temperatura de un proceso

process validation
G Prozeßvalidierung
F validation d'un procédé
S validación de un proceso

process variability
G Prozeßvariabilität
F variabilité du processus
S variabilidad de un proceso

process water
G Prozeßwasser
F eau pour opérations
S agua de procesado

process, in
G im Betriebszustand
F sous condition d'exploitation
S funcionando

process, to
G aufarbeiten
F traiter
S procesar

processable
G verarbeitungsfähig
F traitable
S procesable

processing
G Aufarbeitung, Bearbeitung, Verarbeitung
F fabrication, mise en forme, traitement
S elaboración, proceso, transformación

machine processing
G maschinelle Verarbeitung
F traitement automatique
S elaboración automática, proceso automático, transformación automática

manual processing
G manuelle Verarbeitung
F traitement manuel
S elaboración manual, proceso manual, transformación manual

processing facility
G Prozeßanlage
F installation pour processus
S instalación para proceso

processing instructions
G Verarbeitungsanweisung
F instructions pour le traitement
S instrucción de procesado

processing plant
G Prozeßanlage
F installation pour processus
S instalación para proceso

processing time
G Durchlaufzeit
F temps de traitement
S tiempo de paso

procurement
G Beschaffung
F achats
S adquisición

product analysis
G Produktanalyse
F analyse d'un produit
S análisis del producto

product assay
G Produktanalyse
F analyse d'un produit
S análisis del producto

product contact surface
G produktberührende Oberfläche
F surface au contact d'un produit
S superficie en contacto con el producto

product contamination
G Produktverunreinigung
F contamination d'un produit
S contaminación de un producto

product description
G Produktbeschreibung
F caractérisation d'un produit
S descripción de un producto

product development
G Produktentwicklung
F développement d'un produit
S desarrollo de un producto

product feed
G Produktzufuhr
F alimentation en produit
S suministro de un producto

product launch
G Produkteinführung
F lancement d'un produit
S introducción de un producto (en el mercado)

Product License Application (PLA)
G Antrag auf Vertriebsgenehmigung eines Arzneimittels bei der FDA (USA)
F demande d'autorisation de mise sur le marché (AMM)
S solicitud de permiso a la FDA (EE.UU.) para poner a la venta un medicamento

product origin
G Produktherkunft
F origine du produit
S procedencia del producto

product promotion
G Produktförderung
F mesures propres à favoriser un produit
S promoción de un producto

product purification
G Produktreinigung
F purification d'un produit
S limpieza del producto

product range
G Sortiment
F sortiment
S surtido

product recall
G Produktrückruf
F rappel d'un produit
S retirada de un producto

product release
G Produktfreigabe
F libération de produit
S aprobación del producto

product residue
G Produktrückstand
F résidu d'un produit
S residuo de un producto

product safety
G Produktsicherheit
F sécurité d'un produit
S seguridad de un producto

product scanner
G Füllguttaster
F palpeur de remplissage
S sensor del contenido

product stability
G Produktstabilität
F stabilité d'un produit
S estabilidad de un producto

product yield
G Produktausbeute
F taux de récupération d'un produit
S rendimiento en producto

production
G Gewinnung, Herstellung, Produktion
F fabrication, production
S extracción, fabricación, obtención, producción

production batch
G Produktionscharge
F lot de production
S lote de producción

production data
G Produktionsdaten
F données de production
S datos de producción

production down time (downtime)
G Produktionsausfall, Produktionsausfallzeit
F période d'immobilisation en production
S pérdida de producción, tiempo de pérdida de producción

production facility
G Produktionsbetrieb
F usine de production
S empresa productora

production licence
G Produktionsgenehmigung
F autorisation de production
S permiso de producción

production line
G Produktionslinie
F chaîne de production
S cadena de producción

production output
G Produktionsleistung
F rendement d'une production
S rendimiento de producción

production plant
G Produktionsbetrieb
F usine de production
S empresa productora

production scale
G Produktionsmaßstab
F échelle de production
S escala de producción

laboratory scale
G Labormaßstab
F échelle laboratoire
S escala de laboratorio

production schedule
G Produktionsplan
F schéma de production
S plan de producción

programmable
G programmierbar
F programmable
S programable

programmable logic control (PLC)
G speicherprogrammierbare Steuerung (SPS)
F automate programmable industriel
S control programable mediante memoria

programme control
G Programmsteuerung
F contrôle d'un programme
S control del programa

programmer
G Programmierer
F programmeur
S programador

programming
G Programmierung
F programmation
S programación

project, to
G überhängen, überstehen
F saillir, faire saillir
S pender sobre, sobresalir, resaltar

prolong, to
G verlängern
F prolonger, rallonger
S alargar, prolongar

prolonged release granules
G Retardgranulat
F granules à libération retardée
S granulado retard

proof
G Beweis, Nachweis
F détection, preuve
S demostración, prueba

propellant (gas)
G Treibgas
F gaz propulseur
S propelente

propeller mixer
G Propellermischer
F mélangeur à pales
S mezclador de hélice

property
G Eigenschaft
F propriété, caractéristique
S característica, propiedad

prophylactic
G prophylaktisch
F prophylactique
S profiláctico

prophylaxis
G Prophylaxe
F prophylaxe
S profilaxia

prospective
G prospektiv
F prospective
S prospectivo

protease
G Protease
F protéase
S proteasa

protective clothing
G Schutzkleidung
F vêtement de protection
S ropa protectora

protective gloves
G Schutzhandschuhe
F gants protecteurs
S guantes protectores

protective screen
G Schutzschirm
F écran de protection
S pantalla protectora

protocol, to
G protokollieren
F enregistrer, documenter
S levantar acta, protocolar

prototype
G Erstausführung
F prototype
S prototipo

protozoa
G Protozoen
F protozoaires
S protozoos

protrude, to
G überhängen, überstehen
F saillir, faire saillir
S pender sobre, sobresalir, resaltar

provide with, to
G ausrüsten
F équiper, outiller
S equipar

public liability company
G Aktiengesellschaft
F société anonyme
S sociedad anónima

public water supply
G öffentliche Wasserversorgung
F approvisionnement public en eau
S abastecimiento público de agua

publication
G Veröffentlichung
F publication
S publicación

pull-down cam
G Niederzugsschiene
F came de poinçon descendante
S carril de tracción inferior, corredera de tracción inferior

pulse generator
G Impulsgeber
F générateur d'impulsions
S generador de impulsos

pulverise, to
G pulverisieren
F pulvériser
S pulverizar

pump
G Pumpe
F pompe
S bomba

pump head
G Pumpenkopf
F tête de pompe
S cabeza de bomba

pump inlet
G Pumpeneinlaß
F entrée d'une pompe
S entrada de una bomba

pump valve
G Pumpenventil
F vanne de pompe
S válvula de bomba

punch
G Prägestempel, Stanze, Stempel (zum Tablettieren)
F poinçon
S cuño, estampa, punzonadora, troquel (para comprimidos), troqueladora

lower punch
G Unterstempel
F poinçon inférieur
S troquel inferior

upper punch
G Oberstempel
F poinçon supérieur
S troquel superior

punch chamfer (of tablet punch)
G Fase (am Tablettenstempel)
F biseau (d'un poinçon à comprimés)
S bisel (del troquel de comprimidos)

punch form
G Stempelform
F forme d'un poinçon
S forma del troquel

punch guide
G Stempelführung
F guidage d'un poinçon
S guía del troquel

punch head
G Stempelkopf
F tête d'un poinçon
S cabeza del troquel

punch holder
G Stempelhalter
F support de poinçon
S soporte del troquel

punch neck
G Stempelhals
F collet du poinçon
S cuello de troquel

punch shape
G Stempelform
F forme d'un poinçon
S forma del troquel

punch speed
G Stempelgeschwindigkeit
F vitesse d'un poinçon
S velocidad del troquel

punch station
G Stempelstation
F station de poinçonnage
S estación de troquelado

punch sticking
G Stempelschwergängigkeit
F difficulté de glissement d'un poinçon
S dificultad de deslizamiento del troquel

punch tightness
G Stempeldichtigkeit
F étanchéité d'un poinçon
S estanqueidad del troquel

punch tip
G Stempelkopf
F tête du poinçon
S cabeza de troquel

punch tip length
G Stempelkopflänge
F longueur de la tête du poinçon
S longitud de la cabeza de troquel

punch type
G Stempeltyp
F type de poinçon
S tipo de troquel

punch velocity
G Stempelgeschwindigkeit
F vitesse d'un poinçon
S velocidad del troquel

punch, to
G ausstanzen, einstanzen
F découper à l'emporte-pièce, estamper, poinçonner
S estampar, perforar, punzonar, troquelar

punching station
G Lochstanze
F poinçonneuse
S perforadora, punzonadora, troquel

purchase cost
G Kaufpreis
F prix d'achat
S precio de compra

purchase order number
G Bestellauftragsnummer
F numéro de commande
S número del encargo de pedido

purchase price
G Anschaffungskosten
F frais d'achat
S costes de adquisición

purchase, to
G kaufen
F acheter, acquérir
S comprar

pure steam
G Reindampf, Reinstdampf
F vapeur pure
S vapor puro

pure steam generator
G Reindampferzeuger
F générateur de vapeur pure
S generador de vapor puro

pure water
G Reinstwasser
F eau PPI
S agua purificada

purge gas
G Spülgas
F gas de purge
S gas purgante

purge, to (with)
G begasen, durchströmen (mit)
F rincer (avec), purger
S gasear, inundar (con), purgar (con)

purging
G Begasung
F fumigation
S fumigación

purification
G Aufreinigung (chemisch), Reinigung
F nettoyage, purification
S limpieza, purificación (química)

purified
G gereinigt
F purifié
S purificado

purified steam
G gereinigter Dampf
F vapeur purifiée
S vapor purificado

purified water
G Aqua purificata, gereinigtes Wasser
F eau purifiée
S agua purificada

purity (product)
G Reinheit, Reinheitsgrad
F pureté, niveau de propreté, niveau de pureté
S pureza, grado de pureza

purity test
G Reinheitsprüfung
F test de pureté
S prueba de pureza

put into operation, to
G in Betrieb setzen
F mettre en fonctionnement
S poner en funcionamiento

putrefaction
G Fäulnis
F putréfaction
S putrefacción

pycnometer
G Pyknometer
F pycnomètre
S picnómetro

pyrogen-free
G pyrogenfrei
F dépourvu de pyrogènes
S sin pirógenos

pyrogenicity
G Pyrogenität
F pyrogénicité
S pirogenicidad

pyrogens
G fiebererzeugende Substanzen, Pyrogene
F pyrogènes
S pirógenos

pyrolysis
G Pyrolyse
F pyrolyse
S pirólisis

qualification
G Qualifizierung
F qualification
S cualificación

installation qualification
G Installationsqualifizierung
F qualification de l'installation
S cualificación de una instalación

operational qualification
G Funktionsqualifizierung
F qualification des opérations
S cualificación funcional

performance qualification
G Verfahrensqualifizierung
F qualification des performances
S cualificación de un procedimiento

qualified person
G sachkundige Person, Sachkundiger
F expert, personne compétente, personne qualifiée
S experto, perito, persona cualificada

quality
G Güte, Qualität
F qualité
S calidad, cualidad

consistent quality
G gleichbleibende Qualität
F qualité uniforme
S calidad invariable

quality assurance (QA)
G Qualitätssicherung (QS)
F assurance-qualité
S aseguramiento de la calidad

quality attribute
G Qualitätsmerkmal
F caracteristique de qualité
S característica de calidad

quality control (QC)
G Qualitätskontrolle (QK)
F contrôle-qualité, contrôle de la qualité
S control de calidad

quality control card
G Qualitätsregelkarte
F carte de contrôle de qualité
S ficha de control de calidad

quality grade
G Güteklasse
F degré de qualité
S grado de calidad

quality improvement
G Qualitätsverbesserung
F amélioration de la qualité
S mejora de la calidad

quality management (QM)
G Qualitätsmanagement (QM)
F gestion de la qualité
S gestión de la calidad

total quality management (TQM)
G umfassendes Qualitätsmanagement
F gestion absolue de la qualité
S gestión de la calidad absoluta

quality specification
G Gütebestimmung
F spécification de qualité
S especificación de calidad

quality-determining
G qualitätsbestimmend
F qui détermine la qualité
S determinante de la calidad

quantifiable
G quantitativ bestimmbar
F quantifiable
S cuantificable

quantitative
G quantitativ
F quantitatif
S cuantitativo

quantity
G Menge
F quantité
S cantidad

quantity control
G Füllmengenkontrolle
F contrôle de la quantité de remplissage
S control de la cantidad de relleno

quantity produced
G Produktionsmenge
F quantité produite
S cantidad producida

quantity received
G Liefermenge
F quantité livrée
S cantidad suministrada

quarantine (warehouse)
G Quarantäne, Sperrlager, Sperrung
F quarantaine (entrepôt)
S almacén para cuarentena, bloqueo, cierre, cuarentena

quartz
G Quarz
F quartz
S cuarzo

questionnaire
G Fragebogen, Prüfbogen
F questionnaire
S cuestionario

quick coupling
G Schnellkupplung
F connexion instantanée
S conexión rápida

quick-flange connection
G Schnellverschluß
F connexion à collerette instantanée
S cierre rápido

quotient
G Quotient
F quotient
S cociente

R & S (risk and safety)
G R & S (Risiko und Sicherheit)
F R & S (risque et sécurité)
S R & S (riesgo y seguridad)

R & S phrases
G R & S-Sätze
F phrases de R & S
S frases de R & S

R + D (Research and Development)
G F + E (Forschung und Entwicklung)
F R + D (recherche et développement)
S investigación y desarrollo

racemate
G Razemat
F racémate
S racemado

racemic
G racemisch, razemisch
F racémique
S racémico

rack
G Magazin (für Ampullen)
F plateau
S bandeja (para ampollas)

radiation
G Bestrahlung, Strahlung
F irradiation, radiation
S irradiación, radiación

radiation protection act
G Strahlenschutzgesetz
F loi pour la protection contre les radiations
S ley de protección frente a radiaciones ionizantes

radiation sterilisation
G Strahlensterilisation
F stérilisation par irradiation
S esterilización por irradiación

radioactive decay
G radioaktiver Zerfall
F désintégration radioactive
S desintegración radiactiva

radioactive waste
G radioaktiver Abfall
F résidu radioactif
S residuos radiactivos

radio-label
G radioaktive Markierung
F marquage isotopique
S marcado radiactivo

radio-pharmaceuticals
G Radiopharmazeutika
F produits radiopharmaceutiques
S productos radiofarmacéuticos

rancid
G ranzig
F rance
S rancio

random distribution
G Zufallsverteilung
F distribution randomisée
S distribución aleatoria

random location storage system
G chaotische Lagerhaltung
F entreposage non ordonné
S gestión de stocks caótica

random number generator
G Zufallsgenerator
F générateur de hasard
S generador aleatorio

English German French Spanish

random sample
G Stichprobe
F échantillon prélevé au hasard
S muestra al azar

randomised
G randomisiert
F randomisé
S randomizado

range
G Bandbreite, Bereich
F échelle, intervalle, gamme, zone
S anchura de banda, gama, márgenes, zona

acceptable range
G zulässiger Bereich
F intervalle autorisé
S zona permitida, márgenes permitidos

rare gas
G Edelgas
F gaz inerte, gaz rare
S gas noble

raster
G Raster
F trame
S trama

ratio
G Verhältnis
F rapport, taux
S proporción

rationale
G Begründung
F exposé des motifs, explication
S argumentación, razonamiento

raw data
G Rohdaten
F données brutes
S datos brutos

raw material
G Ausgangsstoff, Rohmaterial, Rohstoff
F matière brute, matériel de départ, matière première
S materia prima, sustancia de partida, sustancia inicial

raw product
G Rohprodukt
F produit brut
S materia prima, producto bruto

raw yield
G Rohausbeute
F rendement brut
S rendimiento bruto

reaction conditions
G Reaktionsbedingungen
F conditions de réaction
S condiciones de reacción

reaction materials
G Ansatz
F matériaux de réaction
S planteamiento, inserción, materiales de reacción

reaction mechanism
G Reaktionsmechanismus
F mécanisme de réaction
S mecanismo de reacción

reaction speed
G Reaktionsgeschwindigkeit
F vitesse de réaction
S velocidad de reacción

reaction velocity
G Reaktionsgeschwindigkeit
F vitesse de réaction
S velocidad de reacción

reaction vessel
G Ansatzbehälter
F container, récipient
S contenedor

mobile vessel, mobile container
G fahrbarer Ansatzbehälter
F cuve sur roues, cuve mobile
S contenedor portátil

reactor
G Reaktor
F réacteur
S reactor

read off, to
G ablesen
F lire, relever
S leer

ready for operation
G betriebsbereit
F prêt au service, prêt à l'utilisation, prêt à l'emploi
S preparado para funcionar

ready-to-use
G gebrauchsfertig
F prêt à l'emploi
S dispuesto para el servicio, listo para el uso

reagent
G Reagenz
F réactif
S reactivo

ready-to-use reagent
G gebrauchsfertiges Reagenz
F réactif prêt à l'emploi
S reactivo listo para el uso

single-component reagent
G Einkomponenten-Reagenz
F réactif à composant unique
S reactivo de componente único

reagent solution
G Reagenzlösung
F solution réactive
S solución reactiva

realisation
G Erfüllung
F réalisation
S cumplimiento, realización

reasoning
G Begründung
F exposé des motifs, explication
S argumentación, razonamiento

re-assembly
G Wiederzusammenbau
F réassemblage
S reensamblaje

recall
G Rückruf
F rappel
S retirada

receipt (of goods)
G Empfangsbestätigung, Wareneingang
F entrée des marchandises, reçu, quittance
S acuse de recibo, entrada de mercancías

receiving code
G Wareneingangscode
F code d'entrée de marchandises
S código de entrada de mercancías

receiving log book
G Wareneingangsbuch
F livre d'entrées de marchandises
S libro de entrada de mercancías

receptor
G Rezeptor
F récepteur
S receptor

recess
G Aussparung, Hohlkehle, Nische, Vertiefung
F cavité, évidure, échancrure, moulure creuse, niche, puits
S canal, cavidad, depresión, garganta, hueco, media caña, nicho, vacío

recirculating air
G Umluft
F air de recirculation
S aire circulante

recirculation
G Umlauf
F recirculation
S circulación, rotación

recombinant
G rekombinant
F recombinant
S recombinante

recommendation
G Empfehlung
F notes explicatives
S recomendación

reconciliation
G Bilanzierung
F vérification, bilancer
S hacer balance

reconstitution
G Wiederherstellung
F rétablissement, reconstitution
S reconstitución, restablecimiento

record
G Aufzeichnung, Protokoll
F enregistrement, référence
S protocolo, registro

record, to (data)
G aufzeichnen, erfassen (Daten), protokollieren
F documenter, enregistrer (des données)
S levantar acta, protocolar, registrar (datos)

recorder
G Schreiber
F enregistreur
S registradora

recorder chart
G Schreiberstreifen
F bande de papier d'enregistreur
S registro de diagramas

recording
G Aufnahme
F enregistrement
S toma, registro

recover, to
G wiedergewinnen
F récupérer
S recuperar

recovery
G Rückgewinnung, Wiedergewinnung
F récupération, rendement
S recuperación

solvent recovery
G Lösungsmittelrückgewinnung
F récupération de solvant
S recuperación de solvente

recovery capability
G Erholungsfähigkeit
F capacité de récupération
S capacidad de recuperación

recovery rate
G Wiederfindungsrate
F taux de récupération, taux de rendement
S tasa de recuperación

recovery time (in clean room)
G Erholzeit (im Reinraum)
F temps de récupération
S tiempo de recuperación (en área estéril)

recruitment phase
G Rekrutierungsphase
F phase de recrutement
S fase de reclutamiento

recrystallisation
G Umkristallisation
F recristallisation
S recristalización

rectal cream
G Rektalcreme
F crème rectale
S crema rectal

rectal foam
G Rektalschaum
F mousse rectale
S espuma rectal

rectal gel
G Rektalgel
F gel rectal
S gel rectal

rectal ointment
G Rektalsalbe
F pommade rectale
S pomada rectal

rectangular
G rechtwinkelig
F rectangulaire
S rectangular

rectified
G rektifiziert
F rectifié
S rectificado

rectifier
G Stromgleichrichter
F redresseur de courant
S rectificador de corriente

re-cycling
G Wiederverwertung
F recyclage
S reciclaje

redistilled water
G Aqua bidest.
F eau pour préparation injectable (PPI)
S agua bidestilada

redox potential
G Redoxpotential
F potentiel redox
S potencial redox

reduce, to (e. g. viruses)
G abreichern (z. B. Viren), reduzieren, senken
F abaisser, baisser, éliminer (par exemple des virus), réduire
S bajar, eliminar (p. ej. virus), reducir

reducer
G Reduzierstück
F réducteur
S reductor

reducing valve
G Druckregler, Reduzierventil
F régulateur de pression, vanne de détente
S regulador de presión, válvula reductora

redundancy
G Entlassung
F licenciement
S despido

reel changes
G Rollenwechsel
F changement de bobine
S cambio de bobina

reel diameter
G Rollendurchmesser
F diamètre de bobine
S diámetro de bobina

re-equip, to
G umrüsten
F moderniser, réorganiser
S modernizar, reorganizar

re-equipping
G Umrüstung
F modernisation, réorganisation
S modernización, reorganización

re-equipping time
G Umrüstzeit
F temps de réorganisation
S tiempo de reequipamiento

refer to, to
G verweisen auf
F faire référence à
S referir a

reference
G Referenzstandard
F standard de référence
S estándar de referencia

reference beam
G Referenzstrahl
F faisceau de référence
S rayo de referencia

reference customers
G Referenzkunden
F clientèle de référence
S clientes de referencia

reference medication (preparation)
G Referenzpräparat
F préparation de référence
S preparado de referencia

Reference Member State (EU) (RMS)
G Erstzulassender (EU) Mitgliedsstaat
F pays rapporteur (UE)
S País Miembro (UE) de Referencia (para registro de medicamentos)

reference point
G Bezugspunkt
F point de référence
S punto de referencia

reference sample
G Bezugsmuster, Rückstellmuster
F échantillon de référence
S muestra de referencia, prueba de referencia

reference solution
G Vergleichslösung
F solution de référence
S solución de referencia

reference to
G Verweis auf
F référence à
S referencia a

refill, to
G umfüllen
F transvaser
S transvasar, trasegar

reflux
G Rückfluß
F reflux
S reflujo

reflux condenser
G Rückflußkühler
F radiateur à reflux
S radiador, refrigerador de reflujo

reformulation
G Umformulierung
F nouvelle formulation
S nueva formulación, reformulación

refractive dispersion
G Brechungsdispersion
F dispersion refractive
S dispersión refringente

refractive index
G Brechungsindex, Brechungszahl
F index de réfraction
S índice de refracción

refractometer
G Refraktometer
F réfractomètre
S refractómetro

refrigerant
G Kühlmittel
F liquide de refroidissement
S medio refrigerante

refrigerate, to
G kühl lagern
F réfrigérer, refroidir
S conservar frío

refrigerating chain
G Kühlkette
F chaîne de réfrigération
S cadena de refrigeración

refrigeration
G Kälteerzeugung
F réfrigération
S refrigeración

refrigerator
G Kühlschrank
F réfrigérateur
S nevera

refringence
G Brechungsvermögen
F réfringence
S refringencia

regeneration
G Regenerierung
F régénération
S regeneración

regional government
G Regierungspräsidium
F gouvernement régional
S gobierno civil

register defect
G Passerfehler
F défaut de registre
S defecto de registro

register difference
G Passerdifferenz
F différence de registre
S diferencia de registro

register, to (data)
G aufzeichnen (Daten)
F enregistrer (des données)
S registrar (datos)

registered name
G Handelsmarke
F marque de commerce
S marca comercial

registration
G Registrierung
F enregistrement
S registro

regulating valve
G Regelventil
F vanne de régulation
S válvula reguladora

regulation
G Verordnung
F décret
S decreto, prescripción

regulations for hazardous goods
G Gefahrstoffverordnung
F décret concernant les matières dangereuses
S decreto sobre sustancias peligrosas

regulatory affairs department
G Zulassungsabteilung
F département des affaires réglementaires
S departamento de registros y licencias sanitarias

regulatory authorities
G Zulassungsbehörde
F autorités compétentes responsables des autorisations de mise sur le marché
S agencia de autorización de licencias sanitarias

reimbursement
G Erstattung
F remboursement
S devolución, restitución

reinforced
G verstärkt
F renforcé
S intensificado, reforzado

reintroduce, to
G wiedereinschleusen
F réintroduire
S reintroducir

reject position
G Ausschußposition, Auswurfstelle
F emplacement de l'éjection, position de rejet
S posición de desecho, zona de expulsión

reject, to
G zurückweisen
F rejeter
S rechazar

rejected materials
G zurückgewiesene Materialien
F matériaux rejetés, matériaux refusés
S materiales rechazados

rejected product
G verworfenes Produkt
F produit rejeté
S producto desechado

English
German
French
Spanish

rejection (e. g. of a patent)
G Ablehnung, Zurückweisung (z. B. eines Patentes)
F refus, rejet (par ex. d'un brevet)
S rechazo (p. ej. de una patente)

rejection number
G Rückweisezahl
F nombre de rejet
S número de rechazo

related substance
G verwandte Substanz
F substance apparentée
S sustancia emparentada

relationship diagram
G Relationsdiagramm
F schéma relationnel
S diagrama de relaciones

relative humidity
G relative Luftfeuchtigkeit
F humidité relative
S humedad atmosférica relativa

relative standard deviation
G relative Standardabweichung
F écart-type relatif
S desviación estándar relativa

relay
G Relais
F relais
S relé, relevador

relay amplifier
G Relaisverstärker
F relais amplificateur
S amplificador de relé

release
G Freigabe, Freisetzung
F libération
S liberación

batch release
G Chargenfreigabe
F libération d'un lot
S liberación de lotes

controlled release
G kontrollierte Freisetzung
F libération contrôlée
S liberación controlada

delayed release
G verzögerte Freisetzung
F libération différée
S liberación retardada

immediate release
G schnelle Freisetzung
F libération immédiate
S liberación rápida

incomplete release
G unvollständige Freisetzung
F libération incomplète
S liberación incompleta

modified release
G modifizierte Freisetzung
F libération modifiée
S liberación modificada

sustained release
G verlängerte Freisetzung
F libération prolongée
S liberación prolongada

release analysis
G Freigabeuntersuchung
F analyse de libération
S análisis de autorización

release behaviour
G Freisetzungsverhalten
F comportement de libération
S comportamiento de liberación

release date
G Freigabedatum
F date de libération
S fecha de liberación

release of medicinal substance
G Arzneistoff-Freisetzung
F libération d'un principe actif
S liberación del principio activo

release procedure
G Freigabeverfahren
F processus de libération
S proceso de autorización

release profile
G Freisetzungsprofil
F profil de libération
S perfil de liberación

release rate
G Freisetzungsrate
F vitesse de libération
S tasa de liberación

release status
G Freigabestatus
F statut de libération
S status de autorización

release, to
G freigeben
F libérer
S liberar

released
G freigegeben
F libéré
S liberado

relevant
G relevant
F pertinent, approprié
S relevante

reliability
G Verläßlichkeit, Zuverlässigkeit
F fiabilité
S fiabilidad, confiabilidad

reliable
G verläßlich, zuverlässig
F fiable
S confiable, digno de confianza, fiable

relief
G Entlastung
F soulagement, décharge
S alivio, descarga

relocate, to
G verlagern
F transférer, déplacer
S desplazar, transferir, trasladar

remote control
G Fernbedienung, Fernsteuerung, Fernüberwachung
F télécontrôle, télécommande
S control remoto, telemando

remote operation
G Fernbedienung
F télécommande
S telemando

removable
G entfernbar, abnehmbar
F amovible, démontable, détachable
S desmontable

removal
G Ausbau, Beseitigung, Demontage, Entfernung
F démontage, élimination
S desmontaje, eliminación

removal of viruses
G Virusabreicherung
F élimination des virus
S eliminación de virus

removal probe
G Entnahmesonde
F sonde d'échantillonnage
S sonda de toma (de muestras)

remuneration
G Vergütung
F rémunération
S remuneración

reorganisation
G Sanierung
F assainissement
S saneamiento

re-pack, to
G umpacken
F changer l'emballage
S envasar de nuevo

re-packaging
G Wiederverpackung
F action de réemballer
S reembalaje

repair
G Instandsetzung, Reparatur
F réparation
S reparación

re-pallet, to
G umpalettieren
F réorganiser les palettes
S cambiar de paleta

repeatability
G Wiederholbarkeit
F répétitivité
S repetitividad

repetition
G Wiederholung
F répétition
S repetición

replace, to
G ersetzen
F remplacer
S reemplazar, sustituir

replaceable
G auswechselbar
F interchangeable
S intercambiable

replacement part
G Austauschteil
F pièce de rechange
S pieza de recambio

replicate analysis
G Wiederholungsanalyse
F analyse répétée
S análisis de repetición

report
G Befund, Bericht
F diagnose, rapport
S diagnóstico, informe

report to someone, to
G jemandem berichten
F rapporter à quelqu'un
S informar a alguien

reprocess, to
G aufarbeiten
F traiter
S procesar

reprocessed product
G wiederaufbereitetes Produkt
F produit recyclé
S producto reciclado

reprocessing
G Aufarbeitung, Nacharbeitung, Wiederaufbereitung
F retouche, retraitement, traitement, traitement complémentaire
S proceso, reprocesado, retocado

reproducibility
G Reproduzierbarkeit
F reproductibilité
S reproductibilidad

reproducible
G reproduzierbar
F reproductible
S reproducible

requalification
G Requalifizierung
F requalification
S recualificación

require, to
G erfordern
F exiger, nécessiter
S exigir, necesitar, requerir

required
G gefordert
F exigé
S exigido, reclamado

required specification
G Pflichtenheft
F spécifications fonctionnelles
S descripción de tareas

required value
G Sollwert
F valeur nominale
S valor nominal

requirement
G Anforderung, Erfordernis
F exigence
S exigencia, necesidad, requerimiento

legal requirement
G gesetzliche Anforderung
F exigence légale
S requerimiento legal

requirements planning
G Bedarfsplanung
F planification des besoins
S planificación de necesidades

research and development
G Forschung und Entwicklung
F recherche et développement
S investigación y desarrollo

reservoir
G Sammelbehälter, Vorratsgefäß, Vorratstank
F collecteur, récipient de stockage, réservoir
S depósito (colector), recipiente de depósito, tanque de depósito

residence time
G Aufenthaltsdauer, Verweilzeit
F temps de résidence
S duración de la permanencia, tiempo de permanencia

mean residence time (MRT)
G mittlere Verweilzeit
F temps de résidence moyen
S tiempo promedio de permanencia

residual hardness (e. g. of water)
G Resthärte (z. B. von Wasser)
F dureté résiduelle (par ex. de l'eau)
S dureza residual (p. ej. del agua)

residual moisture
G Restfeuchte
F humidité résiduelle
S humedad residual

residual volume
G Restvolumen
F volume résiduel
S volumen residual

residue
G Rest, Rückstand, Preßrückstand, Siebrückstand
F résidu, résidu de pressage, résidu de tamisage
S residuo, residuo de prensado, residuo de tamizado, resto

visible residue
G sichtbarer Rückstand
F résidu visible
S residuo visible

residue on annealment
G Glührückstand
F cendres résiduelles
S cenizas residuales

residue on drying
G Trockenrückstand
F résidu de séchage
S residuo seco

residue on evaporating
G Verdampfungsrückstand
F résidus de vaporisation
S residuo de evaporación

residue on ignition
G Verbrennungsrückstand, Glührückstand
F cendres résiduelles, résidu d'ignition
S cenizas residuales, residuo de ignición

resin
G Harz
F résine
S resina

resistance
G Beständigkeit
F stabilité à long terme, résistance
S estabilidad, inalterabilidad

resistance coil
G Widerstandsspule
F bobine de résistance
S bobina de resistencia

resistance to abrasion
G Reibeechtheit
F résistance à l'abrasion
S resistente a la fricción

resistance to bending
G Knickechtheit
F résistance à la plicature
S resistencia al pandeo

resistance to tearing
G Reißfestigkeit
F résistance au déchirement
S resistencia al desgarro

resistance to wear
G Verschleißwiderstand
F résistance à l'usure
S resistencia al desgaste

resistance, electrical
G elektrischer Widerstand
F résistance électrique
S resistencia eléctrica

resistant
G resistent, widerstandsfähig
F résistant
S resistente, tenaz

resistant to abrasion
G abriebfest
F résistant à l'abrasion
S resistente a la abrasión

resistant to corrosion
G korrosionsbeständig
F résistant à la corrosion
S resistente a la corrosión

resistant to fading
G lichtecht
F résistant à la décoloration
S resistente a la decoloración

resorption
G Resorption
F résorption
S resorción

resorption agent
G Resorptionsvermittler
F agent de résorption
S agente de resorción

respiratory protection
G Atemschutz
F masque respiratoire de protection
S protección respiratoria

response time
G Ansprechzeit
F temps de réponse
S tiempo de respuesta

responsibility
G Verantwortlichkeit
F responsabilité
S responsabilidad

responsible person
G Verantwortlicher
F personne responsable
S responsable

rest, at
G im Ruhezustand
F à l'arrêt, immobilisé
S parado

restriction enzyme
G Restriktionsenzym
F enzyme de restriction
S enzima restrictivo

restructuring
G Sanierung
F assainissement
S saneamiento

result
G Ergebnis
F résultats
S resultado

expected results
G erwartete Ergebnisse
F résultats escomptés
S resultados esperados

retain, to
G aufbewahren
F conserver, garder
S conservar, guardar

retained sample
G Rückstellmuster
F échantillon de référence
S muestra de referencia

retaining basket
G Fangkorb
F corbeille
S cesto colector

retaining ring
G Haltering
F anneau de support
S anillo de soporte

retard tablet
G Retardtablette
F comprimé à libération retardée
S comprimido retard

retention
G Aufbewahrung, Retention
F archivage, conservation, rétention, stockage
S almacenaje, conservación, retención

retention efficiency (in filters)
G Rückhaltevermögen (bei Filtern)
F efficacité de rétention (pour un filtre)
S capacidad de retención (de un filtro)

retention factor
G Retentionsfaktor
F facteur de rétention
S factor de retención

retention range
G Rückhaltebereich
F zone de rétention
S márgenes de retención

retention time
G Retentionszeit
F temps de rétention
S tiempo de retención

retentive
G zurückhaltend
F réservé, effacé, réticent
S reservado

re-test
G Wiederholungsprüfung
F essai répété
S ensayo de repetición

reticular
G netzförmig, vernetzt
F réticulaire
S integrado en una red, reticular

retrospective validation
G retrospektive Validierung
F validation rétrospective
S validación retrospectiva

return
G Retoure
F renvoi, rappel
S retorno

return spring
G Rückzugfeder
F ressort de rappel
S muelle de retorno

returnable
G Mehrweg-
F réutilisable
S reutilizable

returned goods
G zurückgegebene Ware
F marchandise retournée
S mercancía devuelta

English German French Spanish

re-usable
G wiederverwendbar, Mehrweg-
F réutilisable
S reutilizable

re-use
G Wiederverwendung
F réutilisation
S reutilización

revalidation
G Revalidierung
F revalidation
S revalidación

reverse flow
G Rücklauf
F retour
S retorno

reverse osmosis (RO)
G Umkehrosmose
F osmose inverse
S ósmosis inversa

reverse osmosis water
G durch Umkehrosmose entsalztes Wasser
F eau désalinisée par osmose inverse
S agua desalinizada mediante ósmosis inversa

reverse-phase chromatography
G Umkehrphasenchromatographie
F chromatographie en phase inverse
S cromatografía en fase inversa

review, to
G revidieren, überarbeiten
F réviser, remanier
S perfeccionar, revisar

reviewed
G überarbeitet
F révisé
S perfeccionado, revisado

revise, to
G revidieren
F réviser
S revisar

revolution counter
G Drehzahlmesser, Umdrehungszähler
F compte-tours, tachymètre
S contador de revoluciones, taquímetro

revolutions (per minute)
G Drehzahl, Umdrehungen (pro Minute), Umdrehungszahl
F nombre de rotations, nombre de tours, rotations (par minute)
S número de revoluciones, revoluciones (por minuto)

revolving brush
G Bürstenwalze, Walzenbürste
F brosse de laminage, brosse rotative
S cepillo rotativo, cepillo rotatorio, cilindro cepillador

revolving plate feeder
G Aufgabedrehteller
F plateau tournant
S placa giratoria

reworking
G Umarbeitung
F retraitement
S adaptación, remodelación, transformación

rheology
G Rheologie
F rhéologie
S reología

right-handed
G rechtsgängig
F droit
S de paso derecho

rigid
G starr, steif
F rigide
S rígido

rim (of a tablet)
G Grat (einer Tablette)
F arête (d'un comprimé)
S borde (de un comprimido)

ring-opening reaction
G Ringöffnungsreaktion
F réaction ouvrant un anneau
S reacción de apertura de anillo

rinse, to
G spülen
F rincer
S enjuagar, irrigar, lavar

rinsing medium
G Spülmedium
F milieu de rinçage
S medio de lavado

rinsing solution
G Spüllösung
F solution de rinçage
S solución de lavado

rinsing water
G Spülwasser
F eau de rinçage
S agua de lavado

rising film evaporator
G Klettererverdampfer
F évaporateur Kestner
S evaporador Kestner

risk analysis
G Risikoanalyse
F analyse des risques
S análisis del riesgo

risk and safety phrases
G Risiko- und Gefahrensätze
F règles concernant les risques et la sécurité
S reglas concernientes a riesgos y peligros

risk of injury
G Verletzungsgefahr
F risque de blessures
S riesgo de lesión

rivet
G Niete
F rivet
S remache

robotic arm
G Roboterarm
F bras d'un robot
S brazo de robot

robotic system
G Robotersystem
F analyseur robot
S sistema robot

robustness
G Robustheit
F robustesse
S robustez

robustness testing
G Prüfung der Robustheit
F test de solidité
S comprobación de la robustez

Rockwell hardness (of tools)
G Rockwell-Härte (von Werkzeug)
F dureté Rockwell (outils)
S dureza Rockwell (de herramientas)

rodent
G Nagetier
F rongeur
S roedor

roll mill
G Walzenmühle
F broyeur à cylindres
S molino de cilindros

roll, to
G walzen
F passer au rouleau
S allanar, aplanar, cilindrar

roller
G Walze
F rouleau, cylindre, tambour
S cilindro, rodillo

room disinfection
G Raumdesinfektion
F désinfection de locaux
S desinfección de la sala

room temperature
G Raumtemperatur
F température ambiante
S temperatura ambiente

rotary basket
G Drehkörbchen
F corbeille rotative
S cesto rotatorio

rotary press
G Rundläuferpresse
F presse rotative
S prensa rotatoria

rotary spray
G Rotationssprühkopf
F tête rotative de pulvérisation
S cabeza rotatoria de pulverización

rotary valve
G Drehschieber
F valve rotatoire
S válvula rotativa

rotary valve pump
G Drehschieberpumpe
F pompe à valve rotatoire
S bomba de válvula rotativa

rotate, to
G rotieren
F tourner
S girar

rotating
G rotierend
F tournant
S girando

rotatory evaporator
G Rotationsverdampfer
F évaporateur rotatif
S evaporador rotatorio

rotor
G Rotor, Laufrad, Flügelrad
F ailette, rotor
S rotor, rueda portante, rueda de aletas

rough
G rauh
F grossier
S áspero

roughness
G Rauhigkeit
F grossièreté
S aspereza

round off, to
G abrunden
F arrondir
S redondear a la cifra inferior

round tablet
G Rundtablette
F comprimé rond
S comprimido redondo

round-bottomed flask
G Rundkolben
F ballon à fond rond
S matraz esférico

rounded off
G abgerundet
F arrondi, arrondi au chiffre inférieur
S redondeado a la cifra inferior

row of perforations
G Lochreihe
F série de perforations
S serie de perforaciones

rubber
G Gummi
F caoutchouc
S goma

rubber gasket
G Gummidichtung
F joint en caoutchouc
S junta de goma

rubber stopper
G Gummistopfen
F bouchon en caoutchouc
S tapón de goma

rubber tube
G Gummischlauch
F tube en caoutchouc
S tubo de goma

rubbish
G Müll
F déchets, résidus
S basura, desechos, residuos

rubbish incineration
G Müllverbrennung
F incinération des déchets
S incineración de desechos

rugged (e. g. instrument, method)
G robust (z. B. Gerät, Methode)
F robuste (par ex. instrument, méthode)
S robusto (p. ej. instrumento, método)

run
G Lauf
F cycle, opération, expérience
S ciclo, marcha, recorrido

run off, to
G auslaufen
F couler, s'écouler
S escaparse, salirse

running time
G Laufzeit
F durée d'opération, durée d'un cycle
S tiempo de funcionamiento

running time meter
G Betriebsstundenzähler
F compteur d'heures de mise en service
S contador de horas de funcionamiento

rupture disk
G Berstscheibe
F disque de rupture
S disco de ruptura

rupture line
G Bruchlinie
F ligne de rupture, ligne de fracture
S línea de ruptura, línea de fractura

rust
G Rost
F rouille
S herrumbre, orín

rust protection
G Rostschutz
F protection contre la rouille
S protección antioxidante

rust, to
G rosten
F rouiller
S oxidarse

rust-free
G rostfrei
F dépourvu de rouille
S sin orín

sachet (as dosage form)
G Beutel (als Darreichungsform), Siegelrandbeutel
F sachet, sachet hermétique
S bolsa hermética, sobre (como forma de administración)

sack filter
G Sackfilter
F sac filtrant
S saco filtrante

safety
G Sicherheit, Unbedenklichkeit
F sécurité
S seguridad

safety at work
G Arbeitssicherheit
F sécurité du travail
S seguridad en el trabajo

safety clothing
G Sicherheitskleidung
F vêtement de sécurité
S ropa de seguridad

English German French Spanish

English German French Spanish

safety data sheet
G Sicherheitsdatenblatt
F feuillet de données sur la sécurité
S pliego de datos de seguridad, hoja de datos de seguridad

safety device
G Sicherheitsvorrichtung
F dispositif de sécurité
S dispositivo de seguridad

safety feature
G Sicherheitsmerkmal
F caractéristique de sécurité
S característica de seguridad

safety glass screen
G Schutzschirm aus Sicherheitsglas
F écran de protection constitué de verre de sécurité
S pantalla protectora de vidrio de seguridad

safety helmet
G Schutzhelm
F casque de protection
S casco protector

safety instructions
G Sicherheitshinweis
F instructions de sécurité
S aviso de seguridad

safety poster
G Plakat mit Sicherheitshinweisen
F affiche avec consignes de sécurité
S cartel con avisos de seguridad

safety precautions
G Sicherheitsmaßnahmen
F précautions de sécurité
S medidas de seguridad

safety regulation
G Sicherheitsvorschriften
F règlement de sécurité
S reglamento de seguridad

safety requirements
G Sicherheitsanforderungen
F consignes de sécurité
S requisito de seguridad

safety risk
G Sicherheitsrisiko
F danger
S riesgo para la seguridad

safety spectacles
G Schutzbrille, Sicherheitsbrille
F lunettes de protection, lunettes de sécurité
S gafas protectoras, gafas de seguridad

safety standards
G Sicherheitsstandards
F normes de sécurité
S estándares de seguridad

safety status
G Sicherheitsstatus
F statut de sécurité
S status de seguridad

safety valve
G Sicherheitsventil
F vanne de sécurité
S válvula de seguridad

sale in pharmacies only, for
G apothekenpflichtig
F vendu uniquement en pharmacie
S de venta sólo en farmacias

sales
G Absatz, Verkauf, Vertrieb, Umsatz
F chiffre d'affaires, ventes
S distribución, movimiento, ventas, volumen de ventas, volumen de negocios

sales channel
G Vertriebsweg
F canal de distribution
S canal de distribución

sales force
G Außendienst
F force de vente
S servicio externo de ventas

sales manager
G Vertriebsleiter
F directeur des ventes
S director de ventas

sales representative
G Außendienstmitarbeiter
F commercial, vendeur
S agente externo de ventas

saline solution
G Kochsalzlösung
F solution saline
S solución salina

salinity
G Salinität, Salzigkeit
F salinité
S salinidad

salt formation
G Salzbildung
F formation de sels
S salificación

sample
G (unverkäufliches) Muster, Probe
F échantillon, spécimen
S espécimen, muestra (gratuita)

composite sample
G Mischprobe
F échantillon du mélange
S muestra mixta

stressed sample
G beanspruchte Probe
F échantillon soumis à un effort
S muestra sometida a carga

sample analysis
G Probenanalyse
F analyse d'échantillon
S análisis de muestras

sample assay
G Probenanalyse
F analyse d'échantillon
S análisis de muestras

sample clean-up
G Probenaufreinigung
F nettoyage d'échantillons
S purificación de muestras

sample injection
G Probeneinspritzung
F injection d'échantillon
S inyección de muestras

sample loop
G Probenschleife
F boucle d'échantillon
S bucle para toma de muestras

sample preparation
G Probenvorbereitung
F préparation d'un échantillon
S preparación de muestras

sample pre-treatment
G Probenvorbehandlung
F prétraitement d'échantillons
S pretratamiento de muestras

sample rack
G Probenständer
F portoir pour échantillons
S estante de muestras

sample spotting (on TLC plate)
G Probenauftrag (als Fleck auf DC-Platte)
F application d'échantillons (sur plaque de CCM)
S depósito de muestras (como mancha sobre la placa de cromatografía en capa fina)

sample storage
G Probenlagerung
F stockage d'échantillons
S almacenamiento de muestras

sample throughput
G Probendurchsatz
F capacité d'analyse d'échantillons
S rendimiento en muestras

sample transfer
G Probenübertragung
F transfert d'échantillons
S transferencia de muestras

sample vessel
G Probengefäß
F récipient pour échantillon
S recipiente para muestras

English German French Spanish

sample vial
G Probenfläschchen
F flacon d'échantillon
S vial de muestras

sampler
G Probenahmegerät, Probengeber
F échantillonneuse, équipement pour le prélèvement d'un échantillon
S aparato de toma de muestras

sampling
G Musterziehung, Probenahme
F échantillonnage, prélèvement d'un échantillon
S toma de muestra

sampling criteria
G Schärfe der Stichprobenanweisung
F critères d'échantillonnage
S rigor de las instrucciones para tomar muestras

sampling device
G Stechheber
F dispositif d'échantillonnage, pipette de prélèvement
S pipeta (de toma de muestras)

sampling equipment
G Probenahmegerät
F équipement pour le prélèvement d'un échantillon
S aparato de toma de muestras

sampling instructions
G Stichprobenanweisung
F instructions d'échantillonnage
S instrucciones para tomar muestras

sampling location
G Probenahmestelle
F point de prélèvement
S lugar de toma de muestras

sampling pipette
G Stechheber
F dispositif d'échantillonnage, pipette de prélèvement
S pipeta (de toma de muestras)

sampling plan
G Probenahmeplan
F programme d'échantillonnage
S plan de toma de muestras

sampling point
G Probenahmestelle
F point de prélèvement
S lugar de toma de muestras

sampling port
G Probeentnahmestutzen
F tubulure de prélèvement d'échantillon
S tubuladura de toma de muestra

sampling probe
G Entnahmesonde
F sonde d'échantillonnage
S sonda de toma (de muestras)

sampling statistics
G Probenahmestatistik
F statistiques de prélèvement
S estadística de toma de muestras

sand-blasted
G sandgestrahlt
F traité au jet de sable
S tratado con chorro de arena

sanitary fittings
G Sanitäranschlüsse
F connections sanitaires
S conexiones sanitarias

sanitary joint
G Sanitärverbindung
F joint sanitaire
S conexión sanitaria

sanitation programme
G Hygieneplan
F programme sanitaire
S plan higiénico, programa sanitario

saponification
G Verseifung
F saponification
S saponificación

saponification value
G Verseifungszahl
F indice de saponification
S índice de saponificación

saponify, to
G verseifen
F saponifier
S saponificar

saturated
G gesättigt
F saturé
S saturado

saturated steam
G gesättigter Wasserdampf, Sattdampf
F vapeur d'eau saturée, vapeur saturée
S vapor de agua saturado, vapor saturado

saturation
G Sättigung
F saturation
S saturación

saturation index
G Sättigungsindex
F indice de saturation
S índice de saturación

scale
G Gradeinteilung, Maßstab, Skala
F échelle, graduation, standard
S escala, estándar, graduación, patrón

measuring scale
G Meßskala
F échelle de mesure
S escala de medida

off-scale
G außerhalb des Anzeigebereichs
F en dehors de l'échelle de mesure
S fuera de la escala de medida

on-scale
G innerhalb des Anzeigebereichs
F dans l'échelle de mesure
S dentro de la escala de medida

scale-up (of a procedure)
G Maßstabsvergößerung (eines Verfahrens)
F extrapolation (d'un procédé)
S aumento a escala (de un proceso)

scaly
G schuppig
F squameux, couvert d'écailles
S escamoso

scanning head
G Tastkopf
F tête d'analyse
S cabeza de exploración

schedule
G Zeitplan
F plan, programme
S horario, calendario

scoop
G Schöpfkelle
F louche
S cazo, vasija

scope
G Geltungsbereich
F champ d'application
S campo de aplicación

scrape off, to
G abkratzen
F racler
S raer, raspar

scrape, to
G schaben
F racler
S raer, rascar, raspar

scraper
G Abstreifer, Schaber
F racloir
S rascador, raspador

scrapie-specific prions (prpsc)
G Scrapie-spezifische Proteine (prpsc)
F prions spécifiques à la scrapie (prpsc)
S priones específicos de la encefalopatía espongiforme ovina

screed
G Ausgleichsestrich, Gefälleestrich
F chape de compensation, chape inclinée
S pavimento compensador, pavimento inclinado

screen
G Bildschirm, Raster
F écran, trame
S pantalla, trama

screening
G Abschirmung, Reihenuntersuchung
F dépistage, screening, série d'analyses, tri
S apantallamiento, examen secuencial, protección, serie de ensayos

screw cap
G Schraubkappe
F bouchon à vis
S cierre de rosca

screw cap glass container
G Schraubglas
F pot fileté
S recipiente de vidrio con cierre de rosca

screw connection
G Schraubverschluß
F fermeture à vis
S cierre de rosca

screw fitting
G Verschraubung
F connexion à filetage
S atornilladura

screw on, to
G aufschrauben
F visser, dévisser
S atornillar

screw thread
G Schraubgewinde
F filetage
S filete de tornillo, rosca de tornillo

screw with nut
G Schraube mit Mutter
F vis avec écrou
S tornillo con tuerca

screw-cap bottle
G Flasche mit Schraubverschluß, Schraubflasche
F bouteille munie d'un bouchon à vis
S botella con cierre de rosca

screw-cap closing machine
G Schraubdeckelverschließmaschine
F machine à serrage de couvercles
S máquina de cierre de rosca

seal
G Dichtung, Plombe, Verschluß, Versiegelung
F bouchon, capuchon, couvercle, fermeture, joint, sceau en plomb
S cierre, empaste, junta, marchamo, precinto, sellado

door seal
G Türdichtung
F joint de porte
S junta de una puerta

seal an ampoule, to
G Ampulle verschließen
F fermer une ampoule, obturer une ampoule
S cerrar una ampolla

seal, to
G abdichten, siegeln, verschließen, versiegeln
F boucher, clore, colmater, étanchéifier, fermer hermétiquement, sceller
S cerrar (herméticamente), precintar, sellar

seal, to (tablets)
G einsiegeln (Tabletten)
F sceller, clore (comprimés)
S estampar (comprimidos)

sealant
G Dichtungsmittel
F matériau d'étanchéité, matériau d'obturation
S material de cierre, material de sellado

sealed
G verplombt
F fermé hermétiquement
S precintado

sealed bag
G Siegelrandbeutel
F sachet hermétique
S bolsa hermética

sealed packaging
G Versiegelungsverpackung
F emballage hermétique
S embalaje sellado

sealer jaws
G Siegelbacken
F mâchoires de fermeture
S mandíbulas de sellado

sealing collar
G Dichtmanschette
F manchette d'étanchéité
S manguito hermético

sealing liquid
G Dichtflüssigkeit
F liquide d'étanchéité
S líquido de cerrado hermético

sealing pressure
G Siegeldruck
F pression de scellage, pression de fermeture
S presión de sellado

sealing ring
G Dichtring
F joint d'étanchéité
S anillo hermético, arandela hermética

sealing station
G Verschlußstation
F station de scellage
S estación de cierre

sealing wax
G Siegellack
F cire à cacheter
S lacre

seam (of a tube)
G Falz (einer Tube), Fuge, Naht, Tubenfalz
F couture, joint (d'un tube), ourlet
S costura, encaje (de un tubo), junta, juntura de un tubo

seamless
G fugenlos
F dépourvu de joint
S sin juntas

seam weld, to
G nahtschweißen
F souder
S soldar

seam, to
G falzen
F plier
S plegar

secondary contamination
G Sekundärkontamination
F contamination secondaire
S contaminación secundaria

secondary crystals
G Sekundärkristalle
F cristaux secondaires
S cristales secundarios

secondary packaging material
G Sekundärpackmittel
F matériel d'emballage secondaire
S material de envase secundario

secondary products
G Sekundärprodukte
F produits secondaires
S productos secundarios

secondary treatment
G Nachbehandlung
F traitement secondaire
S tratamiento subsiguiente

English German French Spanish

secondary yield
G Sekundärausbeute
F rendement secondaire
S rendimiento secundario

second-order reaction
G Reaktion 2. Ordnung
F réaction de second ordre
S reacción de segundo orden

secrecy agreement
G Geheimhaltungsvertrag
F accord de confidentialité
S contrato de confidencialidad

sectional drawing
G Querschnittszeichnung
F croquis de section
S croquis transversal

secure, to
G sicherstellen
F assurer, garantir
S asegurar, garantizar

security
G Sicherheit
F sécurité
S seguridad

safety at work
G Arbeitssicherheit
F sécurité du travail
S seguridad en el trabajo

sedative
G Beruhigungsmittel
F sédatif, calmant
S sedante, tranquilizante

sediment
G Ablagerung, Bodensatz
F dépôt, sédiment
S depósito, sedimento

sediment, to
G sedimentieren
F sédimenter
S sedimentar

seed crystal
G Impfkristall
F germe cristallin
S cristal de sembrado

seed layer
G Kulturrasen
F surface de culture
S superficie de cultivo

see-through scanner
G Durchlichtkontrolleinrichtung
F analyseur à balayage
S dispositivo de control por transiluminación

segregated
G abgetrennt
F séparé, détaché, isolé
S aislado, separado

segregated area
G abgetrennter Bereich
F zone séparée, zone isolée, zone de confinement
S área separada

segregation
G Abtrennung
F séparation, ségrégation
S segregación, separación

selection
G Auslese, Auswahl
F sélection
S selección

selective culture medium
G Selektivnährmedien
F milieu de culture sélectif
S medios de cultivo selectivos

selectivity
G Selektivität
F sélectivité
S selectividad

self-adhesive
G selbstklebend
F auto-adhésif
S autoadhesivo

self-adhesive label
G Haftetikett
F étiquette autoadhésive
S etiqueta autoadhesiva

self-check
G Selbstüberprüfung
F auto-inspection
S autocomprobación

self-inspection
G Selbstinspektion
F auto-inspection
S autoinspección

self-medication
G Selbstmedikation
F automédication
S automedicación

semiconductor
G Halbleiter
F semi-conducteur
S semiconductor

semi-finished product
G Vorprodukt
F produit semi-fini
S producto semiterminado

semi-manufactured product
G Halbfertigware
F produit intermédiaire
S producto semiacabado

semi-permeable membrane
G semipermeable Membran
F membrane semi-perméable
S membrana semipermeable

semi-solid
G halbfest
F semi-solide
S semisólido

sensitising
G allergisierend
F allergisant
S alergizante

sensitive
G empfindlich
F sensible
S sensible

sensitive to corrosion
G korrosionsempfindlich
F sensible à la corrosion
S sensible a la corrosión

sensitivity
G Empfindlichkeit
F sensibilité
S sensibilidad

sensor
G Fühler
F capteur
S sensor

sensor housing
G Sensorgehäuse
F étui du capteur
S caja del sensor

separate, to
G abscheiden
F séparer, sécréter
S precipitar, separar

separated
G abgetrennt
F séparé, détaché, isolé
S aislado, separado

separating funnel
G Scheidetrichter
F entonnoir séparateur
S embudo de separación

separating medium
G Trennmittel
F milieu de séparation
S medio de separación

separating method
G Trennmethode
F méthode de séparation
S método de separación

English German French Spanish

separation
G Abtrennung, Entmischung, Trennung
F démixtion, séparation, ségrégation
S segregación, separación

separation capacity
G Trennungskapazität
F capacité de séparation
S capacidad de separación

separation mechanism
G Trennungsmechanismus
F mécanisme de séparation
S mecanismo de separación

separation media
G Trennmedium
F milieu de séparation
S medio separador

separation performance
G Trennungsleistung
F performance de séparation
S rendimiento separador

separation rate
G Abscheiderate
F vitesse de séparation
S velocidad de separación

separator
G Abscheider
F séparateur
S precipitador, separador

septum
G Septum
F septum
S septo

sequence
G Reihenfolge
F séquence
S secuencia

sequence of operation
G Ablauf (eines Prozesses)
F déroulement d'un procédé
S secuencia (de un proceso)

sequencing
G Sequenzierung
F séquençage
S formación de secuencias, secuenciación

sequencing unit
G Sequenzierungseinheit
F unité de séquençage
S unidad de secuenciación

serial interface
G serielle Schnittstelle
F interface série
S interfase seriada

serial number
G Seriennummer
F numéro de série
S número de serie

series
G Baureihe, Serien
F série(s)
S serie(s)

serum
G Serum
F sérum
S suero

foetal calf serum
G fötales Kälberserum
F sérum fœtal de veau
S suero fetal bovino

serum-free media
G serumfreie Nährmedien
F médium de culture exempt de sérum
S medios de cultivo sin suero

service corridor
G Technikgang
F corridor de service
S corredor de servicio

service technician
G Servicetechniker
F technicien
S técnico de servicio

set of weights
G Gewichtssatz
F série de poids
S juego de pesas

set up, to (a folding carton)
G aufrichten (eine Faltschachtel), einrichten
F dresser, monter (un carton), mettre en place
S montar (una caja plegable), instalar

setting
G Einstellung, Regulierung
F ajustement, réglage
S ajuste, regulación

setting time
G Erstarrungszeit, Abbindezeit
F temps de solidification
S tiempo de solidificación

settlement joint
G Bewegungsfuge
F joint de dilatation
S junta de dilatación

settling plate
G Sedimentationsplatte
F plaque de sédimentation
S placa de sedimentación

set-up
G Zusammenbau
F assemblage, montage
S ensamblaje, montaje

shaft
G Schaft, Welle
F arbre, essieu, tige
S árbol, asta, eje

shake out, to
G ausschütteln
F secouer
S sacudir

shake, to
G rütteln
F secouer
S sacudir, trepidar, vibrar

shaker
G Rüttler, Schüttelmaschine, Schüttler
F secoueuse, secoueur, vibreur
S agitador, vibrador

shaking movement
G Schüttelbewegung
F mouvement d'agitation
S movimiento de agitación

shampoo
G Shampoo
F shampooing
S champú

shape (of particles)
G Form (z. B. von Partikeln)
F forme (de particules)
S forma (por ejemplo de partículas)

sharp
G scharf
F coupant, aiguisé, piquant
S afilado, agudo, cortante

shatter-proof
G bruchfest
F incassable
S irrompible

shear gradient
G Schergefälle
F taux de cisaillement
S gradiente de cizallamiento

shear intensity
G Scherintensität
F intensité de cisaillement
S intensidad de cizallamiento

shear strength
G Scherkraft
F force de cisaillement
S fuerza de cizallamiento

shear stress
G Scherspannung, Schubspannung
F contrainte de cisaillement, contrainte de poussée
S tensión de cizallamiento, tensión de empuje

English German French Spanish

sheath
G Hülle
F douille, coussinet, manchon
S envoltura

shed particles, to
G Partikel abgeben
F libérer des particules
S liberar partículas

sheet (e. g. of foil)
G Bahn (z. B. Folien-), Blech
F bande (d'étoffe), tôle
S rollo, tira (por ejemplo de una lámina), chapa, lámina, plancha

sheet of film
G Folienbahn
F bande d'étoffe
S banda de láminas

shelf
G Lagerregal, Regal
F étagère, étagère de stockage, étagère d'entreposage
S estante, estante de almacén

shelf-life
G Haltbarkeitsdauer, Lagerfähigkeit
F durée de conservation, durée de stockage, stabilité au stockage
S duración de conservación, capacidad de almacenamiento

shift (working)
G (Arbeits-)Schicht
F équipe (de travail), travail en trois-huit
S turno de trabajo

ship, to
G versenden
F expédier
S enviar, expedir

shipment
G Versand
F expédition, envoi
S envío, expedición

shipping
G Versand
F expédition, envoi
S envío, expedición

shipping carton
G Versandkarton
F conteneur
S cartón de envío

shock-resistant
G erschütterungsbeständig
F résistant aux chocs
S resistente a la agitación

short circuit
G Kurzschluß
F court-circuit
S cortocircuito

short weight
G Untergewicht
F insuffisance de poids
S falta de peso

shortcoming
G Qualitätsmangel
F défaut de qualité
S defecto de calidad

short-term stability
G Kurzzeitstabilität
F stabilité à court terme
S estabilidad a corto plazo

shot weight
G Füllgewicht
F poids de remplissage
S peso al envasar

shoulder section (of a bottle)
G Schulter (einer Flasche)
F collet d'une bouteille
S ensanchamiento de una botella

shred, to
G zerkleinern
F hacher
S triturar

shredder
G Zerkleinerer
F hachoir
S trituradora

shrink film
G Schrumpffolie
F feuille rétractable, film rétractable
S lámina retraíble

shrink foil
G Schrumpffolie
F feuille rétractable, film rétractable
S lámina retraíble

shrink, to
G schrumpfen
F rétrécir
S contraerse, retraerse, reducirse

shrinking tunnel
G Schrumpftunnel
F tunnel de rétraction
S túnel de retracción

shut down (of a machine)
G Abschaltung (einer Maschine)
F arrêt (d'une machine)
S desconexión (de una máquina)

shut-off flap
G Absperrklappe
F clapet de fermeture
S válvula de cierre

side effect
G Nebenwirkung
F effet secondaires
S efecto colateral, efecto secundario

side reaction
G Nebenreaktion
F réaction secondaire
S reacción colateral

sieve
G Sieb
F tamis
S cedazo, criba, tamiz

sieve analysis
G Siebanalyse
F granulométrie
S granulometría

sieve fraction
G Siebfraktion
F fraction de tamisage
S fracción de tamizado

sieve insert
G Siebeinsatz
F segment de tamisage
S inserción del tamiz

sieve rupture
G Siebbruch
F rupture de trémie
S ruptura del tamiz

sieve screen
G Siebboden
F tamis
S suelo del tamiz

sieve shaker
G Siebschüttler
F tamis secoueur
S tamiz agitador

sieve tower
G Siebturm
F tour de tamisage
S torre de tamizado

sieve, to
G sieben
F tamiser
S cribar, tamizar

sift, to
G sieben
F tamiser
S cribar, tamizar

signal amplifier
G Signalverstärker
F amplificateur de signal
S amplificador de señal

signature
G (eigenhändige) Unterschrift
F signature, autographe
S firma (autógrafa)

electronic signature
G elektronische Unterschrift
F signature électronique
S firma electrónica

significance
G Bedeutung
F signification
S importancia, significado

sign-in log
G Ankunftsvermerk
F mention de venue
S nota de llegada

sign-out log
G Ausgangsvermerk
F mention d'origine
S mención inicial, nota inicial

silencer
G Schalldämpfer
F silencieux, amortisseur de son
S silenciador

silica
G Siliciumdioxid
F silice
S dióxido de silicio

silica gel
G Kieselgel, Silicagel
F gel de silice
S gel de sílice

silicate
G Silikat
F silicate
S silicato

silicic acid
G Kieselsäure
F silice, acide silicique
S ácido silícico

silicone emulsion
G Silikonemulsion
F émulsion de silicone
S emulsión de silicona

silicone tubing
G Silikonschlauch
F tube de silicone
S tubo de silicona

siliconisation
G Silikonisierung
F siliconisation
S siliconización

silk glossy
G seidenglänzend
F brillant (comme de la soie)
S brillante como seda

simulated test condition
G simulierte Testbedingung
F condition de test simulée
S condiciones simuladas de ensayo

simultaneous
G gleichzeitig
F simultanément
S simultáneo, simultáneamente

single coating process
G Einschichtverfahren
F procédé monocouche
S procedimiento de cubierta simple

single dose
G Einzeldosis
F dose unique
S dosis única

single dose container
G Einzeldosisbehältnis
F récipient monodose
S recipiente de dosis única

single dose form
G monolithische Arzneiform
F forme pharmaceutique monolithique
S formulación monolítica

single dose unit
G einzeldosierte Arzneiform
F une dose d'utilisation, forme d'une unité de prise
S forma farmacéutica de dosis única

single step operation
G in einem Arbeitsgang
F opération en une seule étape
S operación en etapa única

sink
G Ausguß
F évier
S descarga, orificio de descarga

sinker
G Senkkörper
F plomb
S lastre, plomo

sinter, to
G sintern
F fritter
S aglomerar, sinterizar

siphon
G Geruchsverschluß
F siphon
S válvula de hedor

site
G Standort
F emplacement
S emplazamiento, ubicación

site of action
G Angriffspunkt
F site d'application
S lugar de aplicación

site plan
G Lageplan
F schéma, plans du site
S plano del lugar

size
G Format, Größe
F taille, format
S formato, magnitud, tamaño

size changeover
G Formatumstellung
F modification d'un format
S cambio de formato

size exclusion chromatography
G Ausschlußchromatographie
F chromatographie par limite d'exclusion
S cromatografía de exclusión

skilled worker
G Facharbeiter
F ouvrier qualifié
S tabajador cualificado

skirting (of machine)
G Abhängung, Schürze
F tablier
S delantal

sleeve
G Hülse
F douille, coussinet, manchon
S cápsula, cáscara

slide (microscopy)
G Objektträger (Mikroskopie)
F porte-objet (microscopie)
S portaobjetos (microscopio)

sliding door
G Schiebetür
F porte coulissante
S puerta corrediza

slip property
G Gleiteigenschaft
F propriété lubrifiante
S propiedad deslizante

slip, to
G gleiten
F couler, glisser
S deslizar, resbalar

slippage
G Durchschlupf
F décalage
S postigo, puerta falsa

slip-proof
G rutschsicher
F anti-dérapant
S antideslizante

slit
G Schlitz, Spalt, Spalte
F crevasse, fente, fissure, rainure
S fisura, hendidura, raja

slit width
G Spaltbreite
F largeur d'une fissure, largeur d'une fente
S anchura de la fisura

slope
G Gefälle, Neigung, Schräge
F biais, gradient, inclinaison, pente
S declive, gradiente, inclinación, oblicuidad, pendiente

sloped
G geneigt, mit Gefälle
F incliné, avec une pente
S inclinado, con inclinación, con pendiente

sloping
G abgeschrägt, schräg
F biseauté, en biseau, incliné, oblique, taillé en biais
S biselado, inclinado, oblicuo

sloping agar
G Schrägagar
F agar oblique
S agar oblicuo

sloping flooring
G Gefälleestrich
F chape inclinée
S pavimento inclinado

sloping position, in
G Schräglage
F position inclinée
S inclinación

slow fuse
G träge Sicherung
F fusible à action retardée
S fusible lento

smear
G Ausstrich
F ensemencement
S extensión, frotis

smear, to (microbiological colonies)
G ausstreichen (mikrobiol. Kolonien)
F ensemencer (colonies microbiol.)
S sembrar (colonias microbiológicas)

smock
G Kurzkittel
F blouse
S blusa

smoke detector
G Rauchmelder
F détecteur de fumée
S detector de humo

smoke generator
G Raucherzeuger
F générateur de fumée
S generador de humo

smoke tube
G Rauchröhrchen
F tube de fumée
S tubo de humo

smooth
G glatt
F lisse, poli
S liso, pulido, resbaladizo

smooth, to
G glätten
F polir
S alisar, pulir

snap cap
G Schnappdeckel
F couvercle à enclenchement
S tapa de cierre de golpe

snap lid
G Schnappdeckel
F couvercle à enclenchement
S tapa de cierre de golpe

snap, to (an ampoule)
G abknicken (eine Ampulle)
F casser (une ampoule)
S romper por el cuello (ampolla)

soak, to
G imprägnieren, tränken
F imprégner
S impregnar, empapar, embeber

socket
G Buchse, Sockel
F borne, socle
S base, casquillo, hembrilla, manguito, zócalo

sodium hydroxide solution
G Natronlauge
F soude
S sosa alcalina

soft gelatine capsule
G Weichgelatinekapsel
F gélule molle
S cápsula de gelatina blanda

soften, to (water)
G enthärten (Wasser), erweichen
F adoucir (eau), ramollir
S ablandar (agua), reblandecer

softening agent
G Weichmacher
F plastifiant
S plastificante

softening point
G Erweichungspunkt
F point de ramollissement
S punto de reblandecimiento

software qualification
G Softwarequalifizierung
F qualification d'un logiciel
S cualificación de la software

soil
G Boden
F sol, plancher
S suelo

solenoid valve
G elektromagnetisches Ventil, Magnetventil
F vanne solénoïde, vanne magnétique
S válvula electromagnética, válvula magnética

solid
G Feststoff, fest
F solide
S duradero, estable, sólido, sustancia sólida

solid dosage forms
G feste Formen
F forme de dosage solide
S formas sólidas de dosificación

solid extract
G Dickextrakt
F extrait solide
S extracto sólido

solid matter content
G Feststoffgehalt
F teneur en matière solide
S contenido en materia sólida

solid phase
G feste Phase
F phase solide
S fase sólida

solid phase extraction
G Festphasenextraktion
F extraction en phase solide
S extracción en fase sólida

solidification point
G Erstarrungspunkt
F point de solidification
S punto de solidificación

solidification temperature
G Erstarrungstemperatur
F température de solidification
S temperatura de solidificación

solidification time
G Erstarrungszeit, Abbindezeit
F temps de solidification
S tiempo de solidificación

solidify, to
G erstarren
F solidifier
S solidificar

solidity
G Festigkeit
F solidité
S firmeza, solidez

solubiliser
G Lösungsvermittler
F solubilisant
S solubilizante

solubility
G Löslichkeit
F solubilité
S solubilidad

soluble
G löslich
F soluble
S soluble

insoluble
G unlöslich
F insoluble
S insoluble

practically insoluble
G praktisch unlöslich
F pratiquement insoluble
S prácticamente insoluble

readily soluble
G leicht löslich
F facilement soluble
S fácilmente soluble

slightly soluble
G wenig löslich
F peu soluble
S poco soluble

sparingly soluble
G schwer löslich
F difficilement soluble
S difícilmente soluble

very slightly soluble
G sehr schwer löslich
F très difficilement soluble
S muy difícilmente soluble

very soluble
G sehr leicht löslich
F très soluble
S muy fácilmente soluble

solution
G Lösung
F solution
S solución

saturated solution
G gesättigte Lösung
F solution saturée
S solución saturada

supersaturated solution
G übersättigte Lösung
F solution sursaturée
S solución sobresaturada

unsaturated solution
G ungesättigte Lösung
F solution non-saturée
S solución insaturada

solution for haemofiltration
G Hämofiltrationslösung
F solution d'hémofiltration
S solución de hemofiltración

solution for peritoneal dialysis
G Peritonealdialyselösung
F solution pour dialyse péritonéale
S diálisis peritoneal

solvent
G Lösungsmittel
F solvant
S solvente

inorganic solvent
G anorganisches Lösungsmittel
F solvant anorganique
S solvente inorgánico

organic solvent
G organisches Lösungsmittel
F solvant organique
S solvente orgánico

solvent collector
G Lösungsmittelauffangbehälter
F collecteur de solvant
S colector de solvente

solvent evaporation
G Verdampfen des Lösungsmittels
F évaporation du solvant
S evaporación del solvente

solvent front
G Fließmittelfront
F front de migration du solvant
S frente de migración del solvente

solvent recovery
G Lösungsmittelrückgewinnung
F récupération des solvants
S recuperación de solventes

solvent separation
G Lösungsmittelabscheidung
F séparation des solvants
S separación de solventes

solvent storage
G Lösungsmittellager
F stockage de solvants
S almacén de solventes

solvent-resistant
G lösungsmittelbeständig
F résistant aux solvants
S resistente a solventes

sorting belt
G Sortierband
F bande de triage
S cinta clasificadora

sound
G intakt
F intact
S intacto

source
G Quelle
F source
S fuente

source of error (failure)
G Fehlerquelle
F source d'erreur
S fuente de errores

space
G Zwischenraum
F espace
S espacio (intermedio)

spare part
G Austauschteil, Ersatzteil
F pièce de rechange
S pieza de recambio

spare parts list
G Ersatzteilliste
F liste de pièces de rechange
S lista de piezas de recambio

sparks
G Funken
F étincelles
S chispas

spatial folding (e. g. of protein)
G räumliche Faltung (z. B. eines Proteins)
F pliage spatial (par ex. des protéines)
S conformación espacial, plegamiento espacial (p. ej. de una proteína)

spatial structure
G Raumstruktur, Tertiärstruktur
F structure spatiale
S estructura espacial, estructura terciaria (p. ej. de una proteína)

spatula
G Spatel
F spatule
S espátula

English German French Spanish

English German French Spanish

special version
G Sonderausführung
F version spéciale
S construcción especial, versión especial

species
G Art, Gattung, Spezies
F espèce
S género, especie

specific gravity
G spezifisches Gewicht
F poids spécifique
S peso específico

specific gravity meter
G Pyknometer
F pycnomètre
S picnómetro

specific heat
G spezifische Wärme
F chaleur spécifique
S calor específico

specific resistance
G spezifischer Widerstand
F résistance spécifique
S resistencia específica

specific rotation
G spezifische Drehung
F rotation spécifique
S rotación específica

specific surface (area)
G spezifische Oberfläche
F aire spécifique
S superficie específica

specification
G Angabe, Spezifikation, Vorschrift
F donnée, instruction, spécification
S datos, especificación, prescripción

complying with specification
G vorschriftsmäßig
F en conformité avec les spécifications
S conforme a las prescripciones

out of specification (OOS)
G außerhalb der Spezifikation
F hors spécification
S fuera de la especificación

specification limit
G Spezifikationsgrenze
F limite de spécification
S límite de especificación

lower specification limit
G untere Spezifikationsgrenze
F limite inférieure de spécification
S límite inferior de especificación

tight specification limits
G enge Spezifikationsgrenzen
F limites étroites de spécification
S límites estrechos de especificación

upper specification limit
G obere Spezifikationsgrenze
F limite supérieure de spécification
S límite superior de especificación

specificity
G Spezifität
F spécificité
S especificidad

specify, to
G spezifizieren
F spécifier
S especificar

specimen
G Muster
F échantillon, spécimen
S muestra, espécimen

spectrophotometry
G Spektralphotometrie
F spectrophotomètre
S espectrofotometría

spectrum
G Spektrum
F spectre
S espectro

speed adjustment
G Geschwindigkeitseinstellung
F ajustement de la vitesse
S ajuste de la velocidad

speed of solubility
G Lösungsgeschwindigkeit
F vitesse de solubilisation
S velocidad de disolución

spherical
G sphärisch
F sphérique
S esférico

spike
G Spike
F pointe, ajout
S punta

spill, to
G verschütten
F renverser, répandre
S derramar, verter

spiral
G spiralförmig
F en forme d'hélice
S espiraliforme

splash water
G Spritzwasser
F eau de ruissellement
S agua de inyección, agua de rociado

splashes
G Spritzer
F éclaboussures
S inyección, rociado, salpicadura

splice point
G Klebestelle
F aire de collage
S zona de adherencia

splice recognition
G Klebestellenerkennung
F identification de l'aire de collage
S reconocimiento de la zona de adherencia

split bag
G Trennbeutel
F sachet de séparation
S bolsa de separación

spokesman
G Vorsitzender, Obmann
F porte-parole
S portavoz, presidente

sponge
G Schwamm
F éponge
S esponja

spontaneous reaction
G Spontanreaktion
F réaction spontanée
S reacción espontánea

spore former
G Sporenbildner
F producteur de spores
S productor de esporas

spore strip
G Sporenstreifen
F bande de spores
S banda de esporas

spores
G Sporen
F spores
S esporas

sporicide
G sporozid
F sporicide
S esporicida

spot-weld, to
G punktschweißen
F souder par points
S soldar por puntos

spray area
G Sprühbereich
F aire de pulvérisation
S área de pulverización

spray cycle
G Sprühzyklus
F cycle de pulvérisation
S ciclo de pulverización

spray protection
G Spritzschutz
F couvercle anti-éclaboussures
S protección frente al salpicado

spray rate
G Sprührate
F vitesse de pulvérisation
S tasa de pulverización

spray tower
G Rieselturm
F tour d'arrosage
S torre de lavado

spray, to
G aufsprühen
F pulvériser
S pulverizar

spray-dry, to
G sprühtrocknen
F séchage par atomisation
S secar atomizando

spraying system
G Sprühsystem
F système de pulvérisation
S sistema de pulverización

spread (of values)
G Streuung (von Werten)
F diffusion, dispersion (de valeurs)
S dispersión (de valores)

spreadability
G Streichfähigkeit
F aptitude à être étendu
S untabilidad

spreading
G Spreizung
F propagation
S extensión, propagación

spring
G Feder (Sprung-)
F ressort
S resorte

spring balance
G Federwaage
F balance à ressort
S balanza de resorte

spring suspension
G Federaufhängung
F suspension à ressort
S suspensión mediante resorte

sprinkler
G Sprinkleranlage
F réseau de sprinkler
S aspersor

sprinkler can
G Streudose
F flacon saupoudreur
S frasco espolvoreador

sputum
G Sputum
F crachat
S esputo

square root
G Quadratwurzel
F racine carrée
S raíz cuadrada

squeeze bottle
G Quetschflasche
F flacon souple doseur
S recipiente flexible

squeeze, to
G quetschen
F écraser
S aplastar

stabilising agent
G Stabilisator
F agent stabilisant
S estabilizador

stability
G Haltbarkeit
F stabilité
S conservabilidad, estabilidad

stability study
G Stabilitätsuntersuchung
F étude de stabilité
S ensayo de estabilidad

long-term stability
G Langzeitstabilität
F étude de stabilité à long terme
S estabilidad a largo plazo

short-term stability
G Kurzzeitstabilität
F étude de stabilité à court terme
S estabilidad a corto plazo

stability test
G Haltbarkeitsuntersuchung
F test de stabilité
S prueba de estabilidad

stable
G dauerhaft, haltbar
F durable, stable
S consistente, duradero, estable

stack
G Stapel
F pile
S montón, pila

stack, to
G stapeln
F empiler
S almacenar, amontonar, apilar

stacker
G Stapler
F chariot élévateur
S apilador

stacking
G Stapelung
F empilage
S apilamiento

stacking box
G Stapelkasten
F boîte de stockage
S caja de apilamiento

stacking device
G Stapelvorrichtung
F dispositif de stockage
S dispositivo de apilamiento

stacking plan (in warehouse)
G Stapelplan (im Lager)
F plan de stockage (entrepôt)
S plan de almacenamiento

stain
G Färbemittel, Farbe, Fleck
F colorant, pigment, tache, teinture
S color, colorante, mancha, pigmento, tintura

stain, to
G färben
F colorer, teinter, teindre
S colorear, teñir

stainer
G Färbegerät
F appareil à teindre
S teñidor

staining liquid
G Färbelösung
F solution de teinture
S solución colorante

stainless steel
G Edelstahl
F acier inoxydable, inox
S acero inoxidable

stainless steel drum
G Edelstahlfaß
F tonneau en acier inoxydable
S tonel de acero inoxidable

stainless steel piping
G Edelstahlrohrleitung
F tuyauterie en inox
S tubería de acero inoxidable

stairs
G Treppenhaus
F escaliers
S escalera de la casa

stamp (for printing)
G Stempel (zum Drucken)
F tampon (pour imprimer)
S estampadora (para imprimir)

stamp, to
G ausstanzen, prägen, stanzen, stempeln
F découper à l'emporte-pièce, estamper, poinçonner
S acuñar, estampar, perforar, punzonar, troquelar

stand
G Gestell, Stativ
F cadre, support, trépied
S armazón, bastidor, soporte, trípode

standard
G Maßstab, Norm, Referenzstandard
F échelle, norme, standard, standard de référence
S escala, estándar, estándar de referencia, norma, patrón

standard construction
G Grundausführung
F fabrication standard
S versión básica

standard deviation
G Standardabweichung
F déviation standard
S desviación estándar

maximum permitted standard deviation
G maximal zulässige Standardabweichung
F déviation standard maximum permise
S desviación estándar máxima permitida

standard operating procedure (SOP)
G Standardarbeitsanweisung
F procédures opératoires standards
S instrucción estándar de trabajo

standard reference material
G Standardreferenzsubstanz
F substance de référence standard
S sustancia de referencia estándar

standard specification
G Normvorschrift
F spécification standard
S prescripción estándar

standardisation
G Normierung
F standardisation
S normalización, estandarización

standardisation factor
G Standardfaktor
F facteur de standardisation
S factor estándar

standardise, to
G standardisieren
F standardiser
S estandarizar

standardised
G genormt
F standardisé
S estandarizado, normalizado

standing time
G Standzeit
F période d'utilisation
S período de funcionamiento

starch
G Stärke
F amidon
S almidón

start of study
G Studienstart
F démarrage d'un essai clinique
S comienzo del estudio

start of trial
G Studienstart
F démarrage d'un essai clinique
S comienzo del estudio

start speed
G Anfangsgeschwindigkeit
F vitesse initiale
S velocidad inicial

start, to (a process)
G anfahren, starten (Ablauf)
F démarrer (un procédé)
S comenzar (un proceso), poner en marcha

start/stop key
G An/Aus-Taste
F touche marche-arrêt
S interruptor de encendido

starting material
G Ausgangsstoff
F matériel de départ, matière première
S sustancia de partida, sustancia inicial

start-up
G Inbetriebnahme
F mise en service
S puesta en marcha, puesta en servicio

start-up, to
G anfahren
F démarrer
S poner en marcha

state-of-the-art
G Stand der Technik
F dernier cri de la technique
S estado (actual) de la técnica

static charge
G statische Aufladung
F charge statique
S carga estática

static load
G statische Belastung
F charge statique
S carga estática

static stress
G statische Beanspruchung
F stress statique
S tensión estática

stationary phase
G stationäre Phase
F phase stationnaire
S fase estacionaria

statistician
G Statistiker
F statisticien
S estadístico

status report
G Statusbericht
F rapport de situation
S informe de la situación

statute
G Gesetz
F loi
S ley

steam
G Dampf
F vapeur d'eau
S vapor

purified steam
G gereinigter Dampf
F vapeur purifiée
S vapor purificado

steam connection
G Dampfleitungsverbindung
F connexion de conduite à vapeur
S conexión de conducción de vapor

steam consumption
G Dampfverbrauch
F consommation de vapeur
S consumo de vapor

steam generation
G Dampferzeugung
F production de vapeur
S producción de vapor

steam line
G Dampfleitung
F conduite de vapeur
S conducción de vapor

steam pressure
G Dampfdruck
F pression de vapeur
S presión de vapor

steam separator
G Dampfabscheider
F séparateur de vapeur
S separador de vapor

steam sterilisation
G Dampfsterilisation
F stérilisation à la vapeur
S esterilización al vapor

terminal steam sterilisation
G abschließende Dampfsterilisation
F stérilisation finale à la vapeur
S esterilización final al vapor

steam valve
G Dampfventil
F soupape de vapeur
S válvula de vapor

steam-heated
G dampfbeheizt
F chauffé à la vapeur
S calentado al vapor

steel
G Stahl
F acier
S acero

stainless steel
G Edelstahl
F inox, acier inoxydable
S acero inoxidable

steep
G steil
F raide, escarpé
S empinado, escarpado

stem cell bank
G Stammzellbank
F banque de cellules souches
S banco de células germinales

stench trap
G Geruchsverschluß
F siphon
S válvula de hedor

stencil
G Schablone
F matrice, pochoir, patron
S modelo, patrón, plantilla

stepwise
G schrittweise, stufenweise
F étape par étape, par étapes, échelonné
S paso a paso, gradualmente

stereoselective
G stereoselektiv
F stéréosélectif
S estereoselectivo

sterical arrangement
G sterische Anordnung
F configuration stérique
S configuración estérica

sterile
G keimfrei, steril
F stérile
S estéril

sterile clothing
G Sterilraumkleidung
F vêtement pour zone stérile
S vestuario estéril

sterile filtration
G Sterilfiltration
F filtration stérile
S filtración estéril

sterile form
G sterile Zubereitung
F forme stérile
S forma estéril, preparación estéril

sterile gowns
G Sterilraumkleidung
F vêtement pour zone stérile
S vestuario estéril

sterile product
G Sterilprodukt
F produit stérile
S producto estéril

sterile-filter, to
G sterilfiltrieren
F stérile-filtrer
S filtrar estérilmente

sterile-filtered
G sterilfiltriert
F stérile-filtré
S filtrado estérilmente

sterilisability
G Sterilisierbarkeit
F aptitude à être stérilisé
S esterilizabilidad

sterilisation
G Sterilisation
F stérilisation
S esterilización

sterilisation temperature
G Sterilisationstemperatur
F température de stérilisation
S temperatura de esterilización

sterilisation time
G Sterilisationszeit
F temps de stérilisation
S tiempo de esterilización

steriliser
G Sterilisator
F autoclave
S esterilizador

sterility assurance
G Sterilisationssicherheit
F garantie de stérilité
S garantía de esterilización

sterility test
G Steriltest
F test de stérilité
S prueba estéril

steroids
G Steroide
F stéroïdes
S esteroides

stick, to (tablets)
G kleben (bei Tabletten)
F adhérer
S adherir (comprimidos)

sticking plaster
G Heftpflaster, Pflaster
F sparadrap
S esparadrapo

sticky
G klebrig
F collant, gluant
S pegajoso

still
G Destille
F appareil de distillation
S alambique

stir, to
G rühren
F agiter
S agitar

stirrer
G Rührer, Rührwerk
F agitateur
S agitador

stirrer hub
G Rührwerksnabe
F moyeu d'agitateur
S cubo del agitador

stirrer rake
G Rührwerksrechen
F râteau d'agitateur
S rastrillo del agitador

stirring blade
G Rührflügel
F pale d'agitation
S aleta de agitación

stirring speed
G Rührgeschwindigkeit
F vitesse d'agitation
S velocidad de agitación

stirring vessel
G Rührkessel
F récipient de l'agitateur
S caldera de agitación

stock
G Lagerbestand
F inventaire, stock
S existencias en almacén, stocks

stock culture
G Stammkultur (von Organismen)
F culture mère
S cultivo madre (de organismos)

stock management system
G Lagerhaltung
F système de gestion du stockage
S gestión de stocks

stock solution
G Stammlösung
F solution mère
S solución madre

stoichiometry
G Stöchiometrie
F stoichiométrie
S estequiometría

stopcock
G Absperrhahn, Hahn (technisch)
F robinet, robinet d'arrêt
S grifo, grifo de cierre

stopper
G Stopfen
F bouchon, tampon
S tapón

stopper washing machine
G Stopfenwaschmaschine
F machine à laver les bouchons
S máquina de lavado de tapones

storage
G Aufbewahrung, Lagerung
F archivage, conservation, stockage
S almacenaje, almacenamiento, conservación

storage area
G Lager(bereich)
F aire d'entreposage, aire de stockage
S almacén

storage conditions
G Lagerungsbedingungen
F conditions de stockage
S condiciones de almacenamiento

storage precautions
G Vorsichtsmaßnahmen bei der Lagerung
F précautions de stockage
S medidas de precaución al almacenar

storage room
G Lagerraum
F entrepôt
S almacén, depósito

storage space
G Lagerplatz
F espace de stockage
S lugar de almacenamiento

storage stability
G Lagerfähigkeit
F stabilité au stockage
S capacidad de almacenamiento

storage tank
G Aufbewahrungstank
F récipient de stockage
S tanque de conservación

storage vessel
G Lagertank, Vorratstank
F récipient de stockage, cuve de stockage
S tanque (de) depósito

store dry, to
G trocken lagern
F stocker au sec
S almacenar en seco

store, to
G aufbewahren, einlagern
F conserver, garder, stocker
S almacenar, conservar, guardar

stored blood
G Blutkonserve
F sang conservé
S conserva de sangre

straight
G Gerade
F ligne droite
S recta (línea)

straight line
G Gerade
F ligne droite
S recta (línea)

strain (microbiol.)
G Stamm
F lignée
S cepa

stray light
G Lichtstreuung, Streulicht
F dispersion de la lumière, lumière diffuse
S dispersión luminosa, luz difusa

stray range
G Streubreite
F dispersion
S dispersión

streaks
G Schliere
F strie
S estría

street clothing
G Straßenkleidung
F vêtements de ville
S ropa de calle

strength (e. g. of a tablet)
G Stärke (z. B. einer Tablette)
F dureté (par ex. d'un comprimé)
S fuerza (p. ej. de un comprimido)

stress
G Beanspruchung
F soumission à un effort
S carga, tensión

stria
G Schliere
F strie
S estría

strip, to
G ausdampfen
F passer à la vapeur
S evaporar, volatilizar

stroke
G Hub, Kolbenweg
F course de piston
S carrera del émbolo

stroke volume
G Hubvolumen
F volume de course
S volumen de carrera del émbolo

structural analysis
G Strukturaufklärung
F analyse structurelle
S análisis estructural

structural formula
G Strukturformel
F formule développée
S fórmula estructural

stub
G Stichleitung
F bout
S adaptador de guiaondas

study design
G Studiendesign
F design d'un essai clinique
S diseño de un estudio (clínico)

sub-atmospheric pressure
G Atmosphärenunterdruck
F dépression atmosphérique
S presión atmosférica baja

sub-batch
G Teilcharge
F sous-lot
S lote parcial, sublote

sub-culture
G Subkultur
F culture repiquée
S subcultivo

subcutaneous
G subkutan
F sous-cutanée
S subcutáneo

subcutaneous use
G subkutane Anwendung
F utilisation sous-cutanée
S aplicación subcutánea

sublimation
G Sublimierung
F sublimation
S sublimación

sub-lingual spray
G Sublingualspray
F aérosol sublingual
S spray sublingual

submerge, to
G untertauchen
F immerger
S sumergir, sumergirse

submission (of an application for marketing approval)
G Einreichung (eines Zulassungsantrags)
F déposition (d'une demande d'autorisation de mise sur le marché)
S presentación (de una solicitud de autorización)

submission file for marketing authorisation
G Zulassungsdossier
F dossier de demande d'autorisation de mise sur le marché
S dosier de solicitud de autorización

submit, to (application for marketing approval)
G einreichen (Zulassungsantrag)
F soumettre (une demande d'autorisation de mise sur le marché)
S presentar (una solicitud de autorización)

subsequent test
G Nachuntersuchung
F examen supplétif
S examen adicional

subsidiary company
G Tochterfirma
F filiale (société)
S empresa filial, empresa subsidiaria

substance modelling
G Substanzmodellierung
F modelage de substance
S modelado de sustancias

substitution
G Substitution
F substitution
S sustitución

substitution reaction
G Substitutionsreaktion
F réaction de substitution
S reacción de sustitución

substrate
G Substrat
F substrat
S sustrato

sub-strength
G Unterdosierung
F hypo-dose
S infradosificación

suction ventilator
G Luftabsauger
F ventilateur aspirant
S aspirador de aire

sugar-coated tablet
G Dragee, Zuckerdragee
F comprimé dragéifié, dragée
S gragea, gragea azucarada

suitability
G Eignung
F qualification
S aptitud, calificación, idoneidad

suitability test
G Eignungsprüfung
F test de qualification
S prueba de aptitud

suitable
G angemessen, geeignet, passend
F approprié, adéquat, convenable
S adecuado, apropiado, conveniente

suitable for storage
G lagerfähig
F stockable, apte à l'emmagasinage
S adecuado para almacenaje

sulphate ash
G Sulfatasche
F cendre sulfatée
S ceniza sulfatada

sulphuric acid
G Schwefelsäure
F acide sulfurique
S ácido sulfúrico

sum distribution
G Summenverteilung
F distribution des sommes
S distribución de sumas

summary of product characteristics (SPC)
G Zusammenfassung der Produktmerkmale
F résumé des caractéristiques du produit
S resumen de características del producto

sump
G Ölwanne
F carter à huile
S cárter

super-heated steam
G gespannter Wasserdampf
F vapeur surchauffée
S vapor de agua sobrecalentado, vapor sobrecalentado

supernatant
G Überstand
F surnageant
S sobrenadante

supersaturation
G Übersättigung
F sursaturation
S sobresaturación

supervise, to
G überwachen
F contrôler, surveiller
S supervisar, vigilar

supervision
G Aufsicht
F supervision, surveillance
S control, inspección, supervisión

supervisor
G Meister
F maître
S maestro

supplement
G Aufschlag
F supplément, majoration
S aumento, suplemento

supplementation
G Ergänzung
F complément, supplément
S complemento, suplemento

supplier
G Lieferant
F fournisseur
S abastecedor, proveedor

supplier qualification
G Lieferantenqualifizierung
F qualification de fournisseur
S cualificación del abastecedor

supplier's random sample
G Lieferantenstichprobe
F échantillon fortuit du fournisseur
S muestra al azar del abastecedor

supply
G Versorgung
F alimentation
S abastecimiento, suministro

supply connection
G Versorgungsanschluß
F connection de charge
S conexión de abastecimiento

supply input
G Versorgungsanschluß
F connection de charge
S conexión de abastecimiento

supply, to
G liefern, versorgen mit
F fournir, livrer
S abastecer, proveer, suministrar

support
G Halterung, Stutzen
F support, embout
S empalme, soporte, tubuladura

support brace
G Stütze
F support
S apoyo, soporte

support pressure
G Stützdruck
F contre-pression, pression de soutien
S contrapresión, presión de soporte

supporting construction
G Stützkonstruktion
F construction de soutien
S construcción de sostén

supporting structure
G Gerüst
F échafaudage
S andamio, armazón, esqueleto

suppositories
G Suppositorien
F suppositoires
S supositorios

suppository base
G Suppositoriengrundlage
F composant de base d'un suppositoire
S excipiente de un supositorio

suppository machine
G Zäpfchengießmaschine
F machine à mouler des suppositoires
S máquina de moldear supositorios

surface
G Oberfläche
F surface, aire
S superficie

rough surface
G rauhe Oberfläche
F surface rugueuse
S superficie rugosa

smooth surface
G glatte Oberfläche
F surface polie, surface lisse
S superficie lisa

specific surface area
G spezifische Oberfläche
F aire spécifique
S superficie específica

surface activity
G Oberflächenaktivität
F activité de surface
S actividad de superficie

surface binding
G Oberflächenbindung
F liaison superficielle
S ligadura de superficie

surface coating
G Oberflächenbeschichtung
F revêtement de surface
S revestimiento de superficies

surface diameter
G Oberflächendurchmesser
F diamètre d'une surface
S diámetro de una superficie

surface lacquer
G Oberflächenlackierung
F laquage superficiel
S barnizado de superficies

surface properties
G Oberflächenbeschaffenheit
F propriétés de surface
S características de superficie

surface rawness
G Oberflächenrauhigkeit
F rugosité de la surface
S rugosidad de superficie

surface tension
G Oberflächenspannung
F tension superficielle
S tensión superficial

surface treatment
G Oberflächenbehandlung
F traitement de surface
S tratamiento de superficies

surfactant
G grenzflächenaktiver Stoff, oberflächenaktive Verbindung
F tensioactif
S agente tensioactivo, sustancia tensioactiva

susceptible to corrosion
G korrosionsanfällig
F susceptible à la corrosion
S susceptible a la corrosión

suspend, to
G suspendieren
F suspenser
S suspender

suspended ceiling
G abgehängte Decke, Zwischendecke
F faux plafond
S techo intermedio, techo suspendido

suspendibility
G Suspendierbarkeit
F suspensif
S suspensibilidad

suspension
G Aufhängung, Suspendierung, Suspension
F suspension
S suspensión

suspension device
G Aufhängung
F suspension
S suspensión

sustained use
G Dauergebrauch
F utilisation permamente (d'un instrument)
S uso duradero

suture
G Nahtmaterial
F suture
S material de sutura

swab
G Tupfer
F tampon d'ouate, gaze
S torunda

swab test
G Wischtest
F essai de prélèvement par tampon d'ouate
S prueba de prelavado con torunda de algodón

sweetener
G Süßstoff
F édulcorant
S edulcorante

swell, to
G quellen
F gonfler
S brotar, hincharse

swelling capacity
G Quellfähigkeit
F capacité de gonflement
S capacidad de hinchamiento

swing-out device
G Ausschwenkvorrichtung
F dispositif d'orientation
S dispositivo giratorio

switch
G Schalter
F interrupteur
S conmutador, interruptor

switch box
G Schaltkasten
F armoire électrique
S caja de distribución

switch module
G Schaltelement
F élément commutateur
S elemento interruptor

switch off, to
G abschalten
F couper, arrêter
S desconectar

switch on, to
G einschalten
F allumer
S conectar, encender

switching stage
G Schaltstufe
F étape de permutation
S etapa de conmutación

swivel arm
G Schwenkarm
F bras pivotant
S brazo giratorio

swivel lid (e. g. of autoclave)
G Drehdeckel (z. B. eines Autoklaven)
F couvercle pivotant (par ex. d'un autoclave)
S tapa de rosca (p. ej. de autoclave)

swivelled
G ausgeschwenkt
F pivoté
S girado hacia fuera

swivelling device
G Ausschwenkvorrichtung
F dispositif d'orientation
S dispositivo giratorio

synaresis
G Synärese
F synérèse
S sinéresis

synthesis
G Synthese
F synthèse
S síntesis

synthesis route
G Syntheseweg
F voie de synthèse
S vía de síntesis

synthetic granulation
G Aufbaugranulierung
F granulation hors taille
S granulación sintética

synthetic resin
G Kunstharz
F résine synthétique
S resina sintética

synthetic resin screed
G Kunstharzestrich
F couche de résine synthétique
S pavimento de resina sintética

synthetic tissue
G Kunststoffgewebe
F tissu synthétique, tissu en plastique
S tejido sintético

syringe
G Spritze
F seringue
S jeringa

disposable syringe
G Einmalspritze
F seringue à usage unique
S jeringa de uso único

prefilled syringe
G Fertigspritze
F seringue prête à l'emploi
S jeringa lista para el uso

syringe cylinder
G Spritzenzylinder
F cylindre de seringue
S cilindro de jeringa

syrup
G Sirup
F sirop
S jarabe

system specification
G Systemspezifikation
F spécification d'un système
S especificación de un sistema

system suitability test
G Systemeignungstest
F essai d'aptitude d'un système
S ensayo de adecuación de un sistema

tab
G Einstecklasche
F languette, attache, patte
S cubrejunta de pestaña

table
G Tabelle
F tableau, table
S tabla

tablet
G Tablette
F comprimé
S comprimido

faulty tablets
G fehlerhafte Tabletten
F comprimés défectueux
S comprimidos defectuosos

oblong tablet
G längliche Tablette
F comprimé allongé
S comprimido elongado

tablet appearance
G Aussehen der Tablette
F apparence d'un comprimé
S aspecto de un comprimido

tablet category
G Tablettenkategorie
F catégorie du comprimé
S categoría de comprimido

tablet checking
G Tablettenkontrolle
F contrôle d'un comprimé
S control de comprimidos

tablet colour uniformity
G Einheitlichkeit der Tablettenfarbe
F uniformité de la couleur d'un comprimé
S uniformidad del color de los comprimidos

tablet core
G Tablettenkern
F noyau d'un comprimé
S núcleo del comprimido

tablet counter
G Zählbrett (für Tabletten)
F compteur de comprimés
S contador de comprimidos

tablet crushing strength
G Bruchfestigkeit einer Tablette
F résistance à la rupture d'un comprimé
S resistencia a la ruptura de un comprimido

tablet diameter
G Tablettendurchmesser
F diamètre d'un comprimé
S diámetro del comprimido

English German French Spanish

tablet dimensions
G Tablettenabmessungen
F dimensions d'un comprimé
S dimensiones del comprimido

tablet disintegrant
G Sprengmittel
F agent délitant, désintégrant
S desintegrante

tablet dye
G Tablettierfarbe
F couleur de fabrication de comprimés
S color de fabricación de comprimidos

tablet ejection
G Tablettenauswurf
F éjection d'un comprimé
S expulsión de comprimidos

tablet exit chute
G Tablettenablaufrinne
F rigole d'écoulement pour comprimés
S canal de salida de los comprimidos

tablet gate
G Tablettenablaufweichen
F déversoir pour comprimés
S lámina divisoria para comprimidos

tablet hardness
G Tablettenhärte
F dureté d'un comprimé
S dureza del comprimido

tablet inconsistency
G Uneinheitlichkeit von Tabletten
F hétérogénéité des comprimés
S heterogeneidad de los comprimidos

tablet monitoring system
G Tablettenüberwachungssystem
F système de surveillance des comprimés
S sistema de vigilancia de comprimidos

tablet output
G Tablettenausstoß, Tablettierausstoß
F débit de production de comprimés
S rendimiento en comprimidos, rendimiento de la máquina de comprimidos

tablet press
G Tablettenpresse
F presse à comprimés, pastilleuse
S prensa de comprimidos

automated tablet press
G instrumentierte Tablettenpresse
F presse à comprimés avec instruments
S prensa automática de comprimidos

tablet profile
G Tablettenprofil
F profil du comprimé
S perfil de comprimido

tablet surface
G Tablettenoberfläche
F surface d'un comprimé
S superficie del comprimido

tablet thickness
G Tablettendicke
F épaisseur d'un comprimé
S espesor del comprimido

tablet tooling
G Tablettenwerkzeug
F presse-outil pour comprimés
S utensilios para elaborar comprimidos

tablet web height
G Tablettensteghöhe
F hauteur de bande d'un comprimé
S altura de banda de un comprimido

tablet weight
G Tablettengewicht
F poids d'un comprimé
S peso del comprimido

tablet weight variation
G Schwankung des Tablettengewichts
F écart entre les poids d'un comprimé, écart entre les poids d'un cachet
S fluctuación del peso de los comprimidos

tabletting
G Tablettierung
F fabrication de comprimés
S fabricación de comprimidos

computer-integrated tabletting (CIT)
G computerintegrierte Tablettierung
F fabrication de comprimés informatisée
S fabricación informatizada de comprimidos

tabletting machine
G Tablettiermaschine
F machine de fabrication de comprimés
S máquina de fabricación de comprimidos

tabletting mass
G Tablettiermasse
F masse de fabrication pour comprimés
S masa para comprimidos

tabletting punch
G Tablettierstempel
F poinçon de fabrication de comprimés
S troquel para comprimidos

tachometer
G Geschwindigkeitsmesser
F tachymètre
S taquímetro

tachymeter
G Drehzahlmesser
F compte-tours, tachymètre
S contador de revoluciones, taquímetro

tacky
G klebrig
F collant, gluant
S pegajoso

tailings
G Nachlauf
F addition en bout de chaîne
S adición al final de la cadena

take over, to
G übernehmen
F prendre le contrôle de
S adquirir, comprar

tamper-proof seal
G Entnahmesicherung
F sécurité de prélèvement
S precintado de un frasco

tampon
G Tampon
F tampon
S tampón

tangent
G Tangente
F tangente
S tangente

tank aspiration
G Tankbelüftung
F aération du réservoir
S ventilación del tanque

tank wagon
G Tankwagen
F wagon-citerne
S camión cisterna

tanning agent
G Gerbstoff
F tannin
S tanino

tap water
G Leitungswasser
F eau du robinet
S agua corriente

English German French Spanish

tap water feed
G Trinkwasserzufuhr
F arrivée d'eau potable
S abastecimiento de agua potable

tape
G Banderole
F banderole
S precinto

tapered
G verjüngt, konisch
F conique
S disminuido, estrechado, cónico

tapped density
G Stampfdichte
F densité de tassement
S densidad de apisonamiento

tare
G Leergewicht, Tara
F poids à vide, tare
S peso en vacío, tara

tare, to
G austarieren, tarieren
F tarer
S tarar

tarnish, to (metal)
G anlaufen (Metall)
F ternir, se ternir (métal)
S deslustrarse, empañarse (metales)

task force
G Arbeitsgruppe
F groupe de travail
S grupo de trabajo

taste
G Geschmack
F goût
S gusto

taste masking
G Geschmacksüberdeckung
F masquage d'une saveur
S enmascaramiento del sabor

tasteless
G geschmacklos
F insipide, fade
S insípido

tear
G Riß
F déchirure, fissure
S desgarro, fisura

tear strength
G Reißfestigkeit
F résistance au déchirement
S resistencia al desgarro

tear-off tab
G Aufreißlasche
F languette
S lengüeta arrancable

technical acceptance report
G Abnahmebericht
F rapport de réception technique
S informe de recepción técnica

technical floor
G Technikgeschoß
F étage du service technique
S piso de servicio técnico

technical information
G Fachinformation
F information technique
S ficha técnica (de un medicamento)

technique
G Technik, Methode
F technique, méthode
S técnica, método

technology transfer
G Technologietransfer
F transfers de technologie
S transferencia tecnológica

temperature
G Temperatur
F température
S temperatura

temperature controller
G Temperaturregler
F régulateur de température
S regulador de temperatura

temperature decrease
G Temperaturabfall
F baisse de température
S descenso de temperatura

temperature deviation
G Temperaturabweichung
F déviation de température
S desviación de temperatura

temperature equalisation
G Temperaturausgleich
F compensation de température
S compensación de temperatura

temperature fluctuation
G Temperaturschwankung
F variation de température
S fluctuación de la temperatura

temperature gradient
G Temperaturgefälle
F gradient de température
S gradiente de temperatura

temperature increase
G Temperaturerhöhung
F augmentation de température
S aumento de temperatura

temperature recorder
G Temperaturschreiber
F enregistreur de température
S registrador de temperatura

temperature sensor
G Temperaturfühler, Temperatursensor, Wärmefühler
F sonde de température, sonde thermique
S sensor de temperatura, sensor térmico

temperature setting
G Temperatureinstellung
F réglage de la température
S ajuste de temperatura

template
G Schablone
F matrice, pochoir, patron
S modelo, patrón, plantilla

temporary
G vorläufig
F temporaire
S provisional, temporal, transitorio

temporary hardness (of water)
G temporäre Härte (von Wasser)
F dureté temporaire (de l'eau)
S dureza temporal (del agua)

temporary help
G Aushilfe
F stagiaire, aide temporaire
S ayuda temporal

tender
G Ausschreibung
F appel d'offres
S anuncio, concurso, convocatoria

tenside
G oberflächenaktive Verbindung, Tensid
F tensioactif, tenside
S agente tensioactivo

tensile force
G Zugkraft
F force de traction
S fuerza de tracción

tensile strength
G Zerreißfestigkeit
F résistance au déchirement
S resistencia al desgarro

tension
G Spannung, Zug
F tension, traction
S tensión, tracción

teratogenic
G teratogen
F tératogène
S teratógeno

English German French Spanish

terminal
G Klemme
F pince, borne
S borne, pinza, terminal

terminal box
G Klemmkasten
F boîte de bornes
S caja de terminales

terminal sterile filter
G endständiger Sterilfilter
F filtre stérile terminal
S filtro estéril terminal

ternary
G ternär
F ternaire
S ternario

test certificate
G Prüfzertifikat
F certificat d'analyse
S certificado de prueba

test instructions
G Prüfanleitung, Prüfvorschrift
F instructions d'un test, mode opératoire
S instrucciones de prueba, prescripción de prueba

test loop
G Testschleife
F boucle de test
S bucle de pruebas

test method
G Prüfmethode
F méthode analytique, méthode de contrôle
S método de prueba

test organism
G Prüfkeim
F organisme de contrôle
S germen de prueba

test preparation
G Prüfpräparat
F préparation pour test
S preparado de prueba

test protocol
G Prüfprotokoll
F procès-verbal d'un test
S protocolo de prueba

test report
G Prüfbericht
F rapport expérimental
S informe de prueba

test run
G Probelauf
F essai de fonctionnement
S marcha de ensayo

test sample
G Prüfmuster
F échantillon
S muestra de prueba

test strip
G Teststäbchen
F bâtonnet de test
S bastoncillos de prueba

test tube
G Reagenzglas
F tube à essais
S probeta, tubo de ensayo

test, to
G prüfen
F tester
S comprobar, ensayar, examinar, investigar, probar

testing parameter
G Prüfparameter
F paramètre d'analyse
S parámetro de prueba

testing procedure
G Prüfanweisung, Prüfverfahren
F instructions d'un test, procédure de test
S instrucciones de prueba, procedimiento de prueba

testing schedule
G Prüfplan
F protocole opératoire
S plan de prueba, protocolo del ensayo

thaw, to
G auftauen
F dégeler
S descongelar

theoretical yield
G theoretische Ausbeute
F rendement théorique
S rendimiento teórico

therapeutic
G therapeutisch
F thérapeutique
S terapéutico

therapeutic agent
G Heilmittel
F agent thérapeutique
S agente terapéutico

thermal ageing
G thermische Alterung
F vieillissement thermique
S envejecimiento térmico

thermal behaviour
G thermisches Verhalten
F comportement thermique
S comportamiento térmico

thermal conductivity
G Wärmeleitfähigkeit
F conductivité thermique
S conductividad térmica

thermal conversion
G thermische Umwandlung
F conversion thermique
S conversión térmica

thermal expansion
G Wärmeausdehnung
F thermodilatation
S termodilatación

thermal load
G thermische Belastung
F charge thermique
S carga térmica

thermal mass
G thermische Masse
F masse thermique
S masa térmica

thermal reaction
G thermische Reaktion
F réaction thermique
S reacción térmica

thermal shock
G Wärmeschock
F choc thermique
S choque térmico

thermal stability
G thermische Stabilität
F stabilité thermique
S estabilidad térmica

thermocouple
G Thermoelement, Thermofühler
F sonde thermique, thermocouple
S elemento termoeléctrico, pila termoeléctrica, sonda térmica

thermo-elastic
G thermoelastisch
F thermo-élastique
S termoelástico

thermoforming
G Thermoverformung
F emboutissage
S deformación térmica

thermoforming foil
G Tiefziehfolie
F feuille thermoformée
S lámina termoformada

thermoforming machine
G Thermoformmaschine
F emboutisseuse
S máquina de deformación térmica

thermo-plastic
G thermoplastisch
F thermoplastique
S termoplástico

English German French Spanish

thermostat
G Thermostat
F thermostat
S termostato

thick
G dick
F épais
S compacto, espeso, grueso, macizo

thicken, to
G eindicken, verdicken
F épaissir
S concentrar, condensar, espesar

thickener
G Verdickungsmittel
F épaississant
S espesante

thickening agent
G Verdickungsmittel
F épaississant
S espesante

thickness
G Dicke
F épaisseur
S espesor, grosor

thickness gauge
G Dickenmeßgerät
F jauge d'épaisseur, palmer
S calibre de grosores

thin layer chromatography (TLC)
G Dünnschichtchromatographie (DC)
F chromatographie sur couche mince
S cromatografía en capa fina

thin layer chromatography developing chamber
G Dünnschichtchromatographiekammer
F chambre de développement pour chromatographie sur couche mince
S cámara de cromatografía en capa fina

thin-bodied
G dünnflüssig
F fluide, très fluide
S fluido

thorough
G gründlich
F minutieusement
S minucioso, minuciosamente

thoroughness
G Gründlichkeit
F minutie
S minuciosidad

thread
G Faden, Gewinde
F fil, filetage
S filete, hilo, rosca

left-handed
G linksgängig
F à gauche
S de paso izquierdo

right-handed
G rechtsgängig
F à droite
S de paso derecho

thread rupture
G Fadenbruch
F rupture de fil
S ruptura de hilo

three-phase current
G Drehstrom
F courant triphasé
S corriente trifásica

three-phase current motor
G Drehstrommotor
F moteur électrique triphasé
S motor de corriente trifásica

three-way stopcock
G Dreiwegehahn
F robinet d'arrêt à trois voies
S grifo con tres vías

three-way valve
G Dreiwegeventil
F vanne trois voies
S válvula con tres vías

threshold dosage
G Schwellendosis
F dose liminaire
S dosis liminar, dosis umbral

throttle
G Drossel
F régulateur
S estrangulador

throttle check valve
G Drosselrückschlagventil
F soupape de retenue
S válvula estranguladora de retención, válvula activada por reflujo

throttle non-return valve
G Drosselrückschlagventil
F soupape de retenue
S válvula estranguladora de retención, válvula activada por reflujo

throughput
G Durchsatz
F capacité, débit, rendement
S rendimiento

tighten, to
G abdichten
F colmater, boucher, étanchéifier
S cerrar herméticamente

tightly closed
G dicht verschlossen
F hermétiquement fermé
S herméticamente cerrado

tightness
G Dichtigkeit
F étanchéité
S estanqueidad, hermeticidad

tile
G Fliese
F carreau
S baldosa

tilt, to
G kippen
F basculer
S verter, volcar

tiltable
G abklappbar
F pouvant être rabattu, rabattable
S plegable

tilting device
G Kippvorrichtung
F dispositif de basculement
S dispositivo basculante

time constant
G Zeitkonstante
F constante de temps
S constante de tiempo

time lag
G Zeitverzögerung
F retard
S retraso

time limit
G Frist
F délai, terme
S plazo

time required
G Zeitaufwand
F temps requis
S tiempo invertido

timed release
G zeitlich gesteuerte Freigabe
F libération contrôlée
S liberación temporalmente controlada

timer
G Zeitgeber
F minuterie
S sincronizador del tiempo

time-saving
G Zeitersparnis
F économie de temps
S ahorro de tiempo

English
German
French
Spanish

tin
G Dose
F canne
S bote, caja, lata

tincture
G Tinktur
F teinture
S tintura

tincture standard
G Urtinktur
F teinture standard
S tintura madre

tip seal, to (ampoules)
G abschmelzen (Ampullen)
F obturer (des ampoules)
S sellar (ampollas)

tissue
G Gewebe
F tissu
S tejido

tissue cell culture
G Gewebezellkultur
F culture de cellules tissulaires
S cultivo de células tisulares

titration
G Titration
F titration
S titulación

back titration
G Rücktitration
F dosage en retour
S titulación inversa

titration curve
G Titrationskurve
F courbe de titrage, courbe de dosage
S curva de titulación

titre
G Titer
F titre
S título

TLC plate (thin layer chromatography)
G DC-Platte (Dünnschichtchromatographie)
F plaque de CCM (chromatographie en couche mince)
S placa para cromatografía en capa fina (CCF)

tolerance
G Toleranz
F tolérance
S tolerancia

out of tolerance
G außer Toleranz
F hors des limites de tolérance
S fuera de la tolerancia

specified tolerances
G festgelegte Toleranzen
F tolérances spécifiques
S tolerancias prefijadas

tolerance range
G Toleranzbereich
F intervalle de tolérance
S intervalo de tolerancia

tongs
G Tiegelzange, Zange
F pince, pince à creuset, tenailles
S pinza, pinza de crisol

tongue
G Einstecklasche
F languette, attache, patte
S cubrejunta de pestaña

tonicity
G Tonizität
F tonicité
S tonicidad

tool
G Werkzeug
F outil
S instrumento

top punch
G Oberstempel
F poinçon supérieur
S troquel superior

top side
G Oberseite
F face supérieure, côté supérieur
S lado superior

topical
G topisch
F topique
S tópico

torque
G Drehmoment
F couple
S par momento de torsión, par motor

torsion
G Torsionskraft, Verdrillung
F torsion
S fuerza de torsión, torsión

torsion balance
G Torsionswaage
F balance de torsion
S balanza de torsión

torsion force
G Drehkraft
F force de torsion
S fuerza de rotación

torsion spring
G Torsionsfeder
F ressort de torsion
S muelle de torsión

total area
G Gesamtfläche
F surface totale, aire totale
S superficie total

total microbial count
G Gesamtkeimzahl
F nombre total de micro-organismes
S número total de gérmenes

total organic carbon (TOC)
G Gesamtkohlenstoffgehalt, gesamtorganischer Kohlenstoff
F teneur totale en carbone (organique)
S contenido total en carbono (orgánico)

total petroleum hydrocarbon (tph) analysis
G Analyse auf Gesamt-(Petroleum)-Kohlenwasserstoffe
F analyse de la teneur totale du pétrole en hydrocarbures
S análisis de hidrocarburos totales (de petróleo)

total yield
G Gesamtausbeute
F rendement total
S rendimiento total

tough
G zäh
F visqueux, épais
S resistente, tenaz

toughness
G Zähigkeit
F viscosité
S resistencia, tenacidad, viscosidad

toxic
G giftig, toxisch
F toxique
S tóxico, venenoso

toxic by inhalation
G giftig beim Einatmen
F toxique si inhalé
S tóxico si se inhala

toxic if swallowed
G giftig beim Verschlucken
F toxique si ingéré
S tóxico si se ingiere

toxic in contact with skin
G giftig bei Hautkontakt
F toxique au contact de la peau
S tóxico si entra en contacto con la piel

toxic chemical ordinance
G Gefahrstoffverordnung
F décret concernant les matières dangereuses
S decreto sobre sustancias peligrosas

toxic compound
G toxische Verbindung
F substance toxique
S compuesto tóxico

toxicity
G Giftigkeit, Toxizität
F toxicité
S toxicidad

toxicological testing
G toxikologische Prüfung
F étude toxicologique
S prueba toxicológica

toxicology
G Toxikologie
F toxicologie
S toxicología

toxin
G Gift, Giftstoff, Toxin
F poison, toxine
S sustancia venenosa, tóxico, toxina, veneno

trace
G Spur
F trace
S traza, vestigio

trace analysis
G Spurenanalyse
F analyse de traces
S análisis de vestigios

trace elements
G Spurenelemente
F oligoélément
S oligoelementos

traceability
G Rückführbarkeit, Rückverfolgbarkeit
F traçabilité
S trazabilidad, retromarcado

traceable
G rückverfolgbar
F traçable
S de traza determinable

tracer
G Leitsubstanz
F marqueur, traceur
S marcador

tracing system
G Rückverfolgungssystem
F système de suivi, système d'observation
S sistema de retromarcado

traction-compression resistance
G Zug- und Druckfestigekit
F résistance à la traction et à la compression
S resistencia a la tracción y a la presión

trade association
G Berufsgenossenschaft
F association professionelle
S asociación profesional

trade mark
G Warenzeichen
F marque déposée
S marca (de fábrica)

trade name
G Handelsmarke
F marque de commerce
S marca comercial

tradesman
G Handwerker
F ouvrier, artisan
S artesano, trabajador manual

trainee
G Praktikant
F stagiaire
S pasante, practicante

training
G Ausbildung, Schulung
F éducation, entraînement
S adiestramiento, educación, formación, instrucción

transcription
G Transkription
F transcription
S transcripción

transdermal delivery system
G Transdermales Therapeutisches System
F système thérapeutique transdermique
S sistema terapéutico transdérmico

transdermal patch
G transdermales Pflaster
F pansement transcutané
S emplasto transdérmico

transdermal use
G transdermale Anwendung
F utilisation transcutanée
S aplicación transdérmica

transducer
G Meßwertaufnehmer
F capteur, transducteur
S registrador de valores medidos, transductor

transfer
G Übertragung
F transfert
S transferencia

transfer error
G Übertragungsfehler
F erreur de transfer
S error de transferencia

transfer inoculation
G Überimpfung
F repiquage
S sobreinoculación

transfer, to
G übertragen, verlagern
F déplacer, transférer
S desplazar, transferir, trasladar

transferable label
G Abziehetikett
F étiquette prédécoupée
S etiqueta separable

transfusion set
G Transfusionsbesteck
F nécessaire de transfusion
S instrumental de transfusión

translucent
G lichtdurchlässig
F translucide
S translúcido

transmission
G Getriebe
F transmission, engrenage
S engranaje, transmisión

transmittance
G Durchlässigkeit
F perméabilité
S permeabilidad

transparency
G Durchsichtigkeit
F transparence
S transparencia

transparent
G durchsichtig, klar
F transparent
S claro, transparente

transparent foil
G Klarsichtfolie
F feuille transparente
S lámina transparente, película transparente

transport cart
G Transportwagen
F chariot de transport
S carro de transporte

transport damage
G Transportschaden
F dégâts dûs au transport
S daños de transporte

transport regulations
G Transportbestimmungen
F régulations des activités de transport
S especificaciones de transporte

tray
G Blech, Hordenblech, Magazin (für Ampullen), Tablett
F plateau, tôle
S bandeja (para ampollas), chapa, lámina, plancha

tray dryer
G Hordentrockenschrank
F dessicateur à plateaux, dessicateur à claies
S armario de secado en bandeja

tray drying
G Hordentrocknung
F dessication sur claies
S secado en bandeja

tree diagram
G Baumdiagramm
F diagramme arborescent
S diagrama en árbol

trend analysis
G Trendermittlung
F analyse des tendances
S análisis de tendencias

trial
G Versuch
F essai, expérience
S ensayo, experimento, prueba

trial batch
G Versuchscharge
F lot pilote
S lote piloto

trial design
G Studiendesign, Versuchsanordnung
F design d'un essai clinique
S diseño de un estudio (clínico), disposición del ensayo

trial form
G Prüfbogen
F questionnaire
S cuestionario

trial physician
G Prüfarzt
F médecin responsable d'essais cliniques
S médico investigador

trial run
G Probelauf
F essai de fonctionnement
S marcha de ensayo

triangular skirting
G Dreikantsockel
F bordure triangulaire
S zócalo triangular

trickle installation
G Berieselungsanlage
F système de ruissellement
S sistema de lavado

trickle plant
G Berieselungsanlage
F système de ruissellement
S sistema de lavado

trickle, to
G träufeln
F verser au goutte à goutte
S gotear

trituration
G Trituration
F trituration
S trituración

trolley
G Fahrgestell
F chassis mobile
S bastidor, chasis

tropical chamber
G Tropenkammer
F chambre tropicale
S cámara tropical

trouble-shooting
G Fehlerbehebung
F dépannage, action de corriger
S corrección de errores

true density
G wahre Dichte
F densité réelle
S densidad real

true to scale
G maßstabgerecht
F à l'échelle
S a escala

truncated cone
G Kegelstumpf
F troncature d'un cône
S tronco de cono

tube
G Rohrbogen, Schlauch, Tube
F tube, tuyau
S tubo

tube bundle heat exchanger
G Rohrbündelwärmetauscher
F échangeur de chaleur à faisceaux tubulaires
S intercambiador de calor de haces tubulares

tube carriage
G Schlauchwagen
F chariot dévidoir
S transportador de tubos

tube closure
G Tubenverschluß
F bouchon de tube
S cierre de un tubo

tube connector
G Schlauchkupplung
F raccordement de tuyau
S acoplamiento de tubo

tube kink
G Schlauchknick
F coude d'un tuyau
S acodadura de un tubo

tube thread
G Tubengewinde
F filets du tube
S rosca de tubo

tube-filling machine
G Tubenfüllmaschine
F machine de remplissage pour tubes
S máquina de llenado por tubos

tubing
G Schlauchleitung
F tuyauterie
S tubería flexible

tubular bag
G Schlauchbeutel
F poche
S bolsa tubular

tubular film
G Schlauchfolie
F feuille en gaine
S película tubular

tumble blender
G Taumelmischer
F mélangeur culbuteur
S mezclador de volteo

tumbler mixer
G Freifallmischer
F mélangeur culbuteur, malaxeur à chute libre
S mezclador por basculado

tungsten arc lamp
G Wolframbogenlampe
F lampe à arc de tungstène
S lámpara de arco de tungsteno

tunnel steriliser
G Hitzetunnel
F tunnel de stérilisation
S túnel de esterilización

turbid
G trüb
F turbide, trouble
S turbio

turbidity
G Trübung
F turbidité
S turbidez

turbulence
G Turbulenz
F turbulence
S turbulencia

turbulent flow
G turbulente Strömung
F flux turbulent
S flujo turbulento

English
German
French
Spanish

turnkey
G schlüsselfertig
F clé en main
S llave en mano

turnkey plant
G schlüsselfertige Fabrik
F usine clé en main
S fábrica llave en mano

turnover
G Umsatz
F chiffre d'affaires
S movimiento, volumen de negocios

turntable
G Aufgabedrehteller, Drehteller
F plateau tournant
S placa giratoria, plato giratorio

tweezers
G Pinzette
F brucelles
S pinzas

ultrafiltration
G Ultrafiltration
F ultrafiltration
S ultrafiltración

ultra-high throughput screening (UHTS)
G Screenen mit ultrahohem Durchsatz (UHTS)
F screening à ultra-haut rendement
S detención con ultrarrendimiento

ultrapure water
G hochreines Wasser
F eau ultra pure
S agua ultrapurificada

ultrasonic bath
G Ultraschallbad
F bain à ultra-sons
S baño ultrasónico

ultrasound
G Ultraschall
F ultra-son
S ultrasonido

ultraviolet
G ultraviolett
F ultraviolet
S ultravioleta

unambiguous
G eindeutig
F clair, précis
S claro, inequívoco, unívoco

unbreakable
G bruchfest, unzerbrechlich
F incassable
S irrompible

uncertainty
G Unsicherheit
F incertitude
S inseguridad

undamaged
G unbeschädigt
F intact
S indemne

underweight
G Untergewicht
F insuffisance de poids
S falta de peso

unequivocal
G unzweideutig, eindeutig
F non équivoque
S inequívoco

unequivocal code number
G eindeutige Codenummer
F code numérique non équivoque
S número codificador inequívoco

uniform
G einheitlich, gleichmäßig
F uniforme
S constante, homogéneo, uniforme

uniform filling
G gleichmäßige Füllung
F remplissage uniforme
S relleno uniforme

uniform heat transfer
G gleichmäßiger Wärmeübergang
F transition thermique uniforme
S transición térmica uniforme

uniform particle size
G Gleichkorn
F taille des particules uniforme
S tamaño uniforme de las partículas

uniform preconditions
G einheitliche Voraussetzungen
F conditions préalables uniformes
S presupuestos uniformes

uniformity
G Einheitlichkeit, Gleichförmigkeit
F uniformité, consistance
S homogeneidad, uniformidad

uniformity of weight
G Gewichtseinheitlichkeit
F uniformité du poids
S uniformidad del peso

unit
G Einheit
F unité
S unidad

unit of measurement
G Maßeinheit, Meßgröße
F unité de mesure
S dimensión, unidad de medición, unidad de medida

United States Pharmacopoeia (USP)
G Arzneibuch der USA
F pharmacopée américaine
S farmacopea estadounidense

unlock, to
G entriegeln
F déverrouiller
S desbloquear

unmanned
G mannlos
F inoccupé
S desocupado

unmanned operation
G automatischer Betrieb, bedienerloser Betrieb
F fonctionnement automatique, usine automatique
S funcionamiento automático

unpacked
G unverpackt
F non emballé
S no embalado

unsaponifiable matter
G unverseifbare Anteile
F portions insaponifiables
S porciones insaponificables

unsaturated
G ungesättigt
F insaturé
S insaturado

update, to
G aktualisieren
F actualiser
S actualizar

up-front costs
G Vorauskosten
F coûts préalables
S costes preliminares

upgrade, to
G aufrüsten
F moderniser
S modernizar, renovar

upper punch
G Oberstempel
F poinçon supérieur
S troquel superior

upper side
G Oberseite
F face supérieure, côté supérieur
S lado superior

user
G Benutzer
F utilisateur
S usuario

English German French Spanish

English German French Spanish

user requirements
G Lastenheft
F cahier des charges, spécifications de l'usager
S requerimientos del usuario

user specifications
G Lastenheft
F cahier des charges, spécifications de l'usager
S requerimientos del usuario

user-friendly
G bedienerfreundlich
F convivial pour l'utilisateur, adapté à l'utilisateur
S confortable para el usuario

utilities
G Betriebsmittel, Medien
F moyens d'exploitation, moyens de production
S medios de explotación empresarial, medios de producción

UV absorption
G UV-Absorption
F absorption UV
S absorción UV

UV coefficient of absorbance
G UV-Extinktionskoeffizient
F coefficient d'extinction UV
S coeficiente de extinción UV

UV lamp
G UV-Lampe
F lampe UV
S lámpara UV

UV transmittance
G UV-Transmission
F transmission UV
S transmisión UV

UV/VIS detector
G UV/VIS-Detektor
F détecteur UV/VIS
S detector UV/VIS

vaccine
G Impfstoff
F vaccin
S vacuna

vacuum
G Vakuum
F vide
S vacío

vacuum degasification
G Vakuumentgaser
F dégasification à vide
S desgasificador de vacío

vacuum distillation
G Vakuumdestillation
F distillation sous vide
S destilación en vacío

vacuum drying
G Vakuumtrocknung
F dessication sous vide
S secado al vacío

vacuum evaporation
G Vakuumverdampfer
F évaporateur sous vide
S evaporador de vacío

vacuum feed
G Vakuumbeschickung
F alimentation du vide
S alimentación de vacío

vacuum pump
G Vakuumpumpe
F pompe à vide
S bomba de vacío

vacuum test
G Vakuumhaltetest
F test de maintien du vide
S prueba de mantenimiento del vacío

vaginal cream
G Vaginalcreme
F crème vaginale
S crema vaginal

vaginal gel
G Vaginalgel
F gel vaginal
S gel vaginal

vaginal ointment
G Vaginalsalbe
F pommade vaginale
S pomada vaginal

vaginal suppository
G Vaginalzäpfchen
F suppositoire vaginal
S suppositorio vaginal

vaginal tablet
G Vaginaltablette
F comprimé vaginal
S comprimido vaginal

vaginal use
G vaginale Anwendung
F utilisation vaginale
S aplicación vaginal

valency
G Wertigkeit
F valence
S valencia

valid from
G gültig ab
F valide à partir de
S válido a partir de

validatable
G validierbar
F validable
S validable

validation
G Validierung
F validation
S validación

analytical validation
G analytische Validierung
F validation analytique
S validación analítica

concurrent validation
G begleitende Validierung
F validation concurrente
S validación acompañante

prospective validation
G prospektive Validierung
F validation prospective
S validación prospectiva

retrospective validation
G retrospektive Validierung
F validation retrospective
S validación retrospectiva

validation data
G Validierungsdaten
F données de validation
S datos de validación

validation protocol
G Validierungsplan
F protocole de validation
S plan de validación

validation report
G Validierungsbericht
F rapport de validation
S informe de validación

validation review committee
G Steuerungsausschuß zur Validierung
F comité directeur de validation
S comisión fiscal de validación

validation run
G Validierungslauf
F cycle de validation
S ciclo de validación

validity
G Geltungsbereich, Gültigkeit
F champ d'application, validité
S campo de aplicación, validez

valve
G Ventil
F vanne
S válvula

English German French Spanish

ball valve
G Kugelventil
F vanne à billes
S válvula esférica

diaphragm valve
G Membranventil
F vanne à membrane
S válvula de membrana

solenoid valve
G elektromagnetisches Ventil
F vanne solénoïde
S válvula electromagnética

valve setting
G Ventilstellung
F position d'une vanne
S posición de la válvula

vane
G Flügelrad
F ailette
S rueda de aletas, rueda de paletas

vaporisation
G Verdampfung
F vaporisation, évaporisation
S evaporación, vaporización

vaporise, to
G zerstäuben
F atomiser, pulvériser
S atomizar, pulverizar

vapour
G Dampf
F vapeur d'eau
S vapor

vapour phase
G Dampfphase
F phase vapeur
S fase vapor

vapour pressure
G Dampfdruck
F pression de vapeur
S presión de vapor

variability
G Schwankung, Variabilität
F variabilité, variabilité des résultats
S fluctuación, variabilidad

variation
G Änderung
F changement
S cambio, modificación, variación

varnish
G Lack
F vernis
S barniz, laca

varnished cardboard
G lackierte Pappe
F papier vernis
S cartón barnizado

vary, to
G schwanken
F fluctuer
S fluctuar, variar

vaseline
G Vaselin
F vaseline
S vaselina

vegetable dye
G Pflanzenfarbstoff
F pigment végétal
S colorante vegetal, pigmento vegetal

velocimeter
G Geschwindigkeitsmesser
F tachymètre
S taquímetro

vendor
G Lieferant
F fournisseur
S abastecedor, proveedor

vent
G Belüftungsloch
F orifice de ventilation, orifice de purge
S orificio de ventilación

vent filter
G Belüftungsfilter
F filtre de ventilation
S filtro de ventilación

vent flap
G Entlüftungsklappe
F clapet de ventilation, volet de ventilation
S válvula de ventilación

vent, to
G belüften, entlüften
F aérer, désaérer, ventiler
S airear, ventilar

ventilate, to
G belüften, entlüften
F aérer, désaérer, ventiler
S airear, ventilar

ventilated hood
G Abzug
F hotte à flux laminaire, hotte chimique
S escape, campana de extracción de gases

ventilation
G Belüftung
F ventilation
S aireación, ventilación

ventilation system
G Belüftungsanlage, Belüftungssystem, Lüftungsanlage, raumlufttechnische Anlage
F système de ventilation
S sistema de ventilación

ventilation valve
G Belüftungsventil
F valve de ventilation
S válvula de ventilación

ventilator
G Gebläse, Ventilator
F ventilateur
S ventilador

venting line
G Entlüftungsleitung
F canalisation de ventilation, canalisation d'aération
S conducción de ventilación

verification
G Überprüfung, Verifizierung
F vérification
S comprobación, verificación

vermin
G Ungeziefer
F vermine
S bichos

version
G Ausführung, Ausgabe, Version
F édition, version
S edición, modelo, realización, versión

version number
G Versionsnummer
F numéro de version
S número de versión

vertical autoclave
G Vertikalautoklav
F autoclave vertical
S autoclave vertical

vertical electrophoresis
G Vertikalelektrophorese
F électrophorèse verticale
S electroforesis vertical

vertical granulator
G Vertikalgranulator
F granulateur vertical
S granulador vertical

vessel
G Behälter, Gefäß, Kessel
F bac, bouilloire, chaudière, container, cuve, récipient
S caldera, marmita, recipiente

mobile vessel
G fahrbarer Behälter
F cuve mobile, cuve sur roues
S recipiente portátil

vessel emptying
G Gefäßentleerung
F action de vider un flacon, action de vider un récipient
S vaciamiento de un recipiente

vessel manufacturer
G Behälterbauer
F fabricant de cuves
S fabricante de recipientes

vessel wall
G Gefäßwand
F paroi d'un récipient
S pared de un recipiente

vet
G Tierarzt
F vétérinaire
S veterinario

veterinary medicament
G Tierarzneimittel
F médicament à usage vétérinaire
S medicamento de uso veterinario

viability
G Lebensfähigkeit
F viabilité
S viabilidad

viable
G lebensfähig
F viable
S viable

viable particle count
G Zählung lebensfähiger Partikel
F comptage de particules viables
S recuento de partículas viables

viable particles
G lebensfähige Partikel
F particules viables
S partículas viables

vial
G Fläschchen, Gläschen
F fiole, flacon, récipient
S botellín, frasco, vial

vibrate, to
G rütteln
F secouer
S sacudir, trepidar, vibrar

vibrating screen
G Rüttelsieb
F tamis vibrant
S tamiz vibrante

vibrating sieve
G Rüttelsieb
F tamis vibrant
S tamiz vibrante

vibration
G Erschütterung, Schwingung, Vibration
F vibration
S oscilación, trepidación, vibración

vibration-free
G erschütterungsfrei
F exempt de vibration
S sin vibración

vibrator
G Rüttler
F secoueuse, secoueur, vibreur
S vibrador

vigorous stirring
G kräftiges Rühren
F agitation vigoureuse
S agitación intensa

viral agent
G virales Agens
F agent viral
S agente viral

viral vaccine
G Virusimpfstoff
F vaccin viral
S vacuna viral

virology
G Virologie
F virologie
S virología

virus removal
G Virusentfernung
F élimination des virus
S eliminación de virus

viruses
G Viren
F virus
S virus

viscometry
G Viskositätsmessung
F viscosimétrie
S medida de la viscosiad

viscosity
G Viskosität
F viscosité
S viscosidad

viscous
G dickflüssig, viskos, zähflüssig
F visqueux
S espeso, viscoso

viscous solvent
G viskoses Lösungsmittel
F solvant visqueux
S solvente viscoso

visitor tour
G Besuchergang
F circuit de visite
S recorrido de visita

visual control
G optische Kontrolle, Sichtkontrolle
F contrôle visuel
S control óptico, control visual

visual examination
G Sichtprüfung
F examen visuel
S inspección visual

visual inspection
G Durchsichtkontrolle
F inspection visuelle
S inspección visual

visual observation
G visuelle Überwachung
F contrôle visuel
S control visual

visual signal
G optisches Signal
F signal optique
S señal óptica

visualise, to
G sichtbarmachen
F visualiser
S visualizar

vocational training
G Berufsausbildung
F formation professionnelle
S formación profesional

volatile
G flüchtig
F volatile
S volátil

non-volatile
G nicht flüchtig
F non-volatile
S no volátil

volatile components
G flüchtige Bestandteile
F composants volatiles
S componentes volátiles

volatilisation
G Verflüchtigung
F volatilisation
S volatilización

volatilise, to
G sich verflüchtigen
F volatiliser
S volatilizarse

voltage
G Spannung
F tension
S tensión

English German French Spanish

voltage fluctuation
G Spannungsschwankung
F variation de tension
S fluctuación de la tensión

voltage regulator
G Spannungsregler
F régulateur de tension
S regulador de tensión

voltage variation
G Spannungsänderung
F variation de tension
S variación de la tensión

voltmeter
G Spannungsmesser
F voltmètre
S voltímetro

volume
G Fassungsvermögen
F capacité, contenance
S capacidad

volumetric
G volumetrisch
F volumétrique
S volumétrico

volumetric analysis
G volumetrische Analyse
F analyse volumétrique
S análisis volumétrico

volumetric flask
G Meßkolben
F ballon gradué
S matraz graduado

volumetric solution
G Maßlösung
F solution volumétrique
S solución volumétrica

volumetric standard
G Urtiter
F substance standard de titrimétrie
S título estándar

volumetry
G Volumetrie
F volumétrie
S volumetría

voluminous
G voluminös
F volumineux
S voluminoso

volunteer
G Proband
F volontaire
S voluntario

vulcanite
G Hartgummi
F caoutchouc durci, ébonite
S ebonita

vulnerability
G Anfälligkeit
F vulnérabilité
S vulnerabilidad

walk-in
G begehbar
F accessible
S practicable, viable

wall
G Wandung
F paroi
S pared

wall connection
G Wandanschluß
F connexion murale
S conexión de pared

wall duct
G Wanddurchführung
F ouverture dans le mur, conduite
S pasamuros

wall opening
G Wanddurchführung
F ouverture dans le mur, conduite
S pasamuros

wall skirting
G Wandsockel
F bordure d'un mur
S zócalo de la pared

wall thickness
G Wanddicke
F épaisseur d'un mur
S espesor de tabique

warehouse
G Lager(bereich), Lagerraum, Warenlager
F aire d'entreposage, aire de stockage, entrepôt
S almacén, almacén de mercancías, depósito

warehouse stability
G Lagerstabilität
F stabilité de stockage
S estabilidad de almacén

warning
G Warnhinweis
F avertissement
S aviso de alarma

warning letter (from FDA)
G Verwarnung (der FDA)
F lettre d'avertissement (de la FDA)
S carta de aviso (de la FDA)

warranty
G Garantie
F garantie
S garantía

wash basin
G Waschbecken
F évier
S lavabo

wash bottle
G Spritzflasche, Waschflasche
F flacon laveur, pissette
S frasco de lavado, matraz de lavado

washer
G Dichtungsscheibe, Unterlegscheibe
F joint (rondelle), rondelle
S arandela, disco para cierre hermético

washing tower
G Rieselturm
F tour d'arrosage
S torre de lavado

waste
G Abfall, Ausschuß, Müll
F déchets, ordures, résidus
S basura, desechos, residuos

waste avoidance
G Abfallvermeidung
F politique d'élimination des déchets
S evitación de desechos

waste bag
G Abfallbeutel
F sac poubelle
S bolsa de desechos

waste disposal
G Abfallbeseitigung, Abfallentsorgung
F élimination des déchets, élimination des résidus
S eliminación de desechos

waste disposal company
G Abfallentsorgungsfirma
F entreprise d'élimination des résidus, entreprise de traitement des résidus
S empresa de eliminación de desechos

waste disposal vessel
G Abfallbehälter
F récipient d'élimination des déchets, poubelle
S recipiente de desechos

English
German
French
Spanish

waste duct
G Ablaufrinne
F canalisation d'élimination des déchets
S canal de salida

waste gas
G Abgas
F gaz d'échappement, gaz d'évacuation
S gas de escape

waste heat
G Abwärme
F chaleur perdue
S calor de escape, pérdida calórica

waste material
G Abfallprodukt
F déchets
S producto de desecho

waste output
G Entsorgungsanschluß
F conduite destinée aux déchets
S empalme de eliminación

waste regulations
G Abfallbestimmungen
F dispositions (légales) concernant les déchets
S prescripciones sobre desechos

waste water
G Abwasser
F eaux résiduelles, eaux usées, eaux d'égouts
S aguas residuales

waste water line
G Abwasserleitung
F conduite destinée aux eaux résiduelles
S conducción de aguas residuales

waste water pollution
G Abwasserverschmutzung
F pollution des eaux résiduelles
S polución de aguas residuales

waste water treatment plant
G Kläranlage
F station d'épuration
S estación depuradora

water
G Wasser
F eau
S agua

water absorption capacity
G Wasseraufnahmevermögen
F capacité d'absorption d'eau
S capacidad de absorción de agua

water bath
G Wasserbad
F bain-marie
S baño de agua

water column
G Wassersäule
F colonne d'eau
S columna de agua

water content
G Wassergehalt
F teneur en eau
S contenido en agua

water determination
G Wasserbestimmung
F détermination de la teneur en eau
S determinación del contenido en agua

water for injection (WFI)
G Wasser für Injektionszwecke
F eau PPI
S agua para inyección

water hardness
G Wasserhärte
F dureté de l'eau
S dureza del agua

water jacket
G Wassermantel
F chemise d'eau
S camisa de agua

water jet pump
G Wasserstrahlpumpe
F pompe d'une trompe à eau
S bomba de chorro de agua

water of crystallisation
G Kristallwasser
F eau de cristallisation
S agua de cristalización

water piping
G Wasserleitung
F conduite d'eau
S conducción de agua

water purification
G Wasseraufbereitung
F traitement des eaux usées
S purificación de agua

water separator
G Wasserabscheider
F séparateur d'eau
S separador de agua

water softening
G Wasserenthärtung
F adoucissage de l'eau
S reblandecimiento del agua

water supply
G Wasserversorgung
F alimentation en eau
S suministro de agua

water treatment system
G Wasseraufbereitungsanlage
F système de traitement de l'eau
S sistema de tratamiento de agua

water vapour permeability
G Wasserdampfdurchlässigkeit
F perméabilité à la vapeur d'eau
S permeabilidad al vapor de agua

water/oil emulsion
G Wasser-in-Öl-Emulsion
F émulsion d'eau dans l'huile
S emulsión de agua en aceite

waterproof
G wasserdicht
F imperméable à l'eau
S impermeable al agua

waterproof jump-suit
G wasserdichter Anzug
F combinaison imperméable à l'eau
S traje impermeable al agua

water-repellent
G wasserabweisend
F hydrophobe
S hidrófobo, hidrófugo

water-ring pump
G Wasserringpumpe
F pompe à anneau d'eau
S bomba de anillo de agua

water-softener
G Wasserenthärter
F adoucisseur d'eau
S reblandecedor del agua

water-soluble cream
G abwaschbare Salbe
F crème évanescente
S pomada evanescente

water-tight
G wasserdicht
F imperméable à l'eau
S impermeable al agua

wavelength
G Wellenlänge
F longueur d'onde
S longitud de onda

wavelength accuracy
G Wellenlängengenauigkeit
F exactitude de longueur d'onde
S exactitud de la longitud de onda

wavelength programming
G Wellenlängenprogrammierung
F programmation de la longueur d'onde
S programación de la longitud de onda

English German French Spanish

wavelength switching
G Wellenlängenumschaltung
F changement de longueur d'onde
S conmutación de la longitud de onda

wax
G Wachs
F cire
S cera

weak acid
G schwache Säure
F acide faible
S ácido débil

wear and tear
G Abnutzung, Verschleiß, Verschleißerscheinung
F usure
S desgaste, manifestación de desgaste

weigh in, to
G einwiegen
F peser
S pesar

weighing beam
G Wiegebalken
F fléau de balance
S ástil, cruz de la balanza

weighing cubicle
G Wägekabine
F cabine de pesée
S cabina de pesado

weighing facility
G Wiegeanlage
F installation de pesage
S instalación de pesado

weighing pan
G Waagschale
F plateau de balance
S platillo de balanza

weighing scale
G Waagschale
F plateau de balance
S platillo de balanza

weight
G Gewicht
F poids
S peso

weight accuracy
G Gewichtsgenauigkeit
F exactitude d'un poids
S exactitud del peso

weight control
G Gewichtskontrolle
F contrôle du poids
S control del peso

weight loss (on drying)
G Gewichtsverlust (bei der Trocknung)
F perte de poids (lors de la dessication)
S pérdida de peso (al desecar)

weld
G Naht, Schweißnaht
F joint, soudure
S junta, soldadura, sutura

weld, to
G schweißen
F souder
S soldar

welded
G verschweißt
F soudé
S soldado

welding seam
G Schweißnaht
F soudure
S soldadura

well (of blister)
G Napf (beim Blister), Vertiefung
F blister, cavité, emballage à bulles, puits
S cavidad, depresión, pocillo del blíster

wet chemical
G naßchemisch
F chimique humide
S químicamente húmedo

wet chemistry
G Naßchemie
F chimie humide
S química húmeda

wet granulation
G Feuchtgranulierung
F granulation (par voie) humide
S granulación húmeda

wet grinding
G Naßvermahlung
F broyage humide
S molido húmedo

wet sieving
G Naßsiebung
F tamisage humide
S tamizado húmedo

wet, to
G anfeuchten, befeuchten, benetzen
F humidifier, mouiller
S humectar, humedecer, mojar, rociar

wetting agent
G Benetzungsmittel, Feuchthaltemittel, Netzmittel
F mouillant
S humectante

wide-necked bottle
G Weithalsflasche
F bouteille à col large
S botella de cuello ancho

wide-necked vessel
G Weithalsgefäß
F fiole, jarre
S recipiente de cuello ancho

width
G Breite, Weite
F largeur, étendue
S anchura, amplitud, extensión

window
G Fenster
F fenêtre
S ventana

wing screw
G Flügelschraube
F vis à oreilles
S tornillo de aletas

wipe test
G Wischtest
F essai de prélèvement par tampon d'ouate
S prueba de prelavado con torunda de algodón

wiper paddle (e. g. of a mixing vessel)
G Wischblatt (z. B. im Mischbehälter)
F lame d'essuyage (dans la cuve de mélange)
S goma limpia cristales (p. ej. en mezclador)

wire
G Draht
F fil métallique
S alambre

wire mesh
G Drahtgewebe
F toile métallique
S tela metálica

wire sieve
G Drahtsieb
F tamis en toile métallique
S tamiz de alambre

wire strain gauge
G Dehnungsmeßstreifen
F jauge de contrainte
S extensímetro de resistencia

wire, to
G schalten, verdrahten
F enclencher, brancher, connecter
S conectar, conmutar

wiring
G Verkabelung
F câblage
S cables

wiring box
G Schaltkasten
F armoire électrique
S caja de distribución

wiring diagram
G Schaltdiagramm
F diagramme des connexions
S diagrama de circuito

withdrawal
G Entnahme
F retrait
S extracción, toma

wooden case
G Holzkiste
F caisse en bois
S caja de madera

wooden pallet
G Holzpalette
F palette en bois
S paleta de madera

work bench
G Arbeitstisch, Werkbank
F établi, table de travail
S banco de trabajo, mesa de trabajo

work scheduling
G Arbeitsvorbereitung
F planification du travail
S preparación del trabajo

working clothing
G Arbeitskleidung
F vêtement de travail
S ropa de trabajo

working group
G Arbeitsgruppe
F groupe de travail
S grupo de trabajo

working pressure
G Arbeitsdruck, Betriebsdruck
F pression de travail
S presión de trabajo, presión empresarial

working standard
G Arbeitsstandard
F norme de travail
S norma de trabajo

working surface
G Arbeitsoberfläche
F surface de travail
S superficie de trabajo

workman
G Handwerker
F ouvrier, artisan
S artesano, trabajador manual

workshop
G Werkstatt
F atelier
S taller

World Health Organisation (WHO)
G Weltgesundheitsorganisation
F organisation mondiale de la santé (OMS)
S Organización Mundial de la Salud (OMS)

worm drive
G Schneckenförderer
F vis d'Archimède
S transportador de tornillo sin fin

worm gear
G Förderschnecke
F vis sans fin, vis d'Archimède
S tornillo sin fin, tornillo transportador

worm gear box
G Schneckengetriebe
F engrenage à vis sans fin
S engranaje de tornillo sin fin

worm screw
G Förderschnecke, Schnecke
F vis sans fin, vis d'Archimède
S tornillo sin fin, tornillo transportador

worn out
G ausgeleiert
F usé
S desgastado

wound dressing
G Wundauflage
F pansement
S compresa, vendaje de una herida

wrench
G Schraubenschlüssel
F clef de serrage
S cierre de tornillo

wrinkling
G Faltenbildung
F formation de plis, formation de rides
S formación de arrugas, formación de pliegues

X-axis
G X-Achse
F axe des abscisses
S eje X

X-ray contrast medium
G Röntgenkontrastmittel
F produit de contraste aux rayons X
S medio de contraste radiológico

Y-axis
G Y-Achse
F axe des ordonnées
S eje Y

Y-duct
G Hosenrohr
F tube en Y
S tubo en Y

yeast
G Hefe
F levure
S levadura

yield
G Ausbeute, Ertrag
F rendement
S rendimiento

yield calculation
G Ausbeuteberechnung
F calcul du rendement
S cálculo del rendimiento

yield enhancement
G Ausbeutesteigerung
F augmentation du rendement
S aumento del rendimiento

yield point
G Fließgrenze
F limite d'écoulement
S límite de migración (en cromatografía)

yoke
G Gabelarm, Joch
F bras de levier
S brazo de horquilla

zero (in diagram)
G Nullpunkt (beim Diagramm)
F point zéro
S punto cero (en diagrama)

zero adjustment
G Nulleinstellung
F mise à zéro
S posición cero, puesta a cero

zero defect strategy
G Null-Fehler-Strategie
F stratégie zéro défaut
S estrategia de ausencia total de errores

zero drift
G Nullpunktabweichung
F dérive du point zero
S desviación del punto cero

zero line
G Nullinie
F ligne de base, ligne de zéro
S línea de base

zonal concept
G Zonenkonzept
F concept de zones
S concepción por zonas

German A – Z

English
German
French
Spanish

Benutzerhinweise:
S. 10–11

Abbau
E degradation
F dégradation
S degradación

abbaubar
E degradable
F dégradable
S degradable

Abbaugranulierung
E degradation granulation
F granulation de dégradation
S granulación de degradación

Abbauprodukt
E degradation product
F produit de dégradation
S producto de degradación

Abbauweg
E degradation path, metabolic path
F chemin de dégradation
S vía de degradación

Abbindezeit
E solidification time, setting time
F temps de solidification
S tiempo de solidificación

abdampfen
E evaporate, to
F évaporer, faire s'évaporer
S evaporar, volatilizar

Abdampfschale
E evaporating dish
F capsule d'évaporation
S cápsula de evaporación

Abdeckhaube
E cover
F couvercle
S tapadera

Abdeckplatte
E cover glass
F verre de protection, lame
S cubreobjetos

Abdeckung
E cover, hood
F couvercle, capuchon
S casquete, cubierta, sombrerete

abdestillieren
E distil off, to
F distiller
S destilar

abdichten
E tighten, to; seal, to
F colmater, boucher, étanchéifier
S cerrar herméticamente

Abfall
E waste
F déchets, ordures, résidus
S desecho

Abfallbehälter
E waste disposal vessel
F récipient d'élimination des déchets, poubelle
S recipiente de desechos

Abfallbestimmungen
E waste regulations
F dispositions (légales) concernant les déchets
S prescripciones sobre desechos

Abfallbeutel
E waste bag
F sac poubelle
S bolsa de desechos

Abfallentsorgung
E waste disposal
F élimination des déchets, élimination des résidus
S eliminación de desechos

Abfallentsorgungsfirma
E waste disposal company
F entreprise d'élimination des résidus, entreprise de traitement des résidus
S empresa de eliminación de desechos

Abfallprodukt
E waste material
F déchets
S producto de desecho

Abfallvermeidung
E waste avoidance
F politique d'élimination des déchets
S evitación de desechos

Abflachung
E flattening
F aplatissement
S aplanamiento

Abfluß
E drain
F tuyau d'écoulement, drain
S desagüe

Abflußrinne
E drain duct
F rigole d'écoulement
S desaguadero

Abfüllinie
E filling line, bottling line
F ligne de remplissage, rampe de remplissage
S cadena de envasado

Abfüllmaschine
E filling machine
F remplisseuse
S máquina de envasado

Abfüllmenge
E filling quantity
F quantité de remplissage, volume de remplissage
S cantidad envasada

Abfüllnadel
E filling needle
F aiguille de remplissage
S aguja de envasado

Abfüllort
E filling station
F station de remplissage
S estación de llenado

Abfüllrohr
E filling hose, filling pipe
F conduite de remplissage
S conducto de envasado

Abfüllschlauch
E filling tube
F tuyau de remplissage
S tubo de envasado

Abfüllstation
E filling station
F station de remplissage, station de mise en bouteilles, station en bidons
S estación de envasado

Abfüllstraße
E filling line, bottling line
F chaîne de remplissage
S cadena de envasado

Abfüllstrecke
E filling section
F chemin de remplissage
S sección de llenado

Abfüllung
E filling
F remplissage
S envasado, embotellamiento

Abgas
E exhaust gas, waste gas
F gaz d'échappement, gaz d'évacuation
S gas de escape

abgeflacht
E flattened
F aplati
S aplanado

abgehängte Decke
E suspended ceiling
F faux plafond
S techo suspendido

abgerundet
E rounded off
F arrondi, arrondi au chiffre inférieur
S redondeado a la cifra inferior

abgeschrägt
E sloping
F taillé en biais, en biseau, biseauté
S biselado

abgeschwächter Erreger
E attenuated pathogen
F agent pathogène atténué
S agente patógeno atenuado

abgetrennt
E separated, segregated
F séparé, détaché, isolé
S aislado, separado

abgetrennter Bereich
E segregated area
F zone séparée, zone isolée, zone de confinement
S área separada

abgewinkelt
E angled, angular
F à angles, angulaire
S angulado, doblado, escuadrado

abgießen
E decant, to
F décanter, transvaser
S decantar, verter

Abguß
E drain
F conduit d'écoulement, drain
S decantación, vaciado

Abhängung
E skirting, apron (of machine)
F tablier
S delantal

abklappbar
E foldable, tiltable
F pouvant être rabattu, rabattable
S plegable

Abklatschplatte
E contact plate
F plaque de contact
S placa de contacto

Abklatschtest
E direct contact test
F test de contact direct
S prueba de contacto directo

abknicken (eine Ampulle)
E snap, to (an ampoule)
F casser (une ampoule)
S romper por el cuello (ampolla)

Abkochung
E decoction
F décoction
S decocción

Abkommen zur gegenseitigen Anerkennung
E Mutual Recognition Agreement (MRA)
F procédure de reconnaissance mutuelle
S Acuerdo de Reconocimiento Mutuo de Procedimientos Administrativos en la UE

Abkömmling
E derivative
F dérivé
S derivado

abkratzen
E scrape off, to
F racler
S raer, raspar

Abkühlphase
E cooling phase
F phase de refroidissement
S fase de enfriamento

Abkühlung
E cooling
F refroidissement, réfrigération
S enfriamiento

Abkühlungsgeschwindigkeit
E cooling rate
F vitesse de refroidissement
S velocidad de enfriamiento

Abkühlvorrichtung
E cooling device
F dispositif de refroidissement
S dispositivo de enfriamiento

Abkühlzeit
E cool-down time
F temps de refroidissement
S tiempo de enfriamiento

Abkürzung
E abridgement
F raccourci
S abreviatura, abreviación

Ablagerung
E sediment
F dépôt, sédiment
S depósito, sedimento

ablassen (Flüssigkeiten)
E drain, to; discharge, to (liquids)
F faire couler, laisser s'écouler
S dar salida, dejar escapar

Ablaßhahn
E discharge cock, drain cock
F robinet de purge
S grifo de salida

Ablaßstutzen
E discharge nipple, drain nipple, outlet nipple
F manchon d'écoulement, manchon de drainage
S empalme de salida

Ablaßventil
E drain valve, outlet valve
F vanne de purge, vanne de sortie
S válvula de salida

Ablauf (eines Prozesses)
E outlet, drain, sequence (of operation)
F sortie, déroulement (d'un procédé)
S escape, salida, secuencia (de un proceso)

Ablaufrinne
E waste duct
F canalisation d'élimination des déchets
S canal de salida

Ablaufschema
E flow chart
F schéma opérationnel, schéma de marche, schéma de principe, schéma de fabrication
S esquema operacional

Ablaufstutzen
E discharge port, outlet port
F manchon d'écoulement
S empalme de salida

Ablehnung (z. B. eines Patentes)
E rejection (e. g. of a patent)
F refus (par ex. d'un brevet)
S rechazo (p. ej. de una patente)

Ableitung
E ground, earth
F mise à la terre, prise de terre
S derivación, toma de tierra

ablenken
E deflect, to
F dévier
S desviar

Ablenkplatte
E baffle
F plaque déflectrice, chicane
S placa de desviación

ablesen
E read, to; read off, to
F lire, relever
S leer

Abluft
E exhaust air, outlet air
F air d'évacuation, air d'échappement
S aire de escape

Abluftfilter
E exhaust air filter
F filtre à air d'évacuation
S filtro del aire de escape

Abluftkanal
E exhaust air duct
F canal [illegible]uation de l'air
S ca[illegible] de escape

[illegible]
E [illegible] lin[illegible]
F [illegible]te[illegible]tion
S [illegible]cto[illegible]cuación de aire

Ab[illegible]regelklappe
E exhaust valve
F clapet d'évacuation d'air
S válvula de evacuación de aire

Abluftrohr
E exhaust pipe
F conduite d'évacuation d'air
S tubo de evacuación de aire

Abluftschacht
E exhaust air shaft, exhaust air flue
F puits d'évacuation d'air
S pozo de evacuación de aire

abmessen
E meter, to; dose, to
F doser
S medir, dosificar

Abmessungen
E dimensions
F dimensions
S dimensión, medida, cuantía

Abnahme (einer Maschine)
E final acceptance (of a machine)
F réception technique (d'une machine)
S recepción técnica (de una máquina)

Abnahmebericht
E technical acceptance report
F rapport de réception technique
S informe de recepción técnica

abnehmbar
E detachable, removable
F amovible, démontable, détachable
S desmontable

Abnehmer
E customer
F client
S cliente

abnutschen
E filter, to
F filtrer
S filtrar

Abnutzung
E wear and tear
F usure
S desgaste

abpipettieren
E pipette off, to
F pipetter
S pipetear

abreichern (z. B. Viren)
E deplete, to; reduce, to (e. g. viruses)
F éliminer (par exemple des virus)
S eliminar (p. ej. virus)

Abreicherung
E deconcentration
F élimination
S eliminación, reducción

Abrieb
E friability, abrasion
F abrasion
S abrasión

abriebfest
E non-abrasive, resistant to abrasion
F résistant à l'abrasion
S resistente a la abrasión

Abriebfestigkeit
E frictional resistance
F résistance à la friction
S resistencia a la abrasión

abrunden
E round off, to
F arrondir
S redondear a la cifra inferior

English German French Spanish

English
German
French
Spanish

Absatz
E sales
F ventes
S ventas (volumen de)

absaugen
E aspirate, to
F aspirer
S aspirar

Absaugvorrichtung
E aspiration system, evacuation system
F système d'aspiration, système d'évacuation
S sistema de aspiración, sistema de evacuación

abschalten
E switch off, to
F couper, arrêter
S desconectar

Abschalter
E on/off switch
F interrupteur, bouton marche/arrêt
S interruptor

Abschaltung (einer Maschine)
E shut down (of a machine)
F arrêt (d'une machine)
S desconexión (de una máquina)

abscheiden
E separate, to
F séparer, sécréter
S precipitar, separar

Abscheider
E separator
F séparateur
S precipitador, separador

Abscheiderate
E separation rate
F vitesse de séparation
S velocidad de separación

Abschirmer, konischer
E conical screener
F protection cônique
S protector cónico

Abschirmung
E screening
F screening, tri, dépistage
S apantallamiento, protección

abschmelzen (Ampullen)
E tip seal, to (ampoules)
F obturer (des ampoules)
S sellar (ampollas)

Abschmelzhöhe (von Ampullen)
E fusion point (of ampoules)
F point de fusion (d'ampoules)
S punto de fusión (de ampollas)

Abschrägung
E bevel
F biseau
S bisel, faceta

Abschwächung (eines Signals)
E attenuation (of a signal)
F atténuation (d'un signal)
S atenuación (de una señal)

absetzen lassen
E allow to stand, to
F laisser sédimenter, laisser se déposer
S dejar precipitar, dejar sedimentar

absolut
E absolute
F absolu
S absoluto, absolutamente

Absorbens
E absorbent
F absorbant
S absorbente

absorbieren
E absorb, to
F absorber
S absorber

Absorption
E absorption
F absorption
S absorción

Absorptionsfähigkeit
E absorptivity, absorption capacity
F capacité d'absorption
S capacidad de absorción

Absorptionsgeschwindigkeit
E absorption rate
F vitesse d'absorption
S velocidad de absorción

Absorptionsgrundlage (für Salben)
E absorption base (for ointments)
F base d'absorption (pour pommades)
S base de absorción (para pomadas)

Absorptionskoeffizient
E absorption coefficient
F coefficient d'absorption
S coeficiente de absorción

Absorptionsmittel
E absorbent
F absorbant
S medio de absorción

Absorptionsvermögen
E absorbing power, absorbing capacity
F capacité d'absorption
S capacidad de absorción

Abspaltung, endothermische
E endothermic split-off
F scission endothermique
S escisión endotérmica

absperren
E close off, to
F fermer
S cerrar, cortar

Absperrhahn
E stopcock
F robinet d'arrêt
S grifo de cierre

Absperrklappe
E shut-off flap
F clapet de fermeture
S válvula de cierre

Absperrventil
E on/off valve
F valve d'arrêt
S válvula de cierre

Absterberate
E mortality rate
F taux de mortalité
S tasa de extinción, tasa de mortalidad

Abstreifer
E scraper
F racloir
S rascador

Abteilung
E department
F département, service
S departamento

Abteilungsleiter
E head of department
F chef de département, chef de service
S director de departamento

abtöten
E kill, to; destroy, to
F tuer, détruire
S destruir, matar

Abtötung
E killing
F action de tuer
S destrucción

Abtrag
E abrasion
F abrasion
S abrasión

Abtrennung
E segregation, separation
F séparation, ségrégation
S segregación, separación

Abwärme
E waste heat
F chaleur perdue
S calor de escape, pérdida calórica

English
German
French
Spanish

English
German
French
Spanish

abwaschbare Salbe
E water-soluble cream
F crème évanescente
S pomada evanescente

Abwasser
E waste water
F eaux résiduelles, eaux usées, eaux d'égouts
S aguas residuales

Abwasserleitung
E waste water line
F conduite destinée aux eaux résiduelles
S conducción de aguas residuales

Abwasserverschmutzung
E waste water pollution
F pollution des eaux résiduelles
S polución de aguas residuales

Abweichung
E deviation
F déviation, écart
S desviación

Abwesenheit
E absence
F absence
S ausencia

Abziehetikett
E transferable label
F étiquette prédécoupée
S etiqueta separable

Abzug
E ventilated hood, fume cupboard
F hotte à flux laminaire, hotte chimique
S escape, campana de extracción de gases

Acrylharz
E acrylic resin
F résine acrylique
S resina acrílica

Adhärenz
E adherence
F adhérence
S adherencia

adiabatische Reaktionsbedingungen
E adiabatic reaction conditions
F conditions de réaction adiabatiques
S condiciones adiabáticas de reacción

adiabatische Temperatur
E adiabatic temperature
F température adiabatique
S temperatura adiabática

Adsorption
E adsorption
F adsorption
S adsorción

Adsorptionschromatographie
E adsorption chromatography
F chromatographie d'adsorption
S cromatografía de adsorción

Adsorptionsfähigkeit
E adsorptivity, adsorption capacity
F capacité d'adsorption
S capacidad de adsorción

Adsorptionsmittel
E adsorbent
F adsorbant
S medio de adsorción

aerob
E aerobic
F aérobie
S aerobio

aerogen
E airborne
F aéroporté, transporté par l'air, en suspension dans l'air
S aerógeno

Aerosoldose
E aerosol can
F bidon d'aérosol, bombe aérosol
S tubo aerosol

Aerosolmessung
E aerosol measurement
F mesure (de la dose) d'un aérosol
S medida de aerosol

Affinität
E affinity
F affinité
S afinidad

Affinitätschromatographie
E affinity chromatography
F chromatographie d'affinité
S cromatografía de afinidad

Affinitätsdiagramm
E affinity diagram
F diagramme d'affinité
S diagrama de afinidad

Agar
E agar
F agar, agar-agar
S agar

Agglomerat
E agglomerate
F agglomérat
S aglomerado

agglomerieren
E agglomerate, to
F agglomérer
S aglomerar

Agglutination
E agglutination
F agglutination
S aglutinación

Aggregat
E aggregate
F agrégat
S agregado

akkreditieren
E accredit, to
F accréditer
S acreditar

Aktiengesellschaft
E public liability company
F société anonyme
S sociedad anónima

Aktionsgrenze
E action limit
F limite d'action
S límite de acción

Aktivierung
E actuation, activation
F activation
S activación

Aktivierungsenergie
E activation energy
F énergie d'activation
S energía de activación

Aktivkohle
E activated charcoal
F charbon actif
S carbón activado

aktualisieren
E update, to
F actualiser
S actualizar

akustisches Signal
E acoustic signal
F signal acoustique
S señal acústica

Akzeptanzkriterium
E acceptance criterion
F critère d'acceptation
S criterio de aceptación

Akzeptanztest (z. B. für Software)
E acceptance test
(e. g. for software)
F test d'acceptance
(par ex. pour logiciel)
S prueba de aceptación
(p. ej. de software)

Alarm
E alarm, alarm signal
F signal d'alarme
S alarma

Alarmlimit
E alarm limit
F limite d'alarme
S límite de alarma

Alarmsystem
E alarm system
F système d'alarme
S sistema de alarma

Aldehyd
E aldehyde
F aldéhyde
S aldehído

aliquotieren
E aliquot, to
F aliquoter
S alicuotar

Alkalinität
E alkalinity
F alcalinité
S alcalinidad, basicidad

alkalisch
E alkaline
F alcalin
S alcalino, básico

alkalische Behandlung
E alkaline treatment
F traitement alcalin
S tratamiento alcalino

Alkoholauszug
E alcoholate
F alcoolate
S extracto alcohólico

Alkylierung
E alkylation
F alkylation
S alquilación

Allergen
E allergen
F allergène
S alergeno

allergisierend
E sensitising
F allergisant
S alergizante

Alpha-Helix (z. B. eines Proteins)
E alpha helix (e. g. of protein)
F hélice alpha (structure des protéines)
S hélice alfa (p. ej. de proteína)

altern
E age, to
F vieillir
S envejecer

Alterung
E ageing, maturing
F vieillissement
S envejecimiento

beschleunigte Alterung (künstlich)
E forced ageing
F vieillissement (forcé) prématuré
S envejecimiento acelerado (artificial)

thermische Alterung
E thermal ageing
F vieillissement thermique
S envejecimiento térmico

alterungsbeständig
E age-resistant
F résistant au vieillissement
S resistente al envejecimiento

Aluminiumflasche
E aluminium bottle
F bouteille d'aluminium
S botella de aluminio

Aluminiumfolie
E aluminium foil
F feuille d'aluminium
S hoja de aluminio

Aluminiumoxid
E alumina, aluminium oxide
F oxyde d'aluminium
S óxido de aluminio

Alupalette
E aluminium pallet
F alupalette, palette en aluminium
S paleta de aluminio

Amine
E amines
F amines
S aminas

aromatische Amine
E aromatic amines
F amines aromatiques
S aminas aromáticas

primäre Amine
E primary amines
F amines primaires
S aminas primarias

sekundäre Amine
E secondary amines
F amines secondaires
S aminas secundarias

tertiäre Amine
E tertiary amines
F amines tertiaires
S aminas terciarias

Aminosäure
E amino acid
F acide aminé
S aminoácido

essentielle Aminosäure
E essential amino acid
F acide aminé essentiel
S aminoácido esencial

Aminosäurederivat
E amino acid derivative
F dérivé d'acide aminé
S derivado de aminoácido

amorph
E amorphous
F amorphe
S amorfo

Amperemeter
E ammeter
F ampèremètre
S amperímetro

amperometrische Detektion
E amperometric detection
F détecteur ampérométrique
S detección amperométrica

Amplitude
E amplitude
F amplitude
S amplitud

Ampulle
E ampoule
F ampoule
S ampolla

Ampulle aufbrechen
E break an ampoule, to
F casser une ampoule
S romper una ampolla

Ampulle verschließen
E seal an ampoule, to
F fermer une ampoule, obturer une ampoule
S cerrar una ampolla

Ampullenabfüllung
E ampoule filling
F remplissage d'une ampoule
S rellenado de una ampolla

Ampullenfeile
E ampoule file, ampoule cutter
F lime (pour ampoule)
S lima de ampolla

Ampullenhals
E ampoule neck
F col d'une ampoule
S cuello de ampolla

Ampullenschachtel
E ampoule box
F boîte d'ampoules
S caja de ampollas

An/Aus-Taste
E start/stop key
F touche marche-arrêt
S interruptor de encendido

English
German
French
Spanish

anaerob
E anaerobic
F anaérobe
S anaerobio

Analoganzeige
E analogue display
F affichage numérique
S pantalla análoga

Analyse
E analysis
F analyse
S análisis

Analyse auf Gesamt-(Petroleum)-Kohlenwasserstoffe
E total petroleum hydrocarbon (tph) analysis
F analyse de la teneur totale du pétrole en hydrocarbures
S análisis de hidrocarburos totales (de petróleo)

Analyse, coulometrische
E coulometric analysis
F analyse coulométrique
S análisis coulométrico

Analyse, volumetrische
E volumetric analysis
F analyse volumétrique
S análisis volumétrico

Analysengerät
E analytical apparatus
F appareil d'analyses
S aparato de análisis

Analysenwaage
E analytical balance
F balance d'analyse
S báscula de análisis

Analysenzertifikat
E certificate of analysis
F certificat d'analyse
S certificado de análisis

Analyt
E analyte
F analyte, substance à analyser
S sustancia a analizar

analytisch
E analytical
F analytique
S analítico

analytische Säule
E analytical column
F colonne analytique
S columna analítica

analytische Unsicherheit
E analytical uncertainty
F incertitude analytique
S inseguridad analítica

Anbauteil
E attachment, module
F accessoire, dispositif adaptable, module
S pieza de montaje

anbringen
E apply, to; attach, to
F apposer, installer, poser
S instalar, montar

Anbruch
E open case, open package
F emballage ouvert, emballage entamé
S envase abierto

andecken (beim Dragieren)
E precoat, to (tablets)
F pré-enrober
S prerrecubrir (grageas)

Änderung
E change, variation
F changement
S cambio, modificación, variación

Änderungsantrag
E change request
F demande de modification
S solicitud de cambio

Änderungsanzeige
E amendment
F amendement
S anuncio de enmienda

Änderungskontrolle
E change control, change management
F contrôle des changements, contrôle des modifications
S control de modificaciones

Andocksystem
E docking system
F système d'amarrage, système de fixation
S sistema de fijación, sistema de acoplamiento

anfahren
E start, to; start-up, to
F démarrer
S poner en marcha

Anfälligkeit
E vulnerability
F vulnérabilité
S vulnerabilidad

Anfangsgeschwindigkeit
E start speed, initial speed
F vitesse initiale
S velocidad inicial

anfeuchten
E humidise, to; wet, to; moisten, to
F humidifier
S humectar, humedecer

Anforderung
E requirement
F exigence
S exigencia, requerimiento

gesetzliche Anforderung
E legal requirement
F exigence légale
S requerimiento legal

Angaben
E data, specifications
F données, spécifications
S datos, especificaciones

angelieferte Materialien
E incoming goods
F marchandises receptionnées
S materiales suministrados

angemessen
E suitable, appropriate, adequate
F approprié, adéquat
S adecuado, apropiado

angeschlossen
E connected
F connecté
S conectado

falsch angeschlossen
E wrongly connected
F faussement connecté
S mal conectado

Angestellter
E employee
F employé
S empleado

Angriffspunkt
E site of action
F site d'application
S lugar de aplicación

Anhang
E appendix
F appendice
S anexo, apéndice

Anhäufung
E accumulation
F accumulation
S acumulación

Anionenaustauscher
E anion exchanger
F échangeur d'ions anioniques
S intercambiador de aniones

Ankerrührer
E anchor stirrer
F agitateur à ancre
S agitador de ancla

Ankleideraum
E gowning room
F vestiaire
S vestuario

Ankunftsvermerk
E sign-in log
F mention de venue
S nota de llegada

ankuppeln
E couple, to
F accoupler, accrocher
S acoplar

Anlage (Maschine)
E facility, plant (machines)
F usine, établissement industriel, installation
S equipo, instalación (máquina)

Anlage (zur Dokumentation)
E enclosure, appendix
F annexe, appendice
S anexo, apéndice (de un documento)

Anlagensteuerung
E plant control
F système de contrôle d'une installation
S control de plantas e instalaciones

Anlagenwartung
E plant maintenance
F maintenance d'une installation
S mantenimiento de equipo e instalaciones

anlaufen (Metall)
E tarnish, to (metal)
F ternir, se ternir (métal)
S deslustrarse, empañarse (metales)

Annahme
E acceptance
F réception, acceptation, acceptance
S aceptación

Annahmekennlinie
E acceptance graph
F courbe d'acceptance
S característica de aceptación

Annahmezahl
E acceptance number
F indice d'acceptance
S número de aceptación

Annehmbare Qualitätsgrenzlage (AQL)
E acceptable quality level (AQL)
F niveau de qualité acceptable
S límite de calidad aceptable

Einzel-AQL
E individual AQL
F niveau individuel de qualité acceptable
S límite individual de calidad aceptable

Gesamt-AQL
E class AQL
F niveau absolu de qualité acceptable
S límite total de calidad aceptable

anorganisch
E inorganic
F anorganique
S anorgánico

anreichern
E concentrate, to; enrich, to
F concentrer
S concentrar, enriquecer

Anreicherung
E concentration, enrichment
F concentration
S concentración, enriquecimiento

Anreicherungsmedium
E concentration medium, enrichment medium
F médium de concentration
S medio de concentración, medio de enriquecimiento

Ansatz
E reaction materials
F matériaux de réaction
S planteamiento, inserción, materiales de reacción

Ansatzbehälter
E container, reaction vessel
F container, récipient
S contenedor

fahrbarer Ansatzbehälter
E mobile vessel, mobile container
F cuve sur roues, cuve mobile
S contenedor portátil

Ansatzrohr
E extension pipe
F tuyau de rallonge
S tubo de empalme

Ansatzstück
E extension
F rallonge
S pieza de empalme, pieza insertable

ansäuern
E acidify, to
F acidifier
S acidificar

ansaugen
E aspirate, to
F aspirer
S aspirar, succionar

Ansaugstutzen
E aspiration nipple
F manchon d'aspiration
S empalme de aspiración

Ansaugventil
E aspiration valve
F vanne d'aspiration
S válvula de aspiración

Anschaffungskosten
E purchase price
F frais d'achat
S costes de adquisición

anschließen
E connect, to
F connecter
S conectar

Anschluß
E connection
F connexion
S conexión

Anschlußstutzen
E connection port, connection nipple
F douille de connexion, manchon de connexion
S empalme de conexión

Ansprechpartner
E contact person
F interlocuteur
S interlocutor

Ansprechzeit
E response time
F temps de réponse
S tiempo de respuesta

Anstaltspackung
E hospital pack
F emballage pour hôpitaux
S envase clínico

ansteckende Krankheit
E infectious disease
F maladie infectieuse
S enfermedad contagiosa

Antibioticum
E antibiotic
F antibiotique
S antibiótico

Antikörper
E antibody
F anticorps
S anticuerpo

monoklonaler Antikörper
E monoclonal antibody
F anticorps monoclonal
S anticuerpo monoclonal

Antioxidans
E anti-oxidant
F antioxydant
S antioxidante

Antipoden, optische
E optical antipodes
F antipodes optiques
S antípodas ópticos

Antischaummittel
E anti-foaming agent
F agent antimousse
S agente antiespumante

Antistatikum
E anti-static agent
F agent antistatique
S antiestático

Antrag
E application
F requête, demande
S solicitud, instancia

Antrag auf Vertriebsgenehmigung eines Arzneimittels (bei der FDA)
E Product License Application (PLA), Application for Marketing Approval
F demande d'autorisation de mise sur le marché (AMM)
S solicitud de permiso a la FDA (EE.UU.) para poner a la venta un medicamento

Antrag auf Zulassung zum Inverkehrbringen von Arzneimitteln (in der EU)
E Medicines Marketing Authorisation Application (MAA)
F demande d'autorisation de mise sur le marché (AMM)
S solicitud de autorización de venta de medicamentos en la UE

Antrag zur klinischen Prüfung eines Arzneimittels (bei der FDA)
E Investigational New Drug Application (IND)
F demande d'autorisation d'étude clinique d'un nouveau médicament (IND) auprès de la FDA
S solicitud a la FDA (EE.UU.) para investigar clínicamente un nuevo medicamento

Antrag auf Produktzulassung (bei der FDA)
E New Drug Application (NDA)
F demande d'autorisation d'un médicament auprès de la FDA
S solicitud de aprobación de un producto por la FDA

Antrieb
E drive
F entraînement, transmission
S impulso, propulsión, tracción

Antriebseinheit
E drive unit
F unité de transmission
S unidad propulsora

Antriebsgeschwindigkeit
E drive speed, impeller speed
F vitesse de transmission, vitesse de roulement
S velocidad de propulsión, velocidad de rodamiento

Antriebsmotor
E drive motor
F moteur de transmission, moteur propulsif
S motor de propulsión

Antriebswelle
E drive shaft
F arbre de transmission
S árbol motor

Anweisung
E instruction
F instruction, mode d'emploi
S instrucción

Anwendbarkeit
E applicability
F applicabilité
S aplicabilidad

Anwendung
E application
F application
S aplicación

dentale Anwendung
E dental use
F usage dental
S aplicación dental

gastrointestinale Anwendung
E gastro-enteral use
F utilisation gastro-intestinale
S aplicación gastrointestinal

nasale Anwendung
E nasal use
F utilisation nasale
S aplicación nasal

subkutane Anwendung
E subcutaneous use
F utilisation sous-cutanée
S aplicación subcutánea

transdermale Anwendung
E transdermal use
F utilisation transcutanée
S aplicación transdérmica

vaginale Anwendung
E vaginal use
F utilisation vaginale
S aplicación vaginal

zur äußerlichen Anwendung
E for external application
F pour application externe
S para aplicación externa

Anwendung am Auge
E ocular use, ophthalmic use
F pour usage ophtalmique
S uso oftálmico

Anwendung am Ohr
E auricular use
F pour usage auriculaire
S uso otológico

Anwendung am Zahnfleisch
E gingival use
F pour usage gingival
S uso gingival

Anwendung auf der Haut
E cutaneous use
F pour usage cutané
S uso cutáneo

Anwendung in den Nebenhöhlen
E endosinusial use
F pour usage sinusien
S uso endosinusal

Anwendung in der Mundhöhle
E oromucosal use
F usage bucco-mucosal
S uso bucal

Anwendungsgebiet
E area of application
F champ d'application,
domaine d'application
S campo de aplicación

Anwendungssoftware
E application software
F logiciel d'application
S sistema lógico de aplicación,
software de aplicación

Anwesenheit
E presence
F présence
S presencia

Anzeige
E display
F indicateur
S indicación, pantalla

außerhalb des Anzeigebereichs
E off-scale
F en dehors de l'échelle de mesure
S fuera de la escala de medida

innerhalb des Anzeigebereichs
E on-scale
F dans l'échelle de mesure
S dentro de la escala de medida

integrierte Anzeige
E integrated display
F indicateur intégré
S pantalla integrada

English German French Spanish

optische Anzeige
E visual display
F indicateur optique
S pantalla óptica

anzeigen
E display, to; indicate, to
F indiquer, afficher
S indicar, mostrar

Anziehungskraft
E force of attraction
F force d'attraction
S fuerza de atracción

apathogen
E apathogenic
F apathogène
S apatógeno

apothekenpflichtig
E for sale in pharmacies only
F vendu uniquement en pharmacie
S de venta sólo en farmacias

Apotheker
E pharmacist
F pharmacien
S farmacéutico

Applikationsweg
E application route
F voie d'application
S vía de administración

Applikator
E applicator
F applicateur
S aplicador

Aqua bidest.
E redistilled water, double-distilled water
F eau pour préparation injectable (PPI)
S agua bidestilada

Aqua dest.
E distilled water
F eau distillée
S agua destilada

Aqua purificata
E purified water
F eau purifiée
S agua purificada

äquivalent
E equivalent
F équivalent
S equivalente

Äquivalenz
E equivalency
F équivalence
S equivalencia

Arbeitsablauf
E operational cycle
F cycle de fonctionnement
S ciclo de funcionamiento

Arbeitsanweisung
E operating procedure
F procédure opératoire
S instrucción de trabajo

Arbeitsdruck
E working pressure
F pression de travail
S presión de trabajo

Arbeitsfugen
E construction joints
F joints de construction
S juntas de construcción

Arbeitsgang
E operation
F opération
S turno de trabajo

in einem Arbeitsgang
E single step operation
F opération en une seule étape
S operación en etapa única

Arbeitsgruppe
E working group, task force
F groupe de travail
S grupo de trabajo

Arbeitskleidung
E working clothing
F vêtement de travail
S ropa de trabajo

Kleidungsaufnahmebehälter
E clothing receptacle
F corbeille pour vêtements de travail
S cesto para ropa de trabajo

Arbeitsoberfläche
E working surface
F surface de travail
S superficie de trabajo

Arbeitsplatz
E place of work
F poste de travail
S puesto de trabajo, empleo

Arbeitsschicht
E shift (working)
F travail en trois-huit, équipe (de travail)
S turno de trabajo

Arbeitssicherheit
E safety at work
F sécurité du travail, sécurité au travail
S seguridad en el trabajo

Arbeitsstandard
E working standard
F norme de travail
S norma de trabajo

Arbeitsstelle
E employment, job
F emploi
S puesto de trabajo

Arbeitstisch
E bench, work bench
F table de travail, établi
S mesa de trabajo

Arbeitsvorbereitung
E work scheduling
F planification du travail
S preparación del trabajo

Arbeitsvorgänge im Reinraum
E clean room operations
F opérations en zone d'atmosphère contrôlée
S procesos de trabajo en área estéril

Arbeitsvorschrift
E operating procedure, instruction
F procédure opératoire, instruction
S norma de trabajo

Archiv
E archive
F archives
S archivo

Archivierung
E archiving
F archivage
S archivado

Archivierungsmedien
E archiving media
F médium d'archivage
S medios de archivado

arithmetisches Mittel
E arithmetic mean
F moyenne arithmétique
S media aritmética

Armatur
E fitting
F garniture
S armadura, accesorios

Armaturentafel
E panel
F tableau de bord
S cuadro de mandos, tablero de instrumentos

Aromastoff
E aromatic substance
F substance aromatique
S sustancia aromática

arretieren
E lock, to
F fermer à clef
S fijar, parar, retener

English
German
French
Spanish

Arretiervorrichtung (bei Waagen)
E beam arrest (balance)
F relève-plateau
S dispositivo de fijación (en básculas)

Art
E species
F espèce
S especie

Arzneibuch
E pharmacopoeia
F pharmacopée
S farmacopea

Arzneibuch der USA
E United States Pharmacopoeia (USP)
F pharmacopée américaine
S farmacopea estadounidense

Arzneibuchmonographie
E pharmacopoeial monograph
F monographie de la pharmacopée
S monografía de farmacopea

Arzneiform
E dosage form
F forme pharmaceutique
S forma farmacéutica

einzeldosierte Arzneiform
E single dose unit
F une dose d'utilisation, forme d'une unité de prise
S forma farmacéutica de dosis única

monolithische Arzneiform
E single dose form
F forme pharmaceutique monolithique
S formulación monolítica

Arzneimittel
E medicinal product, drug
F médicament, produit pharmaceutique
S medicamento

biotechnologisch hergestelltes Arzneimittel
E biopharmaceutical
F produit biopharmaceutique
S medicamento producido biotecnológicamente

gentechnologisch hergestelltes Arzneimittel
E genetically manufactured medicinal product
F médicament produit par génie génétique
S medicamento producido mediante tecnología genética

Arzneimittelvormischung
E medicinal product premix, drug premix
F préparation pharmaceutique
S elaboración previa del medicamento

Arzneistoff
E medicinal substance, active substance, drug
F principe actif
S principio activo, sustancia medicamentosa

Arzneistoffaufnahme
E absorption of medicinal substance
F adsorption d'un principe actif
S absorción del principio activo

Arzneistoffausscheidung
E excretion of medicinal substance
F élimination d'un principe actif
S eliminación del principio activo

Arzneistoff-Freisetzung
E release of medicinal substance
F libération d'un principe actif
S liberación del principio activo

Ärztemuster
E pharmaceutical sample
F échantillon pharmaceutique
S muestra farmacéutica

ärztliche Untersuchung
E medical examination
F examen médical
S exploración médica

Asbest
E asbestos
F amiante
S asbesto

Asbestfilter
E asbestos filter
F filtre en amiante
S filtro de asbesto

Asche
E ash
F cendre
S ceniza

aseptisch
E aseptic
F aseptique
S aséptico

aseptische Abfüllung
E aseptic filling
F remplissage aseptique
S envasado aséptico

aseptische Herstellung
E aseptic processing
F fabrication aseptique
S fabricación aséptica

aseptische Prozeßtechnik
E aseptic process, aseptic technology
F procédé aseptique, technique aseptique
S técnica de proceso aséptico

Atemschutz
E respiratory protection
F masque respiratoire de protection
S protección respiratoria

ätherisches Öl
E essential oil
F huile essentielle
S aceite etérico

Atmosphärendruck
E atmospheric pressure
F pression atmosphérique
S presión atmosférica

Atmosphärenüberdruck
E excess atmospheric pressure
F surpression atmosphérique
S sobrepresión atmosférica

Atmosphärenunterdruck
E sub-atmospheric pressure
F dépression atmosphérique
S presión atmosférica baja

Atomemissionsspektroskopie
E atomic emission spectroscopy
F spectroscopie par émission atomique
S espectroscopia de emisión atómica

Atomschichtepitaxie
E atomic layer epitaxy (ALE)
F épitaxie d'une couche d'atomes
S epitaxia de un estrato atómico

ätzend
E caustic
F caustique
S cáustico

Audit
E audit
F audit, inspection
S auditoría, inspección

internes Audit
E internal audit
F audit interne
S auditoría interna

Auditfunktion
E audit function
F fonction d'audit
S función de la auditoría

Auditweg
E audit trail
F trace-témoin de l'audit
S traza-testigo de la auditoría

aufarbeiten
E process, to; reprocess, to
F traiter
S procesar

Aufarbeitung
E processing, reprocessing
F traitement
S proceso

Aufbau, instrumenteller
E instrument set-up
F montage des instruments
S montaje de instrumentos

Aufbaugranulierung
E synthetic granulation
F granulation hors taille
S granulación sintética

aufbewahren
E retain, to; store, to
F conserver, garder
S conservar, guardar

Aufbewahrung
E retention, storage, archiving
F conservation, stockage, archivage
S conservación, almacenaje

Aufbewahrungstank
E storage tank
F récipient de stockage
S tanque de conservación

aufblasbar
E inflatable
F gonflable
S hinchable

aufblasbare Silikondichtung
E inflatable silicone seal
F joint de silicone gonflable
S cierre inflable de silicona

aufbringen
E apply, to
F appliquer, étendre
S aplicar, extender

Aufdruck
E imprint
F impression
S impresión

aufdrucken
E imprint, to
F imprimer
S imprimir

Aufenthalt im Magen
E gastric duration, gastric residence
F durée de résidence gastrique
S permanencia en el estómago

Aufenthaltsdauer
E dwell time, residence time
F temps de résidence
S duración de la permanencia

auffangen
E collect, to; entrap, to
F capter, recueillir
S captar, colectar, recoger

Auffanggefäß
E collection vessel
F cuve de collecte,
récipient de collecte
S recipiente colector

Aufgabedrehteller
E revolving plate feeder, turntable
F plateau tournant
S placa giratoria

aufgeben (Probe)
E apply, to (sample)
F appliquer (un échantillon)
S aplicar (una muestra)

Aufguß
E infusion
F infusion
S infusión

Aufhängung
E suspension, suspension device
F suspension
S suspensión

Aufheizspirale
E heating coil
F serpentin chauffant
S serpentín de calentamiento

Aufheizzeit
E heat-up time
F temps de réchauffement
S tiempo de calentamiento

aufkaufen
E acquire, to
F acquérir
S adquirir

aufklären (Struktur)
E elucidate, to (a structure)
F élucider (une structure)
S aclarar, esclarecer (una estructura)

aufkochen
E boil, to
F bouillir
S hervir

Auflösegeschwindigkeit
E dissolution rate, dissolution speed
F vitesse de dissolution
S velocidad de disolución

Auflösemedium
E dissolution medium
F milieu de dissolution
S diluyente, medio de disolución

auflösen
E dissolve, to
F dissoudre
S diluir, disolver

Auflösung
E dissolution
F dissolution
S dilución, disolución

Auflösungsrate
E dissolution rate
F vitesse de dissolution
S tasa de disolución

Auflösungsstudie
E dissolution study
F essai de dissolution
S estudio de dilución

Auflösungsverhalten
E dissolution behaviour
F comportement de dissolution
S comportamiento en disolución

Aufnahme
E recording
F enregistrement
S toma, registro

aufprägen
E emboss, to; imprint, to
F imprimer, empreindre
S estampar, imprimir

Aufrahmung (bei Emulsionen)
E creaming (of emulsions)
F crémage (d'une émulsion)
S cremado (de emulsiones)

Aufreinigung (chemisch)
E purification
F purification
S purificación (química)

Aufreißlasche
E tear-off tab
F languette
S lengüeta arrancable

aufrichten (eine Faltschachtel)
E set up, to (a folding carton)
F dresser, monter (un carton)
S montar (una caja plegable)

aufrüsten
E upgrade, to
F moderniser
S modernizar, renovar

Aufschlag
E supplement, overage
F supplément, majoration
S aumento, suplemento

aufschrauben
E screw on, to
F visser, dévisser
S atornillar

Aufsicht
E supervision
F supervision, surveillance
S control, inspección, supervisión

aufsprühen
E spray, to
F pulvériser
S pulverizar

Aufstellungsort
E installation location
F lieu d'installation
S lugar de instalación

auftauen
E defrost, to; thaw, to
F dégeler
S descongelar

auftragen
E apply, to
F appliquer, étendre
S aplicar, extender, untar

Auftraggeber
E contract provider, principal, client
F donneur d'ordre, commettant, client
S cliente, comitente

Auftragnehmer
E contract acceptor
F preneur d'une commande
S comisionista

Auftragsdicke
E coating thickness
F épaisseur de l'enduit, épaisseur de la couche
S espesor de la capa

Auftragshersteller
E contract manufacturer
F producteur sous-traintant
S fabricante por comisión

Auftragsherstellung
E contract manufacturing
F production par un sous-traitant
S producción por contrata

Auftragslabor
E contract laboratory
F laboratoire sous-traitant
S laboratorio comisionado

Auftragsmenge (beim Coating)
E coating quantity
F quantité (d'enduit) appliquée
S cantidad a aplicar (al recubrir)

Auftragsnummer
E order number
F numéro de commande
S número del encargo

Auftragsproduktion
E contract manufacturing
F production par un sous-traitant
S producción por encargo

Aufwärtskurve
E ascending curve
F courbe ascendante
S curva ascendente

aufzeichnen (Daten)
E log, to; record, to; register, to (data)
F enregistrer (des données)
S registrar (datos)

Aufzeichnung
E record, log
F enregistrement
S registro

Aufzug
E lift, elevator
F ascenseur
S ascensor

Aufzugsschiene (des Oberstempels)
E lifting cam (of upper punch)
F came (de poinçon) ascendante
S carril de ascenso (del troquel superior)

English German French Spanish

Augenbad
E eye lotion
F lotion pour œil
S loción oftálmica

Augencreme
E eye cream
F crème ophtalmique
S crema oftálmica

Augendusche
E eye wash equipment
F douche de rinçage pour les yeux
S equipo de lavado oftálmico

Augengel
E eye gel
F gel pour œil
S gel oftálmico

Augenlid
E eye lid
F paupière
S párpado

Augensalbe
E eye ointment
F pommade pour les yeux
S pomada oftálmica

Augenschutz
E eye protection
F protection oculaire
S protección ocular

Augentropfen
E eye drops
F gouttes ophtalmiques
S gotas oftálmicas

Ausbau
E removal, disassembly
F démontage
S desmontaje

Ausbeute
E yield
F rendement
S rendimiento

tatsächliche Ausbeute
E actual yield
F rendement réel
S rendimiento real

theoretische Ausbeute
E theoretical yield
F rendement théorique
S rendimiento teórico

Ausbeuteberechnung
E yield calculation
F calcul du rendement
S cálculo del rendimiento

Ausbeutesteigerung
E yield enhancement
F augmentation du rendement
S aumento del rendimiento

Ausbildung
E education, training
F éducation
S educación, formación

ausblasen
E blow out, to
F souffler, éteindre
S apagar soplando

ausdampfen
E strip, to; evaporate, to
F passer à la vapeur
S evaporar, volatilizar

Ausdehnung
E expansion
F expansion
S ampliación, dilatación, expansión, extensión

Ausdruck
E printout
F imprimé
S impreso

Papierausdruck
E paper printout, hard copy
F imprimé sur papier
S impreso sobre papel

Ausdünstung
E effluvium
F effluent, efflux
S evaporación, transpiración

Ausfall
E breakdown, downtime (machine), failure
F panne, temps mort, défaillance
S avería, desperfecto, fallo

ausfällen
E precipitate, to
F précipiter
S precipitar

Ausfällung
E precipitation
F précipitation
S precipitación, precipitado

Ausfällungsmittel
E precipitation agent
F agent de précipitation
S agente precipitador

ausflocken
E flocculate, to; flake, to
F floculer
S flocular

Ausführung
E version
F version
S realización, modelo, versión

Ausgabe
E delivery, edition, version, issue
F livraison, édition, version
S distribución, entrega, edición, versión

Ausgangsstoff
E starting material, raw material
F matériel de départ, matière première
S sustancia de partida, sustancia inicial

Ausgangsvermerk
E sign-out log
F mention d'origine
S mención inicial, nota inicial

ausgeben
E dispense, to
F dépenser, distribuer
S distribuir, gastar

ausgelegt für
E designed for
F prévu pour, construit pour
S construido para, diseñado para

ausgeleiert
E worn out
F usé
S desgastado

ausgeschwenkt
E swivelled, pivotted
F pivoté
S girado hacia fuera

Ausgleichsestrich
E screed, floor leveller
F chape de compensation
S pavimento compensador

ausglühen
E ignite, to
F faire rougir, se calciner
S calcinar

Ausguß
E sink
F évier
S descarga, orificio de descarga

aushärten
E cure, to
F tremper
S curar

Aushärtung
E curing
F trempe
S curado

Aushilfe
E temporary help
F stagiaire, aide temporaire
S ayuda temporal

Auskeimung (von Sporen)
E germination
F germination
S germinación (de esporas)

Auskleidung (von Behältern)
E lining (of containers)
F garnissage (de récipients)
S revestimiento (de recipientes)

auskristallisieren
E crystallise out, to
F se cristalliser complètement
S cristalizar completamente

Auskristallisierung
E crystallisation
F cristallisation
S cristalización

Auslaß
E outlet, orifice
F sortie, orifice
S descarga, escape, salida

Auslaßfilter
E outlet filter
F filtre de sortie
S filtro de descarga, filtro de salida

Auslaßöffnung einer Säule
E column outlet
F sortie d'une colonne
S orificio de salida de una columna

Auslaßtemperatur
E outlet temperature
F température de sortie
S temperatura de salida

Auslassung
E omission
F omission
S omisión

Auslaßventil
E outlet valve
F valve de sortie
S válvula de salida

Auslauf
E outlet, discharge outlet
F sortie de vidange, sortie de purge
S desagüe, salida

auslaufen
E run off, to
F couler, s'écouler
S escaparse, salirse

Auslaufen des Patentes
E patent expiry
F expiration d'un brevet
S expiración de una patente

Auslaufstutzen
E outlet nipple
F manchon de purge
S empalme de salida

Auslese
E selection
F sélection
S selección

Auslieferung
E delivery
F livraison
S distribución, entrega

Ausmaß
E dimensions
F dimensions
S cuantía, dimensiones, medidas

auspressen
E express, to
F presser
S exprimir, prensar

Ausreißer
E outlier
F valeur aberrante, anormale
S elemento fuera de los márgenes habituales

ausrichten
E align, to
F aligner, ajuster, centrer
S ajustar, alinear, orientar

English German French Spanish

ausrüsten
E provide with, to; equip, to
F équiper, outiller
S equipar

Ausrüstung
E equipment
F équipement
S equipamiento

für verschiedene Produkte
E multipurpose (equipment)
F (équipement) multi-usage
S para diferentes productos

nur für ein Produkt
E dedicated (equipment)
F (équipement) dédié
S sólo para un producto

Ausrüstungsteil
E accessory
F accessoire
S accesorio

Ausschalter
E on/off switch
F interrupteur, bouton marche/arrêt
S interruptor (de desconexión)

Ausschaltstrom
E breaking current
F courant de coupure
S corriente de desconexión

Ausschlag (eines Zeigers)
E deflection (of pointer)
F déviation (d'une aiguille)
S desviación (de una aguja indicadora)

Ausschlußchromatographie
E size exclusion chromatography
F chromatographie par limite d'exclusion
S cromatografía de exclusión

Ausschlußgrenze
E exclusion limit
F limite d'exclusion
S límite de exclusión

Ausschreibung
E tender
F appel d'offres
S anuncio, concurso, convocatoria

Ausschuß
E waste
F déchets, résidus
S desecho

Ausschußposition
E reject position
F position de rejet
S posición de desecho

ausschütteln
E shake out, to
F secouer
S sacudir

Ausschwenkvorrichtung
E swing-out device, swivelling device
F dispositif d'orientation
S dispositivo giratorio

Aussehen, allgemeines
E general appearance
F apparence générale
S aspecto general

Außendienst
E field force, sales force
F force de vente
S servicio externo de ventas

Außendienstmitarbeiter
E sales representative
F commercial, vendeur
S agente externo de ventas

Außenlack
E outer lacquer
F laque extérieure
S barniz externo

Außenluft
E outside air, external air
F air frais, air libre
S aire fresco, aire libre

Außenmaße
E external dimensions
F dimensions externes
S dimensiones externas

äußerlich
E external
F externe
S externo

Aussparung
E recess
F évidure, échancrure
S hueco, vacío

ausstanzen
E die-cut, to; punch, to; stamp, to
F découper à l'emporte-pièce, poinçonner
S estampar, perforar, punzonar

Ausstoß (Menge)
E ejection, output
F éjection, rejet, niveau de production, niveau de rendement
S eyección, volumen de producción

ausstoßen
E eject, to
F éjecter, expulser, rejeter
S emitir, expeler, expulsar

Ausstoßkraft
E ejection force
F force d'éjection
S fuerza de eyección

Ausstoßzeit
E ejection time
F temps d'éjection
S tiempo de eyección

ausstreichen (mikrobiol. Kolonien)
E smear, to (microbiological colonies)
F ensemencer (colonies microbiol.)
S sembrar (colonias microbiológicas)

Ausstrich
E smear
F ensemencement
S extensión, frotis

austarieren
E tare, to
F tarer
S tarar

austauschbar
E interchangeable, exchangeable
F interchangeable
S intercambiable

Austauscherharz
E ion exchange resin
F résine échangeuse d'ions
S resina de intercambio iónico

Austauschteil
E spare part, replacement part
F pièce de rechange
S pieza de recambio

austragen (Salbe aus Container)
E discharge, to (ointment from container)
F décharger (la pommade du conteneur)
S descargar (pomada del contenedor)

Austritt
E outlet, orifice
F sortie, orifice
S escape, salida

austrocknen
E dry out, to; desiccate, to
F dessiquer
S desecar

Auswahl
E selection
F sélection
S selección

auswechselbar
E exchangeable, replaceable
F interchangeable
S intercambiable

Ausweichmedikation
E alternative medication
F médication alternative
S medicación alternativa

English German French Spanish

Auswerfkurve
E ejector cam
F came d'éjection
S curva de expulsión

Auswertebereich
E evaluation range
F plage d'évaluation
S área de evaluación

Auswertung
E interpretation, evaluation
F interprétation, évaluation
S evaluación, interpretación

Auswurf
E ejection
F éjection, rejet
S eyección

automatischer Auswurf
E automatic ejection
F éjection automatique
S expulsión automática

Auswurfgegenkontrolle
E ejection control
F contrôle de l'éjection
S control de la expulsión

Auswurfkurve (bei der Tablettenpresse)
E ejector cam
F came d'éjection
S curva de expulsión (de prensa de comprimidos)

Auswurfstelle
E reject position
F emplacement de l'éjection
S zona de expulsión

Auszubildender
E apprentice
F apprenti, stagiaire
S aprendiz

Auszug
E extract
F extrait
S extracto

Autoklav
E autoclave
F autoclave
S autoclave

autoklavierbar
E autoclavable
F autoclavable
S esterilizable en autoclave

autoklavieren
E autoclave, to
F autoclaver
S esterilizar en autoclave

Automation
E automation
F automatisation
S automa(tiza)ción

automatisieren
E automate, to
F automatiser
S automatizar

autorisierte Person
E authorised individual
F personne autorisée
S persona autorizada

autorisierter Zugang
E authorised access
F droit d'accès
S acceso autorizado

Azidität
E acidity
F acidité
S acidez

Backe (techn.)
E jaw (tech.)
F mâchoire
S mandíbula, mordaza

Bahn (z. B. Folien-)
E sheet (e. g. of foil)
F bande (d'étoffe)
S rollo, tira (p. ej. de una lámina)

Bajonettverschluß
E bayonet connection
F fermeture à baïonnette
S conexión de bayoneta

Bakterien
E bacteria
F bactérie
S bacterias

Bakterienbelastungstest
E microbial challenge test
F test de stimulation microbien
S prueba de estimulación con bacterias

Bakterienendotoxin
E bacterial endotoxin
F endotoxine bactérienne
S endotoxina bacteriana

bakterizid
E bactericidal
F bactéricide
S bactericida

Bandbreite
E range
F échelle, intervalle, gamme, zone
S anchura de banda, gama, márgenes

Banden, interferierende
E interfering bands
F bandes d'interférence
S bandas de interferencia

Banderole
E band, banderole, tape
F banderole
S precinto

Bandförderer
E conveyor belt
F convoyeur
S transportador de cinta

Bandgeschwindigkeit
E belt speed
F vitesse du tapis
S velocidad de cinta

Bandwaage
E band balance, conveyor balance
F balance de convoyeur
S báscula de cinta

Bandzufuhr
E conveyor
F convoyeur
S suministro por cinta

Base
E base
F base
S base

organische Base
E organic base
F base organique
S base orgánica

Basis
E basis
F base
S base

basisch
E basic, alkaline
F basique, alcalin
S básico, alcalino

Basisformulierung
E basic formulation
F formulation de base
S formulación básica, formulación de base

Basislinie
E baseline
F ligne de base
S línea de base

Basisliniendrift
E baseline drift
F dérive de la ligne de base
S desviación de la línea de base

Basislinienrauschen
E baseline noise
F bruit de fond de la ligne de base
S ruido de fondo de la línea de base

English
German
French
Spanish

Basizität
E basicity
F basicité
S basicidad, alcalinidad

Bauart
E design
F design
S tipo de construcción

Baukastenprinzip
E modular design
F design modulaire
S principio de unidades de montaje

Baumdiagramm
E tree diagram
F diagramme arborescent
S diagrama en árbol

Baumwolle
E cotton
F coton
S algodón

Baureihe
E series
F série
S serie

Bausatz
E kit
F kit, prêt-à-monter
S kit

Baustein
E module
F module
S módulo, piedra de construcción

Beanspruchung
E stress, strain
F soumission à un effort
S carga, desgaste, tensión

statische Beanspruchung
E static stress
F stress statique
S tensión estática

Beanstandung
E complaint
F réclamation
S reclamación

Beanstandungsbericht
E complaint report
F compte-rendu de réclamation
S informe de reclamaciones

Bearbeitung
E processing
F fabrication, mise en forme, traitement
S elaboración, transformación

beauftragt sein mit
E be in charge of, to
F être chargé (d'une affaire)
S estar encargado de

bebrüten
E incubate, to
F incuber
S incubar

Bebrütungszeit
E incubation time
F temps d'incubation
S tiempo de incubación

Becherglas
E beaker
F bécher, gobelet
S probeta

Bedarf, bei
E as required
F sur besoin, sur demande
S en caso necesario

Bedarfsplanung
E requirements planning
F planification des besoins
S planificación de necesidades

Bedeutung
E significance
F signification
S importancia, significado

bedienerfreundlich
E user-friendly
F convivial pour l'utilisateur, adapté à l'utilisateur
S confortable para el usuario

bedienerloser Betrieb
E unmanned operation
F usine automatique
S funcionamiento automático

Bedienhilfen
E operative aids
F aides au fonctionnement
S ayudas de funcionamiento

Bedienpult
E operator console, panel
F pupitre de commande, tableau de commande
S pupitre de mando, tablero de control

Bedienterminal
E control panel
F terminal de contrôle
S terminal de control

Bedienungsanleitung
E operating instructions
F mode d'emploi, instructions opératoires
S instrucción de manejo, instrucción de servicio

Bedienungsbühne
E operating platform
F plate-forme de commande
S plataforma de control

Bedienungselement
E control knob
F bouton de contrôle
S elemento de manejo

Bedienungsfeld
E operating panel
F tableau d'utilisation
S panel de mandos

Bedienungsmodus
E operating mode
F mode d'utilisation
S modo de servicio

Bedienungspersonal
E operating personnel
F personnel de service
S personal de servicio

Bedienungssystem
E operating system
F système d'exploitation
S sistema de servicio

Bedingungen
E conditions
F conditions
S condiciones

bedrucken
E print, to
F imprimer
S imprimir, estampar

Beeinträchtigung
E impairment, damage
F préjudice, dommage
S merma, perjuicio

Beendigung
E completion
F achèvement
S conclusión, terminación

Befehlseingabe
E command, entry
F entrée d'une commande
S entrada de un comando

Befestigung
E fixing, attachment
F fixation
S fijación

befeuchten
E moisten, to; wet, to; humidify, to
F humidifier
S humectar, humedecer

Befeuchter
E humidifier
F humidificateur
S humificador de aire

Befeuchtung
E humidification
F humidification
S humectación, humidificación

Befugnis
E authority
F autorisation
S autorización, competencia

befugte Person
E authorised person
F personne autorisée
S persona autorizada

Befüllrohr
E charge tube
F conduite de charge, conduite d'alimentation
S conducto de carga, conducto de alimentación

Befüllrutsche
E charge chute
F toboggan de charge, toboggan d'alimentation, glissoir de charge
S tobogán de carga

Befüllstutzen
E charge port, nipple
F orifice de charge, orifice d'alimentation
S tubuladura de carga, tubuladura de alimentación

Befund
E diagnosis, report, finding
F diagnose
S diagnóstico

begasen
E purge, to
F purger
S gasear, purgar

Begasung
E fumigation, flushing, purging
F fumigation
S fumigación

Begasungsmittel
E fumigant
F fumigant
S fumigante

begehbar
E accessible, walk-in
F accessible
S practicable, viable

Begründung
E rationale, reasoning
F exposé des motifs, explication
S argumentación, razonamiento

Begutachter
E expert, assessor
F expert
S asesor, experto, perito

Begutachtung
E expert opinion
F opinion d'expert
S dictamen, peritaje

Behälter
E bin, container, vessel
F bac, container, cuve
S recipiente

fahrbarer Behälter
E mobile vessel
F cuve mobile, cuve sur roues
S recipiente portátil

Behälterbauer
E vessel manufacturer
F fabricant de cuves
S fabricante de recipientes

Behältnis
E container
F container, récipient
S recipiente

Endbehältnis
E final container
F container final
S recipiente final

beheizen
E heat, to
F chauffer
S caldear

Beheizung mit externer Dampfzufuhr
E external steam heating
F chauffage avec apport de vapeur externe
S calefacción con suministro de vapor externo

Behörde
E authorities
F autorité réglementaire
S autoridades, organismos oficiales

behördliche Genehmigung
E licence, approval, authorisation
F autorisation d'une autorité réglementaire
S autorización oficial

behördliche Überwachung
E monitoring by the authorities
F surveillance par les autorités
S control oficial

Beilage
E insert
F annexe
S anexo

beimpfen
E inoculate, to
F ensemencer, inoculer
S inocular, sembrar

Beimpfung
E inoculation
F inoculation
S inoculación, siembra

Beipackzettel
E package leaflet, package insert
F notice (d'un emballage)
S prospecto acompañante (del medicamento)

beizen
E marinate, to; pickle, to
F mariner
S adobar, cauterizar, desinfectar

Bekleidungsvorschrift
E gowning procedure
F règles vestimentaires, instructions vestimentaires
S prescripción de vestuario

beladen
E fill, to; charge, to
F charger, alimenter
S envasar, llenar

Beladung
E loading
F charge
S carga

Beladungshöhe (z. B. eines Autoklaven)
E loading height (e. g. of autoclave)
F hauteur de chargement (p. ex. d'un autoclave)
S altura de carga (p. ej. de autoclave)

Beladungsschema
E loading configuration
F schéma de chargement
S esquema de carga

Belag
E coating
F revêtement
S recubrimiento, revestimiento

Belastbarkeit
E load capacity
F capacité de chargement
S capacidad de carga

English German French Spanish

Belastung
E loading
F chargement, charge
S carga

dynamische Belastung
E dynamic load
F charge dynamique
S carga dinámica

mikrobielle Belastung
E microbial load, bioburden
F présence microbienne
S carga microbiana

statische Belastung
E static load
F charge statique
S carga estática

thermische Belastung
E thermal load
F charge thermique
S carga térmica

Belastungsgrenze
E loading limit
F limite de charge
S límite de carga

belastungsstabil
E load-resisting
F stable au chargement
S estable a la carga

Belastungstest
E challenge test
F test de stimulation
S prueba de carga

Beleuchtung
E lighting, illumination
F éclairage
S iluminación

Beleuchtung von hinten
E back illumination
F éclairage par l'arrière
S iluminación desde atrás

Beleuchtungskörper
E light, light fittings
F appareil d'éclairage
S aparato de iluminación

belüften
E vent, to; ventilate, to
F aérer, ventiler
S airear, ventilar

Belüftung
E ventilation
F ventilation
S aireación, ventilación

Belüftungsanlage
E ventilation system
F système de ventilation
S sistema de ventilación

Belüftungsfilter
E vent filter
F filtre de ventilation
S filtro de ventilación

Belüftungsloch
E vent
F orifice de ventilation, orifice de purge
S orificio de ventilación

Belüftungssystem
E ventilation system
F système de ventilation
S sistema de ventilación

Belüftungsventil
E ventilation valve
F valve de ventilation
S válvula de ventilación

Benannte Stelle
E Notified Body
F organisme cité
S departamento citado

benetzen
E wet, to; moisten, to
F humidifier, mouiller
S humedecer, mojar, rociar

Benetzungsmittel
E wetting agent
F mouillant
S humectante

Benutzer
E user
F utilisateur
S usuario

Beobachtung, besondere
E special observation
F observation particulière
S observación especial

Beobachtungsfenster
E observation window
F fenêtre d'observation
S ventana de observación

berechnen
E calculate, to
F calculer
S calcular

Berechnung
E calculation
F calcul
S cálculo

Bereich
E area, range
F intervalle, zone
S área, márgenes, zona

reiner Bereich
E clean area
F zone aseptique
S área limpia

zulässiger Bereich
E acceptable range
F intervalle autorisé
S zona permitida, márgenes permitidos

Bereich mit eingeschränktem Zugang
E limited access area
F zone d'accès limité
S zona de acceso limitado

Bereich mit kontrolliertem Klima
E climate-controlled area
F zone d'atmosphère contrôlée
S zona de atmósfera controlada

Bericht
E report
F rapport
S informe

berichten, jemandem
E report to someone, to
F rapporter à quelqu'un
S informar a alguien

Berichtigung
E correction
F correction
S corrección, enmienda, rectificación

Berieselungsanlage
E trickle installation, trickle plant
F système de ruissellement
S sistema de lavado

Berstdruck
E bursting pressure
F pression d'éclatement
S presión de rotura

Berstdruckfestigkeit
E bursting strength
F résistance à l'éclatement
S resistencia al estallido

bersten
E burst, to
F éclater
S estallar, reventar

Berstscheibe
E bursting disk, rupture disk
F disque de rupture
S disco de ruptura

Berufsausbildung
E vocational training
F formation professionnelle
S formación profesional

English German French Spanish

Berufsgenossenschaft
E trade association
F association professionelle
S asociación profesional

Beruhigungsmittel
E sedative
F sédatif, calmant
S sedante, tranquilizante

beschädigt
E defective, damaged
F défectueux, endommagé
S dañado, estropeado, perjudicado

Beschädigung
E damage
F dommage, dégâts
S daño, perjuicio

Beschaffenheit (einer Substanz)
E nature (of a substance)
F nature (d'une substance)
S naturaleza (de una sustancia)

äußere Beschaffenheit
E appearance
F aspect, apparence
S aspecto externo

Beschaffung
E procurement
F achats
S adquisición

beschichten
E coat, to; laminate, to
F enduire
S laminar, recubrir

Beschichtung
E coating
F couche, enduction
S recubrimiento

Beschickung
E load, feed
F charge
S alimentación, carga

Beschickungsmuster (für Autoklaven)
E load pattern (for autoclaves)
F schéma de charge (pour autoclave)
S esquema de carga (para autoclave)

Beschickungssilo
E feed silo
F trémie de charge
S depósito de carga

Beschickungstrichter
E feed hopper
F trémie de charge
S embudo de carga

beschleunigen
E accelerate, to
F accélérer
S acelerar

Beschleuniger
E accelerator
F accélérateur
S acelerador

beschränkter Zugang
E limited access
F accès limité
S acceso limitado

Beschreibung
E description
F description
S descripción

Beschriftung
E labelling, lettering
F étiquetage, marquage
S etiquetado, marcado, rotulado

Beseitigung
E disposal, removal
F élimination
S eliminación

Abfallbeseitigung
E waste disposal
F élimination de déchets
S eliminación de desechos

Beständigkeit
E durability, resistance
F stabilité à long terme, résistance
S estabilidad, inalterabilidad

Bestandteil
E component, constituent, ingredient
F composant, constituant, ingrédient
S componente, ingrediente

Bestandteile der Packung
E packaging components
F constituants d'un emballage
S componentes del envase

Bestellauftragsnummer
E purchase order number
F numéro de commande
S número del encargo de pedido

Bestellnummer
E order number
F numéro de commande
S número de pedido

Bestellung
E order
F commande
S pedido

bestimmen
E determine, to
F déterminer, évaluer
S averiguar, determinar

bestimmt (für)
E designated (for)
F désigné (pour)
S designado (para)

Bestimmung
E determination
F détermination, évaluation
S análisis, determinación

Bestimmungsgrenze
E limit of quantitation (LOQ)
F limite de quantitation
S límite de análisis,
límite de determinación

obere Bestimmungsgrenze
E upper limit of quantitation
F limite supérieure de quantitation
S límite superior de determinación

untere Bestimmungsgrenze
E lower limit of quantitation
F limite inférieure de quantitation
S límite inferior de determinación

bestrahlen mit
E irradiate, to (with)
F irradier avec
S irradiar con

Bestrahlung
E irradiation, radiation
F irradiation
S irradiación

Bestrahlungsdauer
E duration of exposure to radiation
F durée d'exposition à l'irradiation
S duración de la irradiación

Besuchergang
E visitor tour
F circuit de visite
S recorrido de visita

Betäubungsmittel
E narcotic substance
F substance narcotique
S sustancia narcótica

Betäubungsmittelgesetz
E narcotics regulation
F décret concernant les narcotiques
S decreto sobre narcóticos

Beteiligung
E participation, involvement
F participation
S participación

Betondecke
E concrete ceiling
F plafond en béton
S techo de hormigón

Betrieb setzen, in
E put into operation, to
F mettre en fonctionnement
S poner en funcionamiento

Betrieb, automatischer
E automatic operation, unmanned operation
F fonctionnement automatique
S funcionamiento automático

Betrieb, kontinuierlicher
E continuous operation
F opération continue
S funcionamiento continuo

betriebliche Anpassung
E operational adjustment, process adjustment
F ajustement de fonctionnement, ajustement d'un procédé
S ajuste del funcionamiento, ajuste de un proceso

betriebliches Vorschlagswesen
E employee suggestion scheme
F schéma interne de suggestions pour employés
S sistema empresarial de propuestas

Betriebsanleitung
E operating manual, operating instructions
F mode d'emploi, instructions de service
S instrucciones de funcionamiento

Betriebsbedingungen
E operating conditions
F conditions de service
S condiciones de funcionamiento

betriebsbereit
E ready for operation
F prêt au service, prêt à l'utilisation, prêt à l'emploi
S preparado para funcionar

Betriebsdampf
E plant steam
F vapeur d'une installation
S vapor de una planta

Betriebsdruck
E working pressure
F pression de travail
S presión de trabajo, presión empresarial

Betriebserweiterung
E plant expansion
F agrandissement d'une installation
S ampliación de la empresa

Betriebsfläche
E plant area
F surface d'une installation
S área de las instalaciones empresariales

Betriebsführung
E plant management
F management d'une installation
S gestión empresarial

Betriebsgeheimnis
E company secret
F secret d'entreprise
S secreto empresarial

Betriebsgrenze
E operating limit
F limite de service, limite d'utilisation
S límite de funcionamiento

Betriebshygiene
E plant hygiene, plant sanitation
F hygiène des installations
S higiene de la empresa

Betriebskosten
E operational costs
F coûts de fonctionnement
S costes de funcionamiento

Betriebsleiter
E Plant Manager
F directeur technique
S director técnico de la empresa

Betriebsmittel
E utilities
F moyens d'exploitation, moyens de production
S medios de explotación empresarial, medios de producción

Betriebsparameter
E operational parameter
F paramètre de service
S parámetro de servicio

Betriebsprüfung
E plant audit
F audit d'une installation
S auditoría de empresa

Betriebsspannung
E operating voltage
F voltage, tension de régime
S voltaje de funcionamiento

Betriebsstätte
E plant, factory, facility
F usine, installations, site de fabrication
S plantas empresariales

Betriebsstörung
E breakdown
F perturbation de fonctionnement
S interrupción del funcionamiento

Betriebsstundenzähler
E running time meter
F compteur d'heures de mise en service
S contador de horas de funcionamiento

Betriebszustand, im
E in process
F sous condition d'exploitation
S funcionando

Beugungsfestigkeit
E flexional strength
F résistance à la flexion
S resistencia a la flexión

Beutel
E bag
F poche, sac, sachet
S sobre

in Beutel verpacken
E package in bags, to
F empaqueter en sachets, emballer en sachets
S empaquetar en sobres

Beutel (als Darreichungsform)
E sachet
F sachet
S sobre

Beutel in Außenbeutel
E bag in bag
F sac à double paroi
S sobre de pared doble

bewegliche Teile
E movable parts
F pièces mobiles
S piezas móviles

Bewegungsfuge
E settlement joint
F joint de dilatation
S junta de dilatación

Beweis
E proof
F preuve
S prueba

bewerten
E evaluate, to; assess, to
F évaluer
S evaluar

Bewertung (von Daten)
E evaluation, assessment (of data)
F évaluation (de données)
S evaluación (de datos)

bezeichnen
E label, to; designate, to
F étiqueter
S denominar, marcar, rotular

English
German
French
Spanish

Bezeichnung
E designation
F désignation, appellation
S denominación, marcado, rotulación

Bezugsmuster
E reference sample
F échantillon de référence
S prueba de referencia

Bezugspunkt
E reference point
F point de référence
S punto de referencia

Biegebeanspruchung
E flexional strain
F sollicitation à la flexion
S tensión de flexión

Biegefestigkeit
E flexural strength
F résistance au pliage, résistance au fléchissement
S resistencia a la flexión

Biegespannung
E flexural stress
F tension de pliage, tension de fléchissement
S tensión de flexión

biegsam
E flexible, pliable
F flexible, pliable
S flexible, maleable, plegable

Biegung
E bend, flexure
F courbure, pliage
S flexión, curvatura

Bilanzierung
E reconciliation
F vérification, bilancer
S hacer balance

Bildschirm
E screen
F écran
S pantalla

billigen
E approve, to
F approuver
S aprobar

Billigung
E approval
F approbation
S aprobación

Bimetall
E bimetal
F bimétal
S bimetal

Bindekraft
E adhesive force
F force d'adhésion
S fuerza adhesiva

Bindemittel
E binding agent
F liant
S aglomerante, aglutinante

Bindemitteltyp
E binding agent type
F type de liant
S tipo de aglutinante

Bindung
E bond
F liaison
S enlace

ionische Bindung
E ion bonding
F liaison ionique
S enlace iónico

Bindungsvermögen
E binding capacity
F capacité de fixation
S capacidad de enlace, capacidad de fijación

Bioäquivalenz
E bioequivalence
F bioéquivalence
S bioequivalencia

biochemischer Sauerstoffbedarf (BSB)
E biochemical oxygen demand (bod) analysis
F analyse de la demande biologique d'oxygène (DBO)
S necesidades bioquímicas de oxígeno

Biofilter
E biological filter
F filtre biologique
S filtro biológico

Biogefahr
E biohazard
F danger biologique, risque biologique
S peligro biológico

biogen
E biogenic
F biogène
S biógeno

Biogenerator
E biogenerator
F biogénérateur
S biogenerador

Biogenese
E biogenesis
F biogenèse
S biogénesis

Bioindikator
E bioindicator
F indicateur biologique
S bioindicador

biokompatibel
E biocompatible
F biocompatible
S biocompatible

biologisch abbaubar
E biodegradable
F biodégradable
S degradable biológicamente

biologische Behandlung
E biological treatment
F traitement biologique
S tratamiento biológico

biologische Flüssigkeiten
E biological fluids
F liquides biologiques
S líquidos biológicos

biologische Prüfung
E biological testing
F examens biologiques
S prueba biológica

biologische Sicherheit
E biosafety
F bio-sécurité
S seguridad biológica

biologische Sicherheitsstufe
E biosafety level
F niveau de bio-sécurité
S grado de seguridad biológica

biologischer Abbau
E biodegradation
F biodégradation
S degradación biológica

Biolumineszenz
E bioluminescence
F bioluminescence
S bioluminiscencia

Biomasse
E biomass
F biomasse
S biomasa

Biosicherheitskabinett
E biohazard cabinet
F enceinte de risques biologiques
S gabinete de seguridad biológica

Biosicherheitslabor
E biohazard laboratory, biosafety laboratory
F laboratoire de risques biologiques
S laboratorio de seguridad biológica

English German French Spanish

Biosynthese
E biosynthesis
F biosynthèse
S biosíntesis

Biotechnologie
E biotechnology
F biotechnologie
S biotecnología

biotechnologisch hergestellt
E manufactured biotechnologically
F manufacturé par biotechnologie
S fabricado biotecnológicamente

Bioverfügbarkeit
E bioavailability
F biodisponibilité
S biodisponibilidad

bitter
E bitter
F amer
S amargo

Bitterstoff
E bitter component
F composant amer, substance amère
S sustancia amarga

Blase
E bubble, blister
F bulle
S ampolla, burbuja, vejiga

Blasendrucktest
E bubble point test
F essai de point de bulle
S prueba de presión de vejiga, cistometría

Blasverformung
E blow moulding
F moulage par procédé pressé-soufflé
S moldeo por inyección

Blattrührerapparatur
E paddle stirrer
F pale d'agitation
S pala de agitación

Blaubadtest
E blue dye bath test
F test au bain bleu
S prueba de baño con colorante azul

Blaugel
E blue silica gel
F gel bleu
S gel azul de sílice

Blech
E sheet, plate, tray
F tôle
S chapa, lámina, plancha

Blindprobe
E blank
F valeur témoin, valeur à blanc
S muestra en blanco, testigo

Blindwert
E blank value
F valeur témoin, valeur à blanc
S valor en blanco, valor testigo

Blinklicht
E flash light
F feux clignotant
S luz intermitente

Blister
E blister
F blister
S blíster

Blisterdichtigkeitstest
E blister tightness test
F test d'étanchéité du blister
S prueba de estanqueidad del blíster

Blisterverpackung
E blister pack
F conditionnement à bulles, conditionnement blister, plaquette thermoformée
S embalado en blísters

blockieren
E block, to; jam, to
F bloquer
S bloquear

Blockierung
E blockage
F blocage
S bloqueo

Blutbank
E blood bank
F banque du sang
S banco de sangre

Blüte
E blossom
F fleur
S flor

Blutegel
E leech
F sangsue
S sanguijuela

Blutkonserve
E stored blood
F sang conservé
S conserva de sangre

Blutkörperchen
E blood corpuscle
F globule sanguin
S eritrocito

Blutplasmaderivat
E blood plasma product, blood plasma derivative
F produit d'origine plasmatique
S producto de plasma sanguíneo

Blutprodukt
E blood product
F produit sanguin
S producto sanguíneo

Blutspendewesen
E blood donor service
F banque du sang
S servicio de donantes de sangre

Boden
E floor, soil
F sol, plancher
S suelo

Bodenabfluß
E floor drain
F égoût
S sumidero

Bodenbelag
E flooring, floor finishing
F revêtement de sol
S revestimiento del suelo

Bodenplatte
E bottom plate
F dalle (de sol)
S placa del suelo

Bodensatz
E sediment
F sédiment
S sedimento

Bodensieb
E bottom screen
F tamis bas, crible bas
S tamiz base

Bodenzahl
E plate number
F nombre de plateaux
S número de placa

Bohrung
E bore
F forage, percement
S perforación

Bolzen
E bolt
F boulon, cheville
S clavija, perno

Bördelkappe
E crimping cap
F bouchon, couvercle, calotte
S calota de rebordeo

Bördelmaschine
E capper, crimping machine
F boucheuse, capsuleuse
S máquina de rebordeo

Bördelrand
E bead
F bourrelet
S burlete rebordeado, canto rebordeado

Borosilikatglas
E borosilicate glass
F verre de borosilicate
S vidrio de silicato bórico

Böschungswinkel
E angle of slide
F angle de pente
S ángulo de la pendiente

Brandklasse
E inflammability class
F classe d'inflammables
S clase inflamable

Brandschutz (eines Gerätes)
E flame protector (of instrument)
F ignifugation, ignifugeage (d'un instrument)
S protección frente al fuego (de un aparato)

Brandschutzklappe
E fire protection door
F porte de protection anti-incendie
S puerta de protección contra incendios

Brausetablette
E effervescent tablet
F comprimé effervescent
S comprimido efervescente

Brechampulle
E one-point cut (OPC) ampoule
F ampoule autocassable
S ampolla de apertura manual

Brechpunkt (einer Ampulle)
E cutting point (of an ampoule)
F point de rupture (d'une ampoule)
S punto de ruptura (de una ampolla)

Brechungsdispersion
E refractive dispersion
F dispersion refractive
S dispersión refringente

Brechungsindex
E refractive index
F index de réfraction
S índice de refracción

Brechungsvermögen
E refringence
F réfringence
S refringencia

Brechungswinkel
E angle of refraction
F angle de réfraction
S ángulo de refracción

Brechungszahl
E refractive index
F index de réfraction
S índice de refracción

Breite
E width
F largeur
S anchura

brennbar
E combustible, flammable
F combustible
S combustible, inflamable

nicht brennbar
E non-flammable
F in-inflammable
S no combustible, no inflamable

Brennbarkeit
E flammability
F combustibilité
S combustibilidad, inflamabilidad

Bromierung
E bromination
F bromage
S bromado

Bruch
E debris
F débris
S despojos, restos

bruchfest
E unbreakable, shatter-proof
F incassable
S irrompible

Bruchfestigkeit
E breaking strength, breaking resistance
F résistance à la rupture
S resistencia a la rotura

brüchig
E brittle
F cassant, fragile
S quebradizo

Brüchigkeit
E brittleness
F fragilité
S fragilidad, friabilidad

Bruchkerbe
E break notch
F entaille de rupture
S muesca de ruptura

Bruchlinie
E rupture line, fracture line
F ligne de rupture, ligne de fracture
S línea de ruptura, línea de fractura

Bruchrille
E break notch, break score
F encoche de rupture, entaille de rupture
S ranura de ruptura, surco de ruptura

Bruchstelle
E break point, breaking point
F point de rupture
S lugar de ruptura

Bruchstück
E fragment, piece, fraction
F morceau, fragment
S fragmento

Bruchstückkontrolle
E fragment control
F contrôle des fragments
S control de fragmentos

Brutschrank
E incubator
F incubateur
S incubadora

Bruttomarge
E gross margin
F marge brute
S margen bruto

Buchse
E socket
F borne
S casquillo, hembrilla, manguito

Bügel
E handle, grip
F prise, poignée
S estribo, empuñadura, mango

Bulkmischung
E bulk mixture
F produits en vrac
S mezcla a granel

Bulkware
E bulk (material)
F marchandise en vrac
S mercancía a granel

Bündelmaschine
E bundling machine
F machine d'empaquetage
S máquina de embalaje

bündeln
E bundle, to
F lier ensemble
S enfardar

Bündelpacker
E bundling machine
F lieuse
S enfardador

bündig
E flush
F lié
S enrasado

English German French Spanish

Bunsenbrenner
E Bunsen burner
F bec de gaz, bec de Bunsen
S mechero Bunsen

Bürette
E burette
F burette
S bureta

Bürste
E brush
F brosse
S cepillo

Bürstenwalze
E revolving brush
F brosse de laminage
S cepillo rotativo, cilindro cepillador

cancerogen
E carcinogenic
F cancérogène
S cancerógeno

Carbonsäure
E carboxylic acid
F acide carboxylique
S ácido carbónico

CE-Zeichen
E CE symbol
F symbole CE
S símbolo CE

Charakterisierung (einer Verbindung)
E characterisation (of a compound)
F caractérisation (d'un composé organique)
S caracterización (de un compuesto)

Charge
E batch, lot
F lot
S lote

Teilcharge
E sub-batch, partial batch
F sous-lot, lot partiel
S lote parcial

Chargenbezeichnungsschlüssel
E batch number coding
F système de codage pour les numéros de lot
S código de designación de lotes

Chargencode
E batch code
F codage d'un lot
S código de un lote

Chargendokumentation, elektronische
E electronic batch recording
F documentation électronique
S documentación electrónica de lotes

Chargenfreigabe
E batch release
F libération d'un lot
S liberación de un lote

Chargengröße
E batch size
F taille d'un lot
S tamaño de un lote

Chargenkonsistenz
E batch consistency
F consistance d'un lot
S consistencia de un lote

Chargenkontrolle
E batch control
F contrôle des lots
S control de lotes

Chargennummer
E batch number
F numéro de lot
S número de lote

Chargenprotokoll
E batch record
F relevé d'un lot, enregistrement d'un lot, compte rendu d'un lot
S protocolo de lotes

Chargenrückverfolgbarkeit
E batch traceability
F traçabilité d'un lot
S seguimiento de un lote

chargenspezifisch
E batch-related
F spécifique au lot
S específico del lote

Chelatbildung
E chelate formation
F formation de chélate
S formación de quelatos

Chelatkomplex
E chelate, chelate complex
F chélate, complexe de chélation
S complejo de quelatos

Chelatverbindung
E chelated compound
F composé organique chélaté
S compuesto quelado

Chemie, analytische
E analytical chemistry
F chimie analytique
S química analítica

Chemiebetrieb
E chemical plant
F usine chimique
S planta química

Chemikalien
E chemicals
F produits chimiques
S productos químicos

Chemilumineszenz
E chemiluminescence
F chimiluminescence, chimioluminescence
S quimioluminiscencia

chemisch rein
E chemically pure
F chimiquement pur
S químicamente puro

chemische Agenzien
E chemical agents
F agents chimiques
S agentes químicos

chemische Modifikation
E chemical modification
F modification chimique
S modificación química

chemische Reinheit
E chemical purity
F pureté chimique
S pureza química

chemisches Mittel
E chemical agent
F agent chimique
S agente químico

chemisches Profil
E chemical profile
F profil chimique
S perfil químico

chirale Ligandenaustausch-chromatographie
E chiral ligand exchange chromatography
F chromatographie d'échange de ligands optiquement actifs
S cromatografía de intercambio de ligandos ópticamente activos

chirale Reinheit
E chiral purity
F pureté chirale
S pureza quiral

chiraler Arzneistoff
E chiral medicinal substance
F médicament optiquement actif
S sustancia medicamentosa ópticamente activa

Chiralität
E chirality
F chiralité
S quiralidad

Chlor
E chlorine
F chlor
S cloro

English
German
French
Spanish

chlorieren
E chlorinate, to
F chlorurer
S clorar

Chlorwasser
E chlorinated water
F eau chlorée
S agua clorada

Chromatogramm
E chromatogram
F chromatogramme
S cromatograma

Chromatographie
E chromatography
F chromatographie
S cromatografía

absteigende Chromatographie
E descending chromatography
F chromatographie descendante
S cromatografía descendente

aufsteigende Chromatographie
E ascending chromatography
F chromatographie ascendante
S cromatografía ascendente

Chromatographiekammer
E developing chamber (chromatography)
F chambre de développement (chromatographie)
S cámara cromatográfica

chromatographische Methode
E chromatographic assay
F méthode chromatographique
S método cromatográfico

Chromnickelstahl
E nichrome steel
F acier chromé et nickelé
S acero cromado y niquelado

Chromschwefelsäure
E chromosulphuric acid
F acide sulfurique chromique
S ácido sulfúrico crómico

Chromstahl
E chrome steel
F acier chromé
S acero cromado

Codelesegerät, elektronisches
E electronic code reader
F déchiffreur électronique de codage
S lector electrónico de códigos

Codelesung
E code reading
F lecture du codage
S lectura de códigos

Codestriche
E code bars
F code à barres
S barras de código

Codierung des Verfalldatums
E expiration coding
F codage de la date d'expiration
S codificación de la fecha de caducidad

computergesteuert
E computer-controlled
F contrôlé par ordinateur
S controlado por ordenador

computergestützt
E computerised, computer-assisted
F assisté par ordinateur
S asistido por ordenador

Computersicherheit
E computer security
F sécurité informatique
S seguridad informática

Computervalidierung
E computer validation
F validation d'ordinateur, validation informatique
S validación informática

coulometrische Analyse
E coulometric analysis
F analyse coulométrique
S análisis coulométrico

Creme
E cream
F crème
S crema

Dampf
E steam, vapour
F vapeur d'eau
S vapor

gereinigter Dampf
E purified steam
F vapeur purifiée
S vapor purificado

Dampfabscheider
E steam separator
F séparateur de vapeur
S separador de vapor

dampfbeheizt
E steam-heated
F chauffé à la vapeur
S calentado al vapor

Dampfdruck
E steam pressure, vapour pressure
F pression de vapeur
S presión de vapor

Dampferzeugung
E steam generation
F production de vapeur
S producción de vapor

Dampfleitung
E steam line
F conduite de vapeur
S conducción de vapor

Dampfleitungsverbindung
E steam connection
F connexion de conduite à vapeur
S conexión de conducción de vapor

Dampfphase
E vapour phase
F phase vapeur
S fase vapor

Dampfsterilisation
E steam sterilisation
F stérilisation à la vapeur
S esterilización al vapor

abschließende Dampfsterilisation
E terminal steam sterilisation
F stérilisation finale à la vapeur
S esterilización final al vapor

Dampfventil
E steam valve
F soupape de vapeur
S válvula de vapor

Dampfverbrauch
E steam consumption
F consommation de vapeur
S consumo de vapor

Dampfzufuhr, externe
E external steam
F vapeur externe
S suministro de vapor externo

Darmspülung
E enema
F lavement intestinal
S enema, lavativa

Darreichung (eines Medikaments)
E administration (of a drug)
F administration (d'un médicament)
S administración (de un medicamento)

Darreichungsform
E dosage form, administration form
F forme du dosage, voie d'administration
S forma de administración

Darstellung, grafische
E graph
F graphe
S representación gráfica

Daten
E data
F données
S datos

English German French Spanish

Daten erfassen
E record data, to; log data, to
F enregistrer des données
S registrar datos

Datenaufnahme
E data recording
F enregistrement de données
S registro de datos

Datenbankscreening
E database screening
F screening d'une banque de données
S búsqueda en banco de datos

Datenbanksicherheitskopie
E data base backup
F backup d'une base de données
S copia de seguridad de un banco de datos

Dateneingabe
E data entry
F saisie de données
S entrada de datos

Datensicherheit
E data security
F sécurité des données
S seguridad de datos

Datenspeicherung
E electronic data storage
F sauvegarde électronique de données
S almacenamiento de datos

Datentranskription
E data transcription
F transcription de données
S transcripción de datos

Datenüberprüfung
E collation of data
F collation de données
S comprobación de datos

Datenverarbeitung, elektronische
E electronic data processing
F système de traitement électronique de données
S proceso electrónico de datos

Dauer
E duration
F durée
S duración

Dauerbetrieb
E continuous operation
F fabrication en continu, opération continue
S funcionamiento continuo

Dauergebrauch
E sustained use
F utilisation permamente (d'un instrument)
S uso duradero

dauerhaft
E durable, stable
F durable, stable
S duradero

DC-Platte (Dünnschichtchromatographie)
E TLC plate (thin layer chromatography)
F plaque de CCM (chromatographie en couche mince)
S placa para cromatografía en capa fina (CCF)

Decke
E ceiling
F plafond
S techo

abgehängte Decke
E suspended ceiling
F faux plafond
S techo suspendido

eingezogene Decke
E false ceiling
F faux plafond
S techo falso

Deckel
E lid, cover
F couvercle
S tapa, tapadera

deckeln (Tabletten)
E cap, to (tablets)
F capsuler (comprimés)
S cubrir, recubrir (comprimidos)

Deckelverschließmaschine
E capping machine
F encapsuleur
S máquina para cerrar cápsulas

Deckenbeleuchtung
E ceiling lighting
F éclairage plafonnier
S alumbrado de techo

Deckfolie
E cover foil
F feuille de protection
S hoja de recubrimiento

Deckglas (Mikroskopie)
E cover glass, cover slip (microscopy)
F lame de protection, plaquette en verre (microscopie)
S cubreobjetos (microscopio)

Deckkraft
E covering power, hiding power
F propriété couvrante
S capacidad de cubrir

Decoct
E decoction
F décoction
S decocción

Dehnungsfuge
E expansion joint
F joint dilatable
S junta de dilatación

Dehnungskoeffizient
E coefficient of expansion
F coefficient d'expansion
S coeficiente de dilatación

Dehnungsmeßstreifen
E wire strain gauge
F jauge de contrainte
S extensímetro de resistencia

Dehydratisierung
E dehydration
F déhydratation
S deshidratación

dekantieren
E decant, to
F décanter, transvaser
S decantar

Dekontamination
E decontamination
F décontamination
S descontaminar

demineralisiertes Wasser
E demineralised water
F eau déminéralisée
S agua desmineralizada

Demontage
E disassembly, removal
F démontage
S desmontaje

denaturiert
E denatured
F dénaturé
S desnaturalizado

Denaturierung
E denaturing
F dénaturation
S desnaturalización

Denaturierungsmittel
E denaturing agent
F agent dénaturant
S agente desnaturalizante

dentale Anwendung
E dental use
F usage dental
S uso dental

Depotpräparat
E depot drug
F médicament retard
S preparado retard

Deprotonierung
E deprotonation
F déprotonation
S desprotonización

Derivat
E derivative
F dérivé
S derivado

Desinfektion
E disinfection
F désinfection
S desinfección

Desinfektionsmittel
E disinfectant
F désinfectant
S agente desinfectante

zugelassene Desinfektionsmittel
E approved disinfectants
F désinfectants autorisés
S desinfectantes autorizados

Desinfektionsverfahren
E disinfecting procedure
F procédé de désinfection
S procedimiento de desinfección

desinfizierbar
E disinfectable
F désinfectable
S desinfectable

desinfizieren
E disinfect, to
F désinfecter
S desinfectar

desinfizierende Wirksamkeit
E disinfecting effectiveness
F efficacité de la désinfection
S eficacia desinfectante

Destillat
E distillate
F distillat
S destilado

Destillationsbereich
E distillation range
F intervalle de distillation
S intervalo de destilación

Destillationsboden
E distillation bottom
F bas de la colonne de distillation
S fondo de destilación

Destillationsprozeß
E distillation process
F processus de distillation
S proceso de destilación

Destillationsrückstand
E distillation residue
F résidu de distillation
S residuo de destilación

Destille
E still
F appareil de distillation
S alambique

destillieren
E distil, to
F distiller
S destilar

destilliertes Wasser
E distilled water
F eau distillée
S agua destilada

detektierbar
E detectable
F détectable
S detectable

Detektionsbereich
E detection range
F zone de détection
S zona de detección

Detektionsempfindlichkeit
E detection sensitivity
F sensibilité de détection
S sensibilidad de detección

Detektionsgenauigkeit
E detection precision
F précision de détection
S exactitud de detección

Detektorauslaß
E detector outlet
F sortie de détecteur
S salida del detector

Detektoreinlaß
E detector inlet
F entrée de détecteur
S entrada al detector

Detektorzelle
E detector cell
F cellule de détection
S célula de detección

deutlich
E distinct, clear
F distinct, clair
S claro, distinto

Deutsches Gefahrstoffgesetz
E German Hazardous Substance Act
F législation allemande sur les substances dangereuses
S Ley Alemana de Sustancias Peligrosas

Diagnostica
E diagnostics
F diagnostiques
S agentes diagnósticos

Diagramm
E diagram
F diagramme
S diagrama

Diagrammschreiber
E chart recorder
F enregistreur graphique
S registrador gráfico

dicht
E leak-tight
F étanche
S hermético

dicht verschlossen
E tightly closed
F hermétiquement fermé
S herméticamente cerrado

Dichte
E density
F densité
S densidad

absolute Dichte
E absolute density
F densité absolue
S densidad absoluta

relative Dichte
E relative density
F densité relative
S densidad relativa

scheinbare Dichte
E apparent density
F densité apparente
S densidad aparente

Schüttdichte
E bulk density
F densité de package, densité de damage
S densidad de compresión

Stampfdichte
E tapped density, packed density
F densité de tassement
S densidad de apisonamiento

wahre Dichte
E true density
F densité réelle
S densidad real

dichte Verbindung
E leak-tight connection
F raccordement étanche
S conexión hermética

Dichtflüssigkeit
E sealing liquid
F liquide d'étanchéité
S líquido de cerrado hermético

Dichtigkeit
E tightness
F étanchéité
S estanqueidad, hermeticidad

Dichtigkeitsprüfung
E leak test
F essai d'étanchéité, essai de fuite, essai de perte
S prueba de estanqueidad

Dichtmanschette
E sealing collar
F manchette d'étanchéité
S manguito hermético

Dichtring
E sealing ring
F joint d'étanchéité
S anillo hermético, arandela hermética

Dichtung
E seal, gasket
F joint
S junta

aufblasbare Dichtung
E inflatable gasket
F joint gonflable
S junta hinchable

Türdichtung
E door seal
F joint de porte
S junta de una puerta

Dichtungsführung
E gasket channel
F cannelure pour joint
S guía para la junta

Dichtungsmittel
E sealant
F matériau d'étanchéité, matériau d'obturation
S material de cierre, material de sellado

Dichtungsring
E gasket ring
F joint torique en forme de rondelle
S arandela para junta hermética

Dichtungsscheibe
E washer, gasket
F joint (rondelle)
S disco para cierre hermético

dick
E thick
F épais
S compacto, espeso, grueso, macizo

Dicke
E thickness
F épaisseur
S espesor, grosor

Dickenmeßgerät
E thickness gauge
F jauge d'épaisseur, palmer
S calibre de grosores

Dickextrakt
E solid extract
F extrait solide
S extracto sólido

dickflüssig
E viscous
F visqueux
S viscoso

Differenzdruck
E pressure differential
F pression différentielle
S presión diferencial

Differenzdruckanzeiger
E pressure differential indicator
F indicateur de pression différentielle
S indicador de presión diferencial

Differenzdruckmesser
E differential manometer
F manomètre différentiel
S manómetro diferencial

Diffusion
E diffusion
F diffusion
S difusión

Diffusionsfluß
E diffusion flow
F débit de diffusion
S flujo de difusión

Diffusionsgeschwindigkeit
E diffusion speed
F vitesse de diffusion
S velocidad de difusión

digitale Ausgabe
E digital read out
F édition numérique
S edición digital

diploide Zellkultur
E diploid cell culture
F culture de cellules diploides
S cultivo de células diploides

Dipol-Dipol-Wechselwirkung
E dipole-dipole interaction
F interaction dipolaire
S interacción entre dipolos

Direktbeschickung (zur Keimzahlbestimmung)
E direct inoculation
F inoculation directe
S inoculación directa

Direktor
E director
F directeur
S director

Direkttablettierung
E direct tablet compression
F compression directe
S compresión directa

Diskrepanz
E discrepancy
F disparité, écart
S discrepancia

dispergieren
E disperse, to
F disperser
S dispersar

Dispersion
E dispersion
F dispersion
S dispersión

Dispersionsmittel
E dispersion agent
F agent de dispersion
S agente dispersor

Dissoziation
E dissociation
F dissociation
S disociación

Dokumentation
E documentation
F documentation
S documentación

dokumentieren
E document, to
F documenter
S documentar

doppelblind
E double-blind
F en double aveugle
S doble ciego

Doppelblindversuch
E double-blind study
F essai en double aveugle
S ensayo de doble ciego

Doppelmantel
E double jacket
F double manchon, double manteau
S cubierta doble

Doppelpeak
E double peak
F pic double
S pico doble

Doppelrundläuferpresse
E double rotary press
F presse rotative double
S prensa rotatoria doble

English German French Spanish

Doppelstrahl
E double beam
F double faisceau
S haz doble, rayo doble

Dose
E can, tin
F canne
S bote, caja, lata

Dosieraerosol
E metered dose inhaler
F inhalateur doseur
S aerosol dosificante

Dosiereinheit
E dosage unit
F unité de dosage
S unidad de dosificación

Dosiereinrichtung
E metering device, dosing device
F appareil doseur
S dispositivo dosificante

dosieren
E meter, to; dose, to
F doser
S dosificar, calibrar, medir

Dosiergenauigkeit
E metering accuracy
F exactitude de dosage
S exactitud de la dosificación

Dosierhilfe
E metering aid, dosing aid
F dispositif d'aide au dosage
S dispositivo para dosificar

Dosierkammer
E metering chamber, dosing chamber
F chambre de dosage
S cámara de dosificación

Dosierkolben
E dosing piston
F piston doseur
S matraz de dosificación

Dosierpumpe
E peristaltic pump
F pompe doseuse
S bomba de dosificación

Dosierrad
E dosing wheel
F roue de dosage
S rueda de dosificación

Dosierschleife
E dosing loop
F boucle de dosage
S bucle de dosificación

Dosierschnecke
E dosing screw, feed screw
F vis de dosage
S tornillo dosificante

Dosierstern
E dosing wheel
F roue de dosage
S rueda de dosificación

Dosierung
E dosage
F posologie
S dosificación, posología

Dosierungseinheit
E dosage unit
F dose unitaire
S unidad de dosificación

Dosierungsschema
E dosing pattern
F schéma de dosage
S muestra de dosificación

Dosierungssicherheit
E dosage security
F sécurité de dosage
S seguridad de dosificación

Dosis
E dose
F dose
S dosis

Einzeldosis
E single dose
F dose unique
S dosis única

niedrig dosiert
E low dosed
F à dose faible
S dosis reducida

niedrige Dosis
E low dosage
F dose faible
S dosis baja

tödliche Dosis
E fatal dose
F dose mortelle
S dosis mortal

Dosiskriterium
E dose criterion
F critère de dosage
S criterio de dosificación

Dragee
E sugar-coated tablet
F comprimé dragéifié, dragée
S gragea

dragieren (mit Zuckerüberzug)
E pan-coat, to
F dragéifier
S preparar grageas (con cubierta de azúcar), gragear

Dragierkessel
E coating pan
F dragéification (à la turbine)
S caldera para gragear

Draht
E wire
F fil métallique
S alambre

Drahtgewebe
E wire mesh
F toile métallique
S tela metálica

Drahtnetz
E mesh wire
F tamis métallique
S red de alambre

Drahtsieb
E wire sieve
F tamis en toile métallique
S tamiz de alambre

Drehachse
E axis of rotation
F axe de rotation
S eje de rotación

Drehdeckel (z. B. eines Autoklaven)
E swivel lid (e. g. of autoclave)
F couvercle pivotant (par ex. d'un autoclave)
S tapa de rosca (p. ej. de autoclave)

Drehkörbchen
E rotary basket
F corbeille rotative
S cesto rotatorio

Drehkörbchenmethode
E basket stirring method
F méthode d'agitation à corbeilles
S método de agitación con cesto rotatorio

Drehkraft
E torsion force
F force de torsion
S fuerza de rotación

Drehmoment
E torque
F couple
S momento de torsión, par, par motor

Drehrichtung
E direction of rotation
F direction de rotation
S sentido de la rotación

Drehschieber
E rotary valve
F valve rotatoire
S válvula rotativa

Drehschieberpumpe
E rotary valve pump
F pompe à valve rotatoire
S bomba de válvula rotativa

Drehstrom
E three-phase current
F courant triphasé
S corriente trifásica

Drehstrommotor
E three-phase current motor
F moteur électrique triphasé
S motor de corriente trifásica

Drehteller
E turntable
F plateau tournant
S plato giratorio

Drehung, optische
E optical rotation
F rotation optique
S rotación óptica

Drehzahl
E revolutions
F nombre de rotations
S número de revoluciones

Drehzahlmesser
E revolution counter, tachymeter
F compte-tours, tachymètre
S contador de revoluciones, taquímetro

Dreifachbindung
E trivalent bonding
F triple liaison
S enlace triple

Dreikantsockel
E triangular skirting
F bordure triangulaire
S zócalo triangular

Dreiwegehahn
E three-way stopcock
F robinet d'arrêt à trois voies
S grifo con tres vías

Dreiwegeventil
E three-way valve
F vanne trois voies
S válvula con tres vías

Drossel
E throttle
F régulateur
S estrangulador

Drosselrückschlagventil
E throttle check valve, throttle non-return valve
F soupape de retenue
S válvula estranguladora de retención, válvula activada por reflujo

Drosselventil
E butterfly valve
F vanne papillon
S válvula de mariposa

Druck
E pressure
F pression
S presión

osmotischer Druck
E osmotic pressure
F pression osmotique
S presión osmótica

Überdruck
E positive pressure
F surpression
S sobrepresión

Unterdruck
E negative pressure
F souspression
S presión baja

Druckabfall
E pressure drop
F chute de pression, dépressurisation
S descenso de presión

Druckablaß
E pressure release outlet
F sortie de régulation de pression
S salida de presión

Druckablesung
E pressure reading
F relevé de la pression
S lectura de la presión

Druckanstieg
E pressure increase
F augmentation de pression
S aumento de presión

Druckaufnehmer
E pressure transmitter
F transmetteur de pression
S transmisor de presión

Druckausgleich
E pressure equilibrium
F compensation de pression
S equilibrio de presión

Druckbehälter
E pressurised container
F récipient pressurisé,
récipient soumis à la pression
S recipiente presurizado

Druckbelastung
E pressure loading
F charge de pression
S carga de presión

Druckdifferenz
E pressure differential
F différence de pression
S diferencia de presión

Druckentlastungskanal
E pressure relief duct
F canalisation de décompression
S canal de descompresión

Druckentlastungsklappe
E pressure relief valve
F soupape de sûreté
(pour la pression)
S válvula de descompresión

Druckentlastungsöffnung
E pressure relief opening
F ouverture de décompression
S orificio de descompresión

Drucker
E printer
F imprimante
S impresora

Laserdrucker
E laser printer
F imprimante à laser
S impresora de láser

Tintenstrahldrucker
E ink jet printer
F imprimante à jet d'encre
S impresora de chorro de tinta

Druckerfarbe
E printer ink
F couleur d'imprimante
S impresora a color

Druckerkennung
E print recognition
F identification de l'impression
S identificación del impreso

druckfest
E pressure-resistant
F résistant à la pression
S resistente a la presión

Druckfestigkeit
E pressure resistance
F résistance à la pression
S resistencia a la presión

Druckfreigabe
E print release
F autorisation d'imprimer
S autorización para imprimir

Druckgasflasche
E gas cylinder
F bouteille de gaz
S botella de gas a presión

Druckgefäß
E pressure vessel
F récipient sous pression
S recipiente a presión

Druckhaltetest
E pressure test
F test de pression de retenue
S prueba de retención de la presión

Druckhöhe
E pressurisation level
F niveau de pressurisation
S altura de presión

Druckkolonne
E pressure column
F colonne sous pression
S columna a presión

Druckkolonnendestillationsanlage
E pressure column distillation plant
F appareil de distillation à colonnes multiples
S aparato de destilación a columna de presión

Druckkontrolle (bei Überdruck)
E pressure control (excess pressure)
F contrôle de la pression
S control de presión (en caso de sobrepresión)

Druckkontrolle (von Aufdruckdaten)
E print control (printed matter)
F contrôle de l'impression
S control de impresos

Druckluft
E compressed air
F air comprimé
S aire comprimido

Druckluftanlage
E compressed air plant
F installation servant à la production d'air comprimé
S instalación de aire comprimido

Druckluftzylinder
E compressed air cylinder
F cylindre de compression
S cilindro de aire comprimido

Druckmeßdose
E pressure-measuring point
F point de mesure de la pression
S punto de medida de presión

Druckmeßgerät
E manometer, pressure gauge
F manomètre
S manómetro

Druckreaktionskessel
E pressurised reaction vessel
F cuve à réaction sous pression
S caldera presurizada de reacción

Druckregler
E pressure regulator, reducing valve
F régulateur de pression
S regulador de presión

Druckrolle (an der Tablettenpresse)
E compression roll, compaction roll (tablet press)
F cylindre de compression
S cilindro compresor (en la prensa de comprimidos)

Druckschlauch
E pressure tubing
F tuyauterie apte à la pression
S tubo de presión

Druckschwankung
E pressure fluctuation
F fluctuation de pression
S fluctuación de presión

Druckstation
E compression station
F station de compression
S estación de compresión

Drucksystem
E pressurisation system
F système de pressurisation
S sistema de presurización

Druckwalze
E printing roller
F cylindre à imprimer
S rodillo de imprenta

Duft
E fragrance, odour
F odeur
S aroma, olor

Düngemittel
E fertiliser
F engrais
S abono, fertilizante

dünndarmlöslich
E entero-soluble
F entéro-soluble
S soluble en el intestino delgado

dünnflüssig
E non-viscous, thin, thin-bodied
F fluide, très fluide
S fluido, muy fluido

Dünnschichtchromatographie (DC)
E thin layer chromatography (TLC)
F chromatographie sur couche mince
S cromatografía en capa fina

Dünnschichtchromatographiekammer
E thin layer chromatography developing chamber
F chambre de développement pour chromatographie sur couche mince
S cámara de cromatografía en capa fina

Duplikat
E duplicate
F duplicata
S duplicado

Durchdringung
E penetration, permeation
F pénétration
S penetración

Durchdrückpackung
E blister pack
F plaquette (conditionnement)
S blíster

Durchfluß
E flow
F débit
S paso (de un líquido), flujo

Durchflußgeschwindigkeit
E flow rate
F débit
S velocidad de flujo

Durchflußmesser
E flowmeter
F débimètre
S fluxómetro

Durchflußregulierung
E flow regulation
F régulation du débit
S regulación del flujo

Durchflußzelle
E flow-through cell, flow cell
F cellule de mesure du débit
S célula de fluxometría

Durchflußzytometrie
E flow cytometry
F cytométrie à débit liquide
S citometría de flujo

durchführen
E carry out, to; execute, to
F réaliser, exécuter
S ejecutar, llevar a cabo, realizar

Durchführender
E operator
F exécutant, opérateur
S ejecutante, operador

Durchgang (beim Sieben)
E fines (sieve)
F passant (tamisage)
S tamizado, paso de tamiz

durchlässig
E permeable
F perméable
S permeable

Durchlässigkeit
E transmittance, permeability
F perméabilité
S permeabilidad

Durchlauf
E passage
F passage
S paso

Durchlaufzeit
E processing time
F temps de traitement
S tiempo de paso

Durchlichtkontrolleinrichtung
E see-through scanner
F analyseur à balayage
S dispositivo de control por transiluminación

Durchmesser
E diameter
F diamètre
S diámetro

lichter Durchmesser
E internal diameter
F diamètre interne
S diámetro interno

Durchreiche
E hatch
F porte coupée
S postigo

Durchsatz
E throughput
F capacité, débit, rendement
S rendimiento

Durchschlupf
E slippage
F décalage
S postigo, puerta falsa

Durchschnitt
E average, mean
F moyenne
S media, promedio

durchsichtig
E transparent
F transparent
S transparente

Durchsichtigkeit
E transparency
F transparence
S transparencia

Durchsichtkontrolle
E visual inspection
F inspection visuelle
S inspección visual

durchstechen
E pierce, to
F transpercer
S perforar

Durchstechflasche
E perforable bottle
F bouteille perforable
S botella perforable

durchströmen (mit)
E flush, to (with); purge, to (with)
F rincer (avec), purger
S inundar (con), purgar (con)

Düse
E nozzle
F buse, gicleur, tuyère
S aplicador, inyector, tobera

Düseneinsatz
E nozzle insert
F garniture d'un gicleur
S inserción de la tobera

Düsennadel
E filling nozzle
F aiguille d'injection, injecteur à aiguille
S aguja de inyección

eben
E plane, level
F plat
S liso, llano, plano

ebene Fläche
E flat surface
F surface plane
S superficie plana

Ebene, schiefe
E inclined plane
F plan incliné
S plano inclinado

Ecke
E corner
F coin
S esquina

Edelgas
E inert gas, rare gas
F gaz inerte, gaz rare
S gas noble

Edelmetall
E precious metal
F métal précieux
S metal noble

Edelstahl
E stainless steel
F acier inoxydable, inox
S acero inoxidable

Edelstahlfaß
E stainless steel drum
F tonneau en acier inoxydable
S tonel de acero inoxidable

Edelstahlrohrleitung
E stainless steel piping
F tuyauterie en inox
S tubería de acero inoxidable

EDV (Elektronische Datenverarbeitung)
E EDP (Electronic Data Processing)
F traitement électronique des données, informatique
S proceso electrónico de datos

Effizienz
E efficiency
F efficacité
S eficiencia

EG-GMP-Leitfaden
E EC-GMP Guideline
F directives GMP de la CE
S Líneas directrices de la EC sobre GMP

eichen
E calibrate, to
F calibrer
S calibrar

Eichschein
E calibration certificate
F certificat de calibration
S certificado de calibración

Eichung
E calibration
F calibration
S calibración

Eigenschaft
E property, characteristic
F propriété, caractéristique
S propiedad, característica

Eigentum, intellektuelles
E intellectual property
F propriété intellectuelle
S propiedad intelectual

Eignung
E suitability
F qualification
S aptitud, calificación, idoneidad

Eignungsprüfung
E suitability test
F test de qualification
S prueba de aptitud

einätzen
E etch, to
F corroder, décaper
S grabar (al aguafuerte)

Einbau
E installation, mounting
F installation, montage
S instalación, montaje

einbauen
E fit, to; install, to
F installer
S instalar, montar

English
German
French
Spanish

einbetten
E embed, to
F inclure
S incluir

eindampfen
E evaporate, to
F évaporer
S evaporar

eindeutig
E clear, unambiguous, unequivocal
F clair, précis, non équivoque
S claro, unívoco, inequívoco

eindeutige Codenummer
E unequivocal code number
F code numérique non équivoque
S número codificador inequívoco

eindicken
E concentrate, to; thicken, to
F épaissir
S concentrar, condensar, espesar

eindringen
E penetrate, to
F pénétrer
S penetrar

Eindringtiefe
E penetration depth
F profondeur de pénétration
S profundidad de penetración

einengen (Konzentration)
E concentrate, to
F concentrer
S concentrar, espesar

Einfallswinkel
E angle of incidence
F angle d'incidence
S ángulo de incidencia

einfetten
E grease, to
F graisser
S engrasar

Einfluß
E inlet
F orifice d'entrée de liquide
S orificio de entrada de líquido

Einfuhrerlaubnis
E import licence
F license d'importation
S licencia de importación

Einführung auf den Markt
E launch
F lancement d'un produit
S introducción en el mercado

einfüllen
E fill, to; charge, to
F charger, alimenter
S envasar, llenar

Einfüllklappe
E filling valve, charging valve
F vanne d'alimentation
S válvula de relleno

Einfüllöffnung
E filling port
F ouverture de chargement
S abertura de relleno

Einfüllrohr
E filling tube, charging tube
F conduite d'alimentation
S tubo de relleno

Einfülltrichter
E filling funnel, charging funnel
F trémie de charge
S embudo de relleno

Einfüllvorrichtung
E filling device, charging device
F dispositif d'alimentation,
appareillage d'alimentation
S dispositivo de relleno

Eingangsfilter
E inlet filter
F filtre d'entrée, filtre d'admission
S filtro de entrada

Eingangsprüfung
E examination on receipt
F examen d'entrée
S examen inicial

Eingangstemperatur
E inlet temperature
F température d'entrée, température d'admission
S temperatura de entrada

eingebaut
E fitted
F encastré
S incorporado, instalado, montado

eingeschlossen von
E encased
F enchâssé
S rodeado de

eingeschränkter Zugang
E limited access, restricted access
F accès limité, accès restrictif
S acceso limitado

eingravieren
E engrave, to
F graver
S grabar

Eingriff
E intervention
F intervention
S intervención

Einhaltung
E compliance
F conformité
S cumplimiento, observancia

Einheit
E unit
F unité
S unidad

einheitlich
E uniform
F uniforme
S homogéneo, uniforme

einheitliche Voraussetzungen
E uniform preconditions
F conditions préalables uniformes
S presupuestos uniformes

Einheitlichkeit
E uniformity
F uniformité
S homogeneidad, uniformidad

Einheitlichkeit der Dosierung
E dose uniformity
F uniformité d'une dose
S uniformidad de la dosificación

Einheitlichkeit des Gehaltes
E content uniformity (CU)
F uniformité du contenu
S uniformidad del contenido

Einkomponenten-Reagenz
E single-component reagent
F réactif à composant unique
S reactivo de componente único

einlagern
E store, to
F stocker
S almacenar

Einlaßfilter
E inlet filter
F filtre d'entrée, filtre d'admission
S filtro de entrada

Einlaßtemperatur
E inlet temperature
F température d'entrée, température d'admission
S temperatura de entrada

Einlaßventil
E inlet valve
F vanne d'entrée
S válvula de entrada

Einmalabdeckung
E disposable cover
F couvercle à usage unique, capuchon à usage unique
S cubierta de uso único

English German French Spanish

Einmalanzug
E disposable jump-suit
F combinaison à usage unique
S ropa de uso único

Einmalhandschuhe
E disposable gloves
F gants à usage unique
S guantes de uso único

Einmalhandtücher
E disposable towels
F serviette à usage unique
S toallas de uso único

Einmalspritze
E disposable syringe
F seringue à usage unique
S jeringa de uso único

Einnehmen, zum
E for oral use
F pour administration orale
S para uso oral

einpacken
E pack, to; package, to
F emballer
S embalar, empaquetar, envasar

einprägen
E emboss, to; imprint, to
F empreindre, imprimer
S estampar, imprimir

Einreibemittel
E embrocation, liniment
F beaume, onguent, liniment
S bálsamo, linimento

Einreibung
E embrocation
F embrocation
S fricción, frotamiento

einreichen (Zulassungsantrag)
E submit, to (application for marketing approval)
F soumettre (une demande d'autorisation de mise sur le marché)
S presentar (una solicitud de autorización)

Einreichung (eines Zulassungsantrags)
E submission (of an application for marketing approval)
F déposition (d'une demande d'autorisation de mise sur le marché)
S presentación (de una solicitud de autorización)

einrichten
E set up, to
F mettre en place
S instalar

Einrichtung (in Gebäuden)
E facility, plant
F installation industrielle
S instalación (en edificios)

Einrichtung für einen bestimmten Zweck
E dedicated plant
F installation industrielle dédiée
S instalación para un fin determinado

einschalten
E switch on, to
F allumer
S conectar, encender

Einschichtverfahren
E single coating process
F procédé monocouche
S procedimiento de cubierta simple

Einschluß
E inclusion
F inclusion
S inclusión

Einschlußkristallisation
E inclusion crystallisation
F cristallisation occlusive
S cristalización de inclusión

einschmelzen
E melt, to; fuse, to
F fondre, faire fondre
S fundir

Einschränkung
E limitation
F limitation
S limitación, restricción

einsiegeln (Tabletten)
E seal, to (tablets)
F sceller, clore (comprimés)
S estampar (comprimidos)

Einspritzblock
E injection block
F bloc d'injection
S bloque de inyección

Einspritzdüse
E injection port
F buse d'injection
S inyector

Einspritzung
E injection
F injection
S inyección

Einspritzventil
E injection valve
F vanne d'injection
S válvula de inyección

Einspritzvolumen
E injection volume
F volume d'injection
S volumen de inyección

einstanzen
E punch, to; emboss, to
F estamper
S estampar, troquelar

Einstecklasche
E tab, tongue
F languette, attache, patte
S cubrejunta de pestaña

einstellbar
E adjustable
F ajustable
S ajustable, regulable

einstellen
E adjust, to
F ajuster, régler
S ajustar, regular

Einstellknopf
E adjusting knob
F bouton d'ajustement
S botón de ajuste

Einstellung
E adjustment, setting
F ajustement, réglage
S ajuste, regulación

Einstellungsuntersuchung
E medical examination on starting a new job
F examen médical suite à une embauche
S exploración médica al ser empleado

einstreichen (mit einer Bürste)
E brush coat, to
F enduire à la brosse
S untar con cepillo

einstufen
E grade, to
F classifier
S clasificar

Einstufung
E grade
F classification
S clasificación

eintauchen
E immerse, to; dip, to
F immerger
S sumergir

Eintauchrohr
E dip tube
F tube plongeur
S tubo de inmersión

Eintauchtiefe
E immersion depth
F profondeur d'immersion
S profundidad de inmersión

Eintauchzeit
E immersion period
F période d'immersion
S tiempo de inmersión

eintragen
E enter, to
F inscrire, enregistrer
S inscribir, registrar

Eintragsvorrichtung
E feed system
F système d'alimentation
S sistema de alimentación

eintrichtern
E funnel, to
F remplir à l'aide d'un entonnoir
S llenar con embudo

Eintrittsstutzen
E access port
F tubulure d'accès
S tubuladura de acceso

eintrocknen
E dry, to
F sécher, dessiquer
S desecar, secar

Einwaage
E initial weight
F poids initial
S peso inicial

zentrale Einwaage
E central weighing area
F aire centrale de pesage
S área central de pesado

einwandfrei
E faultless
F irréprochable
S intacto

Einweg-
E disposable
F jetable, à usage unique
S de uso único

Einwegverpackung
E disposable packaging
F conditionnement à usage unique
S embalaje de uso único

einwertig
E monovalent
F monovalent
S monovalente

einwiegen
E weigh in, to
F peser
S pesar

Einwirkung
E effect
F effet
S efecto

Einzeldosis
E single dose
F dose unique
S dosis única

Einzeldosisbehältnis
E single dose container
F récipient monodose
S recipiente de dosis única

Einzelgewicht
E individual weight
F poids individuel
S peso individual

Einzelmerkmal
E individual characteristic
F caractéristique individuelle
S característica individual

Einzelteile
E components
F composants
S componentes

Eispunkt
E freezing point
F point de congélation
S punto de congelación

Eiswasser
E ice water
F eau glacée
S agua helada

elastisch
E elastic
F élastique
S elástico

Elastizität
E elasticity
F élasticité
S elasticidad

elektrische Ladung
E electrical charge
F charge électrique
S carga eléctrica

elektrische Leitfähigkeit
E conductivity
F conductivité électrique
S conductividad eléctrica

elektrische Stromquelle
E electrical power source
F source d'un courant électrique
S fuente de corriente eléctrica

elektrische Zuleitungen
E electrical cables
F câbles électriques
S cables de conducción eléctrica

Elektro-, Meß- und Regeltechnik (EMR)
E measuring and control technology
F électrotechnique et techniques de mesure et de réglage
S electrotécnica y técnicas de medida y regulación

Elektrode
E electrode
F électrode
S electrodo

Elektrolyse
E electrolysis
F électrolyse
S electrólisis

Elektrolyt
E electrolyte
F électrolyte
S electrólito

elektromagnetische Interferenz
E electromagnetic interference
F interférence électromagnétique
S interferencia electromagnética

elektromagnetisches Ventil
E solenoid valve
F vanne solénoïde
S válvula electromagnética

Elektroneneinfangdetektor
E electron capture detector (ECD)
F détecteur à capture électronique
S detector de captura electrónica

Elektronenstrahlbeschleuniger
E electron beam accelerator
F accélérateur de faisceau d'électrons
S acelerador de haz de electrones

elektronische Chargendokumentation
E electronic batch recording system
F système de documentation électronique de lots
S documentación electrónica de lotes

elektronische Datenverarbeitung
E electronic data processing
F traitement électronique des données
S proceso electrónico de datos

elektronische Identifikation (EID)
E electronic identification (EID)
F identification électronique
S identificación electrónica

elektronische Unterschrift
E electronic signature
F signature électronique
S firma electrónica

English
German
French
Spanish

elektro-pneumatischer Betrieb
E electro-pneumatic operation
F opération électro-pneumatique
S funcionamiento electroneumático

elektropoliert
E electro-polished
F électro-poli
S pulido eléctricamente

elektrostatische Aufladung
E electrostatic charge
F charge électrostatique
S carga electrostática

Elementaranalyse
E elementary analysis
F analyse élémentaire
S análisis elemental

eloxiert
E anodised
F oxydé (électrolytiquement)
S oxidado electrolíticamente

Eluat
E eluate
F éluat
S levigado, eluado

Elutionsmittel
E eluant
F éluant
S agente levigante

Email
E enamel
F émail
S esmalte

emailliert
E enamelled
F émaillé
S esmaltado

Emission
E emission
F émission
S emisión

Empfangsbestätigung
E receipt
F reçu, quittance
S acuse de recibo

Empfehlung
E recommendation
F notes explicatives
S recomendación

empfindlich
E sensitive
F sensible
S sensible

Empfindlichkeit
E sensitivity
F sensibilité
S sensibilidad

empirisch
E empirical
F empirique
S empírico

empirische Formel
E empirical formula
F formule empirique
S fórmula empírica

Emulgator
E emulsifier, emulsifying agent
F émulsifiant
S emulsivo

emulgieren
E emulsify, to
F émulsionner
S emulsionar

Emulgiergerät
E emulsifier
F émulseur
S emulsor

Emulsion
E emulsion
F émulsion
S emulsión

Öl-in-Wasser Emulsion
E oil/water emulsion
F émulsion d'huile dans l'eau
S emulsión de aceite en agua

Wasser-in-Öl Emulsion
E water/oil emulsion
F émulsion d'eau dans l'huile
S emulsión de agua en aceite

Enantiomere
E enantiomer
F énantiomère
S enantiómero

enantiomere Reinheit
E enantiomeric purity
F pureté énantiomère
S pureza enantiómera

Endausbeute
E final yield
F rendement final
S rendimiento final

Endbehältnis
E final container
F conditionnement final, conteneur final, récipient final
S recipiente final

Enden, tote
E dead spots
F extrémités
S extremos de desecho

Endlosbahn
E continuous band
F bande continue
S cinta sin fin

endothermische Abspaltung
E endothermic split-off
F scission endothermique
S escisión endotérmica

endothermische Reaktion
E endothermic reaction
F réaction endothermique
S reacción endotérmica

Endotoxin
E endotoxin
F endotoxine
S endotoxina

endozervikale Anwendung
E endocervical use
F usage endo-cervical
S uso endocervical

Endsterilisation
E final sterilisation
F stérilisation finale
S esterilización final

Energieverbrauch
E energy consumption
F consommation d'énergie
S consumo energético

entfernbar
E detachable, removable
F amovible, démontable, détachable
S desmontable

Entfernung
E removal
F élimination
S eliminación

entfetten
E degrease, to
F dégraisser
S desengrasar

entflammbar
E flammable
F inflammable
S inflamable

leicht entflammbar
E highly flammable
F facilement inflammable
S fácilmente inflamable

entgasen
E degas, to; deaerate, to
F dégazer, désaérer
S desgasificar

Entgasung (von Flüssigkeiten)
E degassing, deaeration (of liquids)
F dégazage
S desgasificación (de líquidos)

entgraten
E deburr, to
F ébarber
S desbarbar

Entgrater
E deburrer
F ébarbeur
S desbarbador, desbastador

Entgratung
E deburring
F ébarbage
S desbarbado

enthärten (Wasser)
E soften, to (water)
F adoucir (eau)
S ablandar (agua)

Enthemmer (zur Inaktivierung von Desinfektionsmitteln)
E neutralising substance, inactivating substance (for disinfectant)
F substance neutralisante
S sustancia neutralizante (para inactivar desinfectantes)

entionisiertes Wasser
E deionised water
F eau déionisée
S agua desionizada

entkalken
E decalcify, to
F détartrer
S descalcificar

Entkalker
E decalcifier
F détartrant
S agente descalcificante

entkeimen
E disinfect, to
F désinfecter
S desinfectar

entladen
E discharge, to
F décharger
S descargar

entlassen
E make redundant, to
F renvoyer, licencier, congédier
S despedir

Entlassung
E redundancy
F licenciement
S despido

Entlastung
E relief
F soulagement, décharge
S alivio, descarga

entleeren
E empty, to; evacuate, to
F vider, évacuer
S vaciar

Entleerventil
E emptying valve
F valve de vidange
S válvula de vaciamiento

entlüften
E deaerate, to; ventilate, to; vent, to
F désaérer, ventiler
S airear, ventilar

Entlüftungsklappe
E vent flap
F clapet de ventilation, volet de ventilation
S válvula de ventilación

Entlüftungsleitung
E venting line
F canalisation de ventilation, canalisation d'aération
S conducción de ventilación

entmineralisieren
E deionise, to
F déminéraliser
S desmineralizar

Entmischung
E demixing, separation
F démixtion
S separación

Entnahme
E withdrawal
F retrait
S extracción, toma

Entnahmesicherung
E tamper-proof seal
F sécurité de prélèvement
S precintado de un frasco

Entnahmesonde
E removal probe, sampling probe
F sonde d'échantillonnage
S sonda de toma (de muestras)

Entnahmestelle
E point of withdrawal
F point de retrait
S lugar de extracción

entpyrogenisieren
E depyrogenate, to
F dépyrogéner
S despirogenar, eliminar pirógenos

Entpyrogenisierung
E depyrogenation
F dépyrogénation
S despirogenación,
eliminación de pirógenos

entriegeln
E unlock, to
F déverrouiller
S desbloquear

entsalzen
E desalt, to
F dessaler
S desalinizar

entsäuern
E deacidify, to
F alcaliniser
S alcalinizar, desacidificar

Entschäumer
E anti-foaming agent, defoamer
F antimousse
S agente antiespumante

Entschlüssler
E decoder
F décodeur
S descodificador

Entsorgung
E disposal
F élimination, rejet
S desecho, eliminación

Entsorgungsanschluß
E waste output
F conduite destinée aux déchets
S empalme de eliminación

Entsorgungssystem
E disposal system
F système d'élimination
S sistema de eliminación

Entsorgungsvorschriften
E disposal regulations
F régulations concernant les rejets
S prescripciones de eliminación

entsprechen
E correspond, to
F correspondre (à)
S corresponder

nicht entsprechen
E not corresponding to
F différent de
S no corresponder

entspricht Arzneibuchqualität
E pharmaceutical grade
F qualité pharmaceutique
S calidad farmacéutica

Entstauber
E deduster
F dépoussiéreur
S desempolvante

English
German
French
Spanish

Entstaubung
E dedusting
F action de dépoussiérer, dépoussiérage
S desempolvamiento

Entwicklung
E development
F développement
S desarrollo, evolución

Entwicklung eines neuen Produktes
E new product development
F développement d'un nouveau produit
S desarrollo de un producto nuevo

Entwicklungsanalytik
E analytical development
F développement analytique
S analítica de desarrollo

Entwicklungsbericht
E development report
F rapport de développement
S informe de desarrollo

Entwicklungsstatus
E development status
F état de développement
S status de desarrollo

Entwicklungsstufe
E development stage
F phase de développement
S etapa de desarrollo, nivel de desarrollo

Entwicklungsweg
E development route
F route de développement
S vía de desarrollo, vía evolutiva

Entwurf
E draft
F ébauche
S bosquejo, diseño, esbozo, proyecto

entzündbar
E inflammable, ignitable
F inflammable
S inflamable

Entzündungsreaktion
E inflammatory reaction
F réaction inflammatoire
S reacción inflamatoria

Enzym
E enzyme
F enzyme
S enzima

DNA-modifizierendes Enzym
E DNA-modifying enzyme
F enzyme de modification de l'ADN
S enzima modificador del ADN

epidurale Anwendung
E epidural use
F usage épidural
S uso epidural

Epimerisierung
E eperimisation
F épimérisation
S epimerización

Epoxidharz
E epoxy resin
F résine époxy
S epoxirresina

Eppendorf-Reaktionsgefäß
E Eppendorf reaction vessel
F fiole Eppendorf
S tubo de ensayo Eppendorf

erden
E ground, to; earth, to
F mettre à la terre
S conectar a tierra

Erdung
E ground, grounding, earth, earthing
F mise à la terre, mise la terre, prise de terre
S derivación, toma de tierra

erfordern
E require, to
F exiger, nécessiter
S exigir, necesitar, requerir

Erfordernis
E requirement
F exigence
S exigencia, necesidad, requerimiento

Erfüllung
E fulfilment, realisation
F réalisation
S cumplimiento, realización

Ergänzung
E supplementation
F complément, supplément
S complemento, suplemento

Ergebnis
E result
F résultats
S resultado

erwartete Ergebnisse
E expected results
F résultats escomptés
S resultados esperados

Erhaltungsdosis
E maintenance dosage
F dose de maintien
S dosis de mantenimiento

Erholungsfähigkeit
E recovery capability
F capacité de récupération
S capacidad de recuperación

Erholzeit (im Reinraum)
E recovery time (in clean room)
F temps de récupération
S tiempo de recuperación (en área estéril)

Erlenmeyerkolben
E Erlenmeyer flask
F Erlenmeyer, flacon à fond plat
S matraz de Erlenmeyer

ermitteln
E determine, to
F déterminer, évaluer
S averiguar, determinar

ernten
E harvest, to
F récolter
S cosechar

Erreger (Mikroorganismus)
E pathogen
F pathogène
S agente patógeno (microorganismo)

Ersatzteil
E spare part
F pièce de rechange
S pieza de recambio

Ersatzteilliste
E spare parts list
F liste de pièces de rechange
S lista de piezas de recambio

Erschütterung
E vibration
F vibration
S vibración, trepidación

erschütterungsbeständig
E shock-resistant
F résistant aux chocs
S resistente a la agitación

erschütterungsfrei
E vibration-free
F exempt de vibration
S sin vibración

ersetzen
E replace, to
F remplacer
S reemplazar, sustituir

erstarren
E solidify, to
F solidifier
S solidificar

Erstarrungspunkt
E solidification point
F point de solidification
S punto de solidificación

Erstarrungstemperatur
E solidification temperature
F température de solidification
S temperatura de solidificación

Erstarrungszeit
E solidification time, setting time
F temps de solidification
S tiempo de solidificación

Erstattung
E reimbursement
F remboursement
S devolución, restitución

Erstausführung
E prototype
F prototype
S prototipo

Erste Hilfe
E first aid
F secours d'urgence, premiers secours
S primeros auxilios

erstellen
E compile, to
F compiler, produire
S elaborar, producir, redactar

Erstellung (von Dokumenten)
E compilation (of documents)
F compilation (de documents)
S redacción (de documentos)

Erstzulassender (EU) Mitgliedsstaat
E Reference Member State (EU) (RMS)
F pays rapporteur (UE)
S País Miembro (UE) de Referencia (para registro de medicamentos)

Ertrag
E yield
F rendement
S rendimiento

Erwärmung
E heating
F réchauffement
S calentamiento

erweichen
E soften, to
F ramollir
S reblandecer

Erweichungspunkt
E softening point
F point de ramollissement
S punto de reblandecimiento

Erzeugung
E generation (of)
F engendrement, production
S generación, producción

Esterzahl
E ester number
F nombre d'ester
S número de éster

Ethikkomission
E ethics committee
F commission d'éthique
S comisión ética

ethisch
E ethical
F éthique
S ético

ethische Produkte
E ethical products
F produits éthiques
S productos éticos

Etikett
E label
F étiquette
S etiqueta

Etiketten auf Rollen
E roll-fed labels
F étiquettes en rouleaux
S etiquetas en rollo

lose Etiketten
E loose labels, cut labels
F étiquettes prédécoupées
S etiquetas sueltas

selbstklebende Etiketten, Haftetiketten
E self-adhesive labels
F étiquettes autoadhésives
S etiquetas autoadhesivas

Etikettenbilanzierung
E label reconciliation
F bilan d'étiquettes
S balance de etiquetas

Etikettenzähler
E label counter
F compteur d'étiquettes
S contador de etiquetas

Etikettenzählung
E label count
F comptage d'étiquettes
S recuento de etiquetas

Etikettierung
E labelling
F étiquetage
S etiquetado

Etikettierungsregeln
E labelling rules
F règles d'étiquetage
S reglas de etiquetado

Europäisches Arzneibuch (PhEur)
E European Pharmacopoeia (PhEur)
F pharmacopée européenne (PhEur)
S Farmacopea Europea

Eutektikum
E eutectic point
F point d'eutexie
S punto eutéctico

eutektisch
E eutectic
F eutectique
S eutéctico

Ex-geschützt
E explosion-protected
F protégé contre les explosions
S protegido frente a explosión

Ex-Kanal
E ex-duct, explosion vent
F canal de purge anti-déflagrant, orifice de purge anti-déflagrant
S orificio (válvula) de seguridad (antideflagrante)

Ex-Kanalabdeckung
E explosion relief duct cover
F couvercle de canalisation anti-déflagrant
S cubierta del orificio de seguridad

Ex-Klappen
E explosion panel
F clapet anti-déflagrant
S válvula antideflagrante

Exkretion
E excretion
F excrétion
S excreción

exothermische Reaktion
E exothermic reaction
F réaction exothermique
S reacción exotérmica

expandiertes Polystyrol (EPS)
E expanded polystyrene (EPS)
F polystyrène expansé
S poliesterol expandido

Expertensystem
E expert system
F système expert
S sistema de expertos

Explosionsentlastung
E explosion relief
F décharge d'explosion
S descarga de explosión

Explosionsgefahr
E explosion hazard
F danger d'explosion
S peligro de explosión

explosionsgeschützt
E explosion-protected
F protégé contre une explosion
S protegido contra explosión

English German French Spanish

explosionssicher
E explosion-proof
F anti-déflagrant
S a prueba de explosión

Explosivität
E explosiveness
F explosivité
S explosividad

Exportverpackung
E export package
F emballage à l'export
S embalaje de exportación

Exsiccator
E desiccator
F dessicateur
S desecante, exicante

Extinktion
E absorbance
F absorption
S extinción

Extinktionskoeffizient
E coefficient of absorbance
F coefficient d'absorption
S coeficiente de extinción

extrahierbare Substanz
E extractable substance
F substance extractible
S sustancia extraíble

extrahieren
E extract, to
F extraire
S extraer

Extrakt
E extract
F extrait
S extracto

Dickextrakt
E concentrate
F concentré
S extracto concentrado

Flüssigextrakt
E liquid extract
F extrait liquide
S extracto líquido

Trockenextrakt
E dried concentrate
F concentré sec
S concentrado seco

Extraktion
E extraction
F extraction
S extracción

Extruder
E extruder
F extrudeuse
S extrusor

extrudieren
E extrude, to
F extruder
S extrudir

Extrusion
E extrusion
F extrusion
S extrusión

Exzenterband
E eccentric band
F courroie excentrique
S cinta excéntrica

Exzentermaschine
E eccentric machine
F machine excentrique
S máquina excéntrica

Exzenterpresse
E eccentric tablet press
F presse excentrique à comprimés
S prensa excéntrica

F + E (Forschung und Entwicklung)
E R + D (Research and Development)
F R + D (recherche et développement)
S investigación y desarrollo

Facette
E bevel
F biseau
S bisel, faceta

Facharbeiter
E skilled worker
F ouvrier qualifié
S tabajador cualificado

Fachinformation
E technical information
F information technique
S ficha técnica (de un medicamento)

Faden
E thread
F fil
S hilo

Fadenbruch
E thread rupture
F rupture de fil
S ruptura de hilo

Fadenkreuz
E crosswires
F réticule
S retículo

fahrbar
E mobile
F mobile
S móvil, portátil

Fahrgestell
E trolley
F chassis mobile
S bastidor, chasis

Fallhöhe
E drop height
F hauteur de chute
S altura de caída

Fällung (chemisch)
E precipitation, precipitate
F précipitation, précipité
S precipitación (química), precipitado

Fällungsmittel
E precipitating agent
F agent de précipitation
S agente de precipitación

Fällungstitration
E precipitation titration
F titrage de précipitation, dosage de précipitation
S volumetría de precipitación

Fälschung
E falsification
F falsification
S falsificación

Falte
E fold
F pli
S arruga, pliegue

Faltenbalg
E bellows
F soufflet
S fuelle plegable

Faltenbildung
E wrinkling
F formation de plis, formation de rides
S formación de arrugas, formación de pliegues

Faltenfilter
E fluted filter
F filtre nervuré, filtre cannelé
S filtro acanalado

Faltschachtel
E folding carton
F boîte pliante
S caja plegable

Faltschachtelaufrichtmaschine
E folding carton set-up machine
F plieuse pour boîtes pliantes
S máquina plegadora de cajas

English German French Spanish

Faltschachtelverschließmaschine
E folding carton sealing machine
F machine à sceller les boîtes pliantes
S máquina de cierre de cajas plegables

Falz (einer Tube)
E crimp, seam (of a tube)
F joint (d'un tube)
S encaje (de un tubo)

Falzechtheit
E flexing resistance
F résistance au pliage
S resistencia al plegado

falzen
E fold, to; crimp, to; seam, to
F plier
S plegar

Falzmaschine
E folding machine
F plieuse
S plegadora

Falznaht
E lock seam
F couture de pliage
S soldadura del encaje

Falzstation
E folding station
F station de pliage
S estación de plegado

Falzzange
E crimping tongs
F pincettes, pinces, tenailles
S tenazas para cerrar tubos

Fangkorb
E retaining basket
F corbeille
S cesto colector

Farbabstufung
E colour scale
F gradation de couleurs
S gradación de colores

Farbcodierung
E colour code
F codage de couleurs
S codificación de colores

Farbcodierungsspezifikation
E colour code specification
F spécification du codage de couleurs
S especificación de la codificación de colores

Farbdispersion
E colour dispersion
F dispersion de la couleur
S dispersión cromática

Farbe
E dye, stain, pigment
F colorant, teinture, pigment
S color, pigmento, tintura

Färbegerät
E stainer
F appareil à teindre
S teñidor

Färbelösung
E staining liquid
F solution de teinture
S solución colorante

Färbemittel
E colouring agent, dye, stain
F colorant, teinture
S colorante, tintura

färben
E stain, to
F colorer, teinter, teindre
S colorear, teñir

Färbevermögen
E colour capacity
F capacité de coloration
S capacidad colorante

Färbkraft
E dyeing power
F pouvoir colorant
S poder colorante

farblos
E colourless
F incolore
S incoloro

Farbringleser
E colour ring code reader
F lecteur de codage de couleurs
S lector de anillo cromático

Farbskala
E colour scale
F gamme de couleurs
S escala cromática

Farbstoff
E dye, colouring agent
F colorant, pigment
S colorante

Farbstoffkonzentration
E dye concentration
F concentration d'un colorant
S concentración de colorante

Farbton
E colour shade, hue
F teinte, nuance d'une couleur
S matiz del color

Farbüberzug
E colour coating
F revêtement de couleur
S revestimiento coloreado

Farbumschlag
E colour change
F changement de couleur
S cambio de color

Färbung
E colouration
F coloration, teinture
S coloración

Farbuniformität
E colour uniformity
F uniformité de couleur
S uniformidad cromática

Farbvergleichslösung
E colorimetric solution
F solution colorimétrique
S solución colorimétrica

Fase (am Tablettenstempel)
E punch chamfer (of tablet punch)
F biseau (d'un poinçon à comprimés)
S bisel (del troquel de comprimidos)

Faser
E fibre
F fibre
S fibra

Faserfänger
E fibre catcher
F capteur de fibres
S captador de fibras

Faß
E barrel
F tonneau
S tonel

Fassungsvermögen
E capacity, volume
F capacité, contenance
S capacidad

Fäulnis
E putrefaction
F putréfaction
S putrefacción

Feder (Sprung-)
E spring
F ressort
S resorte

Federaufhängung
E spring suspension
F suspension à ressort
S suspensión mediante resorte

Federwaage
E spring balance
F balance à ressort
S balanza de resorte

English German French Spanish

Fehlcharge
E defective batch, failed batch
F lot défectueux
S lote defectuoso

Fehler
E defect, error, failure, fault, mistake
F défaut, erreur
S error

menschlicher Fehler
E human error
F erreur d'origine humaine
S error humano

zufälliger Fehler
E random error
F erreur aléatoire
S error casual

Fehler beseitigen
E eliminate a failure (fault), to
F éliminer une erreur
S eliminar errores

Fehler finden
E locate a failure (fault), to
F identifier une erreur
S encontrar errores

Fehlerbehebung
E trouble-shooting, failure rectification
F dépannage, action de corriger
S corrección de errores

Fehlerbewertungsliste
E defect (error, failure) evaluation list
F registre d'évaluation d'erreurs
S lista de evaluación de errores

Fehlergrenze
E margin of error
F marge d'erreur
S límite de error, margen de error

fehlerhaft
E defective, faulty
F défectueux
S defectuoso

fehlerhafte Einheiten
E defective units
F unités défectueuses
S unidades defectuosas

Fehlermeldung
E failure message
F message d'erreur
S aviso de errores

Fehlermerkmal
E defect characteristic
F caractéristique du défaut
S característica de defecto

Fehlermöglichkeits- und Einflußanalyse (FMEA)
E failure mode and effect analysis (FMEA)
F analyse de modes et effets des pannes (FMEA)
S análisis de influencia y posibilidad de defectos

Fehlerquelle
E source of error (failure)
F source d'erreur
S fuente de errores

Fehlerrate
E failure rate
F taux d'erreur
S tasa de errores

fehlersicherer Modus
E fail-safe mode
F mode indéréglable
S modo a prueba de errores

Fehleruntersuchung
E error (failure) investigation
F investigation des sources d'une erreur
S investigación de errores

Fehlerursache
E cause of failure
F cause du défaut
S causa de error

Feineinstellung
E fine adjustment
F réglage fin, mise au point précise
S ajuste fino

Feingewebe
E fine tissue
F tissu fragile
S tejido fino

Feinkorn
E fine particle
F particule fine
S partícula fina

feinkörnig
E fine-grained
F à grain fin
S de grano fino

Feinregulierung
E fine adjustment
F réglage fin
S regulación fina

Feinsieb
E fine sieve
F tamis fin
S tamiz fino

Feinstaubfilter
E fine dust filter
F filtre à poussières fines
S filtro de polvo fino

Feinwaage
E precision balance
F balance de précision
S balanza de precisión

Fermentation
E fermentation
F fermentation
S fermentación

Fermentationskessel
E fermentation vessel
F cuve de fermentation
S caldera de fermentación

Fermentationslabor
E fermentation laboratory
F laboratoire de fermentation
S laboratorio de fermentación

Fermentationsraum
E fermentation room
F aire de fermentation
S área de fermentación

Fermenter
E fermenter
F fermenteur
S fermentador

fermentieren
E ferment, to
F faire fermenter
S fermentar

Fernbedienung
E remote control, remote operation
F télécommande
S telemando

Fernsteuerung
E remote control
F télécommande
S control remoto

Fernüberwachung
E remote control
F télécontrôle, télécommande
S control remoto

Fertigarzneimittel
E finished medicinal product
F médicament fini, produit pharmaceutique fini
S medicamento manufacturado, especialidad farmacéutica manufacturada

Fertigpackung
E finished pack
F emballage fini
S envase terminado

Fertigprodukt
E finished product
F produit fini
S producto acabado

English
German
French
Spanish

Fertigspritze
E prefilled syringe
F seringue prête à l'usage
S jeringa dispuesta para el uso

Fertigwaren
E manufactured goods, finished goods
F produits manufacturés
S productos manufacturados

fest
E solid
F solide
S duradero, estable, sólido

fest installiert
E permanently installed
F installé de manière permanente
S instalado fijamente

feste Formen
E solid dosage forms
F forme de dosage solide
S formas sólidas de dosificación

feste Phase
E solid phase
F phase solide
S fase sólida

Festigkeit
E firmness, solidity
F solidité
S firmeza, solidez

Festphasenextraktion
E solid phase extraction
F extraction en phase solide
S extracción en fase sólida

Feststoff
E solid
F solide
S sustancia sólida

Feststoffgehalt
E solid matter content
F teneur en matière solide
S contenido en materia sólida

Fettsalbe
E fatty ointment
F pommade
S pomada con elevado contenido en grasa

Fettsäure
E fatty acid
F acide gras
S ácido graso

feucht
E moist
F humide
S húmedo

Feuchtemesser
E hygrometer
F hygromètre
S higrómetro

Feuchtesensor
E humidity detector
F détecteur d'humidité
S detector de humedad

Feuchtgranulierung
E wet granulation
F granulation (par voie) humide
S granulación húmeda

Feuchthaltemittel
E wetting agent
F mouillant
S humectante

Feuchtigkeit
E humidity, moisture
F humidité
S humedad

gebundene Feuchtigkeit
E bound moisture
F humidité adhérente
S humedad adherente

nicht gebundene Feuchtigkeit
E unbound moisture
F humidité non liée
S humedad no adherente

feuchtigkeitsabweisend
E moisture-repelling
F qui répulse l'humidité
S repelente de la humedad

Feuchtigkeitsaufnahme
E moisture uptake
F absorption d'humidité
S absorción de humedad

feuchtigkeitsbeständig
E moisture-resistant
F résistant à l'humidité
S resistente a la humedad

feuchtigkeitsempfindlich
E moisture-sensitive
F sensible à l'humidité
S sensible a la humedad

Feuchtigkeitsgehalt
E moisture content
F teneur en humidité
S contenido en humedad

Feuchtigkeitsmesser
E hygrometer
F hygromètre
S higrómetro

feuchtigkeitsundurchlässig
E impervious to moisture
F étanche
S impermeable a la humedad

feuerfest
E fire-resistant
F in-inflammable
S ignífugo, resistente al fuego

Feuergefahr
E fire hazard
F risque d'incendie
S peligro de incendio

feuergefährlich
E flammable
F inflammable
S inflamable

feuergeschützt
E fire-proof
F ignifugé, à l'épreuve du feu
S protegido frente al fuego

Feuerlöscher
E fire extinguisher
F extincteur
S extintor (de incendios)

Feuermelder
E fire alarm
F alarme d'incendie
S alarma de incendio

Fiberkarton
E fibre cardboard
F carton à fibres
S cartón de fibra

Fibertrommel
E fibre drum
F tambour à fibres
S tambor de fibras

fiebererzeugende Substanzen
E pyrogens
F pyrogènes
S pirógenos

Filmbeschichtung, wäßrige
E aqueous film coating
F film aqueux, couche aqueuse pelliculaire
S película acuosa de revestimiento

filmbildende Flüssigkeit
E film-forming liquid, collodion
F collodion
S colodión

Filmbildner
E film-forming agent
F agent filmogène
S agente formador de películas

Filmtablette
E coated tablet
F comprimé pelliculé
S gragea

Filmüberzug
E coating
F film de revêtement
S película de revestimiento

Filter
E filter
F filtre
S filtro

endständiger Filter
E terminal filter
F filtre terminal
S filtro terminal

glasfaserverstärkter Filter
E fibre glass-reinforced filter
F filtre renforcé à la fibre de verre
S filtro reforzado con fibra de vidrio

Filterabdichtung
E filter seal
F étanchement d'un filtre
S cierre hermético de un filtro

Filterabreinigungsvorrichtung
E filter cleaning device
F dispositif de nettoyage de filtre
S dispositivo de limpieza de filtros

Filteraufhängevorrichtung
E filter suspension rack
F crémaillère pour filtre
S dispositivo de suspensión de filtros

Filterausbau
E filter removal
F démontage de filtre
S desmontaje de un filtro

Filterbett
E filter bed
F lit de filtre
S lecho filtrante

Filterbeutel
E filter bag
F sac de filtration
S bolsa filtro

Filtereinbau
E filter installation
F installation d'un filtre
S instalación de un filtro

Filtereinsatz
E filter insert
F support de filtre
S inserción del filtro

Filterfläche
E filter surface
F surface d'un filtre
S superficie del filtro

Filtergehäuse
E filter housing
F boîtier de filtre
S armazón del filtro

Filtergestell
E filter stand
F support de filtre
S soporte del filtro

Filterintegrität
E filter integrity
F intégrité d'un filtre
S integridad del filtro

Filterintegritätstest
E filter integrity test
F test d'intégrité de filtre
S prueba de integridad del filtro

Filterkerze
E filter cartridge
F chandelle filtrante
S candela filtrante

Filtermaterialien
E filter materials
F matériaux de filtre
S materiales de filtración

Filteroberfläche
E filter surface
F superficie d'un filtre
S superficie del filtro

Filterpatrone
E filter cartridge
F cartouche de filtre
S cartucho de filtro

Filterrückstand
E filter residue
F résidu de filtration
S residuo de filtración

Filtersack (beim WSG)
E filter bag (for fluidized bed dryer)
F filtre à poches
S bolsa filtro (para infusiones)

Filterwiderstand
E filter resistance
F résistance du filtre
S resistencia del filtro

Filtrat
E filtrate
F filtrat
S filtrado

Filtration
E filtration
F filtration
S filtración

Filtrationsabfall
E filtrate waste
F effluent de filtration
S desecho de filtración

Filtrationsmethode
E filtration method
F méthode de filtration
S método de filtración

Filtrationswiderstand
E filtration resistance
F résistance au filtrage
S resistencia a la filtración

filtrierbar
E filterable
F pouvant être filtré
S filtrable

filtrieren
E filter, to
F filtrer
S filtrar

Filtrierpapier
E filter paper
F papier filtre
S papel de filtro

Firmenzeichen
E logo
F logo
S logotipo

Fixierlösung
E fixing solution
F solution de fixation
S solución fijadora

Flachbeutel
E flat bag
F sachet plat, sachet plan
S bolsa plana

Fläche
E area
F surface, superficie
S superficie

Flamme, offene
E naked flame
F flamme ouverte
S llama abierta

Flammenemissionsspektroskopie
E flame emission spectroscopy
F spectroscopie à émission de flamme
S espectroscopia de emisión de llama

Flammenionisationsdetektor (FID)
E flame ionisation detector (FID)
F détecteur à ionisation de flamme
S detector de ionización de llama

Flammenphotometer
E flame photometer
F photomètre de flamme
S fotómetro de llama

Flammenphotometrie
E flame photometry
F photométrie de flamme
S fotometría de llama

Flammensterilisator
E flame steriliser
F stérilisateur à flammes
S esterilizador a la llama

Flammpistole
E flame gun
F pistolet chalumeau
S pistola de llama

Flammpunkt
E flash point
F point d'inflammation
S punto de ignición

Flansch
E flange
F bride, collerette
S brida, collar

flanschen
E flange, to
F brider
S bridar

Fläschchen
E vial
F flacon, récipient
S botellín, frasco, vial

Flasche
E bottle
F bouteille
S botella

Flasche mit Schraubverschluß
E screw-cap bottle
F bouteille munie d'un bouchon à vis
S botella con cierre de rosca

Flaschenabfüllmaschine
E bottling machine
F machine de remplissage des bouteilles
S embotelladora

Flaschenhals
E bottle neck
F goulot, col de bouteille
S cuello de botella, gollete

Flaschenverschließmaschine
E bottle-closing machine
F machine d'encapsulage
S máquina de cierre de botellas

Flaschenverschluß
E bottle cap
F capsule à bouteilles
S cierre de botella, tapa de botella

Flattermarke
E marker (on leaflet)
F marque inconstante
S marca inconstante

Fleck
E stain
F tache
S mancha

Fliehkraft
E centrifugal force
F force de centrifugation
S fuerza centrífuga

Fliese
E tile
F carreau
S baldosa

Fließband
E conveyor belt
F convoyeur à bande, tapis roulant
S cinta transportadora

Fließdiagramm
E flow chart
F schéma opérationel, schéma de marche, schéma de principe
S diagrama operacional

Fließeigenschaft
E flow property
F propriété d'écoulement
S propiedad fluida

Fließfähigkeit
E flowability
F fluidité
S fluidez

Fließgeschwindigkeit
E flow rate
F débit
S velocidad de flujo

Fließgradient
E flow gradient
F gradient d'écoulement
S gradiente de flujo

Fließgrenze
E yield point
F limite d'écoulement
S límite de migración (en cromatografía)

Fließmittel (in der Chromatographie)
E mobile phase (in chromotography)
F phase mobile
S fase móvil (en cromatografía)

Fließmittel (in der Tablettierung)
E flow promoter (in tabletting)
F fluidifiant
S fluidificante (fabricación de comprimidos)

Fließmittelfront
E solvent front
F front de migration du solvant
S frente de migración del solvente

Flocke
E floc
F bourre
S copo, flóculo

flockig
E flaky
F floconneux
S flocular

Flockung
E flocculation
F floculation
S floculación

flüchtig
E volatile
F volatile
S volátil

flüchtige Bestandteile
E volatile components
F composants volatiles
S componentes volátiles

nicht flüchtig
E non-volatile
F non-volatile
S no volátil

Flügelrad
E fan wheel, blade, impeller, rotor, vane
F ailette
S rueda de aletas, rueda de paletas, rueda portante

Flügelradanemometer
E fan wheel anemometer
F anémomètre à moulinet, anémomètre à ailettes
S anemómetro de rueda de aletas

Flügelrührer
E blade stirrer
F agitateur à pales
S agitador de aletas

Flügelschraube
E wing screw
F vis à oreilles
S tornillo de aletas

Fluoreszenz
E fluorescence
F fluorescence
S fluorescencia

fluoreszierend
E fluorescent
F fluorescent
S fluorescente

Fluorierung
E fluorination
F fluoruration
S fluoración

Fluorometrie
E fluorometry
F fluorométrie
S fluorometría

Flur
E corridor
F corridor
S corredor

Flußdiagramm
E flow chart
F schéma fonctionnel
S diagrama de flujo

flüssig
E liquid
F liquide
S líquido

dickflüssig
E viscous
F visqueux
S viscoso

dünnflüssig
E thin
F (très) fluide
S (muy) fluido

Flüssigabfall
E aqueous waste
F effluent aqueux
S desecho fluido

flüssige Form
E liquid form
F forme liquide (spécialités pharmaceutiques)
S forma líquida de administración

flüssige Phase
E liquid phase
F phase liquide
S fase líquida

Flüssigextrakt
E liquid extract
F extrait liquide
S extracto fluido

flüssig-flüssig-Extraktion
E liquid-liquid extraction
F extraction liquide-liquide
S extracción líquido-líquido

Flüssiggas
E liquid gas
F gaz liquide
S gas líquido

Flüssigkeit
E liquid
F liquide
S líquido

Flüssigkeitsstand
E liquid level
F niveau du liquide
S nivel de líquido

Flüssigkeitsstandsanzeige
E liquid level indicator
F indicateur du niveau de liquide
S indicador de nivel de líquido

Flüssigkristallanzeige
E liquid crystal display (LCD)
F affichage à cristaux liquides
S pantalla de cristal líquido

Flüssigmedien
E liquid media
F milieux liquides
S medios líquidos

Folie
E foil, film
F feuille
S hoja, lámina

beschichtete Folie
E coated foil, coated film
F feuille enduite
S lámina recubierta

endlose Folie
E continuous foil, continuous film
F feuille continue
S lámina continua

Folienbahn
E sheet of film
F bande d'étoffe
S banda de láminas

Folienbedruckung
E film printing
F impression de feuilles
S impresión de láminas

Folienbeschickung
E film supply
F alimentation en feuilles
S abastecimiento de láminas

Foliendicke
E film thickness
F épaisseur de feuille
S espesor de lámina

Folienrißkontrolle
E film tear sensor
F contrôle des déchirures de feuilles
S control de desgarro de láminas

Folienschlupf
E film slippage
F glissement d'une feuille
S deslizamiento de una lámina

Folientastatur
E membrane key pad
F clavier à effleurement
S teclado de membrana plástica

Folienverbundkleber
E film laminating adhesive
F adhésif pour feuilles
S adhesivo para láminas

Folienverformung
E film forming
F façonnage de feuilles
S deformación de láminas

Förder-
E conveyor
F convoyeur
S transportador

Förderband
E conveyor belt
F tapis roulant
S cinta transportadora

fordern
E demand, to
F exiger
S exigir

fördern
E convey, to
F transporter
S fomentar, promover

Förderschnecke
E worm gear, worm screw
F vis sans fin, vis d'Archimède
S tornillo sin fin, tornillo transportador

Form (z. B. von Partikeln)
E shape (of particles)
F forme (de particules)
S forma (p. ej. de partículas)

Format
E format, size
F taille, format
S formato, tamaño

Formatteil (bei einer Tablettenpresse)
E component (of a tablet press)
F composant (d'une presse à comprimés)
S componente formador (de una prensa de comprimidos)

Formatumstellung
E size changeover
F modification d'un format
S cambio de formato

Formblock
E die block
F bloc de moulage
S bloque de moldeo

Formel
E formula
F formule
S fórmula

English German French Spanish

English
German
French
Spanish

Formentrennmittel
E parting agent
F séparateur de formes
S separador de formas

Formgebung
E formulation
F formulation
S formulación (galénica)

Formular
E form
F formulaire
S formulario

Formulierung
E formulation
F formulation
S formulación

Formulierung mit kontrollierter Freisetzung
E controlled release formulation
F formulation avec libération contrôlée
S formulación con liberación controlada

Forschung und Entwicklung
E Research and Development
F recherche et développement
S investigación y desarrollo

fötales Kälberserum
E foetal calf serum (FCS)
F sérum de veau fœtal
S suero bovino fetal

Fragebogen
E questionnaire
F questionnaire
S cuestionario

Fraktion
E fraction
F fraction
S fracción

fraktionieren
E fractionate, to
F fractionner
S fraccionar

Fraktionssammler
E fraction collector
F collecteur de fractions
S colector de fracciones

frei verkäufliches Produkt
E over-the-counter (OTC) product
F produit sans ordonnance, produit en vente libre
S producto de venta libre

Freifallmischer
E tumbler mixer
F mélangeur culbuteur, malaxeur à chute libre
S mezclador por basculado

freifließend
E free flowing
F fluide, s'écoulant librement
S fluyendo libremente

Freigabe
E release
F libération
S liberación

Chargenfreigabe
E batch release
F libération d'un lot
S liberación de lotes

zeitlich gesteuerte Freigabe
E timed release
F libération contrôlée
S liberación temporalmente controlada

Freigabedatum
E release date
F date de libération
S fecha de liberación

Freigabestatus
E release status
F statut de libération
S status de autorización

Freigabeuntersuchung
E release analysis
F analyse de libération
S análisis de autorización

Freigabeverfahren
E release procedure
F processus de libération
S proceso de autorización

freigeben
E release, to
F libérer
S liberar

freigegeben
E released
F libéré
S liberado

Freiheitsgrad
E degree of freedom
F degré de liberté
S grado de libertad

Freiraum
E clearance
F espace libre
S espacio libre

Freisetzung
E release
F libération
S liberación

kontrollierte Freisetzung
E controlled release
F libération contrôlée
S liberación controlada

modifizierte Freisetzung
E modified release
F libération modifiée
S liberación modificada

schnelle Freisetzung
E immediate release
F libération immédiate
S liberación inmediata

unvollständige Freisetzung
E incomplete release
F libération incomplète
S liberación incompleta

verlängerte Freisetzung
E sustained release
F libération prolongée
S liberación prolongada

verzögerte Freisetzung
E delayed release
F libération différée
S liberación retardada

Freisetzungsprofil
E release profile
F profil de libération
S perfil de liberación

Freisetzungsrate
E release rate
F vitesse de libération
S tasa de liberación

Freisetzungsverhalten
E release behaviour
F comportement de libération
S comportamiento de liberación

Freiwilliger, gesunder
E healthy volunteer
F volontaire sain
S voluntario sano

Fremdkörper
E foreign body
F corps étranger
S cuerpo extraño

Frischluftzufuhr
E fresh air inlet
F arrivée d'air frais
S entrada de aire fresco

Frist
E time limit, deadline
F délai, terme
S plazo

Fristverlängerung
E deadline extension
F prolongation d'un délai
S prolongación de un plazo

English
German
French
Spanish

Frontbildung (HPLC)
E fronting (in HPLC)
F formation d'un front (HPLC)
S formación de frente (HPLC)

FTIR-Spektroskopie
E FTIR spectroscopy
F spectroscopie IR par transformation de Fourier
S espectroscopia infrarroja en transformación de Fourier

Fuge
E joint, seam
F joint
S junta

Arbeitsfuge
E construction joint
F joint de construction
S junta de construcción

Bewegungsfuge
E settling joint
F joint de dilatation
S junta de movimiento

Dehnungsfuge
E expansion joint
F joint de compensation
S junta de dilatación

fugenlos
E seamless
F dépourvu de joint
S sin juntas

Fugenmaterial
E jointing material
F matériau pour joint
S material de junta

Fühler
E sensor
F capteur
S sensor

Führungskraft
E executive
F directeur, cadre dirigeant
S directivo, ejecutivo

Führungsrollen
E guide rollers
F rouleaux de guidage
S poleas de guía

Führungsvorrichtung
E guide, guiding device, guiding mechanism
F guide, dispositif de guidage, mécanisme de guidage
S dispositivo de guía, guía

Füllbereich
E filling section
F zone de remplissage
S zona de relleno

Fülleinrichtung
E feed hopper
F trémie de remplissage
S dispositivo de relleno

Füllgewicht
E filling weight, shot weight
F poids de remplissage
S peso al envasar

Füllgut
E contents, charge
F matière de remplissage
S material de relleno

Füllgutkontrolle
E content control
F contrôle du contenu
S control del contenido

Füllguttaster
E product scanner
F palpeur de remplissage
S sensor del contenido

Füllhöhe
E filling level
F niveau de remplissage
S nivel de llenado

Füllkurve (bei der Tablettenpresse)
E filling cam (tablet press)
F came de remplissage
S curva de relleno (prensa de comprimidos)

Füllmenge
E filling quantity
F quantité de remplissage
S cantidad de relleno

Füllmengenkontrolle
E quantity control
F contrôle de la quantité de remplissage
S control de la cantidad de relleno

Füllmittel
E filler
F moyen de remplissage
S medio de relleno

Füllrohr
E feed tube
F tube de remplissage
S tubo de llenado

Füllschuh
E feed shoe
F sabot distributeur
S zueco distribuidor

Füllstand
E level
F niveau
S nivel de relleno

Füllstandsmelder
E level detector
F détecteur de niveau
S detector de nivel de relleno

Füllstandsmesser
E level-measuring device
F dispositif de mesure d'un niveau
S sistema de medida del nivel de relleno

Füllstation
E filling station
F station de remplissage
S estación de llenado

Fülltiefe
E filling depth
F hauteur de remplissage
S altura del relleno

Fülltrichter
E hopper
F trémie
S embudo de llenado

Füllung, gleichmäßige
E uniform filling
F remplissage uniforme
S relleno uniforme

Füllventil
E filling nozzle
F buse de remplissage
S válvula de relleno

Füllvolumen
E filling volume
F volume de charge
S volumen de relleno

fungizid
E fungicidal
F fongicide
S fungicida

Fungizid
E fungicide
F fongicide
S fungicida

Funken
E sparks
F étincelles
S chispas

Funktionsfähigkeit
E operability, functionality
F fonctionnalité
S capacidad funcional

Funktionsqualifizierung
E operational qualification (OQ)
F qualification opérationnelle
S cualificación funcional

Funktionsspezifizierung
E function specification
F spécification de fonctionnement
S especificación funcional

Funktionsstörung
E malfunction
F dysfonctionnement
S disfunción

Funktionstasten
E function keys
F touche de fonctionnement
S botones de operación

Fußbodenabfluß
E floor drain
F bouche d'égout
S sumidero

Fußbodenbelag
E flooring, floor covering
F revêtement de sol
S pavimento, revestimiento del suelo

fusselfreie Kleidung
E lint-free clothes
F vêtement qui ne peluche pas
S ropa sin pelusa

Fütterungsarzneimittel
E drugs for animal feed
F médicament pour nourriture animale
S medicamento para el pienso

Gabelarm
E yoke
F bras de levier
S brazo de horquilla

Gabelstapler
E fork-lift truck
F chariot élévateur
S carretilla elevadora de horquilla

Galenik
E formulation
F formulation
S formulación (galénica)

Galenikabteilung
E galenical development department
F département de développement galénique
S departamento de farmacia galénica

Gammastrahlen
E gamma rays
F rayons gamma
S rayos gamma

Garantie
E guarantee, warranty
F garantie
S garantía

Gärung
E fermentation
F fermentation
S fermentación

Gas
E gas
F gaz
S gas

komprimierte Gase
E compressed gases
F gaz comprimés
S gases comprimidos

unter Druck gelöste Gase
E pressure-dissolved gases
F gaz dissous sous pression
S gas diluido a presión

verflüssigte Gase
E liquified gases
F gaz liquéfiés
S gases licuados

Gasblase
E gas bubble
F bulle de gaz
S burbuja de gas

Gaschromatographie
E gas chromatography
F chromatographie en phase gazeuse
S cromatografía de gases

gasdicht
E gas-tight
F étanche au gaz
S impermeable al gas

Gasdurchströmungsverfahren
E gas flow-through process
F procédé de circulation des gaz
S procedimiento de purga gaseosa

Gasflasche
E gas cylinder
F bouteille de gaz
S botella de gas

gasförmig
E gaseous
F gazeux
S gaseoso

Gasphase
E gaseous phase
F phase gazeuse
S fase gaseosa

Gasraum
E head space
F espace de tête
S espacio para la cabeza

Gassterilisation
E gas sterilisation
F stérilisation au gaz
S esterilización por gas

Gasstrom
E gas flow
F débit de gaz
S corriente gaseosa

Gaszufuhr
E gas supply
F alimentation en gaz
S alimentación de gas

Gattung
E species
F espèce
S género, especie

Gebäude
E building
F bâtiment, édifice
S edificio

Gebäudeplan
E building (facility) floor plan
F plan de l'édifice
S plan del edificio

gebeizt
E pickled
F décapé
S decapado, macerado

gebeizt und gestrahlt
E pickled and blasted
F poncé et décapé
S decapado y pulido

Gebinde
E container, pack
F conditionnement, emballage
S contenedor, haz

eingeschrumpftes Gebinde
E shrink-pack
F emballage sous film rétractable
S haz contraído, haz comprimido

Gebläse
E fan, ventilator
F ventilateur
S ventilador

Gebläserad
E fan wheel
F roue de ventilateur
S rueda de ventilador

Gebrauch, versehentlicher
E inadvertent use
F utilisation par inadvertance
S uso por inadvertencia

Gebrauchsanweisung
E instructions for use, operating instructions
F instructions pour l'utilisation
S instrucción de uso

gebrauchsfertig
E ready-to-use
F prêt à l'emploi
S dispuesto para el servicio, listo para el uso

geeignet
E suitable, appropriate, adequate
F approprié, adéquat
S adecuado, apropiado

Gefahr durch biologische Agenzien
E biohazard
F danger biologique, risque biologique
S peligro biológico

gefährden (Qualität)
E endanger, to (quality)
F mettre en danger, compromettre (la qualité)
S arriesgar, poner en peligro (la calidad)

Gefahrenhinweis
E hazard indication
F mise en garde
S aviso de peligro

gefährdet ungeborene Kinder
E may cause harm to unborn child
F dangereux pour les enfants pendant une grossesse
S peligroso para el feto

giftig bei Hautkontakt
E toxic in contact with skin
F toxique au contact de la peau
S tóxico para la piel

giftig beim Einatmen
E toxic by inhalation
F toxique si inhalé
S tóxico si se inhala

giftig beim Verschlucken
E toxic if swallowed
F toxique si ingéré
S tóxico si se ingiere

kann beim Einatmen Krebs erzeugen
E may cause cancer by inhalation
F cancéreux si inhalé
S cancerógeno si se inhala

kann die Fruchtbarkeit beeinträchtigen
E may impair fertility
F peut altérer la fertilité
S puede dañar la fertilidad

kann Krebs erzeugen
E may cause cancer
F peut provoquer un cancer
S puede causar cáncer

kann vererbliche Genschäden verursachen
E may cause heritable genetic damage
F peut être la cause de dommages génétiques héréditaires
S puede originar daños genéticos hereditarios

reizt die Atemwege
E irritating to respiratory system
F peut irriter le système respiratoire
S irrita las vías respiratorias

reizt die Augen
E irritating to eyes
F peut provoquer des irritations aux yeux
S irrita los ojos

verursacht (schwere) Verbrennungen
E causes (severe) burns
F peut provoquer de (sévères) brûlures
S causa (graves) quemaduras

Gefahrenklasse
E hazard class
F classe de dangers
S clase de peligro

Gefahrenpotential
E hazard potential
F potentiel de danger
S potencial de riesgos

Gefahrensymbol
E hazard symbol
F symbole de danger
S símbolo de peligro

gefährlich
E hazardous, dangerous
F dangereux
S peligroso

Gefahrstoff
E hazardous material, dangerous material
F matériel dangereux
S sustancia peligrosa

Gefahrstoffverordnung
E regulations for hazardous goods, toxic chemical ordinance
F décret concernant les matières dangereuses
S decreto sobre sustancias peligrosas

Gefälle
E gradient, slope
F pente, inclinaison
S declive, gradiente, inclinación, pendiente

mit Gefälle, geneigt
E sloped
F avec une pente, incliné
S con inclinación, inclinado

Gefälleestrich
E sloping flooring, screed
F chape inclinée
S pavimento inclinado

Gefäß
E vessel
F récipient
S recipiente

Gefäßentleerung
E vessel emptying
F action de vider un flacon, action de vider un récipient
S vaciamiento de un recipiente

Gefäßwand
E vessel wall
F paroi d'un récipient
S pared de un recipiente

gefordert
E required
F exigé
S exigido, reclamado

geformt
E moulded
F moulu
S moldeado, comprimido

gefriergetrocknet
E freeze-dried, lyophilised
F lyophilisé
S liofilizado

Gefrierpunkt
E freezing point
F point de congélation
S punto de congelación

Gefrierpunktserniedrigung
E depression of freezing point
F abaissement du point de congélation
S reducción del punto de congelación

Gefrierröhrchen
E cryotube
F tube de congélation
S tubo de congelación

Gefrierschrank
E freezer
F congélateur
S congelador

Gefriertrockner
E freeze dryer, lyophiliser
F lyophilisateur
S liofilizador

Gefriertrocknung
E freeze drying, lyophilisation
F lyophilisation
S liofilización

Gegenanzeige
E contraindication
F contre-indication
S contraindicación

English German French Spanish

Gegendruck (in der Chromatographie)
E back pressure
F contre-pression
S contrapresión (en cromatografía)

Gegenflansch
E counter-flange
F contre-bride
S contrabrida

Gegengewicht
E counter-weight
F contrepoids
S contrapeso

Gegengift
E antidote
F antidote
S antídoto

Gegenion
E counter-ion
F contre-ion, ion complémentaire
S contraión, ion complementario

Gegenseitiges Anerkennungsverfahren bei der Zulassung von Arzneimitteln in der EU
E Mutual Recognition Procedure (MRP)
F procédure de reconnaissance mutuelle
S Procedimiento de Reconocimiento Mutuo en la UE

Gehalt
E content
F contenu
S contenido

Gehaltsbestimmung
E determination of content
F détermination du contenu
S determinación del contenido

Gehaltseinheitlichkeit
E content uniformity (CU)
F uniformité du contenu
S uniformidad del contenido

Gehäuse
E housing
F boîtier
S caja, estuche

Geheimhaltungsvertrag
E secrecy agreement
F accord de confidentialité
S contrato de confidencialidad

Gehörschutz
E ear protector, ear defender
F protection auriculaire
S protección auricular

Geisterpeak
E ghost peak
F pic fantôme
S pico fantasma

Gel
E gel
F gel
S gel

Gel zum Einnehmen
E oral gel
F gel pour administration orale
S gel oral

Gel zur endozervikalen Anwendung
E endocervical gel
F gel pour utilisation endo-cervicale
S gel de uso endocervical

Gelatinekapsel
E gelatine capsule
F capsule de gélatine
S cápsula de gelatina

Hartgelatinekapsel
E hard gelatine capsule
F gélule
S cápsula de gelatina dura

Weichgelatinekapsel
E soft gelatine capsule
F gélule molle
S cápsula de gelatina blanda

Gelbildner
E gel-forming agent
F gélifiant
S gelificante

Gelbildung
E gel formation
F formation de gel
S gelación

Gelchromatographie
E gel chromatography
F chromatographie sur gel
S cromatografía sobre gel

Gelfiltration
E gel filtration
F filtration sur gel
S filtración por gel

gelieren
E gel, to
F geler
S gelar

Geliermittel
E gelling agent, gellant
F gélifiant
S gelificante

gelocht
E perforated
F perforé
S perforado

gelöster Sauerstoff
E dissolved oxygen (DO)
F oxygène dissous
S oxígeno disuelto

Geltungsbereich
E scope, validity
F champ d'application
S campo de aplicación

Gelverschluß
E gel seal
F fermeture pour gel
S cierre por gel

Gemisch
E mixture
F mélange
S mezcla

Gemischtbett-Ionenaustauscher
E mixed bed ion exchange
F échange d'ions sur lit mixte
S intercambiador de iones de lecho mixto

genau
E exact
F exact
S exacto

Genauigkeit (einer Prüfmethode)
E precision
F précision
S exactitud (de un método de prueba)

genehmigen
E authorise, to; approve, to
F autoriser
S autorizar

Genehmigung
E authorisation, approval
F autorisation
S autorización

elektronische Genehmigung
E electronic approval
F autorisation électronique
S autorización electrónica

geneigt
E sloped
F incliné, avec une pente
S inclinado, con pendiente

Generationszeit
E doubling time
F temps de doublement
S tiempo de generación

Generator
E generator
F générateur
S generador

English German French Spanish

English German French Spanish

Genericum
E generic
F générique
S genérico

genetisch veränderte Organismen
E genetically modified organisms (GMO)
F organismes génétiquement modifiés (OGM)
S organismos modificados genéticamente

Genmanipulation
E genetic engineering
F manipulation génétique
S manipulación genética

Genomdaten
E genomic data
F données génomiques
S datos genómicos

Genomlehre
E genomics
F génomique
S teoría del genoma

genormt
E standardised
F standardisé
S estandarizado, normalizado

Gentechnologie
E gene technology
F génie génétique
S tecnología genética

geprägt
E embossed
F estampé
S acuñado, estampado

gepreßt
E moulded
F moulu
S comprimido, moldeado

geprüft
E checked, inspected
F contrôlé, inspecté, vérifié
S comprobado

Gerade
E straight, straight line
F ligne droite
S recta (línea)

Geräte
E apparatus, equipment
F appareillage expérimental
S aparatos

periphere Geräte
E peripheral instrumentation
F appareils périphériques
S aparatos periféricos

Gerätedesinfektion
E instrument disinfection
F désinfection des instruments
S desinfección de instrumentos

Gerätehandbuch
E instrument manual
F manuel d'instructions
S manual de instrucciones

Gerätehersteller
E equipment manufacturer
F fabricant d'équipement
S fabricante de aparatos

Gerätekalibrierung
E instrument calibration
F calibration de l'équipement
S calibración de aparatos

Gerätekennzeichnung
E apparatus designation
F marquage de l'appareil
S caracterización de aparatos

Gerätekonfiguration
E instrument configuration
F configuration de l'instrument
S configuración de aparatos

Geräteoptionen
E instrument options
F options d'un équipement
S opciones del aparato

Geräteschmierung
E instrument lubrication
F lubrification d'un instrument
S lubricación del aparato

Gerätespeicher
E instrument memory
F mémoire d'un instrument
S memoria de un instrumento

Gerätespezifikation
E instrument specification
F spécification de l'instrument
S especificación de aparatos

Gerätetest
E equipment test
F test d'appareils
S comprobación de aparatos

Gerätezubehör
E instrument accessories
F accessoires d'un équipement
S accesorios del aparato

geräuschdämmend
E noise-proof
F insonorisé
S insonorizado

Geräuschentwicklung
E noise development
F émissions sonores
S producción de ruido

Geräuschisolierung
E noise insulation
F insonorisation du bruit
S aislamiento sonoro

Geräuschpegel
E noise level
F niveau du bruit
S nivel sonoro

Gerbstoff
E tanning agent
F tannin
S tanino

gereinigt
E purified
F purifié
S purificado

gereinigter Dampf
E purified steam
F vapeur purifiée
S vapor purificado

gereinigtes Wasser
E purified water
F eau purifiée
S agua purificada

geriffelt
E corrugated
F cannelé, strié
S acanalado, estriado

gerinnen
E coagulate, to
F coaguler
S coagular

Gerinnung
E coagulation
F coagulation
S coagulación

Geruch
E odour
F odeur
S olor

geruchlos
E odourless
F sans odeur
S inodoro

Geruchsverschluß
E stench trap, siphon
F siphon
S válvula de hedor

Gerüst
E supporting structure
F échafaudage
S andamio, armazón, esqueleto

Gesamtabmessungen
E overall dimensions
F dimensions totales
S dimensiones totales

Gesamtausbeute
E total yield
F rendement total
S rendimiento total

Gesamtbreite
E overall width
F largeur totale
S anchura total

Gesamtfläche
E total area
F surface totale, aire totale
S superficie total

Gesamthöhe
E overall height
F hauteur totale
S altura total

Gesamtkeimzahl
E total microbial count
F nombre total de micro-organismes
S número total de gérmenes

Gesamtkohlenstoffgehalt
E total organic carbon (TOC)
F teneur totale en carbone
S contenido total en carbono

Gesamtlänge
E overall length
F longueur totale
S longitud total

gesamtorganischer Kohlenstoff
E total organic carbon (TOC)
F teneur totale en carbone organique
S contenido total en carbono orgánico

gesättigt
E saturated
F saturé
S saturado

Geschäftsführer
E managing director, general manager
F président directeur général (PDG)
S gerente

Geschäftsleitung
E company management
F direction d'une société
S gerencia

geschliffen
E ground
F moulu, poli
S bruñido, pulido, tallado

geschlossener Kreislauf
E closed loop
F circulation fermée
S circulación cerrada

Geschmack
E taste, flavour
F goût
S gusto

geschmacklos
E tasteless, flavourless
F insipide, fade
S insípido

Geschmackstoff
E flavouring agent, flavour
F agent aromatique
S agente saporífero

Geschmacksüberdeckung
E taste masking
F masquage d'une saveur
S enmascaramiento del sabor

Geschwindigkeit, durchschnittliche
E average speed
F vitesse moyenne
S velocidad media

Geschwindigkeitseinstellung
E speed adjustment
F ajustement de la vitesse
S ajuste de la velocidad

Geschwindigkeitsmesser
E tachometer, velocimeter
F tachymètre
S taquímetro

Gesellschaft
E company
F société, compagnie
S sociedad

Gesetz
E law, statute
F loi
S ley

Gesetzesentwurf
E draft bill
F projet de loi
S proyecto de ley

Gesetzgebung
E legislation
F législation
S legislación

Gesichtsschutz
E face protection
F protection faciale
S protección facial

gespannter Wasserdampf
E super-heated steam
F vapeur surchauffée
S vapor sobrecalentado

gesprenkelt
E mottled
F madré
S moteado, salpicado

gesprungen (Glas)
E cracked (glass)
F fêlé
S quebrado (vidrio)

Gestell
E stand, frame
F support, cadre
S armazón, bastidor, soporte

gesunder Freiwilliger
E healthy volunteer
F volontaire sain
S voluntario sano

Gesundheitsprodukte
E health care products
F produits d'hygiène grand public
S productos para la salud

Gesundheitsrisiko
E health risk
F risque pour la santé
S riesgo para la salud

Gesundheitsschaden
E damage to health
F préjudice à la santé
S perjuicio para la salud

gesundheitsschädlich
E harmful
F dangereux
S perjudicial

gesundheitsschädlich bei Hautkontakt
E harmful in contact with skin
F dangereux pour la santé lors d'un contact cutané
S perjudicial para la salud si entra en contacto con la piel

gesundheitsschädlich bei Inhalation
E harmful by inhalation
F dangereux pour la santé si inhalé
S perjudicial para la salud si se inhala

gesundheitsschädlich beim Verschlucken
E harmful if swallowed
F dangereux pour la santé si ingéré
S perjudicial para la salud si se ingiere

Gesundheitsuntersuchung, regelmäßige
E periodic health check
F visite médicale périodique
S inspección médica periódica

English
German
French
Spanish

English

German

French

Spanish

Gesundheitswesen
E health care
F système de santé
S sistema sanitario

Getriebe
E transmission, drive
F transmission, engrenage
S engranaje, transmisión

Gewebe
E tissue
F tissu
S tejido

Gewebezellkultur
E tissue cell culture
F culture de cellules tissulaires
S cultivo de células tisulares

Gewicht
E weight
F poids
S peso

Gewichtsanalyse
E gravimetric analysis
F analyse du poids
S análisis del peso

Gewichtseinheitlichkeit
E uniformity of weight
F uniformité du poids
S uniformidad del peso

Gewichtsgenauigkeit
E weight accuracy
F exactitude d'un poids
S exactitud del peso

Gewichtskonstanz
E constant weight
F constance d'un poids
S constancia del peso

Gewichtskontrolle
E weight control
F contrôle du poids
S control del peso

Gewichtssatz
E set of weights
F série de poids
S juego de pesas

Gewichtsverlust (bei der Trocknung)
E weight loss (on drying)
F perte de poids (lors de la dessication)
S pérdida de peso (al desecar)

Gewinde
E thread
F filetage
S filete, rosca

linksgängig
E left-handed
F à gauche
S de paso izquierdo

rechtsgängig
E right-handed
F à droite
S de paso derecho

Gewinnung
E production, extraction
F production
S extracción, obtención, producción

gewölbt, nach außen
E convex
F convexe
S convexo

gewölbt, nach innen
E concave
F concave
S cóncavo

Gift
E poison, toxin
F poison
S tóxico, veneno

giftig
E poisonous, toxic
F toxique
S tóxico, venenoso

giftig bei Hautkontakt
E toxic in contact with skin
F toxique au contact de la peau
S tóxico si entra en contacto con la piel

giftig beim Einatmen
E toxic by inhalation
F toxique si inhalé
S tóxico si se inhala

giftig beim Verschlucken
E toxic if swallowed
F toxique si ingéré
S tóxico si se ingiere

Giftigkeit
E toxicity
F toxicité
S toxicidad

Giftstoff
E toxin, poison
F toxine
S sustancia venenosa, toxina, veneno

Gitter
E grating
F grille
S retícula

Gitterrost
E grating
F grille
S retícula

Glanz
E gloss
F lustre, brillance
S brillo, lustre

glänzend
E glossy
F brillant, lustré
S brillante, lustrado

Glanzgrad
E grade of gloss, grade of lustre
F degré de lustre
S grado de brillantez

Glas, laminiertes
E laminated glass
F verre stratifié
S vidrio laminado

Glasart
E glass type
F type de verre
S tipo de vidrio

Glasballon
E glass balloon
F ballon de verre
S balón de vidrio

Glasbruch
E breakage of glassware
F débris de verre
S ruptura de vidrio

Gläschen
E vial
F flacon, fiole
S vial

Glaselektrode
E glass electrode
F électrode de verre
S electrodo de vidrio

Glasfaser
E fibreglass
F fibre de verre
S fibra de vidrio

glasfaserverstärkter Filter
E fibreglass-reinforced filter
F filtre renforcé à la fibre de verre
S filtro reforzado con fibra de vidrio

Glasfläschchen
E glass vial
F flacon en verre, fiole en verre
S vial de vidrio

Glasgeräte
E glassware
F verrerie
S instrumental de vidrio

English German French Spanish

Glasküvette
E glass cuvette
F cuvette en verre
S cubeta de vidrio

Glaspartikel
E glass particle
F particule de verre
S partícula de vidrio

Glasröhrchen
E glass tube
F tube de verre
S tubo (de ensayo) de vidrio

Glasschliff
E ground glass
F polissage de verre
S pulido del vidrio

Glassinter
E glass sinter
F fritte de verre
S sínter de vidrio

Glassplitter
E glass splinters
F éclats de verre
S añicos de vidrio

Glasstab
E glass rod
F baguette de verre
S barra de vidrio, bastón de vidrio

glatt
E smooth
F lisse, poli
S liso, pulido, resbaladizo

glätten
E smooth, to
F polir
S alisar, pulir

Gleichförmigkeit
E uniformity, consistency
F uniformité, consistance
S homogeneidad, uniformidad

Gleichgewicht
E equilibrium
F équilibre
S equilibrio

erneutes Gleichgewicht
E re-equilibrium
F rééquilibre
S reequilibrio

Gleichkorn
E uniform particle size
F taille des particules uniforme
S tamaño uniforme de las partículas

gleichmäßig
E uniform
F uniforme
S constante, homogéneo, uniforme

Gleichstrom
E direct current
F courant continu
S corriente continua

Gleichstromquelle
E direct current source
F source de courant continu
S fuente de corriente continua

Gleichung (mathematisch)
E equation
F équation
S ecuación (matemática)

gleichzeitig
E simultaneous
F simultanément
S simultáneo, simultáneamente

Gleiteigenschaft
E slip property
F propriété lubrifiante
S propiedad deslizante

gleiten
E slip, to
F couler, glisser
S deslizar, resbalar

Gleitmittel
E lubricant
F lubrifiant
S lubricante

glühen
E anneal, to
F recuire
S incandescer

Glührückstand
E residue on annealment, residue on ignition
F cendres résiduelles, résidu d'ignition
S cenizas residuales, residuo de ignición

GMP-Entsprechung
E GMP compliance
F conformité aux bonnes pratiques de fabrication
S conformidad con GMP

GMP-gerecht
E GMP-conform
F conforme aux bonnes pratiques de fabrication
S conforme a GMP

GMP-Labor
E GMP-controlled laboratory
F laboratoire conforme aux GMP
S laboratorio controlado para GMP

GMP-Richtlinien
E GMP guidelines
F règles GMP
S directrices de GMP

Befolgung von GMP-Richtlinien
E observance of GMP guidelines
F respect des règles GMP
S observancia de directrices de GMP

Umsetzung von GMP-Richtlinien
E implementation of GMP guidelines
F mise en pratique des règles GMP
S puesta en práctica de directices de GMP

Gradeinteilung
E scale
F graduation
S graduación

Gradient
E gradient
F gradient
S gradiente

Gradientenpumpe
E gradient pump
F pompe à gradient
S bomba de gradiente

graduiert
E graduated
F gradué
S graduado

grafische Darstellung
E graph
F graphe
S representación gráfica

Gramfärbung
E Gram staining
F méthode de coloration de Gram
S tinción de Gram

Gram-negativ
E Gram-negative
F Gram-négatif
S Gram negativo

Gram-positiv
E Gram-positive
F Gram-positif
S Gram positivo

Granulat
E granulate
F granulé
S granulado

Granulat mit veränderter Wirkstoff-Freisetzung
E modified release granules
F libération modifiée de granules
S granulado con liberación modificada de la sustancia activa

English German French Spanish

Granulat, magensaftresistentes
E gastro-resistant granules
F granules gastro-résistantes
S granulado resistente al jugo gástrico

Granulationsleistung
E granulation performance
F rendement de transformation en granulé
S rendimiento de granulación

Granulatkorn
E granule
F granule
S gránulo

granulieren
E granulate, to
F granuler
S granular

Granulierflüssigkeit
E granulating fluid
F liquide de granulation
S líquido de granulación

Granulierverfahren
E granulating process
F procédé de granulation
S procedimiento de granulación

Granulom, Bildung eines
E granuloma formation
F formation d'un granulome
S formación de un granuloma

Grat (einer Tablette)
E rim, bur (of a tablet)
F arête (d'un comprimé)
S borde (de un comprimido)

Gravurrolle
E engraving roll
F rouleau de gravure
S rollo de grabado

Grenzfläche
E interface
F surface de séparation, interface
S interfase, superficie limitante

grenzflächenaktiver Stoff
E surfactant
F tensioactif
S sustancia tensioactiva

Grenzprüfung
E limit test
F test de limites
S prueba de límites

Grenzwert
E limit
F limite
S valor límite

Griff
E handle, grip
F prise, poignée
S asa, empuñadura, estribo, mango

grob
E coarse
F brut, grossier
S grosero, grueso

Grobgranulat
E coarse granules
F granulés grossiers
S granulado grueso

Grobkorn
E coarse particle
F particule grossière
S grano grueso

grobkristallin
E course-grained
F grossièrement cristallin
S groseramente cristalino

Grobsieb
E coarse sieve
F tamis grossier
S tamiz de malla gruesa

Größe
E size
F taille
S magnitud, tamaño

Größenordnung
E order of magnitude
F ordre de magnitude
S orden de magnitud

Grundausführung
E standard construction
F fabrication standard
S versión básica

grundieren
E prime, to
F amorcer
S enderezar, dar la primera capa

gründlich
E thorough
F minutieusement
S minucioso, minuciosamente

Gründlichkeit
E thoroughness
F minutie
S minuciosidad

Grundriß
E plan
F plan (horizontal)
S plano (horizontal)

Gruppenleiter
E group manager
F chef de département
S director de grupo

Gulli
E floor drain
F égoût
S sumidero

gültig ab
E valid from
F valide à partir de
S válido a partir de

Gültigkeit
E validity
F validité
S validez

Gültigkeitsdauer
E period of validity
F durée de validité
S período de validez

Gummi
E rubber
F caoutchouc
S goma

Gummidichtung
E rubber gasket
F joint en caoutchouc
S junta de goma

gummieren
E gum, to
F gommer
S engomar, impermeabilizar

Gummischlauch
E rubber tube
F tube en caoutchouc
S tubo de goma

Gummistopfen
E rubber stopper
F bouchon en caoutchouc
S tapón de goma

Gurgellösung
E gargle
F solution pour gargarisme
S solución para gargarismos

Gutachten
E expertise
F expertise, avis d'expert
S dictamen

Güte
E quality
F qualité
S calidad

Gute Herstellungspraxis (GMP)
E Good Manufacturing Practice (GMP)
F bonnes pratiques de fabrication (GMP)
S Prácticas Correctas de Fabricación (GMP)

Gute Klinische Praxis (GCP)
E Good Clinical Practice (GCP)
F bonnes pratiques cliniques (GCP)
S Prácticas Clínicas Correctas (GCP)

Gute Laborpraxis (GLP)
E Good Laboratory Practice (GLP)
F bonnes pratiques de laboratoire (GLP)
S Prácticas Correctas de Laboratorio (GLP)

Gütebestimmung
E quality specification
F spécification de qualité
S especificación de calidad

Güteklasse
E quality grade
F degré de qualité
S grado de calidad

Güteminderung
E loss of quality
F perte de qualité, baisse de qualité
S pérdida de calidad

Haarhygrometer
E hair hygrometer
F hygromètre à cheveux
S higrómetro capilar

Haarriß
E hairline crack
F fissure capillaire
S fisura capilar

Haarwasser, medizinisches
E medicated hair tonic
F lotion capillaire
S loción capilar

Haftetikett
E self-adhesive label
F étiquette auto-adhésive
S etiqueta autoadhesiva

Haftfähigkeit
E adhesiveness
F pouvoir d'adhésion
S adherencia, adhesividad

Haftkraft
E adhesive power
F force d'adhésion
S fuerza adhesiva

Haftung (physikalisch)
E adhesion
F adhésion
S adhesión (física)

Haftung (rechtlich)
E liability (legal)
F responsabilité (juridique)
S responsabilidad (jurídica)

Hahn (technisch)
E stopcock
F robinet
S grifo

Halbfertigware
E semi-manufactured product
F produit intermédiaire
S producto semiacabado

halbfest
E semi-solid
F semi-solide
S semisólido

Halbleiter
E semiconductor
F semi-conducteur
S semiconductor

Halbwertszeit
E half-life
F demi-vie
S tiempo de vida media

Halogenaustausch
E halogen exchange
F échange d'halogène
S intercambio de halógenos

halogenfreie organische Lösungsmittel
E halogen-free organic solvents
F solvants organiques non halogènes
S diluyentes orgánicos no halogenados

halogenhaltige organische Lösungsmittel
E halogen-containing organic solvents
F solvants organiques halogènes
S diluyentes orgánicos halogenados

halogenierte Verbindungen
E halogenated compounds
F substances halogènes
S compuestos halogenados

Halogenierung
E halogenation
F halogénation
S halogenación

haltbar
E stable
F stable
S consistente, duradero, estable

Haltbarkeit
E stability
F stabilité
S conservabilidad, estabilidad

Haltbarkeitsdauer
E shelf-life
F durée de conservation, durée de stockage
S duración de conservación

Haltbarkeitsuntersuchung
E stability test
F test de stabilité
S prueba de estabilidad

Haltering
E retaining ring
F anneau de support
S anillo de soporte

Halterung
E mount, support
F support
S soporte

Hammermühle
E hammer mill
F broyeur à marteau
S molino triturador

Hämofiltrationslösung
E solution for haemofiltration
F solution d'hémofiltration
S solución de hemofiltración

Handbuch
E instruction manual
F manuel (d'utilisation)
S manual de instrucciones

Händedesinfektion
E hand disinfection
F désinfection des mains
S desinfección de manos

Handelsmarke
E brand name, registered name, trade name
F marque de commerce
S marca comercial

Handelsname
E commercial name
F nom de commerce
S nombre comercial

Handelsware
E commercial product
F produit commercial
S producto comercial

Handhabung
E handling
F maniement, traitement
S manejo, tratamiento

Handpresse
E hand press
F presse manuelle
S prensa manual

Handschuhe
E gloves
F gants
S guante

Handverpackung
E manual packaging
F emballage manuel
S empaquetado manual

Handwaschgelegenheit
E hand wash facility
F possibilité de lavage des mains
S posibilidad de lavar las manos

Handwerker
E workman, tradesman
F ouvrier, artisan
S artesano, trabajador manual

Härte
E hardness
F dureté
S dureza

Härte, permanente (von Wasser)
E permanent hardness (of water)
F dureté permamente (de l'eau)
S dureza permanente (del agua)

Härte, temporäre (von Wasser)
E temporary hardness (of water)
F dureté temporaire (de l'eau)
S dureza temporal (del agua)

Härten
E hardening
F durcissage
S endurecimiento

Härtetester
E hardness tester
F machine à tester la dureté
S máquina de comprobación de dureza

Hartgelatinekapsel
E hard gelatine capsule
F gélule
S cápsula de gelatina dura

Hartgummi
E hard rubber, vulcanite
F caoutchouc durci, ébonite
S ebonita

Harz
E resin
F résine
S resina

Haube
E cover, hood
F couvercle, capuchon
S casquete, cubierta, sombrerete

Haubenhalterung
E cover fitting
F garniture de couvercle
S soporte del casquete

Häufigkeit
E frequency
F fréquence
S frecuencia

Häufigkeitsverteilung
E frequency distribution
F distribution de fréquences
S distribución de frecuencias

Hauptdruckrolle
E main compression roll
F rouleau presseur principal
S rollo principal de prensa

Hauptschalter
E main switch, power switch
F interrupteur principal
S interruptor principal

Hauptstromkreis
E main circuit
F circuit principal
S circuito eléctrico principal

Hausstandard
E internal standard
F standard interne
S estándar interno

hautreizend
E irritating to skin
F irritant pour la peau
S irritante cutáneo

Hebebühne
E lifting platform
F plate-forme de levage
S plataforma elevadora

Hebel
E lever
F levier
S palanca

Hebelpresse
E lever press
F presse à bascule
S prensa de palanca

Hebevorrichtung
E lifting device
F dispositif de levage
S dispositivo elevador

Hefe
E yeast
F levure
S levadura

Heftpflaster
E sticking plaster
F sparadrap
S esparadrapo

Heilmittel
E therapeutic agent
F agent thérapeutique
S agente terapéutico

Heilwasser
E medicinal water
F eau médicinale
S agua medicinal

Heißlagerung
E heated storage
F stockage thermique
S almacenamiento caliente

Heißluftofen
E hot air oven
F four à air chaud
S horno de aire caliente

Heißluftsterilisation
E dry heat sterilisation
F stérilisation à l'air chaud
S esterilización por aire caliente

Heißluftsterilisator
E hot air steriliser
F stérilisateur à air chaud
S esterilizador de aire caliente

Heißsiegelkleber
E heat-sealing adhesive
F adhésif thermofusible
S adhesivo termofusible

Heißsiegellack
E heat-sealing lacquer
F laque thermofusible
S laca termofusible

heißsiegeln
E heat seal, to
F thermosceller
S sellar al calor

Heißwasserberieselung
E hot water spraying
F aspersion d'eau chaude
S rociado con agua caliente

Heizaggregat
E heating aggregate
F appareil de chauffage
S aparato de calefacción

Heizbacke
E heating jaw
F mâchoire chauffante
S mordaza de calefacción

Heizelement
E heating element
F élément chauffant
S elemento calefactor

Heizpilz
E heating mantle
F manteau chauffant
S manguito de caldeo

Heizquelle
E heating source
F source de chauffage,
source de chaleur
S fuente de calor

English German French Spanish

Heizschlange
E heating coil
F serpentin chauffant
S serpentín de calefacción

untergetauchte Heizschlange
E immersed heating coil
F serpentin chauffant immergé
S serpentín de calefacción sumergido

Hemmstoff
E inhibitor
F inhibiteur
S inhibidor

Hemmung
E inhibition
F inhibition
S inhibición

HEPA-Filter
E HEPA (high efficiency particulate air) filters
F filtres HEPA
S filtro HEPA

hermetischer Verschluß
E hermetic seal
F fermeture hermétique
S cierre hermético

Hersteller
E manufacturer
F fabricant
S fabricante

Herstellerangaben
E manufacturer's specification
F spécifications du fabricant
S especificaciones del fabricante

Herstelleraudit
E manufacturer audit
F audit d'un fabricant
S inspección de un fabricante

Herstellerlaubnis
E manufacturing authorisation
F autorisation de fabrication
S permiso de fabricación

Herstellung
E manufacture, production
F fabrication, production
S fabricación

computerintegrierte Herstellung
E computer-integrated manufacturing (CIM)
F fabrication informatisée
S fabricación informatizada

Herstellung im industriellen Maßstab
E industrial scale manufacture
F fabrication à l'échelle industrielle
S fabricación a escala industrial

Herstellung im Lohnauftrag
E contract manufacture
F fabrication en sous-traitance
S fabricación por comisión

Herstellungsanweisung
E manufacturing instructions
F instructions de fabrication
S instrucción de fabricación

Herstellungsauftrag
E manufacturing order
F commande de fabrication
S encargo de producción

Herstellungsbedingungen
E manufacturing conditions
F conditions de production
S condiciones de producción

Herstellungsleiter
E head of production
F directeur de production
S director de producción

Herstellungsprotokoll
E batch processing record
F protocole de fabrication
S protocolo de fabricación

Herstellungsstufe
E manufacturing step
F étape de fabrication
S etapa de producción

Herstellungsumgebung
E manufacturing environment
F zone de fabrication
S entorno de producción

Herstellungsverfahren
E manufacturing procedure
F procédure de fabrication
S procedimiento de fabricación

Herstellungsvorschrift
E master formula, manufacturing instructions
F instructions de fabrication
S prescripciones de fabricación

heteroploide Zellkultur
E heteroploid cell culture
F culture de cellules hétéroploïde
S cultivo celular heteroploide

heterozyklisch
E heterocyclic
F hétérocyclique
S heterocíclico

Hilfsstoff
E excipient, adjuvant
F excipient, adjuvant
S excipiente, sustancia auxiliar

hitzebeständig
E heat-resistant
F résistant à la chaleur
S resistente al calor

Hitzedrahtanemometer
E hot-wire anemometer
F anémomètre à résistance électrique
S anemómetro de resistencia eléctrica

Hitzedurchdringungstest
E heat penetration test
F essai de pénétration thermique
S prueba de penetración térmica

hitzeempfindlich
E heat-sensitive
F sensible à la chaleur
S sensible al calor

hitzelabil
E heat-labile
F sensible à la chaleur
S lábil al calor

hitzestabil
E heat-stable
F stable à la chaleur
S estable al calor

Hitzesterilisation
E heat sterilisation
F stérilisation à la chaleur
S esterilización al calor

Hitzetunnel
E tunnel steriliser
F tunnel de stérilisation
S túnel de esterilización

Hitzeverteilung
E heat distribution
F distribution de chaleur
S distribución del calor

hoch dosiert
E highly dosed
F à haute dose
S altamente dosificado

hochauflösend
E high-resolution
F haute-résolution
S de alta resolución

Hochdruckflüssigkeitschromatographie
E high pressure liquid chromatography (HPLC)
F chromatographie liquide sous haute pression
S cromatografía líquida a alta presión

Hochgeschwindigkeitstablettenpresse
E high-speed tabletting press
F presse à comprimés haute vitesse
S prensa de alta velocidad

hochglanzpoliert
E highly polished
F poli-miroir
S muy pulido

English
German
French
Spanish

English German French Spanish

hochinfektiöses Material
E highly infectious material
F matière hautement infectieuse
S material muy infeccioso

Hochleistungs-
E high performance
F haute performance
S gran rendimiento

Hochleistungspresse
E high-speed press
F presse rapide
S prensa rápida

Hochleistungsschwebstoffilter
E high efficiency particulate air (HEPA) filter
F filtre antipoussières à haute performance
S filtro antipolvo de gran rendimiento

Hochregallager
E high-bay storage
F étagère de stockage
S almacén de estanterías altas

hochreines Wasser
E ultrapure water
F eau ultra pure
S agua ultrapurificada

Höchstdosis
E maximum dosage
F dose maximale
S dosis máxima

Höchstgeschwindigkeit
E maximum speed
F vitesse maximale
S velocidad máxima

Höchstgewicht
E maximum weight
F poids maximum
S peso máximo

Höchstlast
E maximum load
F charge maximale
S carga máxima

hochwirksam
E highly potent, highly effective
F très efficace
S muy eficaz

Höhe
E height
F hauteur
S altura

höhenverstellbar
E height-adjustable
F à hauteur ajustable
S de altura regulable

hohl
E hollow
F creux
S hueco

Hohlkehle
E recess
F moulure creuse
S canal, garganta, media caña

Hohlkehlsockel
E fluted skirting
F plinthe à gorge arrondie
S rodapié en forma de garganta

Hohlkörper
E hollow article, hollow body
F corps creux
S cuerpo hueco

Hohlraum
E cavity, hollow space
F cavité, espace creux
S cavidad, espacio hueco

Holzkiste
E wooden case
F caisse en bois
S caja de madera

Holzpalette
E wooden pallet
F palette en bois
S paleta de madera

homogen
E homogeneous
F homogène
S homogéneo

Homogenisator
E homogeniser
F homogénéiseur
S homogenizador

homogenisieren
E homogenise, to
F homogénéiser
S homogenizar

Homogenität
E homogeneity
F homogénéité
S homogeneidad

homolog
E homologous
F homologue
S homólogo

homöopathische Erzeugnisse
E homeopathic products
F produits homéopathiques
S productos homeopáticos

Hordenblech
E tray
F plateau
S bandeja

Hordentrockenschrank
E tray dryer
F dessicateur à plateaux, dessicateur à claies
S armario de secado en bandeja

Hordentrocknung
E tray drying
F dessication sur claies
S secado en bandeja

Horizontalelektrophorese
E horizontal electrophoresis
F électrophorèse horizontale
S electroforesis horizontal

Hosenrohr
E Y-duct
F tube en Y
S tubo en Y

HPLC-Pumpe
E HPLC pump
F pompe HPLC
S bomba de HPLC

Hub
E stroke
F course de piston
S carrera del émbolo

Hubvolumen
E stroke volume
F volume de course
S volumen de carrera del émbolo

Hubvorrichtung
E lifting device
F appareillage élévateur
S dispositivo elevador

Hubwagen
E lifting truck
F chariot élévateur
S carro elevador

Hülle
E sheath, bush
F douille, coussinet, manchon
S envoltura

Hülse
E sleeve
F douille, coussinet, manchon
S cápsula, cáscara

Hustensaft
E cough syrup
F sirop contre la toux
S jarabe antitusígeno

Hustentropfen
E cough drops
F gouttes antitussives
S gotas antitusivas

English
German
French
Spanish

Hydrat
E hydrate
F hydrate
S hidrato

Hydrogenierung
E hydrogenation
F hydrogénation
S hidrogenación

Hydrolyse
E hydrolysis
F hydrolyse
S hidrólisis

partielle Hydrolyse
E partial hydrolysis
F hydrolyse partielle
S hidrólisis parcial

hydrolytischer Grad
E hydrolytic grade
F degré hydrolytique
S grado hidrolítico

hydrophil
E hydrophilic
F hydrophile
S hidrófilo

hydrophob
E hydrophobic
F hydrophobe
S hidrófobo

Hydroxylzahl
E hydroxyl number
F indice d'hydroxyle
S índice hidroxílico

Hygieneplan
E sanitation programme
F programme sanitaire
S plan higiénico, programa sanitario

Hygienezone
E hygienic area
F zone d'hygiène
S área higiénica

Hygrometer
E hygrometer
F hygromètre
S higrómetro

hygroskopisch
E hygroscopic
F hygroscopique
S higroscópico

Hygroskopizität
E hygroscopicity
F hygroscopie
S higroscopicidad

hypertonisch
E hypertonic
F hypertonique
S hipertónico

hypotonisch
E hypotonic
F hypotonique
S hipotónico

Identifikation
E identification
F identification
S identificación

Identität
E identity
F identité
S identidad

Identitätsprüfung
E identity test
F test d'identité
S prueba de identidad

Immunelektrophorese
E immune electrophoresis
F immunoélectrophorèse
S inmunoelectroforesis

immunologisch
E immunological
F immunologique
S inmunológico

Impfkristall
E seed crystal
F germe cristallin
S cristal de sembrado

Impföse
E inoculating loop
F oeillet d'inoculation
S ojal de inoculación

Impfstoff
E vaccine
F vaccin
S vacuna

Implantat
E implant
F implant
S implantado

Implantatinjektor
E implanter
F injecteur d'implant
S inyector de implantados

implementieren
E implement, to
F implémenter, établir
S establecer, realizar

imprägnieren
E soak, to; impregnate, to
F imprégner
S embeber, empapar, impregnar

Impulsgeber
E pulse generator
F générateur d'impulsions
S generador de impulsos

inaktiviert
E inactivated
F inactivées
S inactivado

Inaktivierung
E inactivation, deactivation
F inactivation
S inactivación

Inaktivierungsgefäß
E inactivation vessel
F récipient servant à l'inactivation
S recipiente de inactivación

Inaktivierungsmittel
E inactivation agent
F agent d'inactivation
S agente inactivador

Inbetriebnahme
E start-up
F mise en service
S puesta en marcha,
puesta en servicio

Inbusschlüssel
E Allen key
F clé BTR
S llave hexagonal

Inbusschraube
E Allen screw
F vis à six pans creux femelle
S tornillo hexagonal

Indikator
E indicator
F indicateur
S indicador

Indikatorkeim
E indicator organism
F organisme indicateur
S germen indicador

inert
E inert
F inerte
S inerte

Inertbegasung
E inert gas purging
F purge au gaz rare
S purga con gases inertes

infektiös
E infectious
F infectieux
S infeccioso

English German French Spanish

Infrarotstrahlung
E infrared radiation
F rayonnement infrarouge
S radiación infrarroja

Infus
E infusion
F infusion
S infusión

Infusionsbesteck
E infusion assembly
F nécessaire pour infusion
S instrumental de infusión

Infusionslösung
E infusion solution
F solution de perfusion
S solución de infusión

Ingenieur
E engineer
F ingénieur
S ingeniero

Ingenieurwesen
E engineering
F ingénieurie
S ingeniería

Inhalation
E inhalation
F inhalation
S inhalación

Inhalt
E content
F contenu
S contenido

inhärente Ungenauigkeit (z. B. einer Technik)
E inherent uncertainty (e. g. of a technique)
F imprécision inhérente (par ex. d'une technologie)
S inexactitud inherente (p. ej. de una técnica)

Initiierung (einer Reaktion)
E initiation (of a reaction)
F initiation (d'une réaction)
S iniciación (de una reacción)

Injektionsflasche
E injection vial
F flacon d'injection
S vial de inyección

Injektionslösung
E injection solution
F solution injectable
S solución inyectable

Injektionsnadel
E injection needle
F aiguille pour injection
S aguja de inyección

Injektionsspitze
E injection tip
F pointe d'injection
S punta de jeringa

Injektionsspritze
E injection syringe
F seringue d'injection
S jeringuilla

Injektor, automatischer
E automatic injector
F injecteur automatique
S inyector automático

injizierbar
E injectible
F injectable
S inyectable

injizieren
E inject, to
F injecter
S inyectar

inkompatibel
E incompatible
F incompatible
S incompatible

Inkompatibilität
E incompatibility
F incompatibilité
S incompatibilidad

Inkubationsdauer
E period of incubation
F période d'incubation
S período de incubación

Inkubationsraum
E incubation room
F chambre d'incubation
S cámara de incubación

inkubieren
E incubate, to
F incuber
S incubar

Innenbeutel
E internal bag
F poche intérieure
S bolsa interior

Innendruck
E internal pressure
F pression interne
S presión interna

Innenlack
E internal lacquer
F laque interne
S barniz interno

Innenlackierung
E internal lacquer
F vernissage interne
S barnizado interno

Innenmaß
E internal dimension
F dimension interne
S dimensión interna

Innenschutzlack
E internal protective lacquer
F laque interne de protection
S barniz protector interno

innovativ
E innovative
F innovant
S innovador

Inokulation
E inoculation
F inoculation
S inoculación

In-Prozeß-Kontrolle
E in-process control (IPC)
F contrôle lors de la fabrication
S control durante el proceso

Insektenbefall
E insect infestation
F invasion d'insectes
S infestación con insectos

Insektenfalle
E insect trap
F piège à insectes
S trampa de insectos

Insektizid
E insecticide
F insecticide
S insecticida

insektizid
E insecticide
F insecticide
S insecticida

in-situ
E in-situ
F in situ
S in situ

In-situ-Dämpfen
E in-situ sterilisation
F stérilisation in situ
S esterilización in situ

Inspektion
E inspection
F inspection
S inspección

Inspektorat
E inspectorate
F inspection (entité admin.)
S inspectoría

English German French Spanish

English German French Spanish

Installation
E installation
F installation
S instalación

Installation vor Ort
E on-site installation
F installation sur site
S instalación in situ

Installationskosten
E installation costs
F coûts d'une installation
S costes de instalación

Installationsqualifizierung
E installation qualification
F qualification de l'installation
S cualificación de una instalación

Instandhaltung
E maintenance
F entretien
S mantenimiento

Instandsetzung
E repair
F réparation
S reparaciones

instrumenteller Aufbau
E instrument set-up
F montage des instruments
S montaje de instrumentos

Instrumententafel
E instrument panel
F tableau d'instruments
S tablero de instrumentos

intakt
E intact, sound
F intact
S intacto

Integrität
E integrity
F intégrité
S integridad

Integritätsprüfung
E integrity testing
F test d'intégrité
S prueba de integridad

Integritätstest
E integrity test
F test d'intégrité
S prueba (test) de integridad

intellektuelles Eigentum
E intellectual property
F propriété intellectuelle
S propiedad intelectual

Interferenz
E interference
F interférence
S interferencia

interferierende Banden
E interfering bands
F bandes d'interférence
S bandas de interferencia

interner Standard
E internal standard
F étalon interne
S estándar interno

internes Audit
E internal audit
F audit interne
S auditoría interna

Inverkehrbringen
E placing on the market
F introduction sur le marché
S introducción en el mercado

Investitionskosten
E investment costs
F coûts d'investissements
S costes de inversión

In-vitro-Diagnose
E in-vitro diagnosis
F diagnostic in-vitro
S diagnóstico in vitro

In-vitro-Freisetzung
E in-vitro release
F libération in-vitro
S liberación in vitro

In-vitro-Freisetzungsrate
E in-vitro release rate
F vitesse de libération in-vitro
S tasa de liberación in vitro

Iodzahl
E iodine number
F indice d'iode, nombre d'iode
S índice de iodo

Iodzahlkolben
E iodine flask
F flacon d'iode
S matraz de índice de iodo

Ion, geladenes
E charged ion
F ion chargé
S ion cargado

Ionenausschlußchromatographie
E ion exclusion chromatography
F chromatographie d'exclusion ionique
S cromatografía de exclusión iónica

Ionenaustausch
E ion exchange
F échange d'ions
S intercambio de iones

Ionenaustauschchromatographie
E ion exchange chromatography
F chromatographie par échange d'ions
S cromatografía de intercambio iónico

Ionenaustauscher
E ion exchanger
F échangeur d'ions
S intercambiador de iones

Ionenpaarchromatographie
E ion pair chromatography
F chromatographie par paires d'ions
S cromatografía de pares de iones

Ionisierung
E ionisation
F ionisation
S ionización

IR-Fingerabdruck
E IR fingerprint
F empreinte digitale IR
S huella dactilar IR

IR-Spektroskopie
E IR spectroscopy
F spectroscopie IR
S espectroscopia IR

IR-Spektrum
E IR spectrum
F spectre infrarouge
S espectro infrarrojo

isokratisch
E isocratic
F isocratique
S isocrático

Isolator
E glove box, isolator
F isolateur
S aislante

Isolierschicht
E insulating layer
F couche d'isolation
S capa aislante

Isolierung
E insulation
F isolation
S aislamiento

isoton
E isotonic
F isotonique
S isotónico

ISO-zertifiziert
E ISO-certificated
F certifié ISO
S ISO-certificado

English German French Spanish

Istwert
E actual value
F valeur actuelle
S valor real

jährlicher Produktbericht
E annual product report
F rapport annuel de production
S informe anual de producción

Joch
E yoke
F bras de levier
S brazo de horquilla

justieren
E adjust, to
F étalonner
S ajustar

Justierschraube
E adjusting screw
F vis de mise au point
S tornillo de ajuste

Justierung
E alignment, adjustment
F étalonnement
S ajuste

Kabel
E cable
F câble
S cable

Kabelkanal
E cable duct
F canal de câbles
S canal de cables

Kabelklemme
E cable terminal
F serre-fils
S terminal de cable

Kabelschelle
E cable clamp
F serre-fils
S abrazadera de cable

Kabelschuh
E cable lug
F cosse de câble
S terminal de cable

kalibrieren
E calibrate, to
F calibrer
S calibrar

Kalibrierintervall
E calibration interval
F intervalle de calibration
S intervalo de calibración

Kalibrierkurve
E calibration curve
F courbe de calibration
S curva de calibración

Kalibrierlabor, akkreditiertes
E accredited calibration laboratory
F laboratoire d'étalonnage homologué
S laboratorio acreditado de calibración

Kalibrierschein
E calibration certificate
F certificat de calibration
S certificado de calibración

Kalibrierung
E calibration
F calibration
S calibración

Ein-Punkt-Kalibrierung
E single point calibration
F calibration par un point de mesure
S calibración por punto único

Kalibrierung anhand mehrerer Meßpunkte
E multiple point calibration
F calibration par points de mesure multiples
S calibración por varios puntos

Kalorimeter
E calorimeter
F calorimètre
S calorímetro

Kälteerzeugung
E refrigeration
F réfrigération
S refrigeración

kältester Punkt (beim Autoklav)
E coldest spot (autoclave)
F point le plus froid (autoclave)
S punto más frío (en autoclave)

Kammer
E chamber
F chambre
S cámara

Kampagne
E campaign
F campagne
S campaña

Kanal
E duct, channel
F canal, canalisation, voie
S canal, tubo, conducto

Kanalnetz
E duct network, ducting
F système de canalisation
S red de canales

Kantine
E canteen
F cantine
S cantina

Kanüle
E cannula, injection needle
F canule
S cánula

Kapazität
E capacity
F capacité
S capacidad

Kapillare
E capillary
F capillaire
S capilar

Kapillarelektrophorese
E capillary electrophoresis
F électrophorèse capillaire
S electroforesis capilar

Kapsel
E capsule
F capsule
S cápsula

Kapselfüllmaschine
E capsule filling machine
F encapsuleuse
S máquina de relleno de cápsulas

Kapselgröße
E capsule size
F taille d'une capsule
S tamaño de una cápsula

Kapselhülse
E capsule shell
F gousse d'une capsule
S cubierta de una cápsula

Kapselmaschine
E encapsulator
F encapsuleuse
S máquina encapsuladora

Karbonstahl
E carbon steel
F acier au carbone
S acero al carbono

Karl-Fischer-Lösung
E Karl Fischer reagent
F réactif de Karl Fischer
S reactivo de Karl Fischer

Karton
E carton
F carton
S cartón

kartonieren
E carton, to
F cartonner
S encartonar

Kartonierer
E cartoning machine
F machine à cartonner
S máquina encartonadora

Kartoniertechnik
E cartoning technology
F technique d'encartonnage
S técnica de encartonar

Kartonierteil
E cartoning section
F aire d'encartonnage
S área de encartonamiento

Kartusche
E cartridge
F cartouche
S cartucho

karzinogen
E carcinogenic
F carcinogène, cancérogène
S carcinógeno

Katalysator
E catalyst
F catalyseur
S catalizador

Katheter
E catheter
F cathéter, sonde
S catéter

Kathode
E cathode
F cathode
S cátodo

Kation
E cation
F cation
S catión

Kationenchromatographie
E cation chromatography
F chromatographie sur résine échangeuse de cations
S cromatografía de cationes

Kationentauscher
E cation exchanger
F échangeur de cations
S intercambiador de cationes

kaufen
E purchase, to
F acheter, acquérir
S comprar

Kaufpreis
E purchase cost
F prix d'achat
S precio de compra

Kaugummi, medizinisches
E medicated chewing gum
F chewing-gum médicamenté
S goma de mascar medicamentosa

Kautablette
E chewing tablet
F comprimé à mâcher
S comprimidos masticables

Kegel
E cone
F cône
S cono

kegelförmig
E conical
F conique
S cónico

Kegelstumpf
E truncated cone
F troncature d'un cône
S tronco de cono

Keilriemen
E fan belt
F courroie trapézoïdale
S correa trapezoidal

Keilriemenantrieb
E belt drive
F entraînement par courroie trapézoïdale
S propulsión por correa trapezoidal

Keim
E organism
F germe, organisme microbien
S germen

Keimbelastung
E bioburden
F teneur en micro-organismes
S carga de gérmenes

Keimdifferenzierung
E microbial differentiation
F différentiation microbienne
S diferenciación de gérmenes

keimfrei
E sterile
F stérile
S estéril

Keimgehalt
E bacterial (microbial) content
F teneur en micro-organismes
S contenido en gérmenes

Keimreduktion
E microbial reduction
F réduction microbienne
S reducción de gérmenes

Keimzahl
E microbial count
F nombre de micro-organismes
S número de gérmenes

Keimzahlbestimmung
E microbial count determination
F détermination du nombre de micro-organismes
S recuento de gérmenes

Kennlinie
E curve
F caractéristique
S característica

kennzeichnen
E mark, to; label, to
F étiqueter, marquer
S etiquetar, marcar

Kennzeichnung
E labelling
F étiquetage, marquage
S etiquetado, marcado

Kerbe
E notch
F fente, gorge
S muesca

Kern
E nucleus
F noyau
S núcleo

Kernresonanzspektroskopie
E nuclear magnetic resonance (NMR) spectroscopy
F spectroscopie nucléaire à résonance magnétique
S espectroscopia de resonancia nuclear

Kessel
E vessel, boiler
F chaudière, bouilloire
S caldera, marmita

Kettenantrieb
E chain drive
F entraînement par chaînes
S propulsión por cadena

Kiesbettfilter
E gravel filter
F filtre de graviers
S filtro de grava

Kieselgel
E silica gel
F gel de silice
S gel de sílice

Kieselsäure
E silicic acid
F silice, acide silicique
S ácido silícico

kindersicher
E child-proof
F inaccessible aux enfants
S inaccesible para niños

English German French Spanish

Kinetik
E kinetics
F cinétique
S cinética

kinetische Reaktion
E kinetic reaction
F réaction cinétique
S reacción cinética

kippen
E tilt, to
F basculer
S verter, volcar

Kippschalter-Kontrollen
E lever switch controls
F interrupteurs à bascule
S controles de interruptor unipolar

Kippvorrichtung
E tilting device
F dispositif de basculement
S dispositivo basculante

Kittel
E lab coat, gown
F blouse
S bata

Klammer
E clamp
F pinces
S pinzas

Klappe
E flap
F clapet, volet
S tapa, válvula

Klappensteller
E flap positioner
F positionneur de clapet
S posicionador de válvulas

Klappensteuerung
E flap control
F guidage de clapet
S control de las válvulas

klar
E clear, transparent
F transparent
S claro, transparente

Kläranlage
E waste water treatment plant
F station d'épuration
S estación depuradora

Klarheit
E clarity
F clareté
S claridad

Klarsichtfolie
E transparent foil
F feuille transparente
S lámina transparente, película transparente

klassieren
E classify, to
F classifier
S clasificar, ordenar

Klebeband
E adhesive tape
F bande adhésive
S cinta adhesiva

Klebefolie
E adhesive film
F film adhésif
S película adhesiva

Klebekraft
E adhesive strength
F force d'adhérence
S fuerza adhesiva

kleben (bei Tabletten)
E adhere, to; stick, to (tablets); glue, to
F adhérer (comprimés), coller
S adherir (comprimidos), encolar, pegar

Kleber
E adhesive, glue
F colle
S sustancia adhesiva

Klebestelle
E splice point
F aire de collage
S zona de adherencia

Klebestellenerkennung
E splice recognition
F identification de l'aire de collage
S reconocimiento de la zona de adherencia

klebrig
E sticky, tacky
F collant, gluant
S pegajoso

Klemme
E terminal
F pince, borne
S borne, pinza, terminal

Klemmkasten
E terminal box
F boîte de bornes
S caja de terminales

Klettererverdampfer
E rising film evaporator
F évaporateur Kestner
S evaporador Kestner

Klimaanlage
E air conditioner
F appareil de climatisation
S aire acondicionado

Klimaprüfkammer
E climatic chamber
F chambre de climatisation
S cámara de aclimat(iz)ación

klimatisiert
E air-conditioned
F air conditionné
S climatizado

Klimatisierung
E air-conditioning
F climatisation
S climatizador

Klinikpackung
E hospital pack
F conditionnement pour hôpitaux
S embalaje para clínica

klinische Forschung
E clinical research
F recherche clinique
S investigación clínica

klinische Prüfeinrichtung
E clinical trial location
F emplacement des essais cliniques
S centro de investigación clínica

klinische Prüfung
E clinical trial
F essai clinique
S ensayo clínico

zur klinischen Prüfung bestimmt
E for clinical trial use
F réservé aux essais cliniques
S reservado para ensayos clínicos

klinisches Prüfmuster
E clinical trial sample
F échantillon clinique
S muestra para ensayos clínicos

Klinke
E latch, door handle
F loquet, poignée de porte
S picaporte, gatillo, trinquete

Klischee
E printing block
F cliché
S cliché

Klistier
E enema
F lavement
S enema, lavativa

Klonierung
E cloning
F clonage
S clonación

English German French Spanish

kneten
E knead, to
F pétrir, malaxer
S amasar

Knickechtheit
E resistance to bending
F résistance à la plicature
S resistencia al pandeo

knicken
E bend, to; buckle, to
F casser, couder
S doblar, quebrar

Knierohr
E pipe bend
F tuyau coudé
S tubo acodado

Koagulation
E coagulation
F coagulation
S coagulación

Koaleszenzfilter
E coalescing filter
F filtre coalescent
S filtro de coalescencia

Kochsalzlösung
E saline solution
F solution saline
S solución salina

Kochsalzlösung, physiologische
E physiological saline
F solution saline physiologique
S solución salina fisiológica

Koenzym
E coenzyme
F coenzyme
S coenzima

kohärent
E coherent
F cohérent
S coherente

Kohäsion
E cohesion
F cohésion
S cohesión

Kohäsionskraft
E cohesive power
F force de cohésion
S fuerza de cohesión

Kohle
E carbon
F carbone
S carbón

Kohlefilter
E carbon filter
F filtre au carbone
S filtro de carbón

Kohlendioxyd
E carbon dioxide
F dioxyde de carbone
S anhídrido carbónico

Kohlenhydrate
E carbohydrates
F hydrates de carbone, glucides
S hidratos de carbono

Kohlenstoff, gesamtorganischer
E total organic carbon (TOC)
F teneur totale en carbone organique
S contenido total en carbono orgánico

Kohlenstoffkette
E carbon chain
F chaîne carbonée
S cadena carbonada

Kohlenwasserstoff
E hydrocarbon
F composé hydrocarboné
S hidrocarburo

Kolben (Glasgefäß)
E flask
F ballon, flacon
S alambique, matraz, retorta

Kolben (technisch)
E piston
F piston
S émbolo, pistón

Kolbenantrieb
E piston drive
F entraînement par piston
S propulsión por émbolo

Kolbenstange
E piston rod
F tige de piston
S barra del émbolo

Kolbenweg
E stroke
F course de piston
S carrera del émbolo

kolieren
E filter, to
F filtrer
S filtrar

Kolloiddispersion
E colloidal dispersion
F dispersion colloïdale
S dispersión coloidal

koloniebildende Einheit (KBE)
E colony-forming unit (CFU)
F unité formant colonie
S unidad formadora de colonias

Kolonne
E column
F colonne
S columna

Kompaktanlage
E compact line
F appareillage compact
S instalación compacta

Kompaktierer
E compactor
F compacteur
S compactador

kompatibel
E compatible
F compatible
S compatible

Kompatibilität
E compatibility
F compatibilité
S compatibilidad

Komplexbildner
E complex former
F substance complexante
S agente secuestrante

Komplexbildung
E complex formation
F formation de complexes
S secuestración

Komplexiermittel
E chelating agent
F agent chélatant
S agente quelante

Kompresse
E compress
F compresse
S compresa

komprimierte Gase
E compressed gases
F gaz comprimés
S gases comprimidos

Kondensat
E condensate
F condensat
S condensado

Kondensation
E condensation
F condensation
S condensación

Kondensator
E condenser
F condenseur
S condensador

English
German
French
Spanish

Kondenswasser
E condense water
F eau condensée
S agua condensada

konfektionieren
E package, to
F emballer
S embalar, empaquetar, envasar

Konfektionierung
E packaging
F conditionnement
S envasado

konfigurierbare Software
E configurable software
F logiciel configurable
S software configurable

Konformationsisomere
E conformation isomers
F isomères de conformation
S isómeros de conformación

Konformität
E conformity
F conformité
S conformidad

Konformitätssicherung
E conformity assurance
F assurance de conformité
S aseguramiento de conformidad

Konformitätszertifikat
E certificate of conformity
F certificat de conformité
S certificado de conformidad

konisch
E tapered, conical
F conique
S disminuido, estrechado, cónico

konischer Abschirmer
E conical screener
F protection cônique
S protector cónico

Konizität
E conicalness, conicity
F amincissement
S disminución, estrechamiento, conicidad

konkav
E concave
F concave
S cóncavo

konservieren
E preserve, to
F conserver
S conservar

konserviert
E preserved
F conservé
S conservado

Konservierung
E preservation
F conservation
S conservación

Konservierungsmittel
E preservative, anti-microbial agent
F conservateur
S medio de conservación

Konservierungsmittelbelastungstest
E anti-microbial effectiveness test
F test d'efficacité anti-microbien
S prueba de eficacia antimicrobiana

Konsistenz
E consistency
F consistance
S consistencia

Kontaktzeit
E contact time
F temps de contact
S tiempo de contacto

Kontaminanten, mikrobielle
E microbial contaminants
F contaminants microbiens
S contaminantes microbianos

Kontamination, aus der Luft stammende
E airborne contamination
F contamination transportée par l'air, contamination aéroportée
S contaminación procedente del aire

Kontaminationsgrad
E contamination level
F niveau de contamination
S grado de contaminación

Kontaminationsprofil (eines Produktes)
E contamination profile (of a product)
F profil de contamination (d'un produit)
S perfil de contaminación (de un producto)

kontaminieren
E contaminate, to
F contaminer
S contaminar

kontaminierende Stoffe
E contaminants
F contaminants
S sustancias contaminantes

kontaminiert
E contaminated
F contaminé
S contaminado

kontinuierliche Kultur
E continuous culture
F culture en continu
S cultivo continuo

Kontraindikation
E contraindication
F contre-indication
S contraindicación

kontraindiziert
E contraindicated
F contre-indiqué
S contraindicado

Kontrastmittel
E contrast medium
F substance de contraste
S medio de contraste

Kontrolle
E control, check
F contrôle
S control

mikrobielle Kontrolle
E microbial control
F contrôle microbien
S control microbiano

optische Kontrolle
E visual control
F contrôle visuel
S control óptico, control visual

Kontrolleiter
E head of quality control
F responsable du contrôle-qualité
S director de control

kontrollierte Freisetzung
E controlled release
F libération contrôlée
S liberación controlada

kontrollierter Zugang
E controlled access
F accès contrôlé
S acceso controlado

kontrollierter Zugangsbereich
E controlled access area
F zone d'accès contrôlé
S zona de acceso controlado

Kontrollinstrumentierung
E control instrumentation
F instruments de contrôle
S instrumentos de control

Kontrollwaage
E control balance
F balance de contrôle
S báscula de control

Konus
E cone
F cône
S cono

konvex
E convex
F convexe
S convexo

Konzentration
E concentration
F concentration
S concentración

Konzern
E company, concern
F compagnie, consortium
S consorcio

Kopfbedeckung
E head covering, headgear
F bonnet
S sombrero

Kopfhaube
E head covering, cap
F bonnet
S capucha, cofia

Kopfraum
E head space
F espace de tête
S espacio para la cabeza

Korbeinsatz für Autoklaven
E autoclave basket
F corbeille d'autoclave
S cesto para autoclave

Korbgerät
E basket apparatus
F appareil à corbeille
S aparato de cesto

Korngröße
E particle size
F taille des particules
S tamaño del grano

Korngrößenverteilung
E particle size distribution
F distribution de la taille des particules
S distribución del tamaño de los granos

körnig
E granular
F granulaire
S granular

Körnung
E grain
F granulation
S granulación

feine Körnung
E fine particles, fine grain
F granulation fine
S granulación fina

körperliche Untersuchung
E physical inspection, physical examination
F inspection physique
S exploración física

Korrektur
E correction
F correction
S corrección

Korrekturmaßnahme
E corrective action
F action corrective
S acción correctora

korrodieren
E corrode, to
F corroder
S corroer

korrodierend
E corrosive
F corrosif
S corroyente

Korrosion
E corrosion
F corrosion
S corrosión

korrosionsanfällig
E susceptible to corrosion
F susceptible à la corrosion
S susceptible a la corrosión

korrosionsbeständig
E resistant to corrosion
F résistant à la corrosion
S resistente a la corrosión

korrosionsempfindlich
E corrodible, sensitive to corrosion
F sensible à la corrosion
S sensible a la corrosión

Kosmetika
E cosmetics
F cosmétiques
S cosméticos

Kosten, laufende
E current cost
F coûts d'exploitation
S costes de explotación

kosteneffizient
E cost-efficient
F économique
S económico

kovalent
E covalent
F covalent
S covalente

Kraft
E force
F force
S fuerza

Kraftaufnehmer
E power absorber
F absorbeur d'énergie
S absorbedor de fuerza

Kraftwerk
E power station
F centrale énergétique
S central energética

Krankheitserreger
E pathogen
F pathogène
S patógeno

krebserregend
E carcinogenic
F carcinogène, cancérogène
S canceróȩgeno

Kreisdiagramm
E pie chart
F diagramme à secteurs
S diagrama circular

Kreislauf, geschlossener
E closed loop
F circulation fermée
S circulación cerrada

Kreuzbalgregler
E cross-bellows controller
F régleur pneumatique
S regulador de fuelle cruzado

Kreuzbruchkerbe
E breaking notch
F encoche de rupture
S muesca de ruptura

Kreuzkontamination
E cross-mix, cross-contamination
F contamination croisée
S contaminación cruzada, mezcla cruzada

Kriechstrom
E leakage current
F courant de cheminement
S corriente de fuga

Kristallaufbau
E crystal structure
F structure cristalline
S estructura cristalina

Kristallgitter
E lattice
F réseau cristallin
S retículo cristalino

kristallin
E crystalline
F cristallin
S cristalino

kristallisieren
E crystallise, to
F cristalliser
S cristalizar

Kristallisierung
E crystallisation
F cristallisation
S cristalización

Kristallwasser
E water of crystallisation
F eau de cristallisation
S agua de cristalización

Kriterium
E criterion
F critère
S criterio

gemäß strengen Kriterien (z. B. Test)
E according to stringent criteria (e. g. testing)
F selon des critères sévères (par ex. un test)
S siguiendo criterios estrictos (p. ej. test)

kritische Micellkonzentration
E critical micelle concentration
F concentration critique de micelles
S concentración crítica de micelas

kritischer Parameter
E critical parameter
F paramètre critique
S parámetro crítico

kritischer Prozeß-Schritt
E critical processing step
F étape critique d'un procédé
S etapa crítica de un proceso

Kubusmischer
E cube mixer
F mélangeur en cube
S mezclador cúbico

Kuchenbildung
E caking, cake formation
F prise en masse
S cuajamiento

Kugeldruckhärte
E ball hardness
F dureté à la bille
S dureza de la bola

Kugeldüse
E ball nozzle
F buse à billes
S aplicador de bola

Kugelfallviskosimeter
E falling sphere viscosimeter
F viscosimètre à sphère descendante
S viscosímetro de esfera descendiente

Kugelgelenk
E ball + socket joint
F rotule, joint à rotule
S articulación de rótula, unión esférica

Kugelkühler
E bulb cooler
F réfrigérant à boules
S refrigerador a bolas

Kugellager
E ball bearing
F roulement à billes
S rodamiento a bolas

Kugelmühle
E ball mill, pebble mill
F broyeur à boulets
S molinillo a bolas

Kugelventil
E ball valve
F clapet à billes, soupape à billes
S válvula esférica

kühl lagern
E refrigerate, to
F réfrigérer, refroidir
S conservar frío

Kühler
E cooler, condenser
F réfrigérant
S refrigerador

Kühlflüssigkeit
E coolant
F réfrigérant
S líquido refrigerante

Kühlkette
E refrigerating chain
F chaîne de réfrigération
S cadena de refrigeración

Kühllager
E cold store, cold storage
F stockage à froid
S almacén frigorífico

Kühlmantel
E cooling jacket
F manteau de refroidissement
S camisa refrigerante

Kühlmittel
E refrigerant, coolant
F liquide de refroidissement
S medio refrigerante

Kühlraum
E cold room
F chambre froide
S cámara frigorífica

Kühlschrank
E refrigerator
F réfrigérateur
S nevera

Kühlturm
E cooling tower
F tour de refroidissement
S torre de refrigeración

Kühlwasser
E cooling water
F eau de refroidissement
S agua de refrigeración

Kühlwasserschleife
E cooling water loop
F boucle d'eau de refroidissement
S serpentín para el agua de refrigeración

Kultur, kontinuierliche
E continuous culture
F culture en continu
S cultivo continuo

Kulturbouillon
E culture broth
F bouillon de culture
S caldo de cultivo

Kulturrasen
E seed layer, culture surface
F surface de culture
S superficie de cultivo

Kunde
E customer
F client
S cliente

Kunstfaser
E artificial fibre
F fibre artificielle
S fibra artificial

Kunstharz
E synthetic resin
F résine synthétique
S resina sintética

Kunstharzestrich
E synthetic resin screed
F couche de résine synthétique
S pavimento de resina sintética

Kunststoff
E plastic, plastic material
F plastique
S plástico

Kunststoffampulle
E plastic ampoule
F ampoule en plastique
S ampolla de plástico

Kunststoffaß
E plastic barrel
F tonneau en plastique
S tonel de plástico

kunststoffbeschichtet
E plastic-coated
F revêtu de plastique
S revestido de plástico

Kunststoffbeschichtung
E plastic coating
F revêtement plastique
S revestimiento plástico

Kunststoff-Flasche
E plastic bottle
F bouteille en plastique
S botella de plástico

Kunststoffgewebe
E synthetic tissue
F tissu synthétique, tissu en plastique
S tejido sintético

Kunststoffpalette
E plastic pallet
F palette en plastique
S paleta de plástico

Kunststoffverpackung
E plastic packaging
F emballage plastique
S embalaje de plástico

Kupfer
E copper
F cuivre
S cobre

Kupplung
E coupling
F couplage
S acoplamiento, embrague

Kurzkittel
E smock
F blouse
S blusa

Kurzschluß
E short circuit
F court-circuit
S cortocircuito

Kurzzeitstabilität
E short-term stability
F stabilité à court terme
S estabilidad a corto plazo

Küvette
E cuvette, cell
F cuvette
S cubeta

Küvettenhalter
E cell mount, cell holder
F support de cuvette
S portacubetas

Küvettenwechsler
E cell changer
F échangeur de cuvette
S intercambiador de cubetas

Labor
E laboratory, lab
F laboratoire
S laboratorio

Laborant
E laboratory assistant
F assistant de laboratoire, laborantin
S asistente de laboratorio

Laborartikel
E lab ware
F matériel de laboratoire
S artículo de laboratorio

Laborinformations- und -management-System (LIMS)
E laboratory information management system (LIMS)
F système de gestion des données de laboratoire (LIMS)
S sistema de gestión de datos de laboratorio (LIMS)

Laborjournal
E laboratory notebook, log book
F cahier de laboratoire
S diario de laboratorio

Laborkittel
E lab coat, gown
F blouse de laboratoire
S bata de laboratorio

Labormaßstab
E laboratory scale
F échelle de laboratoire
S escala de laboratorio

Laborschuhe
E laboratory shoes
F chaussures de laboratoire
S calzado de laboratorio

Labortisch
E bench
F paillasse de laboratoire
S mesa de laboratorio

Lack
E lacquer, varnish
F laque, vernis
S barniz, laca

lackieren
E lacquer, to
F laquer
S barnizar, lacar

Lackiersuspension
E lacquering fluid
F suspension de laquage
S suspensión de lacado

Lackmus
E litmus
F tournesol
S litmus, tornasol

Lackmuspapier
E litmus paper
F papier de tournesol
S papel de tornasol

Lacton
E lactone
F lactone
S lactona

Lactose
E lactose
F lactose
S lactosa

Ladung (Elektrizität)
E load, charge (electricity)
F charge (électricité)
S carga (electricidad)

Lage
E location, layer
F endroit, lieu, couche, phase
S lugar, posición, situación, estrato

Lageplan
E site plan, layout
F schéma, plans du site
S plano del lugar

Lager (Maschinenteil)
E bearing (mach.)
F assise, support
S asiento, cojinete, soporte

Lager(bereich)
E warehouse, storage area
F aire d'entreposage,
aire de stockage
S almacén

Lagerbestand
E inventory, stock
F inventaire, stock
S existencias en almacén, stocks

lagerfähig
E suitable for storage
F stockable, apte à l'emmagasinage
S adecuado para almacenaje

Lagerfähigkeit
E storage stability, shelf-life
F stabilité au stockage
S capacidad de almacenamiento

Lagerhaltung
E stock management system
F système de gestion du stockage
S gestión de stocks

chaotische Lagerhaltung
E random location storage system
F entreposage non ordonné
S gestión de stocks caótica

Lagerplatz
E storage space
F espace de stockage
S lugar de almacenamiento

Lagerraum
E warehouse, storage room
F entrepôt
S almacén, depósito

Lagerregal
E shelf
F étagère de stockage, étagère d'entreposage
S estante de almacén

Lagerstabilität
E warehouse stability
F stabilité de stockage
S estabilidad de almacén

Lagertank
E holding tank, storage vessel
F récipient de stockage, cuve de stockage
S tanque depósito

Lagerung
E storage
F stockage
S almacenamiento

Vorsichtsmaßnahmen bei der Lagerung
E storage precautions
F précautions de stockage
S medidas de precaución al almacenar

Lagerungsbedingungen
E storage conditions
F conditions de stockage
S condiciones de almacenamiento

Lamelle
E lamella
F lamelle
S arandela, disco, laminilla

Lamellenbremse
E multiple disk brake
F frein à disques multiples
S freno de discos múltiples

Laminarfluß
E laminar flow
F flux laminaire
S flujo laminar

Laminarströmung
E laminar air flow
F flux d'air laminaire
S corriente laminar

laminiertes Glas
E laminated glass
F verre stratifié
S vidrio laminado

Länge
E length
F longueur
S longitud

Längenausdehnung
E linear extension
F extension longitudinale
S expansión longitudinal

langkettig
E long-chained
F à chaîne longue
S de cadena larga

längliche Tablette
E oblong tablet
F comprimé allongé
S comprimido elongado

Längsachse
E longitudinal axis
F axe longitudinal
S eje longitudinal

Langzeitstabilität
E long-term stability
F stabilité à long terme
S estabilidad a largo plazo

Langzeittherapie
E long-term therapy
F thérapie à long terme
S terapia a largo plazo

Lärmbelastung
E noise
F pollution par le bruit
S ruido

Laserdrucker
E laser printer
F imprimante à laser
S impresora de láser

Lastenheft
E user requirements, user specifications
F cahier des charges, spécifications de l'usager
S requerimientos del usuario

Lauf
E run
F cycle, opération, expérience
S ciclo, marcha, recorrido

laufend
E current
F courant
S corriente

Laufrad
E rotor, impeller
F ailette
S rueda portante, rueda de aletas

Laufradgeschwindigkeit
E impeller speed, drive speed
F vitesse de roulement, vitesse de transmission
S velocidad de revolución, velocidad de propulsión

Laufrollen
E casters
F rouleau porteur, galet de guidage, poulie de guidage
S polea, roldana

Laufwerk (Computer)
E disk drive (computer)
F minuterie, lecteur (d'un ordinateur)
S unidad (de un ordenador)

Laufzeit
E running time
F durée d'opération, durée d'un cycle
S tiempo de funcionamiento

Lauge
E alkaline solution, lye
F soude
S lejía

Lebendimpfstoff
E live vaccine
F vaccin vivant
S vacuna viva

lebensfähig
E viable
F viable
S viable

Lebensfähigkeit
E viability
F viabilité
S viabilidad

Lebensmittel
E food
F aliment, nourriture
S alimento

lebensmittelecht
E food grade
F qualité alimentaire
S calidad alimenticia

Lebenszyklus
E life cycle
F cycle de vie
S ciclo vital

Leck
E leak, leakage
F fuite
S escape

Lecktest
E leak test
F essai d'étanchéité
S prueba de escape

LED-Anzeige
E LED readout
F affichage électroluminescent
S pantalla electroluminiscente

Leergewicht
E dead weight, net weight, tare
F poids à vide
S peso en vacío, tara

Leerwert
E blank value
F valeur à blanc
S valor en blanco

Legierung
E alloy
F alliage
S aleación

Lehre
E apprenticeship
F apprentissage
S aprendizaje, enseñanza

Lehrling
E apprentice
F apprenti
S aprendiz

Leim
E glue
F colle
S cola

leimen
E glue, to
F coller
S encolar, pegar

Leistung
E capacity, performance
F performance
S rendimiento

Leistungsaufnahme
E power input
F puissance absorbée
S absorción de potencia

Leistungsqualifizierung
E performance qualification
F qualification des performances (d'un procédé)
S cualificación del rendimiento

Leistungsverbrauch
E power consumption
F consommation d'énergie
S consumo de energía

Leitblech
E baffle, deflector
F déflecteur
S deflector, disruptor

leiten
E guide, to
F diriger
S conducir, dirigir

Leiter (als Person)
E head
F directeur
S director

leitfähig
E conductive
F conducteur
S conductor

Leitfähigkeit
E conductivity
F conductivité
S conductibilidad

Leitfähigkeitsmesser
E conductivity meter, conductivity sensor
F conductimètre, capteur de conductivité
S conductímetro, sensor de conductividad

Leitfähigkeitsmeßzelle
E conductivity cell
F cellule de mesure de conductivité
S célula de medida de la conductividad

Leitlinie
E policy, guideline
F directive
S directiva

Leitsubstanz
E marker, tracer
F marqueur, traceur
S marcador

Leitsystem
E control system
F système de contrôle
S sistema de control

Leitung (Gas, Wasser)
E piping (gas, water)
F conduite (de gaz, d'eau)
S conducción, tubería (gas, agua)

Leitungswasser
E tap water
F eau du robinet
S agua corriente

Lenkrollen
E casters
F rouleau porteur, galet de guidage, poulie de guidage
S polea, roldana

lesbar
E legible
F lisible
S legible

letztes Spülwasser
E final rinse
F rinçage final
S agua del lavado final

lichtbeständig
E light-fast
F résistant à la lumière
S resistente a la luz

Lichtbeständigkeit
E light-fastness
F résistance à la lumière
S resistencia a la luz

Lichtbeugung
E diffraction
F diffraction de la lumière
S difracción luminosa

lichtdurchlässig
E translucent
F translucide
S translúcido

Lichtdurchlässigkeit
E light transmittance
F transparence
S transparencia para la luz

lichtecht
E resistant to fading
F résistant à la décoloration
S resistente a la decoloración

lichtempfindlich
E light-sensitive
F photo-sensible, sensible à la lumière
S fotosensible

Lichtquelle
E light source
F source de lumière
S fuente luminosa

Lichtschranke
E optical barrier, light barrier
F barrière optique
S barrera luminosa, barrera óptica

Lichtstreuung
E light scattering, stray light
F dispersion de la lumière
S dispersión luminosa

lichtundurchlässig
E opaque
F opaque
S opaco

Lieferant
E supplier, vendor
F fournisseur
S abastecedor, proveedor

Lieferantenqualifizierung
E supplier qualification
F qualification de fournisseur
S cualificación del abastecedor

Lieferantenstichprobe
E supplier's random sample
F échantillon fortuit du fournisseur
S muestra al azar del abastecedor

Lieferdatum
E due date, delivery date
F date de livraison
S fecha de entrega

Liefermenge
E quantity received
F quantité livrée
S cantidad suministrada

liefern
E supply, to
F fournir, livrer
S abastecer, proveer, suministrar

Lieferschein
E delivery note
F bordereau de livraison
S talón de entrega

Liefertermin
E delivery date
F date de livraison
S fecha de entrega

Lieferung
E delivery
F livraison
S entrega

Ligandenaustauschchromatographie, chirale
E chiral ligand exchange chromatography
F chromatographie par échange de ligands optiquement actifs
S cromatografía de intercambio de ligandos ópticamente activos

Linearbereich
E linear range
F intervalle linéaire
S área lineal

Linearität
E linearity
F linéarité
S linealidad

Linienabnahme (an der Verpackungslinie)
E line clearance (at a packaging line)
F ligne de dégagement (d'une chaîne de conditionnement)
S punto de descarga (de la cadena de envasado)

Liniment
E liniment
F liniment
S linimento

linksdrehend
E laevo-rotary
F lévogyre
S levógiro

linksgängig
E left-hand
F à pas gauche
S de paso izquierdo

Linse
E lens
F lentille
S lente

Lipid
E lipid
F lipide
S lípido

lipophil
E lipophilic
F lipophile
S lipófilo

lipophob
E lipophobic
F lipophobe
S lipófobo

Lizenz
E licence
F licence
S licencia

Lizenzabkommen
E licensing agreement
F contrat de licence
S acuerdo de licencia

Lochblende
E aperture, diaphragm
F diaphragme
S diafragma

Lochboden
E perforated base
F base perforée
S suelo perforado

Lochreihe
E row of perforations
F série de perforations
S serie de perforaciones

Lochstanze
E punching station
F poinçonneuse
S perforadora, punzonadora, troquel

Logbuch
E log book
F cahier de route
S cuaderno de bitácora

Logistik
E logistics
F logistique
S logística

logistische Systeme
E logistic systems
F systèmes logistiques
S sistemas logísticos

Logo
E logo
F logo
S logotipo

Lohnabpacker
E contract packager
F empaqueteur
S empaquetador comisionado

Lohnauftrag
E manufacturing contract
F contrat de fabrication
S negocio de comisión

Lohnherstellung
E contract manufacture
F fabrication par sous-traitance
S fabricación por comisión

Lohnherstellungsauftrag
E contract manufacturer order
F commande de fabrication par sous-traitance
S encargo de fabricación por comisión

Lohnverpackung
E contract packaging
F empaquetage par sous-traitance
S embalaje por comisión

Lösemedium
E dissolution medium
F milieu de dissolution
S disolvente

lösen
E dissolve, to
F dissoudre
S disolver, diluir

loses Pulver
E loose powder
F poudre en vrac
S polvo suelto

Losgröße
E batch size
F taille d'un lot
S tamaño de un lote

löslich
E soluble
F soluble
S soluble

English German French Spanish

leicht löslich
E readily soluble
F facilement soluble
S fácilmente soluble

praktisch unlöslich
E practically insoluble
F pratiquement insoluble
S prácticamente insoluble

schwer löslich
E sparingly soluble
F difficilement soluble
S difícilmente soluble

sehr leicht löslich
E very soluble
F très soluble
S muy fácilmente soluble

sehr schwer löslich
E very slightly soluble
F très difficilement soluble
S muy difícilmente soluble

unlöslich
E insoluble
F insoluble
S insoluble

wenig löslich
E slightly soluble
F peu soluble
S poco soluble

Löslichkeit
E solubility
F solubilité
S solubilidad

Lösung
E solution
F solution
S solución

gesättigte Lösung
E saturated solution
F solution saturée
S solución saturada

übersättigte Lösung
E supersaturated solution
F solution sursaturée
S solución sobresaturada

ungesättigte Lösung
E unsaturated solution
F solution non-saturée
S solución insaturada

Lösungsgeschwindigkeit
E speed of solubility
F vitesse de solubilisation
S velocidad de disolución

Lösungsherstellung
E preparation of solution
F préparation d'une solution
S preparación de una solución

Lösungsmittel
E solvent
F solvant
S solvente

anorganisches Lösungsmittel
E inorganic solvent
F solvant inorganique
S solvente inorgánico

organisches Lösungsmittel
E organic solvent
F solvant organique
S solvente orgánico

viskoses Lösungsmittel
E viscous solvent
F solvant visqueux
S solvente viscoso

Lösungsmittelabscheidung
E solvent separation
F séparation des solvants
S separación de solventes

Lösungsmittelauffangbehälter
E solvent collector
F collecteur de solvant
S colector de solvente

lösungsmittelbeständig
E solvent-resistant
F résistant aux solvants
S resistente a solventes

Lösungsmittellager
E solvent storage
F stockage de solvants
S almacén de solventes

Lösungsmittelrückgewinnung
E solvent recovery
F récupération des solvants
S recuperación de solventes

Lösungsvermittler
E solubiliser
F solubilisant
S solubilizante

Lotion
E lotion
F lotion
S loción

Luftabsauger
E suction ventilator
F ventilateur aspirant
S aspirador de aire

Luftabsaugung
E air aspiration, air exhaust system
F système d'évacuation d'air
S aspiración de aire

Luftansaugstutzen
E air suction connection port
F tubulure d'aspiration d'air
S empalme para aspiración de aire

Luftaustrittsöffnung
E air outlet
F sortie d'air
S orificio de salida del aire

Luftbefeuchter
E humidifier
F humidificateur
S humidificador de aire

Luftblase, eingeschlossene
E entrapped air bubble
F bulle d'air piégée
S burbuja de aire capturada

luftdicht
E air-tight
F étanche à l'air
S hermético, impermeable al aire

Luftdichtheit
E air tightness
F imperméabilité à l'air
S hermeticidad para el aire

Luftdruck
E air pressure
F pression d'air
S presión de aire

Luftdruckfühler
E air pressure sensor
F détecteur de pression atmosphérique
S sensor de presión atmosférica

luftdurchlässig
E permeable to air
F perméable à l'air
S permeable al aire

Luftdurchlässigkeit
E air permeability
F perméabilité à l'air
S permeabilidad al aire

Luftdurchsatz
E air throughput
F débit d'écoulement d'air
S rendimiento de aire

Lufteinschluß
E air entrapment
F inclusion d'air
S inclusión de aire

Luftfeuchtigkeit
E humidity
F humidité
S humedad del aire

relative Luftfeuchtigkeit
E relative humidity
F humidité relative
S humedad atmosférica relativa

Luftfilter
E air filter
F filtre à air
S filtro de aire

Luftführung
E air flow pattern
F modèle d'écoulement d'air
S patrón de conducción de aire

Luftgeschwindigkeit
E air velocity
F vitesse de l'air
S velocidad del aire

luftgetrocknet
E air-dried
F séché à l'air
S secado al aire

Luftkeimsammler
E microbial collector
F échantillonneur d'air
S colector de gérmenes del aire

Luftkeimzahl
E air microbial count
F nombre de micro-organismes de l'air
S número de gérmenes del aire

Luftkonvektion
E air convection
F convection de l'air
S convección de aire

Luftschacht
E air duct, air shaft
F canalisation d'air
S canalización de aire

Luftstrahl
E air jet
F jet d'air
S chorro de aire

Luftstrahlmühle
E air attrition mill, fluid energy mill
F microniseur à jet d'air
S micronizador del chorro de aire

Luftstrahlsiebung
E air sieving
F tamisage d'air
S tamizado del aire

Luftstrom
E air current
F écoulement d'air
S corriente de aire

Luftströmung
E air flow
F circulation d'air
S flujo de aire

Luftströmungsrichtung
E air flow direction
F direction de l'écoulement d'air
S dirección del flujo aéreo

Luftstromwächter
E air flow controller
F régulateur d'écoulement d'air
S controlador de la corriente de aire

luftundurchlässig
E impermeable to air
F imperméable à l'air
S impermeable al aire

Luftundurchlässigkeit
E air impermeability
F imperméabilité à l'air
S impermeabilidad al aire

Lüftungsanlage
E ventilation system
F système de ventilation
S sistema de ventilación

Luftversorgung
E air supply
F alimentation en air
S abastecimiento de aire

Luftverwirbelung
E air turbulence
F turbulence d'air
S turbulencia del aire

Luftwechsel
E air exchange
F renouvellement d'air
S renovación del aire

Luftwechselrate
E air exchange rate
F taux de renouvellement d'air
S tasa de renovación de aire

Lumineszenztaster
E luminescence scanner
F scanner à luminescence
S sensor de luminiscencia

Lupe
E magnifying glass
F loupe
S lupa

Lutschtablette
E lozenge, pastille
F pastille, tablette à sucer
S comprimido para chupar

Lyophilisat
E lyophilisate
F lyophilisat
S liofilizado

Lyophilisation
E freeze drying, lyophilisation
F lyophilisation
S liofilización

Lysat
E lysate
F lysat
S lisado

Magazin (für Ampullen)
E rack, tray
F plateau
S bandeja (para ampollas)

Magensaft
E gastric juice, gastric fluid
F suc gastrique
S jugo gástrico

magensaftresistent
E gastro-resistant
F résistant au suc gastrique
S resistente al jugo gástrico

magensaftresistent überzogen
E enteric-coated
F à enrobage entérique
S con cubierta resistente al jugo gástrico

magensaftresistentes Granulat
E gastro-resistant granules
F granules gastro-résistantes
S granulado resistente al jugo gástrico

Magnetband
E magnetic tape
F bande magnétique
S cinta magnética

Magnetkupplung
E magnetic clutch
F embrayage magnétique
S acoplamiento magnético

Magnetrührer
E magnetic stirrer
F agitateur magnétique
S agitador magnético

Magnetventil
E solenoid valve
F vanne magnétique
S válvula magnética

mahlen
E mill, to; crush, to; grind, to
F broyer
S moler

Maisstärke
E corn starch
F amidon du maïs
S almidón de maíz

Makromolekül
E macromolecule
F macro-molécule
S macromolécula

Makroporen
E macropores
F macropores
S macroporos

MAK-Wert
E MAC value
F taux de concentration maximal de travail
S valor de concentración máxima de trabajo

Mangel
E deficiency
F déficience, carence, insuffisance
S carencia, defecto, deficiencia, insuficiencia

Mängelprotokoll
E deficiency protocol
F procès-verbal des défauts
S protocolo de deficiencias

Mängelrüge
E deficiency report
F compte-rendu des insuffisances
S reclamación por vicios

Mannloch
E manhole
F trou d'homme
S registro

mannlos
E unmanned
F inoccupé
S desocupado

Manometer
E manometer
F manomètre de pression
S manómetro

Manschette
E collar
F collier, bague, anneau
S manguito

Mantelkühlung
E cooling jacket
F chemise de refroidissement
S camisa de refrigeración

Manteltablette
E laminated tablet
F comprimé multicouche
S comprimido de cubierta estratificada

manuell
E manual
F manuel
S manual

Markenname
E brand name
F nom commercial
S nombre comercial

Markteinführung
E launch
F introduction sur le marché
S introducción en el mercado

Marktzulassung
E marketing authorisation/approval
F autorisation de mise sur le marché (A.M.M.)
S autorización de (para) venta en el mercado

Maschenweite
E mesh size
F ouverture de maille
S tamaño del orificio de la malla

maschinell
E mechanical
F mécanique
S mecánico

Maschinenabdeckung
E machine cover
F couvercle de machine
S cubierta de la máquina

Maschinenausfall
E machine breakdown
F défaillance de machine
S avería de una máquina

Maschinengeschwindigkeit
E machine speed
F vitesse de machine
S velocidad de una máquina

Maschinenraum
E machine room
F salle des machines
S sala de máquinas

Maschinenstillstand
E machine stoppage
F arrêt de machine
S detención de la máquina

Maske
E mask
F masque
S máscara

maskieren
E mask, to
F masquer
S enmascarar

Maskierung
E masking
F masque
S enmascaramiento

Masse, thermische
E thermal mass
F masse thermique
S masa térmica

Maßeinheit
E unit of measurement
F unité de mesure
S unidad de medida

Maßlösung
E volumetric solution
F solution volumétrique
S solución volumétrica

Maßnahme
E measure
F mesure
S medida

Maßstab
E scale, standard
F échelle, standard
S escala, estándar, patrón

maßstabgerecht
E true to scale
F à l'échelle
S a escala

Maßstabsvergößerung (eines Verfahrens)
E scale-up (of a procedure)
F extrapolation (d'un procédé)
S aumento a escala (de un proceso)

Materialbeanspruchung
E material stress
F sollicitation du matériel
S tensión sobre el material

Materialbewegung
E material movement
F mouvement des matériaux
S movimiento de material

Materialermüdung
E material fatigue
F fatigue du matériel
S fatiga del material

Materialfluß
E material flow
F flux des matériaux
S flujo de material

Materialschleuse
E material lock
F sas réservé au matériel
S esclusa de material

Materialspezifikationen
E material specifications
F spécifications des matériaux
S especificaciones del material

Materialverschwendung
E material wastage
F gaspillage
S derroche de material

Materialverträglichkeit
E material compatibility
F compatibilité des matériaux
S compatibilidad de materiales

Materialwirtschaft
E materials handling, materials management
F manipulation des matériaux
S administración del material

Matrixdatenanalyse
E matrix data analysis
F analyse de données matricielles
S análisis de datos en matriz

Matrixdiagramm
E matrix diagram
F diagramme matriciel
S diagrama en matriz

Matrize (an der Tablettenpresse)
E die (of tabletting machine)
F matrice (d'une presse à comprimés)
S matriz (de una prensa de comprimidos)

Matrize für Mehrfachwerkzeug
E multi-bore die
F matrice pour outil multiple
S matrices para herramientas de uso múltiple

Matrizenausrichtung
E die alignment
F ajustage de la matrice
S disposición de matrices

Matrizenbohrung
E pitch die
F forure d'une matrice
S orificio de matriz

Matrizenöffnung
E die bore, die opening
F cavité de matrice, ouverture d'une matrice
S abertura de matriz

Matrizenscheibe
E die plate
F plateau d'une matrice
S disco matriz

Matrizenscheibendurchmesser
E die plate diameter
F diamètre du plateau d'une matrice
S diámetro del disco matriz

Matrizentisch
E die table
F table d'une matrice
S mesa para matriz

Matrizentischgeschwindigkeit
E die plate speed
F vitesse de la table d'une matrice
S velocidad de la mesa para matriz

Matrizentischhöhe
E die plate height
F hauteur du plateau d'une matrice
S altura de la mesa para matriz

Matrizenwand
E die wall
F paroi d'une matrice
S pared de matriz

matt
E mat
F mat
S mate

maximal zulässige Verdünnung (MZV)
E maximum valid dilution (MVD)
F dilution maximale autorisée
S dilución máxima permitida

maximale Arbeitsplatzkonzentration (MAK)
E maximum allowable concentration (MAC)
F concentration maximale de postes de travail
S concentración máxima de puestos de trabajo

Mazeration
E maceration
F macération
S maceración

Medien
E utilities
F moyens d'exploitation, moyens de production
S medios de explotación empresarial, medios de producción

Mediensterilisator
E media steriliser
F stérilisateur de milieu
S esterilizador de medios

Medikation
E medication
F médication
S medicación

Medium
E medium
F milieu
S medio

Medizinische Wissenschaft
E medical science
F science médicale
S ciencia médica

Medizinprodukt
E medical device
F produit à usage médical
S producto médico

Mehrdosenbehältnis
E multiple-dose container
F conditionnement multi-doses
S recipiente de dosis múltiple

Mehrgewicht
E excess weight
F excédent de poids
S excedente de peso

Mehrkanalschreiber
E multi-channel recorder
F enregistreur à canaux multiples
S registradora de canales múltiples

Mehrstufendestillationsanlage
E multi-stage distillation unit
F unité de distillation à plusieurs étages
S unidad de destilación a etapas múltiples

Mehrweg-
E returnable, re-usable
F réutilisable
S reutilizable

mehrwertig
E multivalent
F polyvalent
S polivalente

Mehrzweckanlage
E multi-purpose equipment
F installation technique multi-usages
S instalación de uso múltiple

Meinungsbildner
E opinion leader
F leader d'opinion
S líder de opinión

Meister (als Ausbildung)
E foreman, supervisor
F maître
S maestro

Membran
E membrane, diaphragm
F membrane
S membrana

permeable Membran
E permeable membrane
F membrane perméable
S membrana permeable

semipermeable Membran
E semi-permeable membrane
F membrane semi-perméable
S membrana semipermeable

Membranfilter
E membrane filter
F filtre à membrane, filtre microporeux
S filtro de membrana

English German French Spanish

Membranfiltration
E membrane filtration
F filtration par membrane
S filtración por membrana

Membranfläche
E membrane area
F surface de membrane
S superficie de la membrana

Membrantyp
E membrane type
F type de membrane
S tipo de membrana

Membranvakuum
E membrane vacuum
F vide à diaphragme
S vacío de membrana

Membranventil
E diaphragm valve
F vanne à membrane
S válvula de membrana

Menge
E quantity, amount
F quantité
S cantidad

menschlicher Fehler
E human error
F erreur humaine
S error humano

menügesteuert
E menu-controlled
F commandé par menu
S dirigido por minuta

Merkmal
E feature
F caractéristique, particularité
S característica

Mesoporen
E mesopores
F mésopores
S mesoporos

meßbar
E measurable
F mesurable
S medible, mensurable

Meßbecher
E graduated beaker
F coupe, gobelet
S vaso graduado

Meßbereich
E measuring range
F gamme de mesure
S zona de medición

messen
E measure, to
F mesurer
S medir

Meßfehler
E measuring error
F erreur de mesure
S error de medición

Meßgerät
E measuring instrument
F instrument de mesure
S aparato de medición

Meßgröße
E unit of measurement
F unité de mesure
S unidad de medición, dimensión

Meßkolben
E volumetric flask
F ballon gradué
S matraz graduado

Meßlehre
E gauge
F jauge
S galga, gálibo, calibre

Meßlöffel
E measuring spoon
F cuillère-mesure
S cuchara de medida

Meßmittel
E measuring device
F instrument de mesure
S dispositivo de medición

Meßpunkt
E measuring point
F point de mesure
S punto de medida

Meß-Steuer-Regel (MSR) -Technik
E measuring and control technology
F techniques de mesure, de réglage et de contrôle
S técnica de medición, regulación y control

Meßumformer
E measurement converter
F convertisseur
S convertidor de mediciones

Messung
E measurement
F mesure
S medición, medida

Meßwertaufnehmer
E transducer
F capteur, transducteur
S registrador de valores medidos, transductor

Meßzylinder, graduierter
E graduated measuring cylinder
F éprouvette graduée
S probeta graduada

Metall
E metal
F métal
S metal

Metallbruch
E metal fracture
F fracture du métal
S fractura de un metal

metallorganische Verbindung
E organo-metallic compound
F composé organo-métallique
S compuesto organometálico

Metallsuchgerät
E metal detector
F détecteur de métaux
S detector de metales

Methode
E technique, method
F technique, méthode
S técnica, método

Migration
E migration
F migration
S migración

mikrobiell
E microbial
F microbien
S microbiano

mikrobielle Kontaminanten
E microbial contaminants
F contaminants microbiens
S contaminantes microbianos

mikrobielle Kontrolle
E microbial control
F contrôle microbien
S control microbiano

mikrobielle Nebenprodukte
E microbial by-products
F produits secondaires microbiens
S productos colaterales microbianos

Mikrobiologie
E microbiology
F microbiologie
S microbiología

mikrobiologisch
E microbiological
F microbiologique
S microbiológico

Mikrofiltration
E micro-filtration
F micro-filtration
S microfiltración

Mikrofiltrationsmembran
E micro-filtration membrane
F membrane de micro-filtration
S membrana de microfiltración

mikrokristallin
E microcrystalline
F microcristallin
S microcristalino

Mikrometerschraube
E fine adjusting screw, micrometer screw
F micromètre, vis micromètre
S tornillo micrométrico

Mikronisierung
E micronisation
F micronisation
S micronización

Mikroorganismen
E microorganisms
F micro-organismes
S microorganismos

apathogene Mikroorganismen
E non-pathogenic microorganisms
F micro-organismes non-pathogènes
S microorganismos apatógenos

lebensfähige Mikroorganismen
E viable microorganisms
F micro-organismes viables
S microorganismos viables

pathogene Mikroorganismen
E pathogenic microorganisms
F micro-organismes pathogènes
S microorganismos patógenos

Mikropipettierung
E micro-pipetting
F micro-pipettage
S micropipetado

Mikroplasma
E micro-plasma
F micro-plasma
S microplasma

Mikroskop
E microscope
F microcospe
S microscopio

mikroverkapselt
E micro-encapsulated
F micro-encapsulé
S microencapsulado

Mikrowelle
E microwave
F micro-onde
S microonda

Mikrowellentrocknung
E microwave drying
F séchage à micro-ondes
S desecación por microondas

minderwertig
E inferior
F de mauvaise qualité
S de menor calidad

Mindestinhalt
E minimum contents
F contenu minimal
S contenido mínimo

mischbar
E miscible
F miscible
S miscible

nicht mischbar
E immiscible
F non miscible
S no miscible

Mischbett
E mixed bed
F lit mixe
S lecho mixto

Mischbettionentauscher
E mixed bed ion exchanger
F échangeur d'ions à lit mixte
S intercambiador de iones de lecho mixto

mischen
E blend, to; mix, to
F mélanger
S mezclar

Mischer
E blender, blending apparatus
F mélangeur, malaxeur
S mezclador

Mischer mit hohem Scherkraftanteil
E high shear mixer
F mélangeur avec forces de cisaillements importantes
S mezclador de cizallamiento intenso

Taumelmischer
E tumble blender
F mélangeur turbulent
S mezclador de turbulencia

Zwangsmischer
E forced-circulation mixer
F mélangeur excentrique
S mezclador de circulación forzada

Mischgut
E blending mixture
F mélange homogénéisé
S mezcla homogeneizada

Mischmuster
E composite sample
F échantillon mixte
S muestra mixta

Mischung
E blend, mixture
F mixture, mélange
S mezcla, mixtura

Mischungsverhältnis
E blending ratio
F dosage, proportions de mélange, titration
S proporción de mezcla

Mischzyklus
E blending cycle
F cycle de mélange
S ciclo de mezcla

Mißbrauch
E abuse
F abus
S abuso

Mitbewerber
E competitor
F compétiteur
S competidor

Mitgliedstaat
E member state
F état membre
S estado miembro

Mizellkonzentration, kritische
E critical micelle concentration
F concentration critique de micelles
S concentración micelar crítica

mm Wassersäule
E mm water
F mm de pression d'eau
S mm de presión de agua

Modifikation, chemische
E chemical modification
F modification chimique
S modificación química

modifiziert
E modified
F modifié
S modificado

Modularbauweise
E modular design
F design modulaire
S diseño modular

Mol
E mole
F mole
S mol

molar
E molar
F molaire
S molar

Molarität
E molarity
F molarité
S molaridad

molekular
E molecular
F moléculaire
S molecular

Molekularbiologie
E molecular biology
F biologie moléculaire
S biología molecular

Molekularformel
E molecular formula
F formule brute
S fórmula molecular

Molekulargewicht
E molecular weight
F poids moléculaire
S peso molecular

Molekularmodellierung
E molecular modelling
F modelage moléculaire
S modelado molecular

Molekülgröße
E molecular size
F taille moléculaire
S tamaño molecular

Mono-Anlage
E dedicated equipment
F équipement dédié
S instalación para uso único

monochrom
E monochromatic
F monochromatique
S monocromo

Monochromator
E monochromator
F monochromateur
S monocromador

monolithisches Material
E monolithic material
F matériau monolithique
S material monolítico

Monomer
E monomer
F monomère
S monómero

Montage
E assembly, mounting
F assemblage, montage
S montaje

Montagewagen
E mounting trolley
F chariot de montage
S carro de montaje

Moorzubereitung
E mud pack preparation
F préparation de tourbe
S preparación de turba

Mörser
E mortar
F mortier
S mortero

Mörtelbett
E mortar bed
F lit de mortier
S lecho de mortero

Motordrehzahl
E motor revolutions
F vitesse de rotation d'un moteur
S número de revoluciones del motor

Motorgehäuse
E motor housing
F carter d'un moteur
S cárter del motor

Motorleistung
E motor performance
F performance d'un moteur
S rendimiento de un motor

Muffe
E bush, bushing (mach.)
F manchon, collet
S manguito

Muffelofen
E muffle furnace
F four à moufle
S horno de manguito

Mühle
E mill
F broyeur
S molino

Mull
E gauze
F gaze
S gasa

Müll
E rubbish, waste
F déchets, résidus
S basura, desechos, residuos

Mullbinde
E gauze bandage
F bande de gaze
S venda de gasa

Müllverbrennung
E rubbish incineration
F incinération des déchets
S incineración de desechos

multizentrisch
E multicentric
F multicentrique
S multicéntrico

Mundschutz
E face mask
F masque de protection facial
S protección bucal

Mundspüllösung
E mouthwash
F solution pour bain de bouche
S solución de enjuague bucal

Mundstück
E mouthpiece
F embout
S boquilla, embocadura

Mündung
E orifice
F orifice
S desembocadura, orificio

Mundwasser
E mouthwash
F bain de bouche
S enjuague bucal

Muster
E sample, specimen
F échantillon, spécimen
S muestra, espécimen

unverkäufliches Muster
E sample
F échantillon
S muestra gratuita

Musterziehung
E sampling
F échantillonnage
S toma de muestras

mutagen
E mutagenic
F mutagène
S mutágeno

Mutter
E nut
F écrou
S tuerca

Mutterfirma
E parent company
F société mère
S sociedad matriz

Mutterlauge
E mother liquor
F eau mère, lessive-mère
S lejía madre

English German French Spanish

English
German
French
Spanish

Nacharbeitung
E reprocessing
F traitement complémentaire, retouche
S reprocesado, retocado

Nachbehandlung
E secondary treatment
F traitement secondaire
S tratamiento subsiguiente

Nachgeschmack
E after-taste
F arrière-goût
S regusto

Nachlauf
E tailings
F addition en bout de chaîne
S adición al final de la cadena

Nachlegestapel
E back-up stack
F empilement de réserve
S montón de reserva

Nachtrocknen
E final drying
F séchage final
S secado final

Nachuntersuchung
E subsequent test
F examen supplétif
S examen adicional

Nachweis
E detection, evidence, proof
F détection, preuve
S demostración, prueba

nachweisbar
E detectable
F détectable
S detectable

nicht nachweisbar
E undetectable
F indétectable
S no detectable

Nachweisgrenze
E limit of detection (LOD)
F limite de détection
S límite de detección

Nadellöcher
E pin holes
F perforations d'aiguille
S perforaciones de aguja

Nagetier
E rodent
F rongeur
S roedor

Nährboden
E culture medium
F milieu de culture
S medio de cultivo

Nährbouillon
E culture broth
F bouillon de culture
S caldo de cultivo

Nährlösung
E culture broth
F bouillon de culture
S solución de cultivo, solución nutritiva

Nährmedienabfüllung
E culture medium filling, media fill
F remplissage des milieux de culture
S relleno con medio de cultivo

Nährmedienherstellung
E culture media preparation
F préparation des milieux de culture
S preparación de medio de cultivo

Nährmedienküche
E culture media preparation room
F salle de préparation des milieux de culture
S sala de preparación de medios de cultivo

Nährmedium
E culture medium, nutrient medium
F milieu de culture
S medio de cultivo

Trockennährmedium
E dehydrated medium
F milieu de culture déhydraté
S medio de cultivo deshidratado

Nährstoff
E nutrient
F aliment, produit nutritif, nutriment
S alimento, nutriente, sustancia nutricia

Nahrungsergänzungsmittel
E food additive
F additif alimentaire
S aditivo alimentario

Naht
E joint, seam, weld
F couture, joint, ourlet
S costura, junta, soldadura, sutura

nahtlos
E seamless
F dépourvu de joint
S sin sutura

Nahtmaterial
E suture
F suture
S material de sutura

nahtschweißen
E seam weld, to
F souder
S soldar

Namenszeichen
E initials
F initiales
S iniciales

Napf (beim Blister)
E well, cup (of blister)
F blister, emballage à bulles
S pocillo del blíster

Nasencreme
E nasal cream
F crème nasale
S crema nasal

Nasengel
E nasal gel
F gel nasal
S gel nasal

Nasenolive
E nasal applicator
F applicateur nasal
S aplicador nasal

Nasensalbe
E nasal ointment
F pommade nasale
S pomada nasal

Nasentropfen
E nose drops
F gouttes nasales
S gotas nasales

Naßchemie
E wet chemistry
F chimie humide
S química húmeda

naßchemisch
E wet chemical
F chimique humide
S químicamente húmedo

Naßsiebung
E wet sieving
F tamisage humide
S tamizado húmedo

Naßvermahlung
E wet grinding
F broyage humide
S molido húmedo

Natronlauge
E sodium hydroxide solution
F soude
S sosa alcalina

Naturprodukt
E natural product
F produit naturel
S producto natural

English German French Spanish

Nebel
E fog
F brouillard
S niebla

Nebelgenerator
E atomiser
F atomiseur
S atomizador

Nebenbereich
E auxilary area
F zone auxiliaire
S área auxiliar

Nebenprodukt
E by-product
F sous-produit, produit secondaire
S producto colateral, producto secundario

mikrobielle Nebenprodukte
E microbial by-products
F produits secondaires microbiens
S productos colaterales microbianos

Nebenreaktion
E side reaction
F réaction secondaire
S reacción colateral

Nebenwirkung
E side effect
F effet secondaires
S efecto colateral, efecto secundario

Neigung
E slope, gradient
F pente, gradient
S inclinación, pendiente

Neigungswinkel
E angle of slope, angle of gradient
F angle de pente
S ángulo de inclinación

Nenngröße
E nominal size
F taille nominale
S tamaño nominal

Nennvolumen
E nominal volume
F volume nominal
S volumen nominal

Nennweite
E nominal width
F largeur nominale
S anchura nominal

Nennwert
E nominal value
F valeur nominale
S valor nominal

Netz
E net, grid
F grille
S red

netzförmig
E reticular, net-like
F réticulaire
S reticular

Netzgerät
E power supply
F alimentation en courant électrique
S alimentador a la red

Netzmittel
E wetting agent
F mouillant
S humectante

Netzschalter
E power switch, main switch
F interrupteur de courant
S interruptor a la red

Netzschwankungen
E power supply fluctuation
F variations de l'intensité du courant
S fluctuaciones del suministro eléctrico, fluctuaciones de la intensidad de corriente eléctrica

Netzspannung
E line voltage
F tension du secteur
S tensión de la red

Netzwerk
E network
F réseau
S malla, obra de malla, retículo

Neuheitsgrad (z. B. eines Produktes)
E novelty (e. g. of a product)
F degré d'innovation (par ex. d'un produit)
S grado de novedad (p. ej. de un producto)

Neutronenaktivierungsanalyse
E neutron activation analysis
F analyse par activation neutronique
S análisis de activación de neutrones

Nichteinhaltung
E non-compliance
F non conformité
S no observancia

nichtflüchtig
E non-volatile
F non volatile
S no volátil

nichtlinear
E non-linear
F non linéaire
S no lineal

nicht-wäßrig
E non-aqueous
F non aqueux
S no acuoso

Niederschlag
E precipitate
F précipité
S precipitado

Niederzugsschiene
E pull-down cam
F came de poinçon descendante
S carril de tracción inferior, corredera de tracción inferior

Niete (techn.)
E rivet
F rivet
S remache

Nische
E niche, recess
F niche
S nicho

Nivellierung
E levelling
F nivellement
S nivelación

Nocke
E cam
F came
S leva

Nockenwelle
E camshaft
F arbre à cames
S árbol de levas

Norm
E standard
F norme, standard
S norma

Normalität (einer Lösung)
E normality (of a solution)
F normalité (d'une solution)
S normalidad (de una disolución)

Normierung
E standardisation
F standardisation
S normalización, estandarización

Normvorschrift
E standard specification
F spécification standard
S prescripción estándar

Not-Aus
E emergency off
F arrêt d'urgence
S interruptor de emergencia

Notfall
E emergency
F urgence
S caso de urgencia

Notstromaggregat
E emergency power supply
F générateur de courant d'urgence
S generador eléctrico de emergencia

nukleasefreies Wasser
E nuclease-free water
F eau dénuée de nucléase
S agua sin nucleasas

Nukleinsäure
E nucleic acid
F acide nucléique
S ácido nucleico

nukleophile Substitution
E nucleophilic substitution
F substitution nucléophilique
S sustitución nucleófila

Nulleinstellung
E zero adjustment
F mise à zéro
S posición cero, puesta a cero

Null-Fehler-Strategie
E zero defect strategy
F stratégie zéro défaut
S estrategia de ausencia total de errores

Nullinie
E zero line
F ligne de base, ligne de zéro
S línea de base

Nullpunkt (beim Diagramm)
E zero (in diagram)
F point zéro
S punto cero (en diagrama)

Nullpunktabweichung
E zero drift
F dérive du point zero
S desviación del punto cero

Nut
E groove
F cannelure, sillon, rainure
S muesca, ranura

Nutsche
E Buchner funnel
F entonnoir de Büchner
S embudo de Buechner

Nutzungsvolumen
E effective volume
F volume effectif
S volumen efectivo

Oberfläche
E surface
F surface, aire
S superficie

glatte Oberfläche
E smooth surface
F surface polie, surface lisse
S superficie lisa

rauhe Oberfläche
E rough surface
F surface rugueuse
S superficie rugosa

spezifische Oberfläche
E specific surface area
F aire spécifique
S superficie específica

oberflächenaktive Verbindung
E surfactant, tenside
F tensioactif
S agente tensioactivo

Oberflächenaktivität
E surface activity
F activité de surface
S actividad de superficie

Oberflächenbehandlung
E surface treatment
F traitement de surface
S tratamiento de superficies

Oberflächenbeschaffenheit
E surface properties
F propriétés de surface
S características de superficie

Oberflächenbeschichtung
E surface coating
F revêtement de surface
S revestimiento de superficies

Oberflächenbindung
E surface binding
F liaison superficielle
S ligadura de superficie

Oberflächendurchmesser
E surface diameter
F diamètre d'une surface
S diámetro de una superficie

Oberflächenlackierung
E surface lacquer
F laquage superficiel
S barnizado de superficies

Oberflächenrauhigkeit
E surface rawness
F rugosité de la surface
S rugosidad de superficie

Oberflächenspannung
E surface tension
F tension superficielle
S tensión superficial

Oberseite
E upper side, top side
F face supérieure, côté supérieur
S lado superior

Oberstempel
E upper punch, top punch
F poinçon supérieur
S troquel superior

Objektlinse
E object lens
F lentille objet
S lente del objetivo

Objektträger (Mikroskopie)
E slide (microscopy)
F porte-objet (microscopie)
S portaobjetos (microscopio)

Oblate
E capsule, cachet
F capsule, cachet
S oblea, gragea

Oblatenkapsel
E cachet
F cachet
S cápsula amilácea

obligatorisch
E compulsory
F obligatoire
S obligatorio

Oblongtablette
E oblong tablet
F comprimé oblong
S comprimido oblongo

Obmann
E chairman, spokesman
F porte-parole
S portavoz, presidente

offene Flamme
E naked flame
F flamme ouverte
S llama abierta

Öffnung
E opening
F ouverture
S abertura

Ohrencreme
E ear cream
F crème auriculaire
S crema auricular

Ohrengel
E ear gel
F gel auriculaire
S gel auricular

English
German
French
Spanish

Ohrensalbe
E ear ointment
F pommade auriculaire
S pomada auricular

Ohrenspüllösung
E ear wash
F solution de lavage auriculaire
S solución de lavado auricular

Ohrentropfen
E ear drops
F gouttes auriculaires
S gotas auriculares

Okklusivverband
E occlusive dressing
F bandage d'occlusion
S vendaje oclusivo

Okular
E ocular
F occulaire
S ocular

Ölabscheidefilter
E oil-separating filter
F filtre de retenue d'huile
S filtro de separación de aceite

Ölabscheider
E oil separator, oil trap
F siphon de dépôt d'huile, séparateur d'huile, déshuileur
S separador de aceite

Ölbad
E oil bath
F bain d'huile
S baño de aceite

ölig
E oily
F huileux
S oleaginoso, oleoso

Oligomere
E oligomers
F oligomères
S oligómero

Öl-in-Wasser-Emulsion
E oil/water emulsion
F émulsion d'huile dans l'eau
S emulsión de aceite en agua

Ölwanne
E sump
F carter à huile
S cárter

Opaleszenz
E opalescence
F opalescence
S opalescencia

Ophthalmica
E ophthalmic products
F produits ophtalmiques
S productos oftálmicos

Optimierung
E optimisation
F optimisation
S optim(iz)ación

optische Antipoden
E optical antipodes
F antipodes optiques
S antípodas ópticos

optische Anzeige
E display
F indication visuelle
S señal óptica

optische Drehung
E optical rotation
F rotation optique
S rotación óptica

optische Kontrolle
E visual control
F contrôle visuel
S control óptico, control visual

optische Reinheit
E optical purity
F pureté optique
S pureza óptica

optisches Signal
E visual signal
F signal optique
S señal óptica

oral
E oral
F oral
S oral

orbital geschweißt
E orbitally welded
F soudé par soudure orbitale
S soldado orbitalmente

Orbitalschweißen
E orbital fusion welding
F soudure orbitale
S soldadura orbital

Organigramm
E organisation chart, organogram
F organigramme
S organigrama

organische Base
E organic base
F base organique
S base orgánica

organische Phase
E organic phase
F phase organique
S fase orgánica

organisches Lösungsmittel
E organic solvent
F solvant organique
S diluyente orgánico

Orginalpackung
E original package
F conditionnement d'origine
S envase original

O-Ring
E O-ring
F joint torique
S anillo tórico

Ort
E location
F endroit, lieu
S lugar, posición, situación

Ortsbesichtigung
E on-site visit
F visite sur site
S visita del lugar

Öse
E eye, eyelet
F œillet
S ojal

Osmolalität
E osmolality
F osmolalité
S osmolalidad

Osmometer
E osmometer
F osmomètre
S osmómetro

Osmose
E osmosis
F osmose
S ósmosis

osmotischer Druck
E osmotic pressure
F pression osmotique
S presión osmótica

Oszillation
E oscillation
F oscillation
S oscilación

OTC-Produkt
E over-the-counter (OTC) product
F produit sans ordonnance, produit en vente libre
S producto de venta libre

Ovalität
E ovality
F forme ovale
S ovalidad

English German French Spanish

Oxigenierung
E oxygenation
F oxygénation
S oxigenación

Oximbildung
E oximation
F oximation
S oximación

Oximierung
E oximation
F oximation
S oximación

Oxydationsmittel
E oxidising agent
F oxydant
S oxidante

oxydierbar
E oxidisable
F oxydable
S oxidable

Oxydierung
E oxidation
F oxydation
S oxidación

Ozon
E ozone
F ozone
S ozono

Ozonisierung
E ozonisation
F ozonisation, ozonation
S ozon(iz)ación

Packguteinschub
E package loading
F passage intercalé de conditionnements
S inserción de embalajes

Packhilfsmittel
E packaging aids
F auxiliaires de conditionnement
S materiales auxilares para envasado

Packmaterial
E packaging material
F matériel d'emballage
S material de embalaje

bedrucktes Packmaterial
E printed packaging material
F matériel d'emballage imprimé
S material impreso de embalaje

unbedrucktes Packmaterial
E unprinted packaging material
F conditionnement non-imprimé
S medio de envasado no impreso

Packmittel
E packaging material
F matériel d'emballage
S material de embalaje

primäres Packmittel
E primary packaging material
F conditionnement primaire
S medio de envasado primario

sekundäres Packmittel
E secondary packaging material
F conditionnement secondaire
S medio de envasado secundario

Packmittelausgabe
E packaging material dispensary
F distribution du matériel d'emballage
S distribución de material de embalaje

Packmittelhersteller
E packaging material manufacturer
F fabricant de matériel d'emballage
S fabricante de material de embalaje

Packmittel-Lager
E packaging warehouse
F magasin d'articles de conditionnement
S almacén de medios de envasado

Packung
E package, pack
F emballage, conditionnement
S embalaje, envase, envoltura

kindergesicherte Verpackung
E child-resistant pack
F conditionnement de sécurité pour enfants
S envase a prueba de niños

Packungsbeilage
E package insert, package leaflet
F notice explicative
S prospecto informativo del medicamento

vorgefaltete Packungsbeilage
E pre-folded package insert
F notice explicative dépliante
S prospecto informativo del medicamento previamente plegado

Packungsgröße
E package size
F taille de l'emballage
S tamaño del envase

Packungsstapelung
E package stacking
F empilage de conditionnement
S apilamiento de envases

Palette
E pallet
F palette
S paleta

Alupalette
E aluminium pallet
F alupalette, palette en aluminium
S paleta de aluminio

Holzpalette
E wooden pallet
F palette en bois
S paleta de madera

Kunststoffpalette
E plastic pallet
F palette en plastique
S paleta de plástico

Palettenstellplatz
E pallet store
F dépôt de palettes
S almacén para paletas

palettieren
E palletise, to
F palettiser
S cargar con paleta

Palettiermaschine
E palletiser
F palettiseur
S máquina de carga con paleta

Panne
E breakdown, failure
F panne
S avería

Papierausdruck
E paper printout, hard copy
F imprimé sur papier
S impreso (en, sobre papel)

Pappe
E pasteboard, cardboard
F carton
S cartón

lackierte Pappe
E varnished cardboard
F papier vernis
S cartón barnizado

Pappschachtel
E carton
F carton
S caja de cartón

Parallelschaltung
E parallel connection
F connection parallèle
S conexión paralela

Parameter, kritischer
E critical parameter
F paramètre critique
S parámetro crítico

Parenteralia
E parenterals
F préparations injectables
S inyectables

großvolumige Parenteralia
E large volume parenterals (LVP)
F préparations injectables de grand volume
S inyectables voluminosos

kleinvolumige Parenteralia
E small volume parenterals (SVP)
F préparations injectables de petit volume
S inyectables de escaso volumen

Partialdruck
E partial pressure
F pression partielle
S presión parcial

Partikel
E particle, particulate matter
F particule
S partícula

aus der Luft stammende Partikel
E airborne particles
F particules aéroportées
S partículas procedentes del aire

lebensfähige Partikel
E viable particles
F particules viables
S partículas viables

Partikel abgeben
E shed particles, to
F libérer des particules
S liberar partículas

partikelabgebendes Material
E particle-releasing material
F matériau libérant des particules
S material que desprende partículas

Partikelabscheiderate
E particle separation rate
F taux de retenue des particules
S tasa de separación de partículas

Partikelansammlung
E accumulation of particles
F accumulation de particules
S acumulación de partículas

Partikelerzeugung
E particle generation
F génération de particules
S producción de partículas

Partikelfilter
E particle filter
F filtre à particules
S filtro de partículas

Partikelform
E particle form
F forme d'une particule
S forma de las partículas

partikelfrei
E particle-free
F libre de particules
S sin partículas

Partikelgröße
E particle size
F taille des particules
S tamaño de las partículas

Partikelmeßgerät
E particle measuring instrument
F appareil de mesure des particules
S aparato de medición de partículas

Partikelmonitoring
E particle monitoring
F contrôle des particules
S control de partículas

Partikelverteilung
E particle distribution
F distribution des particules
S distribución de partículas

Partikelzahlen
E particle count
F nombre de particules
S número de partículas

Partikelzähler
E particle counter
F compteur de particules
S contador de partículas

passend
E suitable
F convenable
S adecuado, conveniente

Passerdifferenz
E register difference
F différence de registre
S diferencia de registro

Passerfehler
E register defect
F défaut de registre
S defecto de registro

Paßfeder (des Stempels)
E key (of punch)
F clavette, ressort d'ajustage (de poinçon)
S llave (de troquel)

passiviert
E passivated
F passivé
S pasivado

Passivierung (z. B. von Stahl)
E passivation (e. g. of steel)
F passivation (par ex. de l'acier inoxydable)
S pasivación (p. ej. de acero)

Paßwort
E password
F mot de passe
S consigna

Paste
E paste
F pâte
S pasta

Paste zum Einnehmen
E oral paste
F pâte pour utilisation orale
S pasta oral

Paste zur Anwendung auf der Haut
E cutaneous paste
F pâte pour utilisation cutanée
S pasta cutánea

pastenartig
E pasty, paste-like
F pâteux
S pastoso

Pasteurisierung
E pasteurisation
F pasteurisation
S paste(u)rización

Pastille
E pastille
F pastille
S pastilla

pastös
E pasty
F pâteux
S pastoso

Patent
E patent
F brevet
S patente

Erteilung eines Patentes
E patent approval
F approbation de brevet
S aprobación de patente

Verletzung eines Patentes
E infringement of a patent
F violation de brevet
S violación de patente

Patentamt
E patent office
F office des brevets
S oficina de patentes

Patentanmeldung
E patent filing
F dépôt de demande de brevet
S solicitud de patente

Patentanspruch
E patent claim
F droits liés à un brevet
S reclamación de patente

English German French Spanish

Patentbeantragung
E patent application
F demande de brevet
S solicitud de patente

Patenteinreichung
E patent filing
F dépôt de demande de brevet
S solicitud de patente

Patentfristerneuerung
E patent prolongation
F prorogation d'un brevet
S prolongación del plazo de patente

Patentgültigkeitsdauer
E patent duration, patent life
F durée de validité d'un brevet
S duración de la validez de una patente

patentiert
E patented
F breveté
S patentado

Patentschutz
E patent protection
F protection d'un brevet
S protección de patentes

Patentumfang
E patent scope
F étendue d'un brevet
S extensión de una patente

pathogen
E pathogenic
F pathogénique
S patógeno

Pathogene
E pathogens
F pathogènes
S agentes patógenos

pathologisch
E pathological
F pathologique
S patológico

Patient
E patient
F patient
S paciente

Patientenbroschüre
E patient information leaflet
F brochure d'information pour patient
S folleto de información del paciente

Patientennummer
E patient identification number
F numéro d'identification d'un patient
S número de identificación del paciente

Patrone
E cartridge
F cartouche
S cartucho

Patronendichtung
E cartridge gasket
F joint de cartouche
S junta de cartucho

Peak
E peak
F pic
S pico

nicht zugehöriger Peak
E extraneous peak
F pic étranger
S pico extraño

Peakbreite
E peak width
F largeur de pic
S anchura del pico

Peakfläche
E peak area
F surface de pic
S superficie del pico

Peakhöhe
E peak height
F hauteur de pic
S altura del pico

Peakreinheit
E peak purity
F pureté de pic
S pureza del pico

Peakschulter
E peak shoulder
F épaulement de pic
S hombro del pico

Peakverbreiterung
E peak spreading
F étalement de pic
S ensanchamiento del pico

Pegel
E level
F niveau
S nivel

Pegelmesser
E level sensor
F détecteur de niveau
S sensor de nivel

Pegelstand
E level
F niveau
S nivel

Peilung
E bearing
F sondage, coussinet
S sondeo

Pellet
E pellet
F pellet
S pellet

pelletieren
E pelletise, to
F pastiller, transformer en pastilles
S transformar en pellets

Penetration
E penetration
F pénétration
S penetración

Pepton
E peptone
F peptone
S peptona

perforieren
E perforate, to
F perforer
S perforar

Perforierung
E perforation
F perforation
S perforación

Perforierwerkzeug
E perforation tool
F outil de perforation
S instrumentos de perforación

periphere Geräte
E peripheral instrumentation
F appareils périphériques
S aparatos periféricos

Peritonealdialyselösung
E solution for peritoneal dialysis
F solution pour dialyse péritonéale
S diálisis peritoneal

Perkolation
E percolation
F percolation
S percolación

perkolieren
E percolate, to
F extrahir par percolation
S percolar

permanente Härte (von Wasser)
E permanent hardness (of water)
F dureté permamente (de l'eau)
S dureza permanente (del agua)

permeabel
E permeable
F perméable
S permeable

English German French Spanish

Permeabilität
E permeability
F perméabilité
S permeabilidad

permeable Membran
E permeable membrane
F membrane perméable
S membrana permeable

perorale Darreichung
E oral administration
F administration orale
S administración peroral

Peroxydzahl
E peroxide number, peroxide index
F index de peroxyde
S índice de peróxido

Personal in Schlüsselstellung
E key personnel
F personnel occupant un poste à responsabilités
S personal en posición clave

Personalabteilung
E personnel department
F service de personnel
S departamento de personal

Personalakte
E personnel file
F acte du personnel
S acta personal

Personalfluß
E personnel flow
F flux du personnel
S flujo de personal

Personalhygiene
E personnel hygiene
F hygiène du personnel
S higiene personal

Personalkosten
E personnel cost
F coûts du personnel
S costes del personal

Personalschleuse
E personnel lock
F sas réservé au personnel
S entrada para el personal

Personalschulung
E personnel training
F formation du personnel
S formación del personal

Personenschutz
E personnel safety, personnel protection
F sécurité du personnel
S seguridad del personal

Pestizid
E pesticide
F pesticide
S pesticida

Petrischale
E Petri dish
F boîte de Petri
S placa de Petri

petrochemische Substanzen
E petrochemicals
F substances pétrochimiques
S sustancias petroquímicas

Pflanzenfarbstoff
E vegetable dye
F pigment végétal
S colorante vegetal, pigmento vegetal

pflanzlich
E plant, plant-based, phyto-
F végétal
S vegetal

pflanzliches Arzneimittel
E herbal medicine
F phytopharmaceutique
S fitofármaco

Pflaster
E sticking plaster
F sparadrap
S esparadrapo

transdermales Pflaster
E transdermal patch
F pansement transcutané
S emplasto transdérmico

Pflichtenheft
E required specification
F spécifications fonctionnelles
S descripción de tareas

Pflugscharmischer
E high shear mixer
F mélangeur à forces de cisaillement
S mezclador de cizallamiento

Pharmakokinetik
E pharmacokinetics
F pharmacocinétique
S farmacocinética

Pharmakologie
E pharmacology
F pharmacologie
S farmacología

pharmakologische Aktivität
E pharmacological activity
F activité pharmacologique
S actividad farmacológica

Pharmakopöe
E pharmacopoeia
F pharmacopée
S farmacopea

Pharma-Sparte
E pharmaceutical division
F division pharmaceutique
S sector farmacéutico

Pharma-Wasser
E pharmaceutical water
F eau pharmaceutique
S agua farmacéutica

pharmazeutischer Unternehmer
E pharmaceutical manufacturer
F industriel de la pharmacie
S fabricante farmacéutico

Phase, feste
E solid phase
F phase solide
S fase sólida

Phase, flüssige
E liquid phase
F phase liquide
S fase líquida

Phase, organische
E organic phase
F phase organique
S fase orgánica

Phase, stationäre
E stationary phase
F phase stationnaire
S fase estacionaria

Phase, wäßrige
E aqueous phase
F phase aqueuse
S fase acuosa

Phasendiagramm
E phase diagram
F diagramme de phases
S diagrama de fases

Phasenübergang
E phase transition
F transition de phase
S transición de fase

Phasenverteilung
E phase distribution
F distribution de phases
S distribución de fases

pH-Meter
E pH meter
F pH-mètre
S pH metro

Phosphoreszenz
E phosphorescence
F phosphorescence
S fosforescencia

photochemisch
E photochemical
F photochimique
S fotoquímico

Photolyse
E photolysis
F photolyse
S fotólisis

Photometer
E photometer
F photomètre
S fotómetro

Photometrie
E photometry
F photométrie
S fotometría

Photozelle
E photo cell, photoelectric cell
F cellule photoélectrique
S célula fotoeléctrica

pH-Wert
E pH
F pH
S pH

pH-Wert-Einstellung
E pH adjustment
F ajustement du pH
S ajuste del pH

physikalisch-chemische Eigenschaften
E physical-chemical characteristics
F caractéristiques physico-chimiques
S propiedades fisicoquímicas

physikalische Eigenschaften
E physical characteristics
F caractéristiques physiques
S propiedades físicas

physiologische Kochsalzlösung
E physiological saline
F solution saline physiologique
S solución salina fisiológica

physiologische Prüfung
E physiological testing
F examen physiologique
S prueba fisiológica

Phytochemie
E phytochemistry
F phytochimie
S fitoquímica

Phytopharmaka
E phytopharmaceuticals, herbal medicines
F phytopharmaceutiques
S fitofármacos

piezoelektrische Zündung
E piezo ignition
F allumage piezoélectrique
S encendido piezoeléctrico

Pigment
E pigment
F pigment
S pigmento

Pille
E pill
F pilule
S píldora

pilzabtötend
E anti-fungal
F antifongique
S antifúngico, fungicida

Pilze
E fungi, moulds
F champignons
S hongos

Pinzette
E tweezers
F brucelles
S pinzas

Pipette
E pipette
F pipette
S pipeta

Pipettenflasche
E pipette bottle
F flacon de pipette
S frasco de pipeteo

Pipettenspitze
E pipette tip
F pointe de pipette
S punta de pipeta

Pipettierhilfe
E pipetting aid
F système d'aide au pipettage
S sistema de ayuda para pipetear

Pipettiersystem
E pipetting system, pipettor
F système de pipettage
S sistema de pipeteo

Pistill
E pestle
F pilon
S pistilo

Pixel
E pixel
F pixel
S píxel

Placebo
E placebo
F placebo
S placebo

placebokontrolliert
E placebo-controlled
F contrôlé par placebo
S controlado por placebo

Plakat mit Sicherheitshinweisen
E safety poster
F affiche avec consignes de sécurité
S cartel con avisos de seguridad

Planetenmischer
E planetary mixer
F mélangeur planétaire
S mezclador planetario

Plastikfolie
E plastic film
F film plastique
S lámina de plástico

plastisch
E plastic
F plastique
S plástico

Plastizität
E plasticity
F plasticité
S plasticidad

Platine
E circuit board
F platine
S platino

Plattenabstand
E plate spacing
F distance entre plateaux
S distancia entre placas

Plattengußverfahren (Mikrobiologie)
E plate method
F coulage de plaques
S método de placas

Plazierung
E placement
F placement
S colocación

Plexiglas
E Plexiglas, acrylic glass
F plexiglas
S plexiglás

Plombe
E seal
F sceau en plomb
S empaste, marchamo, precinto

pneumatisch
E pneumatic
F pneumatique
S neumático

English German French Spanish

polar
E polar
F polaire
S polar

Polarimeter
E polarimeter
F polarimètre
S polarímetro

Polarisator
E polariser
F polariseur
S polarizador

Polarität
E polarity
F polarité
S polaridad

polieren
E polish, to
F polir
S bruñir, pulir

Poliermittel
E polish
F produit de polissage
S producto para pulir

polyaromatische Kohlenwasserstoffe (PAK)
E polyaromatic hydrocarbons (PAH)
F hydrocarbures polyaromatiques
S hidrocarburos poliaromáticos

polycyclisch
E polycyclic
F polycyclique
S policíclico

Polyethylenbeschichtung
E polyethylene coating
F couverture en polyéthylène
S cubierta de polietileno

polymer
E polymer
F polymère
S polímero

Polymer, wäßriges
E aqueous polymer
F polymère aqueux
S polímero acuoso

Polystyrol-Einsatz
E polystyrene insert
F insert en polystyrène
S inserción de poliestirol

Polyvinylchlorid (PVC)
E polyvinyl chloride (PVC)
F chlorure de polyvinyl (PVC)
S cloruro de polivinilo

Polyvinylidenfluorid
E polyvinylidene fluoride (PVDF)
F fluorure de polyvinylidène (PVDF)
S fluoruro de polivinilideno

Porendurchmesser
E pore diameter
F diamètre d'un pore
S diámetro de poro

porenfrei
E pore-free
F dépourvu de pores
S sin poros

Porengröße
E pore size
F taille d'un pore
S tamaño del poro

Porenvolumen
E pore volume
F volume d'un pore
S volumen del poro

porös
E porous
F poreux
S poroso

Porosität
E porosity
F porosité
S porosidad

portionierte Abpackung
E portioned packaging
F conditionnement en plusieurs phases
S envase porcionado

potentielle Anwendungen
E potential applications
F applications potentielles
S aplicaciones potenciales

Potentiometer
E potentiometer
F potentiomètre
S potenciómetro

Potenzierung
E potentation
F potentialisation
S potenciación

Präformulierung
E pre-formulation
F préformulation
S preformulación

Prägefolie
E embossed film
F feuille estampée
S lámina de estampado

prägen
E stamp, to; emboss, to
F poinçonner, estamper
S acuñar, estampar, troquelar

Prägestation
E embossing station, coding station
F station d'estampage
S estación de troquelado

Prägestempel
E hob, punch
F poinçon
S cuño, troquel

Prägung
E embossment
F estampage
S acuñado, estampado, troquelado

Praktikant
E trainee
F stagiaire
S pasante, practicante

präzise
E precise
F précis
S preciso

Präzision
E precision
F précision
S precisión

Präzisionswaage
E precision balance
F balance de précision
S balanza de precisión

Preßdruck
E moulding pressure
F pression de pressage, pression de moulage
S presión de prensado

Preßeigenschaften
E compression characteristics
F caractéristiques de compression
S características de compresión

preßfertige Mischung
E compactible mixture
F mélange comprimable
S mezcla comprimible

Preßformat
E compression format
F format de compression
S formato de compresión

Preßgeschwindigkeit
E compression speed
F vitesse de compression
S velocidad de compresión

Preßgranulat
E moulding granulate
F granule moulée
S granulado de compresión

English German French Spanish

Preßkammer
E compression chamber
F chambre de compression
S cámara de compresión

Preßkraft
E compaction force
F force de compression
S fuerza de compresión

Preßling
E pellet, compressed core
F implant, pastille, boulette
S masa comprimida

Preßluft
E compressed air
F air comprimé
S aire comprimido

Preßmasse
E compression material, moulding compound
F composé comprimable, matière moulée
S masa comprimible

Preßmaterial
E pressing material
F matériel de moulage, matériel de pressage
S material de prensado

Preßrückstand
E residue
F résidu de pressage
S residuo de prensado

Preßtabletten
E compressed tablets
F comprimés
S comprimidos

Preßversuch
E moulding trial
F essai de compression
S ensayo de compresión

Preßwerkzeug
E compaction device, compression mould
F outil de compression
S instrumental de compresión

Primärdampf
E primary steam
F vapeur primaire
S vapor primario

Primärformulierung
E primary formulation
F formulation primaire
S formulación primaria

Primärkontamination
E primary contamination
F contamination primaire
S contaminación primaria

Primärpackmittel
E primary packaging material
F matériel d'emballage primaire
S material primario de envase

Prion, zelluläres
E cellular prion (prpc)
F prion cellulaire (prpc)
S prión celular (prpc)

Prionproteine
E prion proteins (prp)
F protéines-prions (prp)
S proteína priónica (prp)

Proband
E volunteer
F volontaire
S voluntario

Probe
E sample
F échantillon, spécimen
S muestra

beanspruchte Probe
E stressed sample
F échantillon soumis à un effort
S muestra sometida a carga

Mischprobe
E composite sample
F échantillon du mélange
S muestra mixta

Probeentnahmestutzen
E sampling port
F tubulure de prélèvement d'échantillon
S tubuladura de toma de muestra

Probelauf
E trial run, test run
F essai de fonctionnement
S marcha de ensayo

Probenahme
E sampling
F échantillonnage, prélèvement d'un échantillon
S toma de muestra

Probenahmegerät
E sampling equipment, sampler
F équipement pour le prélèvement d'un échantillon
S aparato de toma de muestras

Probenahmeplan
E sampling plan
F programme d'échantillonnage
S plan de toma de muestras

Probenahmestatistik
E sampling statistics
F statistiques de prélèvement
S estadística de toma de muestras

Probenahmestelle
E sampling location, sampling point
F point de prélèvement
S lugar de toma de muestras

Probenanalyse
E sample assay, sample analysis
F analyse d'échantillon
S análisis de muestras

Probenaufreinigung
E sample clean-up
F nettoyage d'échantillons
S purificación de muestras

Probenauftrag (als Fleck auf DC-Platte)
E sample spotting (on TLC plate)
F application d'échantillons (sur plaque de CCM)
S depósito de muestras (como mancha sobre la placa de cromatografía en capa fina)

Probendurchsatz
E sample throughput
F capacité d'analyse d'échantillons
S rendimiento en muestras

Probeneinspritzung
E sample injection
F injection d'échantillon
S inyección de muestras

Probenfläschchen
E sample vial
F flacon d'échantillon
S vial de muestras

Probengeber
E sampler
F échantillonneuse
S aparato de toma de muestras

Probengefäß
E sample vessel
F récipient pour échantillon
S recipiente para muestras

Probenlagerung
E sample storage
F stockage d'échantillons
S almacenamiento de muestras

Probenschleife
E sample loop
F boucle d'échantillon
S bucle para toma de muestras

Probenständer
E sample rack
F portoir pour échantillons
S estante de muestras

Probenübertragung
E sample transfer
F transfert d'échantillons
S transferencia de muestras

Probenvorbehandlung
E sample pre-treatment
F prétraitement d'échantillons
S pretratamiento de muestras

Probenvorbereitung
E sample preparation
F préparation d'un échantillon
S preparación de muestras

Problementscheidungsplan
E problem decision plan
F plan de solutionnement d'un problème
S plan para decidir problemas

Produktanalyse
E product assay, product analysis
F analyse d'un produit
S análisis del producto

Produktausbeute
E product yield
F taux de récupération d'un produit
S rendimiento en producto

Produktbericht, jährlicher
E annual product report
F rapport annuel de production
S informe anual de producción

produktberührende Oberfläche
E product contact surface
F surface au contact d'un produit
S superficie en contacto con el producto

Produktbeschreibung
E product description
F caractérisation d'un produit
S descripción de un producto

Produkteinführung
E product launch
F lancement d'un produit
S introducción de un producto (en el mercado)

Produktentwicklung
E product development
F développement d'un produit
S desarrollo de un producto

Produktförderung
E product promotion
F mesures propres à favoriser un produit
S promoción de un producto

Produktfreigabe
E product release
F libération de produit
S aprobación del producto

Produktherkunft
E product origin
F origine du produit
S procedencia del producto

Produktion
E production, manufacture
F production
S producción

Produktion im Versuchsmaßstab
E pilot scale production
F production à l'échelle pilote
S producción a escala piloto

Produktionsanlagen
E process equipment
F équipement d'un procédé de fabrication
S equipo de instrumentos para el proceso de producción

Produktionsausfall
E production downtime
F période d'immobilisation en production
S pérdida de producción

Produktionsausfallzeit
E production down time
F période d'immobilisation en production
S tiempo de pérdida de producción

produktionsbegleitende Validierung
E concurrent validation
F validation concurrente
S validación concomitante a la producción

Produktionsbetrieb
E production facility, production plant
F usine de production
S empresa productora

Produktionscharge
E production batch
F lot de production
S lote de producción

Produktionsdaten
E production data
F données de production
S datos de producción

Produktionsgenehmigung
E production licence
F autorisation de production
S permiso de producción

Produktionsleistung
E production output
F rendement d'une production
S rendimiento de producción

Produktionslinie
E production line
F chaîne de production
S cadena de producción

Produktionsmaßstab
E production scale
F échelle de production
S escala de producción

Produktionsmenge
E quantity produced
F quantité produite
S cantidad producida

Produktionsort
E manufacturing location/site
F lieu de production
S lugar de producción

Produktionsplan
E production schedule
F schéma de production
S plan de producción

Produktionsstätte
E manufacturing site
F site de production
S lugar de producción

Produktreinigung
E product purification
F purification d'un produit
S limpieza del producto

Produktrückruf
E product recall
F rappel d'un produit
S retirada de un producto

Produktrückstand
E product residue
F résidu d'un produit
S residuo de un producto

Produktsicherheit
E product safety
F sécurité d'un produit
S seguridad de un producto

Produktstabilität
E product stability
F stabilité d'un produit
S estabilidad de un producto

Produktverunreinigung
E product contamination
F contamination d'un produit
S contaminación de un producto

Produktzufuhr
E product feed
F alimentation en produit
S suministro de un producto

Produktzulassungsantrag
E application for marketing authorisation
F demande d'autorisation de mise sur le marché
S solicitud de autorización de un producto (para la venta)

programmierbar
E programmable
F programmable
S programable

English German French Spanish

Programmierer
E programmer
F programmeur
S programador

Programmierung
E programming
F programmation
S programación

Programmsteuerung
E programme control
F contrôle d'un programme
S control del programa

Prokurist
E executive with power of procuration
F fondé de pouvoirs
S apoderado general

promoviert
E graduate (with doctorate), PhD
F titulaire d'un doctorat
S doctorado

Propellermischer
E propeller mixer
F mélangeur à pales
S mezclador de hélice

prophylaktisch
E prophylactic
F prophylactique
S profiláctico

Prophylaxe
E prophylaxis
F prophylaxe
S profilaxia

prospektiv
E prospective
F prospective
S prospectivo

prospektive Validierung
E prospective validation
F validation prospective
S validación prospectiva

Prospektzuführung
E leaflet feed
F approvisionnement en dépliants
S suministro de prospectos

Protease
E protease
F protéase
S proteasa

Protokoll
E record
F enregistrement, référence
S protocolo

protokollieren
E protocol, to; record, to; document, to
F enregistrer, documenter
S levantar acta, protocolar

Protozoen
E protozoa
F protozoaires
S protozoos

Prozeßabluft
E exhaust air
F air d'évacuation
S aire de escape de un proceso

Prozeßanlage
E processing facility, processing plant
F installation pour processus
S instalación para proceso

Prozeßanpassung
E operational adjustment, process adjustment
F ajustement de fonctionnement, ajustement d'un procédé
S ajuste del funcionamiento, ajuste de un proceso

Prozeßautomatisierung
E process automation
F automatisation d'un procédé
S automa(tiza)ción de un proceso

Prozeßdokumentation
E process documentation
F documentation d'un procédé
S documentación de un proceso

Prozeßflußdiagramm
E process flow diagram (PFD)
F schéma fonctionnel
S diagrama de flujo de procesos

Prozeßleitsystem
E process control system
F système de gestion d'un procédé
S sistema de gestión de un proceso

Prozeßschritt, kritischer
E critical processing step
F étape critique d'un procédé
S etapa crítica de un proceso

Prozeßsteuerung
E process control
F contrôle d'un procédé
S control de un proceso

Prozeßtemperatur
E process temperature
F température d'un procédé
S temperatura de un proceso

Prozeßumgebung
E process environment
F environnement d'un procédé
S entorno de un proceso

Prozeßvalidierung
E process validation
F validation d'un procédé
S validación de un proceso

Prozeßvariabilität
E process variability
F variabilité du processus
S variabilidad de un proceso

Prozeßwasser
E process water
F eau pour opérations
S agua de procesado

Prüfanleitung
E test instructions
F mode opératoire
S instrucciones de prueba

Prüfanweisung
E testing procedure
F instructions d'un test
S instrucciones de prueba

Prüfarzt
E trial physician, investigator
F médecin responsable d'essais cliniques
S médico investigador

Prüfbericht
E test report
F rapport expérimental
S informe de prueba

Prüfbogen
E questionnaire, trial form, case report form
F questionnaire
S cuestionario

prüfen
E test, to
F tester
S comprobar, ensayar, examinar, investigar, probar

Prüfkeim
E test organism
F organisme de contrôle
S germen de prueba

Prüfmethode
E test method, analytical method
F méthode analytique, méthode de contrôle
S método de prueba

Prüfmittel (zur Kalibrierung)
E calibrating equipment
F équipement de calibration
S sistema de prueba (para calibrar)

Prüfmuster
E test sample
F échantillon
S muestra de prueba

English German French Spanish

English German French Spanish

Prüfparameter
E testing parameter
F paramètre d'analyse
S parámetro de prueba

Prüfplan
E testing schedule
F protocole opératoire
S plan de prueba, protocolo del ensayo

Prüfpräparat
E test preparation
F préparation pour test
S preparado de prueba

Prüfprotokoll
E test protocol
F procès-verbal d'un test
S protocolo de prueba

Prüfung
E analysis, control test
F analyse, test de contrôle
S examen, ensayo, prueba, test

biologische Prüfung
E biological testing
F examens biologiques
S prueba biológica

physiologische Prüfung
E physiological testing
F examen physiologique
S prueba fisiológica

toxikologische Prüfung
E toxicological testing
F étude toxicologique
S prueba toxicológica

Prüfung der Robustheit
E robustness testing
F test de solidité
S comprobación de la robustez

Prüfverfahren
E analytical procedure, testing procedure
F procédure de test
S procedimiento de prueba

Prüfvorschrift
E test instructions
F instructions d'un test
S prescripción de prueba

Prüfzertifikat
E test certificate
F certificat d'analyse
S certificado de prueba

Puder
E powder
F poudre
S polvo

pudrig
E powdery
F poudreux
S pulverulento

Puffer
E buffer
F tampon
S tampón

Pufferkapazität
E buffering capacity
F capacité d'un tampon
S capacidad de tamponamiento

Pufferlösung
E buffer solution
F solution tampon
S solución de tamponamiento

Pulver
E powder
F poudre
S polvo

loses Pulver
E loose powder
F poudre en vrac
S polvo suelto

Pulver zum Einnehmen
E oral powder
F poudre à utilisation orale
S polvo oral

Pulverbett
E powder bed
F lit de poudre
S lecho de polvo

Pulverdichte
E powder density
F densité d'une poudre
S densidad del polvo

Pulverdosierschnecke
E powder feeder
F vis doseuse pour poudre
S tornillo sin fin dosificador de polvo

Pulverfraktion
E powder fraction
F fraction de poudre
S fracción de polvo

pulverisieren
E pulverise, to; powder, to; grind, to
F pulvériser
S pulverizar

Pulvermischung
E powdered mixture
F mélange de poudre
S mezcla de polvo

Pumpe
E pump
F pompe
S bomba

Pumpeneinlaß
E pump inlet
F entrée d'une pompe
S entrada de una bomba

Pumpenkopf
E pump head
F tête de pompe
S cabeza de bomba

Pumpenventil
E pump valve
F vanne de pompe
S válvula de bomba

Punktschreiber
E dotted-line recorder
F enregistreur par ligne pointillée
S registradora de línea de puntos

punktschweißen
E spot-weld, to
F souder par points
S soldar por puntos

Pyknometer
E pycnometer, specific gravity meter
F pycnomètre
S picnómetro

Pyrogene
E pyrogens
F pyrogènes
S pirógenos

pyrogenfrei
E pyrogen-free
F dépourvu de pyrogènes
S sin pirógenos

Pyrogenität
E pyrogenicity
F pyrogénicité
S pirogenicidad

Pyrolyse
E pyrolysis
F pyrolyse
S pirólisis

Quadratwurzel
E square root
F racine carrée
S raíz cuadrada

Qualifizierung
E qualification
F qualification
S cualificación

Funktionsqualifizierung
E operational qualification
F qualification des opérations
S cualificación funcional

English
German
French
Spanish

Installationsqualifizierung
E installation qualification
F qualification de l'installation
S cualificación de una instalación

Verfahrensqualifizierung
E performance qualification
F qualification des performances
S cualificación de un procedimiento

Qualifizierung der Ausrüstung
E equipment qualification
F qualification de l'équipement
S cualificación del equipamiento

Qualität
E quality
F qualité
S calidad

gleichbleibende Qualität
E consistent quality
F qualité uniforme
S calidad invariable

qualitätsbestimmend
E quality-determining
F qui détermine la qualité
S determinante de la calidad

Qualitätskontrolle (QK)
E quality control (QC)
F contrôle-qualité,
contrôle de la qualité
S control de calidad

Qualitätsmanagement (QM)
E quality management (QM)
F gestion de la qualité
S gestión de la calidad

umfassendes Qualitätsmanagement
E total quality management (TQM)
F gestion absolue de la qualité
S gestión de la calidad absoluta

Qualitätsmangel
E defect, shortcoming
F défaut de qualité
S defecto de calidad

Qualitätsmerkmal
E quality attribute
F caracteristique de qualité
S característica de calidad

Qualitätsregelkarte
E quality control card
F carte de contrôle de qualité
S ficha de control de calidad

Qualitätssicherung (QS)
E quality assurance (QA)
F assurance-qualité
S aseguramiento de la calidad

Qualitätsverbesserung
E quality improvement
F amélioration de la qualité
S mejora de la calidad

quantitativ
E quantitative
F quantitatif
S cuantitativo

quantitativ bestimmbar
E quantifiable
F quantifiable
S cuantificable

Quarantäne
E quarantine
F quarantaine
S cuarentena

Quarz
E quartz
F quartz
S cuarzo

Quelle
E source
F source
S fuente

quellen
E swell, to
F gonfler
S brotar, hincharse

Quellfähigkeit
E swelling capacity
F capacité de gonflement
S capacidad de hinchamiento

Querschnitt
E cross-section
F section transversale, coupe transversale
S sección transversal

Querschnittszeichnung
E sectional drawing
F croquis de section
S croquis transversal

Querstange
E cross bar
F tige transversale
S barra transversal

Quervernetzung
E cross-linking
F connexion latérale
S conexión lateral

Querverweis
E cross reference
F référence
S referencia

quetschen
E pinch, to; squeeze, to
F écraser
S aplastar

Quetschflasche
E squeeze bottle
F flacon souple doseur
S recipiente flexible

Quotient
E quotient
F quotient
S cociente

R & S (Risiko und Sicherheit)
E R & S (risk and safety)
F R & S (risque et sécurité)
S R & S (riesgo y seguridad)

R & S-Sätze
E R & S phrases
F phrases de R & S
S frases de R & S

R+I-Schema
E installation scheme, piping and instrument diagram; piping and instrument diagram (P&ID)
F schéma de l'installation, des canalisations et diagrammes des instruments; schéma fonctionnel et instrumental
S esquema de instalación, de canalización y diagramas de instrumentos; esquema de procesos e instrumentos

racemisch
E racemic
F racémique
S racémico

radioaktive Markierung
E radio-label
F marquage isotopique
S marcado radiactivo

radioaktiver Abfall
E radioactive waste
F résidu radioactif
S residuos radiactivos

radioaktiver Zerfall
E radioactive decay
F désintégration radioactive
S desintegración radiactiva

Radiopharmazeutika
E radio-pharmaceuticals
F produits radiopharmaceutiques
S productos radiofarmacéuticos

Rand
E edge
F arête, bord
S arista, borde

Rändelmutter
E knurled nut
F écrou moleté
S tuerca moleteada

English
German
French
Spanish

Rändelschraube
E knurled screw
F vis moletée
S tornillo moleteado

randomisiert
E randomised
F randomisé
S randomizado

randvoll
E brimful
F plein à ras-bord
S lleno a rebosar

ranzig
E rancid
F rance
S rancio

Raster
E raster, screen
F trame
S trama

rauchende Säure
E fuming acid
F acide fumant
S ácido fumante

Raucherzeuger
E smoke generator
F générateur de fumée
S generador de humo

Rauchmelder
E smoke detector
F détecteur de fumée
S detector de humo

Rauchröhrchen
E smoke tube
F tube de fumée
S tubo de humo

rauh
E rough
F grossier
S áspero

Rauhigkeit
E roughness
F grossièreté
S aspereza

Raumabluft
E exhaust air
F air d'évacuation
S aire de escape

Raumbegasung
E fumigation
F fumigation
S fumigación

Raumdesinfektion
E room disinfection
F désinfection de locaux
S desinfección de la sala

räumliche Faltung (z. B. eines Proteins)
E spatial folding (e. g. of protein)
F pliage spatial (par ex. des protéines)
S conformación espacial, plegamiento espacial (p. ej. de una proteína)

räumliche Trennung
E physical segregation
F ségrégation physique
S separación espacial

Räumlichkeiten
E premises
F locaux
S locales

raumlufttechnische Anlage
E ventilation system
F système de ventilation
S sistema de ventilación

Raumstruktur
E spatial structure
F structure spatiale
S estructura espacial, estructura terciaria (p. ej. de una proteína)

Raumtemperatur
E room temperature, ambient temperature
F température ambiante
S temperatura ambiente

Rauschen
E noise
F bruit
S ruido (de fondo)

Basislinienrauschen
E baseline noise
F bruit de fond d'une ligne de base
S ruido (de fondo) en la línea de base

Rauschmittel
E narcotic
F narcotique
S narcótico

Razemat
E racemate
F racémate
S racemado

razemisch
E racemic
F racémique
S racémico

Reagenz
E reagent
F réactif
S reactivo

gebrauchsfertiges Reagenz
E ready-to-use reagent
F réactif prêt à l'emploi
S reactivo listo para el uso

Reagenzglas
E test tube
F tube à essais
S probeta, tubo de ensayo

Reagenzlösung
E reagent solution
F solution réactive
S solución reactiva

Reaktion 1. Ordnung
E first-order reaction
F réaction de premier ordre
S reacción de primer orden

Reaktion 2. Ordnung
E second-order reaction
F réaction de second ordre
S reacción de segundo orden

Reaktion, endothermische
E endothermic reaction
F réaction endothermique
S reacción endotérmica

Reaktion, exothermische
E exothermic reaction
F réaction exothermique
S reacción exotérmica

Reaktion, kinetische
E kinetic reaction
F réaction cinétique
S reacción cinética

Reaktion, thermische
E thermal reaction
F réaction thermique
S reacción térmica

Reaktion, unerwünschte
E adverse reaction
F réaction indésirable, effet adverse
S reacción indeseable

Reaktionsbedingungen
E reaction conditions
F conditions de réaction
S condiciones de reacción

Reaktionsgeschwindigkeit
E reaction speed, reaction velocity
F vitesse de réaction
S velocidad de reacción

Reaktionsmechanismus
E reaction mechanism
F mécanisme de réaction
S mecanismo de reacción

reaktionsträge
E poorly reactive
F inerte
S inerte

Reaktionsverlauf
E course of a reaction
F déroulement d'une réaction
S transcurso de la reacción

Reaktionswärme
E heat of reaction
F chaleur due à la réaction
S calor de reacción

Reaktor
E reactor
F réacteur
S reactor

Rechenfehler
E calculation error
F erreur de calcul
S error de cálculo

Rechnung
E calculation
F calculation, calcul
S cálculo

rechtsdrehend
E dextro-rotatory
F dextrogyre
S dextrógiro

rechtsgängig
E right-handed
F droit
S de paso derecho

rechtwinkelig
E rectangular
F rectangulaire
S rectangular

Redoxpotential
E redox potential
F potentiel redox
S potencial redox

reduzieren
E reduce, to
F réduire
S reducir

Reduzierstück
E reducer
F réducteur
S reductor

Reduzierventil
E reducing valve
F vanne de détente
S válvula reductora

Referenzkunden
E reference customers
F clientèle de référence
S clientes de referencia

Referenzpräparat
E reference medication (preparation)
F préparation de référence
S preparado de referencia

Referenzstandard
E reference, standard
F standard de référence
S estándar de referencia

Referenzstrahl
E reference beam
F faisceau de référence
S rayo de referencia

Reflektionswinkel
E angle of reflection
F angle de réflexion
S ángulo de reflexión

Refraktometer
E refractometer
F réfractomètre
S refractómetro

Regal
E shelf
F étagère
S estante

regelbar
E adjustable
F ajustable
S regulable

Regelgenauigkeit
E control accuracy
F exactitude de réglage, exactitude de contrôle
S exactitud de la regulación

Regelklappe
E control flap, control valve
F clapet de réglage
S válvula reguladora

Regelkreis
E control loop
F boucle d'asservissement
S circuito regulador

Regelventil
E regulating valve
F vanne de régulation
S válvula reguladora

Regelwerk, regionales
E local code
F code régional
S código regional

Regenerierung
E regeneration
F régénération
S regeneración

Regierungspräsidium
E regional government
F gouvernement régional
S gobierno civil

Registrierung
E registration
F enregistrement
S registro

Regler
E controller, control valve
F régulateur
S regulador

Reglereinstellung
E controller set point
F réglage d'un régulateur
S ajuste de un regulador

regulierbar
E controllable, adjustable
F ajustable
S regulable

Regulierung
E adjustment, setting
F ajustement, réglage
S ajuste, regulación

Reibeechtheit
E resistance to abrasion
F résistance à l'abrasion
S resistente a la fricción

Reibschale
E mortar
F mortier
S mortero

Reibung
E friction
F friction
S fricción, frotamiento

Reibungskoeffizient
E coefficient of friction
F coefficient de friction, coefficient de frottement
S coeficiente de fricción

Reibungskraft
E frictional force
F force de friction, force de frottement
S fuerza de fricción

Reibungswiderstand
E frictional resistance
F résistance à la friction, résistance au frottement
S resistencia a la fricción

Reihenfolge
E sequence
F séquence
S secuencia

English German French Spanish

Reihenuntersuchung
E screening
F screening, série d'analyses
S examen secuencial, serie de ensayos

Reindampf
E pure steam
F vapeur pure
S vapor puro

Reindampferzeuger
E pure steam generator
F générateur de vapeur pure
S generador de vapor puro

Reinheit
E purity
F pureté
S pureza

chemische Reinheit
E chemical purity
F pureté chimique
S pureza química

chirale Reinheit
E chiral purity
F pureté chirale
S pureza quiral

enantiomere Reinheit
E enantiomeric purity
F pureté énantiomère
S pureza enantiómera

optische Reinheit
E optical purity
F pureté optique
S pureza óptica

Reinheitsgrad
E cleanliness grade (e. g. room), purity (product)
F niveau de propreté, niveau de pureté
S grado de pureza

Reinheitsklasse
E cleanliness class, cleanliness grade
F classe d'environnement
S nivel de pureza

Reinheitsprüfung
E purity test
F test de pureté
S prueba de pureza

Reinigung
E cleaning, purification
F nettoyage
S limpieza

Reinigung (von Anlagen) im geschlossenen System
E cleaning in-place (CIP)
F nettoyage en place (CIP)
S limpieza (de instalaciones) en sistema cerrado

Reinigungsfirma
E contract cleaner
F entreprise de nettoyage
S empresa de limpieza

Reinigungsgerät
E cleaning equipment
F équipement de nettoyage
S aparato de limpieza

Reinigungsgrad
E cleanliness grade
F niveau de propreté
S grado de limpieza

Reinigungsmittel
E cleansing agent, detergent
F agent de nettoyage
S detergente, producto de limpieza

Reinigungsplan
E cleaning schedule
F programme de nettoyage
S plan de limpieza

Reinigungstuch
E cleaning cloth, cleaning tissue
F chiffon, serpillière
S paño de limpieza

Reinigungsvalidierung
E cleaning validation
F validation du nettoyage
S validación de la limpieza

Reinigungsvorschrift
E cleaning procedure
F procédure de nettoyage
S instrucción de limpieza

Reinluft
E clean air
F air filtré
S aire limpio

Reinraum
E clean room, clean area
F zone d'atmosphère contrôlée
S área estéril

Reinraumklasse
E clean room grade, clean room class
F niveau de stérilité
S nivel de esterilidad

Reinraumkleidung
E clean room clothing
F vêtement protecteur pour zone d'atmosphère contrôlée
S ropa para área estéril

Reinraumtechnik
E clean room engineering
F ingénierie des zones d'atmosphère contrôlée
S técnica para el área estéril

Reinstdampf
E clean steam, pure steam
F vapeur pure
S vapor puro

Reinstwasser
E pure water, high purity water
F eau PPI, eau de haute pureté
S agua purificada, agua ultrapurificada

Reißfestigkeit
E resistance to tearing, tear strength
F résistance au déchirement
S resistencia al desgarro

reizende Substanz
E irritating substance
F substance irritante
S sustancia irritante

reizt die Atemwege
E irritating to respiratory system
F irritant pour le système respiratoire
S irrita las vías respiratorias

reizt die Augen
E irritating to eyes
F irritant pour les yeux
S irrita los ojos

Reizung (chemisch)
E irritation (chem.)
F irritation (chimique)
S irritación (química)

Reklamation
E complaint
F réclamation
S reclamación

rekombinant
E recombinant
F recombinant
S recombinante

Rekrutierungsphase
E recruitment phase
F phase de recrutement
S fase de reclutamiento

Rektalcreme
E rectal cream
F crème rectale
S crema rectal

Rektalgel
E rectal gel
F gel rectal
S gel rectal

Rektalsalbe
E rectal ointment
F pommade rectale
S pomada rectal

Rektalschaum
E rectal foam
F mousse rectale
S espuma rectal

rektifiziert
E rectified
F rectifié
S rectificado

Relais
E relay
F relais
S relé, relevador

Relaisverstärker
E relay amplifier
F relais amplificateur
S amplificador de relé

Relationsdiagramm
E relationship diagram
F schéma relationnel
S diagrama de relaciones

relevant
E relevant, pertinent
F pertinent, approprié
S relevante

Reparatur
E repair
F réparation
S reparación

reproduzierbar
E reproducible
F reproductible
S reproducible

Reproduzierbarkeit
E reproducibility
F reproductibilité
S reproductibilidad

Requalifizierung
E requalification
F requalification
S recualificación

resistent
E resistant
F résistant
S resistente

Resistenzentwicklung
E development of resistance
F développement d'une résistance
S desarrollo de resistencia

Resorption
E resorption
F résorption
S resorción

Resorptionsvermittler
E resorption agent
F agent de résorption
S agente de resorción

Rest
E residue
F résidu
S residuo

Restfeuchte
E residual moisture
F humidité résiduelle
S humedad residual

Resthärte (z. B. von Wasser)
E residual hardness (e. g. of water)
F dureté résiduelle (par ex. de l'eau)
S dureza residual (p. ej. del agua)

Restriktionsenzym
E restriction enzyme
F enzyme de restriction
S enzima restrictivo

Restvolumen
E residual volume
F volume résiduel
S volumen residual

Retardgranulat
E prolonged release granules
F granules à libération retardée
S granulado retard

Retardtablette
E retard tablet, delayed action tablet
F comprimé à libération retardée
S comprimido retard

Retention
E retention
F rétention
S retención

Retentionsfaktor
E retention factor
F facteur de rétention
S factor de retención

Retentionszeit
E retention time
F temps de rétention
S tiempo de retención

Retoure
E return
F renvoi, rappel
S retorno

retrospektive Validierung
E retrospective validation
F validation rétrospective
S validación retrospectiva

Revalidierung
E revalidation
F revalidation
S revalidación

revidieren
E revise, to; review, to
F réviser
S revisar

Rezept
E prescription
F ordonnance
S receta

Rezeptor
E receptor
F récepteur
S receptor

rezeptpflichtig
E prescription only
F disponible seulement sur ordonnance
S con receta médica

Rezeptur
E formulation
F formulation
S formulación

Rheologie
E rheology
F rhéologie
S reología

Richtigkeit (einer Prüfmethode)
E accuracy
F exactitude
S corrección, exactitud (de un método de prueba)

Richtlinie
E directive, guideline
F directive
S directriz

abteilungsübergreifende Richtlinie
E cross-functional guideline
F lignes directrices générales
S directriz general

Riemenantrieb
E belt drive
F entraînement par courroie
S propulsión por correa

rieselfähig
E capable of flowing, flowable
F capable d'écoulement
S capaz de fluir

Rieselfähigkeit
E flowing property, fluidity
F propriété d'écoulement
S capacidad de fluir

Rieselturm
E washing tower, spray tower
F tour d'arrosage
S torre de lavado

riffeln
E corrugate, to
F canneler, strier
S acanalar, estriar

English
German
French
Spanish

Riffelung
E corrugation
F cannelure, striage
S acanaladura, estría, ranura

Rille
E groove
F cannelure, rainure, sillon
S acanaladura, estría, ranura

Rinderprion
E bovine prion
F prion bovin
S prión bovino

Ringleitung
E main ring
F boucle de recirculation
S cañería en anillo, red anular

Ringöffnungsreaktion
E ring-opening reaction
F réaction ouvrant un anneau
S reacción de apertura de anillo

Rinne
E gutter
F gouttière
S canal, reguera, surco

Risiko- und Gefahrensätze
E risk and safety phrases
F règles concernant les risques et la sécurité
S reglas concernientes a riesgos y peligros

Risikoanalyse
E risk analysis
F analyse des risques
S análisis del riesgo

Riß
E crack, tear
F déchirure, fissure
S desgarro, fisura

rißüberbrückend
E crack-filling
F colmatant (une fissure)
S rellenante de una fisura

Ritzel
E pinion
F pignon
S piñón

Roboterarm
E robotic arm
F bras d'un robot
S brazo de robot

Robotersystem
E robotic system
F analyseur robot
S sistema robot

robust (z. B. Gerät, Methode)
E rugged (e. g. instrument, method)
F robuste (par ex. instrument, méthode)
S robusto (p. ej. instrumento, método)

Robustheit
E robustness
F robustesse
S robustez

Robustheit des Prozesses
E process robustness
F robustesse d'un procédé
S robustez del proceso

Rockwell-Härte (von Werkzeug)
E Rockwell hardness (of tools)
F dureté Rockwell (outils)
S dureza Rockwell (de herramientas)

Rohausbeute
E raw yield
F rendement brut
S rendimiento bruto

Rohdaten
E raw data
F données brutes
S datos brutos

Rohling
E blank
F ébauche, pièce brute
S pieza bruta

Rohmaterial
E raw material
F matière brute
S materia prima

Rohprodukt
E crude product, raw product
F produit brut
S materia prima, producto bruto

Rohrbogen
E tube
F tube
S tubo

Rohrbündelwärmetauscher
E tube bundle heat exchanger
F échangeur de chaleur à faisceaux tubulaires
S intercambiador de calor de haces tubulares

Rohrleitung
E pipe(work), pipeline
F canalisation
S canalización

Rohrleitungskennzeichnung
E piping designation
F marquage des tuyaux
S caracterización de cañerías

Rohrleitungssystem
E piping system
F système de canalisation
S sistema de canalización

Rohrzucker
E cane sugar
F sucre de canne
S azúcar de caña

Rohstoff
E raw material
F matière brute
S materia prima

inaktiver Rohstoff
E inactive raw material
F matière première inactive
S materia prima inactiva

Rollendurchmesser
E reel diameter
F diamètre de bobine
S diámetro de bobina

Rollenwechsel
E reel changes
F changement de bobine
S cambio de bobina

Röntgenkontrastmittel
E X-ray contrast medium
F produit de contraste aux rayons X
S medio de contraste radiológico

Rost
E rust
F rouille
S herrumbre, orín

rosten
E rust, to
F rouiller
S oxidarse

rostfrei
E rust-free
F dépourvu de rouille
S sin orín

Rostschutz
E rust protection
F protection contre la rouille
S protección antioxidante

Rotationssprühkopf
E rotary spray
F tête rotative de pulvérisation
S cabeza rotatoria de pulverización

Rotationsverdampfer
E rotatory evaporator
F évaporateur rotatif
S evaporador rotatorio

rotieren
E rotate, to
F tourner
S girar

rotierend
E rotating
F tournant
S girando

Rotor
E rotor
F rotor
S rotor

Rückfluß
E back flow, reflux
F reflux
S reflujo

Rückflußkühler
E reflux condenser
F radiateur à reflux
S radiador, refrigerador de reflujo

Rückführbarkeit
E traceability
F traçabilité
S trazabilidad, retromarcado

Rückgewinnung
E recovery
F récupération
S recuperación

Lösungsmittelrückgewinnung
E solvent recovery
F récupération de solvant
S recuperación de solvente

Rückhaltebereich
E retention range
F zone de rétention
S márgenes de retención

Rückhaltevermögen (bei Filtern)
E retention efficiency (in filters)
F efficacité de rétention (pour un filtre)
S capacidad de retención (de un filtro)

Rücklauf
E reverse flow
F retour
S retorno

Rückruf
E recall
F rappel
S retirada

Rückschlagklappe
E flap trap
F clapet anti-retour
S válvula de retención

Rückschlagventil
E non-return valve, check valve
F vanne anti-retour
S válvula de retención

Rückstand
E residue
F résidu
S residuo, resto

sichtbarer Rückstand
E visible residue
F résidu visible
S residuo visible

Rückstauklappe
E back flow preventer, back flow flap
F clapet antirefouleur
S válvula de retención

Rückstellmuster
E retained sample, reference sample
F échantillon de référence
S muestra de referencia

Rücktitration
E back titration
F dosage en retour
S titulación retrógrada

rückverfolgbar
E traceable
F traçable
S de traza determinable

Rückverfolgbarkeit
E traceability
F traçabilité
S trazabilidad, retromarcado

Rückverfolgungssystem
E tracing system
F système de suivi, système d'observation
S sistema de retromarcado

Rückweisezahl
E rejection number
F nombre de rejet
S número de rechazo

Rückzugfeder
E counter-spring, return spring
F ressort de rappel
S muelle de retorno

Ruhezustand, im
E at rest
F à l'arrêt, immobilisé
S parado

rühren
E stir, to
F agiter
S agitar

Rühren, kräftiges
E vigorous stirring
F agitation vigoureuse
S agitación intensa

Rührer
E stirrer
F agitateur
S agitador

Rührfisch
E magnetic stirring bar
F agitateur magnétique, barreau aimanté
S agitador magnético

Rührflügel
E stirring blade
F pale d'agitation
S aleta de agitación

Rührgeschwindigkeit
E stirring speed, agitating speed
F vitesse d'agitation
S velocidad de agitación

Rührkessel
E stirring vessel
F récipient de l'agitateur
S caldera de agitación

Rührwerk
E stirrer, agitator
F agitateur
S agitador

Rührwerksnabe
E stirrer hub
F moyeu d'agitateur
S cubo del agitador

Rührwerksrechen
E stirrer rake
F râteau d'agitateur
S rastrillo del agitador

Rundkolben
E round-bottomed flask
F ballon à fond rond
S matraz esférico

Rundläuferpresse
E rotary press
F presse rotative
S prensa rotatoria

Rundtablette
E round tablet
F comprimé rond
S comprimido redondo

Rutsche
E chute
F toboggan
S tobogán

rutschsicher
E slip-proof, non-slip
F anti-dérapant
S antideslizante

rütteln
E shake, to; vibrate, to
F secouer
S sacudir, trepidar, vibrar

Rüttelsieb
E vibrating sieve, vibrating screen
F tamis vibrant
S tamiz vibrante

Rüttler
E vibrator, shaker
F secoueuse, secoueur, vibreur
S vibrador

Sachbearbeiter
E person responsible, clerk
F responsable
S encargado, ponente

sachkundige Person
E qualified person
F personne qualifiée
S persona cualificada

Sachkundiger
E qualified person
F personne compétente, expert
S experto, perito

Sachverständiger
E expert
F expert
S experto, perito

Sackfilter
E sack filter
F sac filtrant
S saco filtrante

Saft
E juice
F jus
S jugo (animal), zumo (vegetal)

Salbe
E ointment
F pommade
S pomada, ungüento

Salbengrundlage
E ointment base
F ingrédient de base d'une pommade
S excipiente de una pomada

Salbenmühle
E ointment mill
F broyeur à pommade
S molino de pomada

Salinität
E salinity
F salinité
S salinidad

Salpetersäure
E nitric acid
F acide nitrique
S ácido nítrico

Salzbildung
E salt formation
F formation de sels
S salificación

Salzigkeit
E salinity
F salinité
S salinidad

Salzsäure
E hydrochloric acid
F acide chlorhydrique
S ácido clorhídrico

Sammelbehälter
E reservoir, collector
F réservoir, collecteur
S depósito (colector)

Sammelsystem
E collection system
F système de collecte
S sistema colector

sandgestrahlt
E sand-blasted
F traité au jet de sable
S tratado con chorro de arena

Sanierung
E reorganisation, restructuring
F assainissement
S saneamiento

Sanitäranschlüsse
E sanitary fittings
F connections sanitaires
S conexiones sanitarias

Sanitärverbindung
E sanitary joint
F joint sanitaire
S conexión sanitaria

Sattdampf
E saturated steam
F vapeur saturée
S vapor saturado

Sättigung
E saturation
F saturation
S saturación

Sättigungsindex
E saturation index
F indice de saturation
S índice de saturación

Sauberkeit
E cleanliness
F propreté
S limpieza

sauer
E acid
F acide
S ácido

Sauerstoff
E oxygen
F oxygène
S oxígeno

gelöster Sauerstoff
E dissolved oxygen (DO)
F oxygène dissous
S oxígeno disuelto

Sauerstoffbedarf, biochemischer (BSB)
E biochemical oxygen demand (bod) analysis
F analyse de la demande biologique d'oxygène (DBO)
S necesidades bioquímicas de oxígeno

Sauerstoffentwicklung
E oxygen release
F évolution de la teneur en oxygène
S liberación de oxígeno

Sauerstoffgehalt
E oxygen content
F teneur en oxygène
S contenido en oxígeno

Säugetierzellinie
E mammalian cell line
F lignée de cellule de mammifère
S línea de células de mamífero

Säugetierzellkultur
E mammalian cell culture
F culture de cellules de mammifère
S cultivo de células de mamífero

Saugfähigkeit
E absorptive capacity
F capacité d'absorption
S capacidad de absorción

Saugflasche
E aspirator bottle
F biberon
S biberón

Säule
E column
F colonne
S columna

Säulendurchmesser
E column diameter
F diamètre de colonne
S diámetro de la columna

Säulenfüllmaterial
E column filler
F matériel de remplissage d'une colonne
S material de relleno de la columna

Säulenfüllung
E column packing
F package de colonne
S llenado de la columna

English German French Spanish

Säulenkonditionierung
E column conditioning
F conditionnement d'une colonne
S acondicionamiento de la columna

Säulenlänge
E column length
F longueur de colonne
S longitud de la columna

Säulenofen
E column oven
F four pour colonne
S horno de columna

Säulenüberladung
E column overloading
F surcharge de la colonne
S sobrecarga de columna

Säulenverbindung
E column coupling
F couplage de colonnes
S acople de columna

Säure
E acid
F acide
S ácido

schwache Säure
E weak acid
F acide faible
S ácido débil

starke Säure
E concentrated acid
F acide concentré
S ácido concentrado

säurebeständig
E acid-resistant
F résistant aux acides
S resistente a los ácidos

Säurezahl
E acid value
F indice d'acide
S índice de ácido

schaben
E scrape, to
F racler
S raer, rascar, raspar

Schaber
E scraper
F racloir
S rascador, raspador

Schablone
E stencil, template
F matrice, pochoir, patron
S modelo, patrón, plantilla

Schacht
E duct
F conduite, bouche
S conducto, pozo

Schachtel
E box, carton
F carton, boîte
S caja

Schachtsystem
E ducting system
F système de canalisation
S sistema de conducciones

schädlich
E harmful, hazardous
F nocif
S dañino, nocivo

schädliches Mittel
E harmful agent
F agent nocif
S agente nocivo

Schädlingsbekämpfung
E pest control
F lutte antiparasitaire
S control de plagas, lucha antiparasitaria

Schädlingsvertilgungsmittel
E pesticide
F pesticide
S pesticida

Schaft
E shaft
F arbre, essieu, tige
S árbol, asta, eje

Schalldämpfer
E silencer, attenuator
F silencieux, amortisseur de son
S silenciador

Schaltbild
E circuit diagram
F schéma de montage, schéma des connexions
S diagrama de circuito

Schaltdiagramm
E wiring diagram
F diagramme des connexions
S diagrama de circuito

Schaltelement
E switch module
F élément commutateur
S elemento interruptor

schalten
E wire, to
F enclencher, brancher, connecter
S conectar, conmutar

Schalter
E switch
F interrupteur
S conmutador, interruptor

Schaltkasten
E switch box, control box, wiring box
F armoire électrique
S caja de distribución

Schaltstufe
E switching stage
F étape de permutation
S etapa de conmutación

Schalttafel
E control panel
F pupitre de commande, tableau de commande
S cuadro de distribución, cuadro de mando

Schaltung (elektrisch)
E circuit (electrical)
F circuit, connexion (électrique)
S conexión (eléctrica)

scharf
E sharp
F coupant, aiguisé, piquant
S afilado, agudo, cortante

Schaufel
E blade
F pale, pelle
S pala

Schauglas
E observation window, observation port
F fenêtre d'observation
S ventana de observación

Schaum
E foam
F mousse
S espuma

Schaum zur Anwendung auf der Haut
E cutaneous foam
F mousse pour utilisation cutanée
S espuma cutánea

Schaumbildung
E foam formation, foaming
F formation de mousse, moussage, production de mousse
S formación de espuma

schäumen
E foam, to
F mousser
S espumar

schäumend
E effervescent
F effervescent
S espumante

Schaumspray
E foam spray
F aérosol pour mousse
S aerosol de espuma

English German French Spanish

Schaumstoff
E foam plastic
F mousse en plastique
S espuma

Scheidetrichter
E separating funnel
F entonnoir séparateur
S embudo de separación

scheinbare Dichte
E apparent density
F densité apparente
S densidad aparente

Schelle
E clip
F collier
S abrazadera, collar

Schergefälle
E shear gradient
F taux de cisaillement
S gradiente de cizallamiento

Scherintensität
E shear intensity
F intensité de cisaillement
S intensidad de cizallamiento

Scherkraft
E shear strength
F force de cisaillement
S fuerza de cizallamiento

Scherspannung
E shear stress
F contrainte de cisaillement
S tensión de cizallamiento

Schicht
E layer, shift (working)
F couche, phase, équipe (de travail)
S estrato, turno de trabajo

Schieber
E cursor
F curseur
S compuerta, corredera, cursor

Schiebetür
E sliding door
F porte coulissante
S puerta corrediza

schiefe Ebene
E inclined plane
F plan incliné
S plano inclinado

Schikane
E baffle
F chicane
S vejación

Schimmel
E mould
F moisissure
S moho

Schimmelbefall
E mould growth
F formation de moisissure
S crecimiento de moho

schimmelig
E mouldy, mildewed
F moisi
S enmohecido, mohoso

Schimmelpilz
E fungus, mould
F champignon
S moho

Schlag
E impact
F impact, coup
S choque, golpe, impacto

Schlagfestigkeit
E impact resistance
F résistance au choc
S resistencia a los choques

Schlagkraft
E impact force
F force de frappe, force d'impact
S fuerza impactante, fuerza de percusión

Schlangenkühler
E cooling coil
F serpentin de refroidissement
S serpentín refrigerador

Schlauch
E tube
F tube, tuyau
S tubo

Schlauchbeutel
E tubular bag
F poche
S bolsa tubular

Schlauchfolie
E tubular film, film tube
F feuille en gaine
S película tubular

Schlauchknick
E tube kink
F coude d'un tuyau
S acodadura de un tubo

Schlauchkupplung
E tube connector
F raccordement de tuyau
S acoplamiento de tubo

Schlauchleitung
E tubing
F tuyauterie
S tubería flexible

Schlauchpumpe
E peristaltic pump
F pompe péristaltique
S bomba peristáltica

Schlauchwagen
E tube carriage
F chariot dévidoir
S transportador de tubos

Schleifenvolumen
E loop volume
F volume de la boucle
S volumen de bucle

Schleim
E mucilage
F mucilage, mucus
S mucosidad

Schleimhaut
E mucous membrane
F muqueuse
S mucosa

Schleimhautgewebe
E mucosal tissue
F tissu d'une muqueuse
S tejido mucoso

schleimig
E mucous
F muqueux
S mucoso, mucilaginoso

Schleuse
E lock
F sas
S esclusa

Materialschleuse
E material lock
F sas réservé aux fournitures
S esclusa de material

Personenschleuse
E personnel lock
F sas réservé au personnel
S esclusa de personal

Schliere
E streaks, stria
F strie
S estría

Schliffkolben
E ground-joint flask
F ballon rodé
S matraz esmerilado

Schliffstopfen
E ground stopper
F bouchon rodé
S tapón esmerilado

English German French Spanish

English German French Spanish

Schlitz
E slit
F fente, fissure, rainure
S fisura, hendidura, raja

Schlüssel (des Stempels)
E key (of punch)
F clavette, ressort d'ajustage (de poinçon)
S llave (de troquel)

schlüsselfertig
E turnkey
F clé en main
S llave en mano

schlüsselfertige Fabrik
E turnkey plant
F usine clé en main
S fábrica llave en mano

Schlüsselkomponente
E key component
F composant clé
S componente clave

Schmelzbereich
E melting range
F plage de fusion
S márgenes de fusión

Schmelze
E melt
F fusion
S fundición, fusión

schmelzen
E melt, to
F fondre
S fundir

Schmelzindex
E melting index
F indice de fusion
S índice de fusión

Schmelzofen
E furnace
F four
S horno fundidor

Schmelzpunkt
E melting point
F point de fusion
S punto de fusión

Sofortschmelzpunkt
E instant melting point
F point de fusion instantané
S punto de fusión inmediata

schmieren
E grease, to; lubricate, to
F graisser, lubrifier
S engrasar, lubri(fi)car

Schmierfett
E grease
F graisse
S grasa lubri(fi)cante

Schmiermittel
E lubricant
F lubrifiant
S lubri(fi)cante

Schmiernippel
E lubricating nipple
F bouchon graisseur
S boquilla lubri(fi)cante

Schmierstoffpumpe
E lubrication pump
F pompe lubrifiante
S bomba de lubri(fi)cante

Schnappdeckel
E snap cap, snap lid
F couvercle à enclenchement
S tapa de cierre de golpe

Schnecke
E worm screw
F vis sans fin
S tornillo sin fin

Schneckendosiermaschine
E dosing screw conveyor
F convoyeur à vis doseuse
S máquina dosificadora de tornillo sin fin

Schneckenförderer
E worm drive
F vis d'Archimède
S transportador de tornillo sin fin

Schneckengetriebe
E worm gear box
F engrenage à vis sans fin
S engranaje de tornillo si fin

schnell freisetzend
E immediate release
F à libération immédiate
S de liberación rápida

Schnellkupplung
E quick coupling, instant coupling
F connexion instantanée
S conexión rápida

Schnellspannvorrichtung
E fast-clamping device
F dispositif de serrage rapide
S dispositivo tensor rápido

Schnellverschluß
E quick-flange connection
F connexion à collerette instantanée
S cierre rápido

Schnittstelle, serielle
E serial interface
F interface série
S interfase seriada

Schokoladenagar
E chocolate agar
F gélose chocolat
S agar chocolate

Schöpfkelle
E ladle, scoop
F louche
S cazo, vasija

Schottverschraubung
E bulkhead connection
F connexion étanche
S atornillado hermético

schräg
E sloping
F incliné, oblique
S inclinado, oblicuo

Schrägagar
E sloping agar
F agar oblique
S agar oblicuo

Schräge
E slope
F biais
S inclinación, oblicuidad

Schräglage
E sloping position, in
F position inclinée
S inclinación

Schraubdeckelverschließmaschine
E screw-cap closing machine
F machine à serrage de couvercles
S máquina de cierre de rosca

Schraube mit Mutter
E screw with nut
F vis avec écrou
S tornillo con tuerca

Schraubenmutter
E nut
F écrou
S tuerca

Schraubenschlüssel
E wrench
F clef de serrage
S cierre de tornillo

Schraubflasche
E screw-cap bottle
F bouteille munie d'un bouchon à vis
S botella con cierre de rosca

Schraubgewinde
E screw thread
F filetage
S filete de tornillo, rosca de tornillo

Schraubglas
E screw cap glass container
F pot fileté
S recipiente de vidrio con cierre de rosca

Schraubkappe
E screw cap
F bouchon à vis
S cierre de rosca

Schraubverschluß
E screw connection
F fermeture à vis
S cierre de rosca

Schreiber
E recorder, chart recorder
F enregistreur
S registradora

Schreiberausdruck
E print-out
F imprimé
S impreso

Schreiberstreifen
E recorder chart
F bande de papier d'enregistreur
S registro de diagramas

schrittweise
E stepwise
F étape par étape
S paso a paso

schrumpfen
E shrink, to
F rétrécir
S contraerse, retraerse, reducirse

Schrumpffolie
E shrink foil, shrink film
F feuille rétractable, film rétractable
S lámina retraíble

Schrumpftunnel
E shrinking tunnel
F tunnel de rétraction
S túnel de retracción

Schubspannung
E shear stress
F contrainte de poussée
S tensión de empuje

Schulter (einer Flasche)
E shoulder section (of a bottle)
F collet (d'une bouteille)
S ensanchamiento (de una botella)

Schulung
E training
F éducation, entraînement
S adiestramiento, instrucción

schuppig
E scaly
F squameux, couvert d'écailles
S escamoso

Schürze
E skirting, apron (of machine)
F tablier
S delantal

Schüttdichte
E bulk density
F densité apparente
S densidad de la masa comprimida

Schüttelbewegung
E shaking movement
F mouvement d'agitation
S movimiento de agitación

Schüttelmaschine
E shaker
F secoueuse
S agitador

Schüttelmixtur
E mixture to be shaken
F mixture devant être agitée
S mezcla a agitar

Schüttgut
E bulk material
F matériau en vrac
S carga a granel

Schüttler
E shaker
F secoueuse, secoueur
S agitador

Schütt-Trichter
E hopper, funnel
F trémie d'alimentation, entonnoir d'alimentation
S tolva

Schütz (elektrisch)
E fuse (electrical)
F protection (électrique)
S protección (eléctrica)

Schutzbrille
E safety spectacles
F lunettes de protection
S gafas protectoras

Schutzgas
E inert gas
F gaz inerte
S gas inerte

Schutzgasverpackung
E inert gas packaging
F emballage avec gaz inerte
S embalaje con gas inerte

Schutzhandschuhe
E protective gloves
F gants protecteurs
S guantes protectores

Schutzhelm
E safety helmet, hard hat
F casque de protection
S casco protector

Schutzkleidung
E protective clothing
F vêtement de protection
S ropa protectora

Schutzschirm
E protective screen
F écran de protection
S pantalla protectora

Schutzschirm aus Sicherheitsglas
E safety glass screen
F écran de protection constitué de verre de sécurité
S pantalla protectora de vidrio de seguridad

schwache Säure
E weak acid
F acide faible
S ácido débil

Schwamm
E sponge
F éponge
S esponja

schwanken
E vary, to; fluctuate, to
F fluctuer
S fluctuar, variar

Schwankung
E variability
F variabilité
S fluctuación

Schwankung des Tablettengewichts
E tablet weight variation
F écart entre les poids d'un comprimé, écart entre les poids d'un cachet
S fluctuación del peso de los comprimidos

Schwefelsäure
E sulphuric acid
F acide sulfurique
S ácido sulfúrico

schweißen
E weld, to
F souder
S soldar

Schweißnaht
E welding seam, weld
F soudure
S soldadura

Schwellendosis
E threshold dosage
F dose liminaire
S dosis liminar, dosis umbral

Schwenkarm
E swivel arm
F bras pivotant
S brazo giratorio

schwenkbar
E hinged, pivotable
F pivotable
S giratorio

Schwerkraft
E gravity
F force de gravité
S fuerza de gravedad

Schwermetall
E heavy metal
F métal lourd
S metal pesado

Schwerpunkt
E centre of gravity
F centre de gravité
S baricentro, centro de gravedad

Schwingung
E vibration
F vibration
S oscilación, vibración

Scrapie-spezifische Proteine (prpsc)
E scrapie-specific prions (prpsc)
F prions spécifiques à la scrapie (prpsc)
S priones específicos de la encefalopatía espongiforme ovina

Screenen mit ultrahohem Durchsatz (UHTS)
E ultra-high throughput screening (UHTS)
F screening à ultra-haut rendement
S detención con ultrarrendimiento

Sedimentationsplatte
E settling plate
F plaque de sédimentation
S placa de sedimentación

sedimentieren
E sediment, to
F sédimenter
S sedimentar

seidenglänzend
E silk glossy
F brillant (comme de la soie)
S brillante como seda

Sekundärausbeute
E secondary yield
F rendement secondaire
S rendimiento secundario

Sekundärkontamination
E secondary contamination
F contamination secondaire
S contaminación secundaria

Sekundärkristalle
E secondary crystals
F cristaux secondaires
S cristales secundarios

Sekundärpackmittel
E secondary packaging material
F matériel d'emballage secondaire
S material de envase secundario

Sekundärprodukte
E secondary products
F produits secondaires
S productos secundarios

Selbstinspektion
E self-inspection
F auto-inspection
S autoinspección

selbstklebend
E self-adhesive
F auto-adhésif
S autoadhesivo

Selbstmedikation
E self-medication
F automédication
S automedicación

Selbstmedikationsprodukt
E over-the-counter (OTC) product
F produit sans ordonnance
S producto para automedicación

Selbstüberprüfung
E self-check
F auto-inspection
S autocomprobación

Selektivität
E selectivity
F sélectivité
S selectividad

Selektivnährmedien
E selective culture medium
F milieu de culture sélectif
S medios de cultivo selectivos

semipermeable Membran
E semi-permeable membrane
F membrane semi-perméable
S membrana semipermeable

senken
E lower, to; reduce, to
F abaisser, baisser
S bajar, reducir

Senkkörper
E sinker
F plomb
S lastre, plomo

Senkniete
E countersunk rivet
F rivet conique
S remache avellanado

Senkschraube
E countersunk screw
F vis conique
S tornillo avellanado

Sensorgehäuse
E sensor housing
F étui du capteur
S caja del sensor

Septum
E septum
F septum
S septo

Sequenzierung
E sequencing
F séquençage
S formación de secuencias, secuenciación

Sequenzierungseinheit
E sequencing unit
F unité de séquençage
S unidad de secuenciación

Seren, tierische
E animal sera
F sérums d'origine animale
S sueros de origen animal

serielle Schnittstelle
E serial interface
F interface série
S interfase seriada

Serien
E series
F séries
S series

Seriennummer
E serial number
F numéro de série
S número de serie

Serum
E serum
F sérum
S suero

fötales Kälberserum
E foetal calf serum
F sérum fœtal de veau
S suero fetal bovino

serumfreie Nährmedien
E serum-free media
F médium de culture exempt de sérum
S medios de cultivo sin suero

English German French Spanish

English
German
French
Spanish

Servicetechniker
E service technician
F technicien
S técnico de servicio

Shampoo
E shampoo
F shampooing
S champú

Sicherheit
E safety, security
F sécurité
S seguridad

Arbeitssicherheit
E safety at work
F sécurité du travail
S seguridad en el trabajo

Sicherheitsanforderungen
E safety requirements
F consignes de sécurité
S requisito de seguridad

Sicherheitsbrille
E safety spectacles
F lunettes de sécurité
S gafas de seguridad

Sicherheitsdatenblatt
E safety data sheet, material safety data sheet (MSDS)
F feuille(t) de données de sécurité
S hoja de datos de seguridad, pliego de datos de seguridad

Sicherheitshinweis
E safety instructions
F instructions de sécurité
S aviso de seguridad

Sicherheitskleidung
E safety clothing
F vêtement de sécurité
S ropa de seguridad

Sicherheitskopie
E back-up file
F copie de sauvegarde
S copia de seguridad

Sicherheitsmaßnahmen
E safety precautions
F précautions de sécurité
S medidas de seguridad

Sicherheitsmerkmal
E safety feature
F caractéristique de sécurité
S característica de seguridad

Sicherheitsrisiko
E safety risk
F danger
S riesgo para la seguridad

Sicherheitsstandards
E safety standards
F normes de sécurité
S estándares de seguridad

Sicherheitsstatus
E safety status
F statut de sécurité
S status de seguridad

Sicherheitsventil
E safety valve
F vanne de sécurité
S válvula de seguridad

Sicherheitsvorrichtung
E safety device
F dispositif de sécurité
S dispositivo de seguridad

Sicherheitsvorschriften
E safety regulation
F règlement de sécurité
S reglamento de seguridad

sicherstellen
E guarantee, to; secure, to; ensure, to
F assurer, garantir
S asegurar, garantizar

Sicherung (elektrisch)
E fuse
F fusible
S cortacircuito, fusible

flinke Sicherung
E fast fuse
F fusible à action instantanée
S fusible rápido

träge Sicherung
E slow fuse
F fusible à action retardée
S fusible lento

Sicherungskasten
E fuse box
F boîte de fusibles
S caja de fusibles

sichtbarmachen
E visualise, to
F visualiser
S visualizar

sichten
E classify, to
F classifier
S clasificar, ordenar

Sichtfenster
E observation window
F fenêtre de visée
S ventana visual

Sichtkontrolle
E visual control
F contrôle visuel
S control visual

Sichtprüfung
E visual examination
F examen visuel
S inspección visual

Sieb
E sieve
F tamis
S cedazo, criba, tamiz

Siebanalyse
E sieve analysis
F granulométrie
S granulometría

Siebboden
E sieve screen
F tamis
S suelo del tamiz

Siebbruch
E sieve rupture
F rupture de trémie
S ruptura del tamiz

Siebdurchgang
E fines
F passant
S paso de tamiz, tamizado

Siebeinsatz
E sieve insert
F segment de tamisage
S inserción del tamiz

sieben
E sieve, to; sift, to
F tamiser
S cribar, tamizar

Siebfraktion
E sieve fraction
F fraction de tamisage
S fracción de tamizado

Siebrückstand
E overs, residue
F résidu de tamisage
S residuo de tamizado

Siebschüttler
E sieve shaker
F tamis secoueur
S tamiz agitador

Siebturm
E sieve tower
F tour de tamisage
S torre de tamizado

Siedekapillare
E boiling capillary
F capillaire d'ébullition
S capilar de ebullición

sieden
E boil, to
F bouillir
S hervir

Siedepunkt
E boiling point
F point d'ébullition
S punto de ebullición

Siedestein
E boiling chip
F pierre facilitant l'ébullition
S piedra de ebullición

Siedeverzug
E boiling retardation
F retardement de l'ébullition
S retraso de la ebullición

Siegelbacken
E sealer jaws
F mâchoires de fermeture
S mandíbulas de sellado

Siegeldruck
E sealing pressure
F pression de scellage, pression de fermeture
S presión de sellado

Siegellack
E sealing wax
F cire à cacheter
S lacre

siegeln
E seal, to
F sceller, clore
S precintar, sellar

Siegelrandbeutel
E sealed bag, sachet
F sachet hermétique
S bolsa hermética

Signal, akustisches
E acoustic signal
F signal acoustique
S señal acústica

Signal, optisches
E visual signal
F signal optique
S señal óptica

Signallampe
E control lamp
F lampe de contrôle
S lámpara de señales

Signalverstärker
E signal amplifier
F amplificateur de signal
S amplificador de señal

Silicagel
E silica gel
F gel de silice
S gel de sílice

Siliciumdioxid
E silica
F silice
S dióxido de silicio

Silikat
E silicate
F silicate
S silicato

Silikonemulsion
E silicone emulsion
F émulsion de silicone
S emulsión de silicona

Silikonisierung
E siliconisation
F siliconisation
S siliconización

Silikonschlauch
E silicone tubing
F tube de silicone
S tubo de silicona

Sinkkasten
E catch basin, drain
F bassin de descente
S fuente (descendente) de recogida

Sinnesprüfung
E organoleptic testing
F test organoleptique
S prueba organoléptica

Sinterglas
E fused glass
F verre fritté
S vidrio sinterizado

Sinterglasteilchen
E fused glass particles
F particules de verre fritté
S partículas de vidrio sinterizado

sintern
E sinter, to
F fritter
S aglomerar, sinterizar

Sirup
E syrup
F sirop
S jarabe

Skala
E scale
F échelle
S escala

Meßskala
E measuring scale
F échelle de mesure
S escala de medida

Skaleneinteilung
E graduation
F graduation
S graduación de una escala

Sockel
E base, socket
F socle
S base, casquillo, zócalo

Sofortschmelzpunkt
E instant melting point
F point de fusion instantané
S punto de fusión instantánea

Software, konfigurierbare
E configurable software
F logiciel configurable
S software configurable

Softwarequalifizierung
E software qualification
F qualification d'un logiciel
S cualificación de la software

Sollwert
E required value
F valeur nominale
S valor nominal

Sonde
E probe
F sonde
S sonda

Sonderausführung
E special version
F version spéciale
S construcción especial, versión especial

Sortierband
E sorting belt
F bande de triage
S cinta clasificadora

Sortiment
E product range
F sortiment
S surtido

Spalt
E slit
F fissure, fente
S fisura, hendidura

Spaltbreite
E slit width
F largeur d'une fissure, largeur d'une fente
S anchura de la fisura

Spalte
E slit, cleft
F fissure, fente, crevasse
S fisura

English
German
French
Spanish

Spannung (elektrisch)
E voltage
F tension
S tensión

Spannungsänderung
E voltage variation
F variation de tension
S variación de la tensión

Spannungsmesser
E voltmeter
F voltmètre
S voltímetro

Spannungsregler
E voltage regulator
F régulateur de tension
S regulador de tensión

Spannungsschwankung
E voltage fluctuation
F variation de tension
S fluctuación de la tensión

Sparte
E division
F département, section
S especialidad, rama, sector

Spatel
E spatula
F spatule
S espátula

speicherprogrammierbare Steuerung (SPS)
E programmable logic control (PLC)
F automate programmable industriel
S control programable mediante memoria

Speisewasser
E feed water
F eau d'alimentation
S agua de alimentación

Spektralphotometrie
E spectrophotometry
F spectrophotomètre
S espectrofotometría

Spektrum
E spectrum
F spectre
S espectro

Spender (als Person)
E dispenser, donor (person)
F distributeur, donneur (personne)
S distribuidor, donante (persona)

Sperrflüssigkeit
E barrier fluid
F barrière fluidique
S barrera líquida

Sperrlager
E quarantine (warehouse)
F quarantaine (entrepôt)
S almacén para cuarentena

Sperrschicht
E barrier layer
F couche de barrage
S estrato barrera

Sperrung
E quarantine
F quarantaine
S bloqueo, cierre, cuarentena

Sperrventil
E blocking valve
F vanne de verrouillage
S válvula de bloqueo

Spezies
E species
F espèce
S especie

Spezifikation
E specification
F spécification
S especificación

außerhalb der Spezifikation
E out of specification (OOS)
F hors spécification
S fuera de la especificación

Spezifikationsgrenze
E specification limit
F limite de spécification
S límite de especificación

enge Spezifikationsgrenzen
E tight specification limits
F limites étroites de spécification
S límites estrechos de especificación

obere Spezifikationsgrenze
E upper specification limit
F limite supérieure de spécification
S límite superior de especificación

untere Spezifikationsgrenze
E lower specification limit
F limite inférieure de spécification
S límite inferior de especificación

spezifische Drehung
E specific rotation
F rotation spécifique
S rotación específica

spezifische Oberfläche
E specific surface (area)
F aire spécifique
S superficie específica

spezifische Wärme
E specific heat
F chaleur spécifique
S calor específico

spezifischer Widerstand
E specific resistance
F résistance spécifique
S resistencia específica

spezifisches Gewicht
E specific gravity
F poids spécifique
S peso específico

Spezifität
E specificity
F spécificité
S especificidad

spezifizieren
E specify, to
F spécifier
S especificar

sphärisch
E spherical
F sphérique
S esférico

Spießampulle
E glass ampoule
F ampoule de verre
S ampolla de vidrio

Spike
E spike
F pointe, ajout
S punta

Spind
E locker
F placard de vestiaire
S armario estrecho

Spindraum
E locker room
F vestiaire
S vestuario

spiralförmig
E spiral
F en forme d'hélice
S espiraliforme

Spitzkolben
E conical flask
F ballon conique
S matraz cónico

Spontanreaktion
E spontaneous reaction
F réaction spontanée
S reacción espontánea

Sporen
E spores
F spores
S esporas

English German French Spanish

Sporenbildner
E spore former
F producteur de spores
S productor de esporas

Sporenstreifen
E spore strip
F bande de spores
S banda de esporas

sporozid
E sporicide
F sporicide
S esporicida

Spreizung
E spreading
F propagation
S extensión, propagación

Sprengmittel
E disintegrant, tablet disintegrant
F agent délitant, désintégrant
S desintegrante

Sprinkleranlage
E sprinkler
F réseau de sprinkler
S aspersor

Spritze
E syringe
F seringue
S jeringa

Einmalspritze
E disposable syringe
F seringue à usage unique
S jeringa de uso único

Fertigspritze
E prefilled syringe
F seringue prête à l'emploi
S jeringa lista para el uso

Spritzenzylinder
E syringe cylinder
F cylindre de seringue
S cilindro de jeringa

Spritzer
E splashes
F éclaboussures
S inyección, rociado, salpicadura

Spritzflasche
E wash bottle
F pissette, flacon laveur
S matraz de lavado

Spritzgußteil
E injection-moulded component
F composant moulé par injection
S componente moldeado por inyección

Spritzschutz
E spray protection
F couvercle anti-éclaboussures
S protección frente al salpicado

Spritzwasser
E splash water
F eau de ruissellement
S agua de inyección, agua de rociado

spröde
E brittle
F cassant, fragile
S frágil, quebradizo

Sprühbereich
E spray area
F aire de pulvérisation
S área de pulverización

Sprühkopf
E nozzle head
F gicleur, buse
S cabeza del inyector

Sprührate
E spray rate
F vitesse de pulvérisation
S tasa de pulverización

Sprühsystem
E spraying system
F système de pulvérisation
S sistema de pulverización

sprühtrocknen
E spray-dry, to
F séchage par atomisation
S secar atomizando

Sprühzyklus
E spray cycle
F cycle de pulvérisation
S ciclo de pulverización

spülen
E rinse, to
F rincer
S enjuagar, irrigar, lavar

Spülgas
E purge gas
F gas de purge
S gas purgante

Spüllösung
E rinsing solution
F solution de rinçage
S solución de lavado

Spülmedium
E rinsing medium
F milieu de rinçage
S medio de lavado

Spülwasser
E rinsing water
F eau de rinçage
S agua de lavado

Spur
E trace
F trace
S traza, vestigio

Spurenanalyse
E trace analysis
F analyse de traces
S análisis de vestigios

Spurenelemente
E trace elements
F oligoélément
S oligoelementos

Sputum
E sputum
F crachat
S esputo

Stabilisator
E stabilising agent
F agent stabilisant
S estabilizador

Stabilität, thermische
E thermal stability
F stabilité thermique
S estabilidad térmica

Stabilitätsuntersuchung
E stability study
F étude de stabilité
S ensayo de estabilidad

Kurzzeitstabilität
E short-term stability
F étude de stabilité à court terme
S estabilidad a corto plazo

Langzeitstabilität
E long-term stability
F étude de stabilité à long terme
S estabilidad a largo plazo

Stadtwasser
E public water supply
F approvisionnement public en eau
S abastecimiento público de agua

Stahl
E steel
F acier
S acero

Edelstahl
E stainless steel
F inox, acier inoxydable
S acero inoxidable

Stamm (mikrobiol.)
E strain
F lignée
S cepa

English German French Spanish

Stammkultur
E stock culture
F culture mère
S cultivo madre

Stammlösung
E stock solution
F solution mère
S solución madre

Stammzellbank
E stem cell bank
F banque de cellules souches
S banco de células germinales

Stampfdichte
E packed density, tapped density
F densité de tassement
S densidad de apisonamiento

Stand der Technik
E state-of-the-art
F dernier cri de la technique
S estado (actual) de la técnica

Standard, interner
E internal standard
F étalon interne
S estándar interno

Standardabweichung
E standard deviation
F déviation standard
S desviación estándar

maximal zulässige Standardabweichung
E maximum permitted standard deviation
F déviation standard maximum permise
S desviación estándar máxima permitida

relative Standardabweichung
E relative standard deviation
F écart-type relatif
S desviación estándar relativa

Standardarbeitsanweisung
E standard operating procedure (SOP)
F procédures opératoires standards
S instrucción estándar de trabajo

Standardfaktor
E standardisation factor
F facteur de standardisation
S factor estándar

standardisieren
E standardise, to
F standardiser
S estandarizar

Standardreferenzsubstanz
E standard reference material
F substance de référence standard
S sustancia de referencia estándar

Standort
E site, location
F emplacement
S emplazamiento, ubicación

Standortwechsel
E change of site, change of location
F déménagement
S cambio de emplazamiento

Standzeit (von Filtern)
E standing time, period of use (of filters)
F période d'utilisation (de filtres)
S período de funcionamiento, período de uso (de filtros)

Stanze
E punch
F poinçon
S estampa, punzonadora, troqueladora

stanzen
E stamp, to; emboss, to
F poinçonner, estamper
S estampar, punzonar, troquelar

Stanzstation
E die-cutting station
F station de poinçonnage
S estación de troquelado

Stapel
E stack, pile
F pile
S montón, pila

Stapelkasten
E stacking box
F boîte de stockage
S caja de apilamiento

stapeln
E stack, to
F empiler
S almacenar, amontonar, apilar

Stapelplan (im Lager)
E stacking plan (in warehouse)
F plan de stockage (entrepôt)
S plan de almacenamiento

Stapelung
E stacking
F empilage
S apilamiento

Stapelvorrichtung
E stacking device
F dispositif de stockage
S dispositivo de apilamiento

Stapler
E stacker
F chariot élévateur
S apilador

Stärke (Substanz)
E starch
F amidon
S almidón

Stärke (z. B. einer Tablette)
E strength
F dureté
S fuerza

starr
E rigid
F rigide
S rígido

starten (Ablauf)
E start, to (a process)
F démarrer (un procédé)
S comenzar (un proceso)

stationäre Phase
E stationary phase
F phase stationnaire
S fase estacionaria

statische Aufladung
E static charge
F charge statique
S carga estática

statische Beanspruchung
E static stress
F stress statique
S tensión estática

statische Belastung
E static load
F charge statique
S carga estática

Statistiker
E statistician
F statisticien
S estadístico

Stativ
E stand
F trépied
S soporte, trípode

Statusbericht
E status report
F rapport de situation
S informe de la situación

Staubabsauganlage
E dust exhausting device, dust extraction
F système d'aspiration de la poussière
S sistema de aspiración de polvo

Staubanteil
E dust concentration
F concentration en poussière
S proporción de polvo

English German French Spanish

staubdicht
E dust-tight
F étanche à la poussière
S hermético para el polvo

Staubentwicklung
E dust production
F production de poussière
S producción de polvo

staubgeschützt
E dustproof
F imperméable à la poussière
S protegido frente al polvo

Staubkontrolle
E dust control
F contrôle de la poussière
S control de polvo

Staubmaske
E dust mask
F masque contre la poussière
S máscara contra el polvo

Staubpartikel
E dust particles
F particules de poussière
S partícula de polvo

Staubschutz
E dust guard
F protection contre les poussières
S protección contra el polvo

Stechheber
E powder sampler, sampling device, sampling pipette
F dispositif d'échantillonnage, pipette de prélèvement
S pipeta (de toma de muestras)

Steckkapsel
E hard capsule
F gélule
S cápsula gelatinosa dura

Steckkupplung
E plug connection
F connexion à fiche(s)
S conexión de enchufe

Steghöhe (bei Tabletten)
E band height (of tablets)
F hauteur de bande (de comprimés)
S altura de banda (de comprimidos)

steif
E rigid
F rigide
S rígido

Steigrohr
E dip tube
F colonne d'ascension
S tubo ascensional, tubo montante

steil
E steep
F raide, escarpé
S empinado, escarpado

Stellenbeschreibung
E job description
F description d'un emploi
S descripción de un puesto de trabajo

Stellvertreter
E deputy
F suppléant, remplaçant
S suplente, sustituto

Stellvertretung
E deputisation
F suppléance
S suplencia, sustitución

Stellwand
E partition
F mur de partage
S pantalla protectora

Stempel (zum Drucken)
E stamp
F tampon
S estampadora

Stempel (zum Tablettieren)
E punch
F poinçon
S troquel

Oberstempel
E upper punch
F poinçon supérieur
S troquel superior

Unterstempel
E lower punch
F poinçon inférieur
S troquel inferior

Stempeldichtigkeit
E punch tightness
F étanchéité d'un poinçon
S estanqueidad del troquel

Stempelform
E punch shape, punch form
F forme d'un poinçon
S forma del troquel

Stempelführung
E punch guide
F guidage d'un poinçon
S guía del troquel

Stempelgeschwindigkeit
E punch speed, punch velocity
F vitesse d'un poinçon
S velocidad del troquel

Stempelhals
E punch neck
F collet du poinçon
S cuello de troquel

Stempelhalter
E punch holder
F support de poinçon
S soporte del troquel

Stempelkopf
E punch head, punch tip
F tête du poinçon
S cabeza de troquel

Stempelkopflänge
E punch tip length
F longueur de la tête du poinçon
S longitud de la cabeza de troquel

Stempelleichtgängigkeit
E easy punch sliding
F facilité de glissement d'un poinçon
S facilidad de deslizamiento del troquel

stempeln
E mark, to; stamp, to
F poinçonner
S troquelar

Stempelschwergängigkeit
E punch sticking
F difficulté de glissement d'un poinçon
S dificultad de deslizamiento del troquel

Stempelstation
E punch station
F station de poinçonnage
S estación de troquelado

Stempeltyp
E punch type
F type de poinçon
S tipo de troquel

stereoselektiv
E stereoselective
F stéréosélectif
S estereoselectivo

steril
E sterile
F stérile
S estéril

sterile Zubereitung
E sterile form
F forme stérile
S forma estéril, preparación estéril

Sterilfilter, endständiger
E terminal sterile filter
F filtre stérile terminal
S filtro estéril terminal

Sterilfiltration
E sterile filtration
F filtration stérile
S filtración estéril

sterilfiltrieren
E sterile-filter, to
F stérile-filtrer
S filtrar estérilmente

sterilfiltriert
E sterile-filtered
F stérile-filtré
S filtrado estérilmente

Sterilisation
E sterilisation
F stérilisation
S esterilización

Sterilisationssicherheit
E sterility assurance
F garantie de stérilité
S garantía de esterilización

Sterilisationstemperatur
E sterilisation temperature
F température de stérilisation
S temperatura de esterilización

Sterilisationszeit
E duration of sterilisation, sterilisation time
F durée de stérilisation, temps de stérilisation
S tiempo de esterilización

Sterilisator
E autoclave, steriliser
F autoclave
S esterilizador

Sterilisierbarkeit
E sterilisability
F aptitude à être stérilisé
S esterilizabilidad

Sterilisierkammer
E autoclave (sterilisation) chamber
F chambre d'autoclave
S cámara de esterilización

Sterilprodukt
E sterile product
F produit stérile
S producto estéril

Sterilraumkleidung
E sterile gowns, sterile clothing
F vêtement pour zone stérile
S vestuario estéril

Steriltest
E sterility test
F test de stérilité
S prueba estéril

sterische Anordnung
E sterical arrangement
F configuration stérique
S configuración estérica

Steroide
E steroids
F stéroïdes
S esteroides

Steuerung
E control
F contrôle
S control

Steuerungsausschuß zur Validierung
E validation review committee
F comité directeur de validation
S comisión fiscal de validación

Stichleitung
E stub
F bout
S adaptador de guiaondas

Stichprobe
E random sample
F échantillon prélevé au hasard
S muestra al azar

Stichprobenanweisung
E sampling instructions
F instructions d'échantillonnage
S instrucciones para tomar muestras

Schärfe der Stichprobenanweisung
E sampling criteria
F critères d'échantillonnage
S rigor de las instrucciones para tomar muestras

Stickstoff
E nitrogen
F azote
S nitrógeno

Stickstoff-Phosphor-Detektor
E nitrogen-phosphorous detector (NPD)
F détecteur d'azote phosphorisé
S detector de nitrógeno fosforado

Stift (technisch)
E pin
F broche, pointeau, goupille
S clavija, perno, pivote

Stiftmühle
E pin mill
F broyeur à broches
S molino de clavija

Stöchiometrie
E stoichiometry
F stoichiométrie
S estequiometría

Stockwerksplan
E floor plan
F plan d'étage
S plano de los pisos

Stopfen
E plug, stopper
F bouchon, tampon
S tapón

Stopfen aus Butylgummi
E butyl rubber stoppers
F bouchon en caoutchouc butyle
S tapón de caucho butílico

Stopfenwaschmaschine
E stopper washing machine
F machine à laver les bouchons
S máquina de lavado de tapones

Stopgrenze
E action limit
F limite d'action
S límite de acción

Störanzeige
E fault (failure) display
F affichage d'une erreur
S pantalla de aviso de avería

Störbanden
E interfering bands
F bandes d'interférence
S bandas de interferencia

Störfall
E fault, failure, accident
F panne, incident
S avería, fallo, incidente

Störung
E malfunction, interference
F perturbation, dérangement
S avería, fallo

elektrische Störung
E electrical interference
F interférence électrique
S avería eléctrica

Störungsmeldung
E malfunction indication, malfunction alarm, failure alarm
F alarme de mauvais fonctionnement
S aviso de avería

Stoß
E impact
F impact, choc, coup
S choque, golpe, impacto

stoßfest
E impact-resistant
F résistant aux chocs
S resistente a los golpes

Stoßschutz
E impact protection
F protection anti-chocs
S protección frente a la colisión

Strahlenschutzgesetz
E radiation protection act
F loi pour la protection contre les radiations
S ley de protección frente a radiaciones ionizantes

English German French Spanish

Strahlensterilisation
E radiation sterilisation
F stérilisation par irradiation
S esterilización por irradiación

Strahlung
E radiation
F radiation
S radiación

Strangpresse
E extruder
F extrudeuse
S prensa extrusora

Straßenkleidung
E street clothing
F vêtements de ville
S ropa de calle

Streichfähigkeit
E spreadability
F aptitude à être étendu
S untabilidad

Streßtest
E accelerated stability test
F test de stabilité accéléré
S estudio acelerado de estabilidad

Streubreite
E dispersion, stray range
F dispersion
S dispersión

Streudose
E sprinkler can
F flacon saupoudreur
S frasco espolvoreador

Streulicht
E stray light
F lumière diffuse
S luz difusa

Streulicht-Detektor
E light-scattering detector
F détecteur de lumière diffuse
S detector de luz dispersa

Streupulver
E dusting powder
F poudrage
S polvo vulnerario

Streuung (von Werten)
E spread, distribution (of values)
F diffusion, dispersion (de valeurs)
S dispersión (de valores)

Strichmarkierung
E graduation mark
F marque de graduation
S marca de graduación

Strom
E current, electricity
F courant, électricité
S corriente eléctrica

Stromaufnahme
E power consumption
F consommation d'électricité
S consumo de electricidad

Stromausfall
E power failure
F coupure de courant
S corte de corriente

zeitweiser Stromausfall
E intermittent power interruption
F coupure de courant intermittente
S corte intermitente de coriente, corte transitorio de corriente

Stromgleichrichter
E rectifier
F redresseur de courant
S rectificador de corriente

Stromkreis
E circuit, loop
F circuit
S circuito eléctrico

Strommesser
E ammeter
F ampèremètre
S amperímetro

Stromquelle
E power source
F source d'électricité
S fuente de electricidad

Stromstärke
E amperage
F ampérage
S amperaje, intensidad de corriente

Strömung, laminare
E laminar flow
F flux laminaire
S flujo laminar

Strömung, turbulente
E turbulent flow
F flux turbulent
S flujo turbulento

Strömungsgeschwindigkeit
E flow rate
F débit
S velocidad del flujo

Strömungswächter
E flow meter
F débitmètre
S fluxómetro

Stromversorgung
E power supply
F alimentation en courant électrique
S suministro eléctrico

Stromversorgungsschwankungen
E power supply fluctuation
F variations de l'intensité du courant
S fluctuaciones de la intensidad de corriente eléctrica

Strukturaufklärung
E structural analysis
F analyse structurelle
S análisis estructural

Strukturformel
E structural formula
F formule développée
S fórmula estructural

Stückgut
E itemised goods
F colis
S bultos sueltos

Stückliste
E bill of materials, list of items
F liste-inventaire, liste détaillée
S especificación, lista detallada, inventario

Stückzahl
E number of items
F nombre de pièces
S número de piezas

Studie, klinische
E clinical study, clinical trial
F essai clinique
S estudio clínico

Studiendauer
E duration of trial
F durée d'un essai
S duración de prueba

Studiendesign
E study design, trial design
F design d'un essai clinique
S diseño de un estudio (clínico)

Studienende
E end of study, end of trial
F fin d'un essai clinique
S fin del estudio

Studienstart
E start of study, start of trial
F démarrage d'un essai clinique
S comienzo del estudio

stufenlos
E continuous
F continu
S continuo

Stufenplan
E graduated plan
F plan échelonné
S plan escalonado, plan graduado

English
German
French
Spanish

Stufenplanbeauftragter
E pharmaco-vigilance manager, drug safety manager
F personne responsable de la pharmaco-vigilance
S responsable de farmacovigilancia

stufenweise
E stepwise
F par étapes, échelonné
S gradualmente

Stuhluntersuchung
E faeces test
F analyse des selles
S examen de heces

stumpfschweißen
E butt-weld, to
F souder par rapprochement
S soldar a tope

Stundenleistung
E output per hour
F rendement horaire, débit horaire
S rendimiento horario

Stützdruck
E support pressure
F contre-pression, pression de soutien
S contrapresión, presión de soporte

Stütze
E support brace
F support
S apoyo, soporte

Stutzen
E support
F support, embout
S empalme, tubuladura

Stützkonstruktion
E supporting construction
F construction de soutien
S construcción de sostén

Subkultur
E sub-culture
F culture repiquée
S subcultivo

subkutan
E subcutaneous
F sous-cutanée
S subcutáneo

Sublimierung
E sublimation
F sublimation
S sublimación

Sublingualspray
E sub-lingual spray
F aérosol sublingual
S spray sublingual

Substanzmodellierung
E substance modelling
F modelage de substance
S modelado de sustancias

Substitution
E substitution
F substitution
S sustitución

Substitutionsreaktion
E substitution reaction
F réaction de substitution
S reacción de sustitución

Substrat
E substrate
F substrat
S sustrato

Sucht
E addiction
F accoutumance
S adicción

Sulfatasche
E sulphate ash
F cendre sulfatée
S ceniza sulfatada

Summenverteilung
E sum distribution
F distribution des sommes
S distribución de sumas

Suppositorien
E suppositories
F suppositoires
S supositorios

Suppositoriengrundlage
E suppository base
F composant de base d'un suppositoire
S excipiente de un supositorio

Suspendierbarkeit
E suspendibility
F suspensif
S suspensibilidad

suspendieren
E suspend, to
F suspenser
S suspender

Suspendierung
E suspension
F suspension
S suspensión

Suspension
E suspension
F suspension
S suspensión

Süßstoff
E sweetener
F édulcorant
S edulcorante

Synärese
E synaresis
F synérèse
S sinéresis

Synthese
E synthesis
F synthèse
S síntesis

Syntheseweg
E synthesis route
F voie de synthèse
S vía de síntesis

Systemeignungstest
E system suitability test
F essai d'aptitude d'un système
S ensayo de adecuación de un sistema

Systemspezifikation
E system specification
F spécification d'un système
S especificación de un sistema

Tabelle
E table
F tableau, table
S tabla

Tablett
E tray
F plateau
S bandeja

Tablette
E tablet
F comprimé
S comprimido

Aussehen der Tablette
E tablet appearance
F apparence d'un comprimé
S aspecto de un comprimido

Bruchfestigkeit einer Tablette
E tablet crushing strength
F résistance à la rupture d'un comprimé
S resistencia a la ruptura de un comprimido

Einheitlichkeit der Tablettenfarbe
E tablet colour uniformity
F uniformité de la couleur d'un comprimé
S uniformidad del color de los comprimidos

fehlerhafte Tabletten
E faulty tablets
F comprimés défectueux
S comprimidos defectuosos

längliche Tablette
E oblong tablet
F comprimé allongé
S comprimido elongado

Uneinheitlichkeit von Tabletten
E tablet inconsistency
F hétérogénéité des comprimés
S heterogeneidad de los comprimidos

Tablettenablaufrinne
E tablet exit chute
F rigole d'écoulement pour comprimés
S canal de salida de los comprimidos

Tablettenablaufweichen
E tablet gate
F déversoir pour comprimés
S lámina divisoria para comprimidos

Tablettenabmessungen
E tablet dimensions
F dimensions d'un comprimé
S dimensiones del comprimido

Tablettenausstoß
E tablet output
F débit de production de comprimés
S rendimiento en comprimidos

Tablettenauswurf
E tablet ejection
F éjection d'un comprimé
S expulsión de comprimidos

Tablettendicke
E tablet thickness
F épaisseur d'un comprimé
S espesor del comprimido

Tablettendurchmesser
E tablet diameter
F diamètre d'un comprimé
S diámetro del comprimido

Tablettengewicht
E tablet weight
F poids d'un comprimé
S peso del comprimido

Tablettenhärte
E tablet hardness
F dureté d'un comprimé
S dureza del comprimido

Tablettenkategorie
E tablet category
F catégorie du comprimé
S categoría de comprimido

Tablettenkern
E tablet core
F noyau d'un comprimé
S núcleo del comprimido

Tablettenkontrolle
E tablet checking
F contrôle d'un comprimé
S control de comprimidos

Tablettenoberfläche
E tablet surface
F surface d'un comprimé
S superficie del comprimido

Tablettenpresse
E tablet press
F presse à comprimés, pastilleuse
S prensa de comprimidos

instrumentierte Tablettenpresse
E automated tablet press
F presse à comprimés avec instruments
S prensa automática de comprimidos

Rundläuferpresse
E rotary press
F presse rotative
S prensa rotatoria

Tablettenprofil
E tablet profile
F profil du comprimé
S perfil de comprimido

Tablettensteghöhe
E tablet web height
F hauteur de bande d'un comprimé
S altura de banda de un comprimido

Tablettenüberwachungssystem
E tablet monitoring system
F système de surveillance des comprimés
S sistema de vigilancia de comprimidos

Tablettenwerkzeug
E tablet tooling
F presse-outil pour comprimés
S utensilios para elaborar comprimidos

Tablettierausstoß
E tablet output
F débit de production de comprimés
S rendimiento de la máquina de comprimidos

Tablettierfarbe
E tablet dye
F couleur de fabrication de comprimés
S color de fabricación de comprimidos

Tablettiermaschine
E tabletting machine
F machine de fabrication de comprimés
S máquina de fabricación de comprimidos

Tablettiermasse
E tabletting mass
F masse de fabrication pour comprimés
S masa para comprimidos

Tablettierstempel
E tabletting punch
F poinçon de fabrication de comprimés
S troquel para comprimidos

Tablettierung
E tabletting, compression, compaction
F fabrication de comprimés
S fabricación de comprimidos

computerintegrierte Tablettierung
E computer-integrated tabletting (CIT)
F fabrication de comprimés informatisée
S fabricación informatizada de comprimidos

Tablettierwerkzeug
E compaction device
F instrument de fabrication de comprimés
S instrumentos para fabricar comprimidos

Tagesdosis
E daily dosage
F dose journalière
S dosis diaria

täglich
E daily
F journalier
S diario

Taktzahl
E cycle number
F cadence
S número de ciclos

Tampon
E tampon
F tampon
S tampón

Tangente
E tangent
F tangente
S tangente

Tankbelüftung
E tank aspiration
F aération du réservoir
S ventilación del tanque

Tankwagen
E tank wagon
F wagon-citerne
S camión cisterna

English German French Spanish

Tara
E tare
F tare
S tara

tarieren
E tare, to
F tarer
S tarar

Tastatur(feld)
E key board
F clavier
S teclado

Taste
E key
F touche
S tecla

Tastkopf
E scanning head
F tête d'analyse
S cabeza de exploración

Tauchbad
E immersion bath
F bain d'immersion
S baño de sumersión

Tauchlack
E immersion lacquer
F laque par immersion
S barniz de inmersión

Tauchrohr
E dip tube
F colonne d'immersion
S tubo de inmersión

Tauchschwert
E immersion sword
F lame d'immersion
S lámina de inmersión

Tauchsieder
E immersion heater
F chauffe-liquide
S calentador de inmersión

Tauchverfahren, im
E by immersion
F procédé par immersion
S en procedimiento de inmersión

Taumelmischer
E tumble blender
F mélangeur culbuteur
S mezclador de volteo

Taupunkt
E dewpoint
F point de rosée
S punto de descongelación

Technik
E technique, method
F technique, méthode
S técnica, método

Technik (als Abteilung)
E engineering
F ingénierie
S departamento técnico

Technikgang
E service corridor
F corridor de service
S corredor de servicio

Technikgeschoß
E technical floor
F étage du service technique
S piso de servicio técnico

technische Zeichnung
E engineering drawing
F dessin technique
S dibujo técnico

Technischer Leiter
E head of engineering department
F directeur du département d'ingénierie
S director del departamento técnico

Technologietransfer
E technology transfer
F transfers de technologie
S transferencia tecnológica

teigartig
E doughy, pasty
F pâteux
S pastoso

Teil
E part, moiety
F partie, portion
S parte

Teilcharge
E partial batch, sub-batch
F sous-lot
S lote parcial, sublote

Teilchen
E particle
F particule
S partícula

Teilchenform
E particle form, particle shape
F forme d'une particule
S forma de la partícula

Teilchengröße
E particle size
F taille des particules
S tamaño de la partícula

Teilchenspektrometer
E particle spectrometer
F spectomètre de particules
S espectrometría de partículas

Teilstrich
E graduation mark
F marque de graduation
S marca de graduación

Teilzeitkraft
E part-time employee
F employé à mi-temps
S empleado a tiempo parcial

Temperatur
E temperature
F température
S temperatura

adiabatische Temperatur
E adiabatic temperature
F température adiabatique
S temperatura adiabática

Temperaturabfall
E temperature decrease
F baisse de température
S descenso de temperatura

Temperaturabweichung
E temperature deviation
F déviation de température
S desviación de temperatura

Temperaturausgleich
E temperature equalisation
F compensation de température
S compensación de temperatura

Temperatureinstellung
E temperature setting
F réglage de la température
S ajuste de temperatura

Temperaturerhöhung
E temperature increase
F augmentation de température
S aumento de temperatura

Temperaturfühler
E temperature sensor
F sonde de température
S sensor de temperatura

Temperaturgefälle
E temperature gradient
F gradient de température
S gradiente de temperatura

Temperaturregler
E temperature controller
F régulateur de température
S regulador de temperatura

Temperaturschreiber
E temperature recorder
F enregistreur de température
S registrador de temperatura

English German French Spanish

Temperaturschwankung
E temperature fluctuation
F variation de température
S fluctuación de la temperatura

Temperatursensor
E temperature sensor
F sonde thermique
S sensor de temperatura

Temperaturverteilung
E heat distribution
F répartition de la température
S distribución de temperatura

temporäre Härte (von Wasser)
E temporary hardness (of water)
F dureté temporaire (de l'eau)
S dureza temporal (del agua)

Tensid
E tenside
F tenside
S agente tensioactivo

teratogen
E teratogenic
F tératogène
S teratógeno

ternär
E ternary
F ternaire
S ternario

Tertiärstruktur
E spatial structure
F structure spatiale
S estructura espacial, estructura terciaria (p. ej. de una proteína)

Testbedingung, simulierte
E simulated test condition
F condition de test simulée
S condiciones simuladas de ensayo

Testergebnis
E analytical result
F résultat d'analyse
S resultado de la prueba

Testschleife
E test loop
F boucle de test
S bucle de pruebas

Teststäbchen
E test strip
F bâtonnet de test
S bastoncillos de prueba

theoretische Ausbeute
E theoretical yield
F rendement théorique
S rendimiento teórico

therapeutisch
E therapeutic
F thérapeutique
S terapéutico

thermische Alterung
E thermal ageing
F vieillissement thermique
S envejecimiento térmico

thermische Belastung
E thermal load
F charge thermique
S carga térmica

thermische Masse
E thermal mass
F masse thermique
S masa térmica

thermische Reaktion
E thermal reaction
F réaction thermique
S reacción térmica

thermische Stabilität
E thermal stability
F stabilité thermique
S estabilidad térmica

thermische Umwandlung
E thermal conversion
F conversion thermique
S conversión térmica

thermisches Verhalten
E thermal behaviour
F comportement thermique
S comportamiento térmico

thermoelastisch
E thermo-elastic
F thermo-élastique
S termoelástico

Thermoelement
E thermocouple
F thermocouple
S elemento termoeléctrico, pila termoeléctrica

Thermoformmaschine
E thermoforming machine
F emboutisseuse
S máquina de deformación térmica

Thermofühler
E thermocouple, heat sensor
F sonde thermique
S sonda térmica

thermoplastisch
E thermo-plastic
F thermoplastique
S termoplástico

Thermostat
E thermostat
F thermostat
S termostato

Thermoverformung
E thermoforming
F emboutissage
S deformación térmica

Tiefenfilter
E depth filter
F filtre profondeur
S filtro de profundidad

tieffrieren
E deep-freeze, to
F congeler
S congelar

tiefgefroren
E deep-frozen
F congelé
S congelado

Tiefkühllager
E frozen storage
F stockage à très basse température
S almacén congelador

Tiefkühlung
E deep freezing
F surgélation
S congelación

tiefziehen
E deep draw, to
F emboutir
S embutir a profundidad

Tiefziehfolie
E thermoforming foil
F feuille thermoformée
S lámina termoformada

Tiefziehmaschine
E blister (forming) line
F machine pour conditionnements thermoformés
S máquina para troquelar en caliente

Tiefziehverpackung
E blister pack
F conditionnement thermoformé, conditionnement sous blister
S envase termoformado, envase blíster

Tiegel
E crucible
F creuset
S crisol

Tiegelzange
E tongs
F pince à creuset
S pinza de crisol

Tierarzneimittel
E veterinary medicament
F médicament à usage vétérinaire
S medicamento de uso veterinario

Tierarzt
E doctor of veterinary medicine, vet
F vétérinaire
S veterinario

tierische Seren
E animal sera
F sérums d'origine animale
S sueros de origen animal

Tierversuch
E animal experiment
F expériences réalisées sur animaux
S experimento con animales

Tinktur
E tincture
F teinture
S tintura

Tinte
E ink
F encre
S tinta

Tintenstrahldrucker
E ink jet printer
F imprimante à jet d'encre
S impresora de chorro de tinta

Titer
E titre
F titre
S título

Titration
E titration
F titration, dosage
S titulación

Rücktitration
E back titration
F dosage en retour
S titulación inversa

Titrationskurve
E titration curve
F courbe de titrage, courbe de dosage
S curva de titulación

Tochterfirma
E subsidiary company
F filiale (société)
S empresa filial, empresa subsidiaria

tödliche Dosis
E fatal dose
F dose mortelle
S dosis mortal

Toleranz
E tolerance
F tolérance
S tolerancia

außer Toleranz
E out of tolerance
F hors des limites de tolérance
S fuera de la tolerancia

festgelegte Toleranzen
E specified tolerances
F tolérances spécifiques
S tolerancias prefijadas

Toleranzbereich
E tolerance range
F intervalle de tolérance
S intervalo de tolerancia

Tonizität
E tonicity
F tonicité
S tonicidad

topisch
E topical
F topique
S tópico

Torsionsfeder
E torsion spring
F ressort de torsion
S muelle de torsión

Torsionskraft
E torsion
F torsion
S fuerza de torsión

Torsionswaage
E torsion balance
F balance de torsion
S balanza de torsión

tote Enden
E dead spots
F extrémités
S extremos de desecho

Totraum
E dead space
F espace mort
S espacio muerto

totraumfrei
E dead volume-free
F dépourvu de volume mort
S sin espacios muertos

Totvolumen
E dead volume
F volume mort
S volumen muerto

Totzeit
E dead time
F temps mort
S tiempo muerto

Toxikologie
E toxicology
F toxicologie
S toxicología

toxikologische Prüfung
E toxicological testing
F étude toxicologique
S prueba toxicológica

Toxin
E toxin, poison
F toxine
S toxina, veneno

toxisch
E toxic, poisonous
F toxique
S tóxico

toxische Verbindung
E toxic compound
F substance toxique
S compuesto tóxico

Toxizität
E toxicity
F toxicité
S toxicidad

Trägergas
E carrier gas
F gaz porteur
S gas portador

Tragfähigkeit
E loading capacity
F limite de charge, force portante
S capacidad de carga

Tränenflüssigkeit
E lacrimal fluid
F liquide lacrymal
S líquido lacrimal

tränken
E soak, to; impregnate, to
F imprégner
S embeber, empapar, impregnar

transdermales Pflaster
E transdermal patch
F pansement transcutané
S emplasto transdérmico

Transdermales Therapeutisches System
E transdermal delivery system
F système thérapeutique transdermique
S sistema terapéutico transdérmico

Transfusionsbesteck
E transfusion set
F nécessaire de transfusion
S instrumental de transfusión

Transkription
E transcription
F transcription
S transcripción

English German French Spanish

Transportband
E conveyor belt
F tapis roulant, convoyeur à bande
S cinta transportadora

Transportbestimmungen
E transport regulations
F régulations des activités de transport
S especificaciones de transporte

Transportschaden
E transport damage
F dégâts dûs au transport
S daños de transporte

Transportwagen
E transport cart
F chariot de transport
S carro de transporte

träufeln
E drip, to; trickle, to
F verser au goutte à goutte
S gotear

Treibgas
E propellant (gas)
F gaz propulseur
S propelente

Trendermittlung
E trend analysis
F analyse des tendances
S análisis de tendencias

Trennbeutel
E split bag
F sachet de séparation
S bolsa de separación

Trennfuge
E joint
F joint
S junta

Trennleistung der Säule
E column performance
F performance d'une colonne
S rendimiento separador de la columna

Trennmedium
E separation media
F milieu de séparation
S medio separador

Trennmethode
E separating method
F méthode de séparation
S método de separación

Trennmittel
E separating medium
F milieu de séparation
S medio de separación

Trennung
E separation
F séparation
S separación

Trennungskapazität
E separation capacity
F capacité de séparation
S capacidad de separación

Trennungsleistung
E separation performance
F performance de séparation
S rendimiento separador

Trennungsmechanismus
E separation mechanism
F mécanisme de séparation
S mecanismo de separación

Trennwand
E partition
F mur de séparation
S tabique (de separación)

Treppenhaus
E stairs
F escaliers
S escalera de la casa

Trichter
E funnel, hopper
F entonnoir, trémie
S embudo, tolva

Trichteröffnung
E funnel opening
F ouverture d'un entonnoir, ouverture d'un trémie
S abertura del embudo

Trinkampulle
E oral ampoule
F ampoule buvable
S ampolla bebible

Trinkwasser
E drinking water, potable water
F eau potable
S agua corriente potable, agua potable

Trinkwasserzufuhr
E tap water feed
F arrivée d'eau potable
S abastecimiento de agua potable

trittsicher
E non-crushing, hard-wearing
F sûr à la marche
S de paso seguro

Trituration
E trituration
F trituration
S trituración

trocken lagern
E store dry, to
F stocker au sec
S almacenar en seco

Trockenextrakt
E dry extract, dried concentrate
F extrait sec, concentré sec
S concentrado seco

Trockengewicht
E dry weight
F poids sec, extrait sec
S peso seco

Trockengewichtanalyse
E dry weight analysis
F analyse à poids sec
S análisis de peso seco

Trockengranulierung
E dry granulation
F granulation par séchage
S granulación en seco

Trockenhitzesterilisator
E dry heat steriliser
F stérilisateur à chaleur sèche
S esterilizador de calor seco

Trockenmittel
E drying agent
F agent de dessication
S agente desecante

Trockennährmedium
E dehydrated culture medium
F milieu déhydraté
S medio de cultivo deshidratado

Trockenofen
E dry heat oven
F étuve
S estufa de secado, horno de secado

Trockenrückstand
E residue on drying
F résidu de séchage
S residuo seco

Trockenschrank
E drying oven
F séchoir
S secador

trocknen
E dry, to; desiccate, to
F sécher
S desecar, secar

Trocknungsmittel
E desiccant
F déshydratant, desséchant
S desecante, deshidratante

Trocknungsverlust
E loss on drying
F pertes dues au séchage
S pérdidas por desecación

Trocknungszeit
E drying time
F temps de séchage
S tiempo de desecación

Trocknungszyklus
E drying cycle
F cycle de séchage
S ciclo de desecación

Trommel
E drum
F tambour
S tambor

Trommelcoater
E pan coater
F machine d'enrobage à tambour
S máquina de tambor para gragear

Trommelmischer
E drum mixer
F mélangeur à tambour
S mezclador de tambor

Tropenkammer
E tropical chamber
F chambre tropicale
S cámara tropical

Tröpfchen
E droplet
F gouttelettes
S gotita

Tröpfchenabscheidung
E drop-collection
F collecte de gouttelettes
S separación de gotitas

Tropfeinsatz
E dropper insert
F bouchon à compte-gouttes
S tapón cuentagotas

tropfen
E drop, to
F fuire
S gotear

Tropfen zum Einnehmen
E oral drops
F gouttes pour voie orale
S gotas orales

Tropfenzähler
E drop counter
F compte-gouttes
S cuentagotas

Tropfflasche
E dropping bottle
F flacon compte-gouttes, flacon doseur
S frasco cuentagotas

Tropfpunkt
E dropping point
F point de goutte, température de liquéfaction
S punto de goteo

Tropfschutz
E drop protection
F protection anti-gouttes
S protección frente al goteo

Tropfverschluß
E drop closure
F obturateur doseur
S tapón cuentagotas

trüb
E turbid, cloudy
F turbide, trouble
S turbio

Trübung
E turbidity
F turbidité
S turbidez

Trümmer
E debris
F débris
S escombros

Tube
E tube
F tube
S tubo

Tubenfalz
E crimp, seam
F joint d'un tube
S juntura de un tubo

Tubenfüllmaschine
E tube-filling machine
F machine de remplissage pour tubes
S máquina de llenado por tubos

Tubengewinde
E tube thread
F filets du tube
S rosca de tubo

Tubenverschluß
E tube closure
F bouchon de tube
S cierre de un tubo

Tupfer
E swab, gauze, pad
F tampon d'ouate, gaze
S torunda

turbulente Strömung
E turbulent flow
F flux turbulent
S flujo turbulento

Turbulenz
E turbulence
F turbulence
S turbulencia

Türdichtung
E door seal
F joint de porte
S junta de una puerta

Türklinke
E door handle
F poignée de porte
S picaporte

Tyndallisation
E fractional sterilisation
F tyndallisation
S tindalización

überarbeiten
E review, to
F réviser, remanier
S perfeccionar, revisar

überarbeitet
E reviewed
F révisé
S perfeccionado, revisado

überdosiert
E overdosed
F surdosé, surdosage
S sobredosificado

Überdosierung
E overdose
F surdosage, surdose
S sobredosificación

Überdruck
E positive pressure, excess pressure
F surpression
S sobrepresión

übereinstimmen mit
E conform with, to
F être en conformité avec
S coincidir con

Übereinstimmung
E conformity
F conformité
S concordancia, coincidencia

Überfüllung
E overfill(ing)
F quantité en excès
S repleción

überhängen
E project, to; protrude, to
F saillir, faire saillir
S pender sobre, sobresalir, resaltar

überholt
E obsolete, out-dated
F obsolète, périmé, suranné, vieillot
S obsoleto, envejecido

Überimpfung
E transfer inoculation
F repiquage
S sobreinoculación

Überlastung
E overload, overloading
F surcharge
S sobrecarga

Überlauf
E overflow
F débordement
S desbordamiento, rebosadero

Überlaufgefäß
E overflow vessel
F récipient de débordement
S recipiente de desbordamiento

übernehmen
E take over, to
F prendre le contrôle de
S adquirir, comprar

überprüfen
E control, to; check, to
F contrôler, vérifier
S comprobar

Überprüfung
E verification, check
F vérification
S comprobación

Übersättigung
E supersaturation
F sursaturation
S sobresaturación

Überschneidung
E overlap
F chevauchement, recouvrement
S entrecruzamiento, interferencia

Überschreibfunktion
E overwrite function
F fonction d'écrasement
S función sobreescribir

überschreiten
E exceed, to
F excéder
S exceder

Überschuhe
E overshoe
F couvre-chaussure
S chanclos

Überschuß
E excess
F excès
S excedente, sobrante

Übersetzung (im Getriebe)
E gear ratio
F transmission
S transmisión

Überstand
E supernatant
F surnageant
S sobrenadante

überstehen
E project, to; protrude, to
F saillir, faire saillir
S sobresalir, pender sobre

Übertrag
E carryover
F report, somme intermédiaire
S transporte

übertragen
E transfer, to
F transférer
S transferir

Übertragung
E transfer
F transfert
S transferencia

Übertragungsfehler
E transfer error
F erreur de transfer
S error de transferencia

überwachen
E monitor, to; supervise, to
F contrôler, surveiller
S supervisar, vigilar

Überwachung
E monitoring
F contrôle, surveillance
S supervisión, vigilancia

ständige Überwachung
E continuous monitoring
F contrôle continu
S vigilancia continua

Überwachungseinrichtung
E monitoring device
F appareil de contrôle, appareil de surveillance
S dispositivo de vigilancia

Überwachungssystem
E monitoring system
F système de contrôle, système de surveillance
S sistema de vigilancia

überziehen (Tabletten)
E coat, to (tablets)
F enrober (comprimés)
S recubrir (comprimidos)

überzogen (Tabletten)
E coated (tablets)
F enduit, enrobé (comprimés)
S recubierto (comprimidos)

Überzug
E coat, film
F couche, pellicule
S cubierta, revestimiento

Überzugslack
E coating lacquer
F vernis de couverture
S barniz de cobertura

Uhrzeigersinn, gegen
E anticlockwise
F contre le sens des aiguilles d'une montre
S sentido antihorario

Uhrzeigersinn, im
E clockwise
F dans le sens des aiguilles d'une montre
S sentido horario

Ultrafiltration
E ultrafiltration
F ultrafiltration
S ultrafiltración

Ultraschall
E ultrasound
F ultra-son
S ultrasonido

Ultraschallbad
E ultrasonic bath
F bain à ultra-sons
S baño ultrasónico

ultraviolett
E ultraviolet
F ultraviolet
S ultravioleta

Umarbeitung
E reworking
F retraitement
S adaptación, remodelación, transformación

umbördeln
E flange, to; bead, to; border, to
F sertir
S bordear, rebordear, redondear

Umdrehungen (pro Minute)
E revolutions (per minute)
F rotations (par minute)
S revoluciones (por minuto)

Umdrehungszahl
E revolutions
F nombre de tours
S número de revoluciones

Umdrehungszähler
E revolution counter
F tachymètre
S taquímetro

English German French Spanish

Umfang
E circumference
F circonférence, périmètre, étendue
S circunferencia, perímetro, extensión

Umformulierung
E reformulation
F nouvelle formulation
S nueva formulación, reformulación

umfüllen
E refill, to
F transvaser
S transvasar, trasegar

Umgang (mit)
E handling (of)
F maniement, traitement
S trato (con)

umgeben von
E encased
F enchâssé
S rodeado de

Umgebung
E environment
F environnement
S entorno

nicht kontrollierte Umgebung
E uncontrolled environment
F environnement non controlé
S entorno no controlado

nicht-wäßrige Umgebung
E non-aqueous environment
F milieu non aquatique
S entorno no acuoso

Umgebungsbedingungen
E environmental conditions
F conditions de l'environnement
S condiciones ambientales

Umgebungskontrolle
E environmental monitoring
F contrôle de l'environnement
S control del entorno

Umgebungstemperatur
E ambient temperature
F température ambiante
S temperatura ambiental

Umkarton
E outer carton
F boîte, carton, carton d'expédition
S caja, cartón, cartón externo

Umkehrosmose
E reverse osmosis (RO)
F osmose inverse
S ósmosis inversa

Umkehrphasenchromatographie
E reverse-phase chromatography
F chromatographie en phase inverse
S cromatografía en fase inversa

Umkleide
E changing room
F vestiaire
S vestuario

Umkristallisation
E recrystallisation
F recristallisation
S recristalización

Umlauf
E recirculation
F recirculation
S circulación, rotación

Umlenkblech
E baffle
F chicane de déviation
S chapa desviadora

Umluft
E recirculating air
F air de recirculation
S aire circulante

Umlufttrockner
E circulatory dryer
F séchoir à circulation d'air
S secador de circulación de aire

Ummantelung
E jacket, mantle
F gaine, enveloppe
S revestimiento

umpacken
E re-pack, to
F changer l'emballage
S envasar de nuevo

umpalettieren
E re-pallet, to
F réorganiser les palettes
S cambiar de paleta

Umrechnung
E conversion
F conversion
S conversión

umrüsten
E re-equip, to
F moderniser, réorganiser
S modernizar, reorganizar

Umrüstung
E re-equipping
F modernisation, réorganisation
S modernización, reorganización

Umrüstzeit
E re-equipping time
F temps de réorganisation
S tiempo de reequipamiento

Umsatz
E turnover, sales
F chiffre d'affaires
S movimiento, volumen de negocios

Umschlagpaste
E poultice
F cataplasme
S cataplasma

Umverpackung
E outer packaging
F emballage externe
S embalaje externo

Umwälzpumpe
E circulatory pump
F pompe de circulation
S bomba de circulación

Umwandler
E converter
F convertisseur
S transformador

Umwandlung, thermische
E thermal conversion
F conversion thermique
S conversión térmica

Umwandlungsfähigkeit (einer Substanz in einer Reaktion)
E convertibility (of a substance in a reaction)
F convertibilité (d'une substance en une réaction)
S convertibilidad (de una sustancia en una reacción)

Umwelt
E environment
F environnement
S entorno, medio ambiente

Umweltanalyse
E environmental analysis
F analyse de l'environnement
S análisis del medio ambiente

Umweltbewußtsein
E environmental awareness
F conscience de l'environnement
S conciencia del medio ambiente

Umwelteinfluß
E environmental influence
F influence de l'environnement
S influencia del medio ambiente

umweltfreundlich
E environmentally friendly, non-polluting
F écologique
S ecológico

Umweltkontrolle
E environmental control
F contrôle de l'environnement
S control ecológico

Umweltschaden
E environmental damage
F atteinte à l'environnement
S daño ecológico

Umweltschutzbehörde
E environmental protection agency (EPA)
F agence pour la protection de l'environnement
S autoridades de protección del medio ambiente

Umweltschutzbericht
E environmental report
F rapport sur l'écologie
S informe ecológico

Umweltschützer
E environmentalist, ecologist
F écologiste
S ecologista

Umweltschutzmanagement
E environmental management
F gestion de l'environnement
S gestión ecológica

umweltverschmutzend
E polluting, harmful
F polluant
S polucionante

Umweltverschmutzung
E environmental waste
F pollution de l'environnement
S desgaste ecológico, degradación ecológica

unauslöschbar
E indelible
F indélébile
S indeleble

Unbedenklichkeit
E safety
F sécurité
S seguridad

unbeschädigt
E undamaged
F intact
S indemne

undicht
E leaky
F non étanche
S permeable

Undichtigkeit
E leak, leakage
F fuite
S permeabilidad

undurchlässig
E impermeable, impervious
F imperméable
S impermeable

Undurchlässigkeit
E impermeability, imperviousness
F imperméabilité
S impermeabilidad

undurchsichtig
E opaque
F opaque
S opaco

Uneinheitlichkeit von Tabletten
E tablet inconsistency
F hétérogénéité des comprimés
S heterogeneidad de comprimidos

unerwünschte Reaktion
E adverse reaction
F réaction indésirable, effet adverse
S reacción indeseable

Unfall
E accident
F accident
S accidente

unfallsicher
E accident-proof
F protégé contre les accidents
S a prueba de accidentes

Ungenauigkeit, inhärente (z. B. einer Technik)
E inherent uncertainty (e. g. of a technique)
F imprécision inhérente (par ex. d'une technologie)
S inexactitud inherente (p. ej. de una técnica)

ungesättigt
E unsaturated
F insaturé
S insaturado

Ungeziefer
E vermin
F vermine
S bichos

ungültig
E invalid
F non valable
S inválido

Unkrautvernichtungsmittel
E herbicide
F herbicide
S herbicida

unlöslich
E insoluble
F insoluble
S insoluble

unpolar
E non-polar
F non polaire
S no polar

unschädliche Mittel
E harmless products
F produits inoffensifs
S productos inocuos

Unsicherheit
E uncertainty
F incertitude
S inseguridad

Unsterilität
E non-sterility
F fécondité
S fertilidad, fecundidad

Unterbrechung (einer Reaktion)
E interruption, cessation (of a reaction)
F interruption (d'une réaction)
S interrupción (de una reacción)

Unterdosierung
E sub-strength
F hypo-dose
S infradosificación

Unterdruck
E negative pressure
F sous-pression, depression
S depresión, hipotensión

Untergestell
E base
F socle
S pie, soporte

Untergewicht
E short weight, underweight
F insuffisance de poids
S falta de peso

Unterlegscheibe
E washer
F rondelle
S arandela

Untermischung
E cross-mix, cross-contamination, mix in, mix
F contamination croisée, mélange
S contaminación cruzada, mezcla cruzada, entremezcla

Unternehmer, pharmazeutischer
E pharmaceutical manufacturer
F industriel de la pharmacie
S fabricante farmacéutico

Unterschrift
E signature
F signature
S firma

eigenhändige Unterschrift
E signature
F autographe
S firma autógrafa

English German French Spanish

elektronische Unterschrift
E electronic signature
F signature électronique
S firma electrónica

Unterschrift zur Genehmigung
E approval signature
F signature d'autorisation
S firma autorizante

Unterseite
E base
F face inférieure
S lado inferior

Unterstempel
E lower punch
F poinçon inférieur
S troquel inferior

untersuchen
E investigate, to
F inspecter
S examinar, explorar, investigar

Untersuchung
E investigation
F inspection
S examen, exploración, investigación

ärztliche Untersuchung
E medical examination
F examen médical
S exploración médica

körperliche Untersuchung
E physical inspection, physical examination
F inspection physique
S exploración física

untertauchen
E submerge, to; immerse, to
F immerger
S sumergir, sumergirse

unverkäufliches Muster
E sample
F échantillon
S muestra gratuita

unverpackt
E unpacked
F non emballé
S no embalado

Unversehrtheit
E integrity
F intégrité
S integridad

Unversehrtheit der Verpackung
E package integrity
F intégrité d'un conditionnement
S integridad de un embalaje

unverseifbare Anteile
E unsaponifiable matter
F portions insaponifiables
S porciones insaponificables

Unverträglichkeit
E incompatibility
F incompatibilité
S incompatibilidad, intolerancia

unvollständig
E incomplete
F incomplet
S incompleto

unzerbrechlich
E unbreakable
F incassable
S irrompible

unzugänglich
E inaccessible
F inaccessible
S inaccesible

unzugängliche Stellen
E inaccessible points
F endroits inaccessibles
S lugares inaccesibles

unzweideutig
E unequivocal
F non équivoque
S inequívoco

Urkunde
E certificate
F certificat
S documento

Ursprungsart
E origin of species
F espèce d'origine
S especie de origen

Urtinktur
E tincture standard
F teinture standard
S tintura madre

Urtiter
E volumetric standard
F substance standard de titrimétrie
S título estándar

UV/VIS-Detektor
E UV/VIS detector
F détecteur UV/VIS
S detector UV/VIS

UV-Absorption
E UV absorption
F absorption UV
S absorción UV

UV-Extinktionskoeffizient
E UV coefficient of absorbance
F coefficient d'extinction UV
S coeficiente de extinción UV

UV-Lampe
E UV lamp
F lampe UV
S lámpara UV

UV-Transmission
E UV transmittance
F transmission UV
S transmisión UV

Vaginalcreme
E vaginal cream
F crème vaginale
S crema vaginal

Vaginalgel
E vaginal gel
F gel vaginal
S gel vaginal

Vaginalsalbe
E vaginal ointment
F pommade vaginale
S pomada vaginal

Vaginaltablette
E vaginal tablet
F comprimé vaginal
S comprimido vaginal

Vaginaltampon
E medicated vaginal tampon
F tampon vaginal
S tampón vaginal

Vaginalzäpfchen
E vaginal suppository, pessary
F suppositoire vaginal
S supositorio vaginal

Vakuum
E vacuum
F vide
S vacío

Vakuumbeschickung
E vacuum feed
F alimentation du vide
S alimentación de vacío

Vakuumdestillation
E vacuum distillation
F distillation sous vide
S destilación en vacío

Vakuumentgaser
E vacuum degasification
F dégasification à vide
S desgasificador de vacío

Vakuumhaltetest
E vacuum test
F test de maintien du vide
S prueba de mantenimiento del vacío

English German French Spanish

Vakuumpumpe
E vacuum pump
F pompe à vide
S bomba de vacío

Vakuumtrocknung
E vacuum drying
F dessication sous vide
S secado al vacío

Vakuumverdampfer
E vacuum evaporation
F évaporateur sous vide
S evaporador de vacío

validierbar
E validatable
F validable
S validable

Validierung
E validation
F validation
S validación

analytische Validierung
E analytical validation
F validation analytique
S validación analítica

begleitende Validierung
E concurrent validation
F validation concurrente
S validación acompañante

prospektive Validierung
E prospective validation
F validation prospective
S validación prospectiva

retrospektive Validierung
E retrospective validation
F validation retrospective
S validación retrospectiva

Validierungsbericht
E validation report
F rapport de validation
S informe de validación

Validierungsdaten
E validation data
F données de validation
S datos de validación

Validierungslauf
E validation run
F cycle de validation
S ciclo de validación

Validierungsplan
E validation protocol
F protocole de validation
S plan de validación

Variabilität
E variability
F variabilité des résultats
S variabilidad

Variationskoeffizient
E coefficient of variation
F coefficient de variation
S coeficiente de validación

Vaselin
E vaseline
F vaseline
S vaselina

Ventil
E valve
F vanne
S válvula

elektromagnetisches Ventil
E solenoid valve
F vanne solénoïde
S válvula electromagnética

Kugelventil
E ball valve
F vanne à billes
S válvula esférica

Membranventil
E diaphragm valve
F vanne à membrane
S válvula de membrana

Ventilator
E ventilator, fan
F ventilateur
S ventilador

Ventilstellung
E valve setting
F position d'une vanne
S posición de la válvula

Verabreichung
E administration
F administration
S administración

veraltet
E obsolete
F obsolète
S envejecido, obsoleto

Verantwortlicher
E responsible person
F personne responsable
S responsable

Verantwortlichkeit
E responsibility
F responsabilité
S responsabilidad

Verarbeitung
E processing
F fabrication, mise en forme, traitement
S elaboración, transformación

manuelle Verarbeitung
E manual processing
F traitement manuel
S elaboración manual, transformación manual

maschinelle Verarbeitung
E machine processing
F traitement automatique
S elaboración automática, transformación automática

Verarbeitungsanweisung
E processing instructions
F instructions pour le traitement
S instrucción de procesado

verarbeitungsfähig
E processable
F traitable
S procesable

Veraschung
E ashing
F incinération
S incineración

verbacken (Säule)
E bake off, to (column)
F agglutiner (colonne)
S preparar (columna)

Verband
E bandage
F pansement, bandage
S vendaje

Verbandwatte
E cotton wool
F ouate à pansement
S algodón de vendaje

verbessern
E improve, to
F améliorer
S mejorar

verbindlich
E binding
F obligatoire
S obligatorio

unverbindlich
E without obligation
F ne comportant aucune obligation
S no obligatorio

Verbindlichkeit (finanz.)
E liability (financial)
F passif (finance)
S obligación, pasivo (contabilidad)

Verbindung (techn.)
E connection
F connexion
S conexión

English
German
French
Spanish

Verbindung, chemische
E chemical compound
F combinaison chimique
S compuesto químico

Verbindung, toxische
E toxic compound
F substance toxique
S compuesto tóxico

Verbindungsmaterial
E bonding material
F substance de liaison
S material de unión

Verbindungsstück
E connector
F raccord
S pieza de unión

verblassen
E fade, to
F perdre sa couleur, se défraîchir
S empalidecer

Verblindung
E blinding
F préparation pour essai en aveugle
S preparación para ensayo ciego

verbördeln
E crimp, to; cap, to
F capsuler
S rebordear cantos

Verbrauch
E consumption
F consommation
S consumo

Verbraucher
E consumer
F consommateur
S consumidor

Verbrauchsmaterial
E consumables
F consommables
S material consumible

Verbreitung von (Staub)
E dissemination of (dust)
F dissémination de (poussière)
S diseminación de (polvo)

Verbrennung
E combustion, incineration
F combustion, incinération
S combustión, incineración

Verbrennungsanlage
E incinerator
F incinérateur
S crematorio

Verbrennungsrückstand
E residue on ignition
F cendres résiduelles
S cenizas residuales

Verbundfolie
E laminated foil, composite foil
F feuille stratifiée
S hoja laminada, lámina estratificada

verchromt
E chromium plated
F chromé
S cromado

verdampfen
E evaporate, to
F évaporer, faire s'évaporer
S evaporar, evaporarse

Verdampfen des Lösungsmittels
E solvent evaporation
F évaporation du solvant
S evaporación del solvente

Verdampfer
E evaporator
F évaporateur
S evaporador

Verdampfung
E vaporisation
F vaporisation, évaporisation
S evaporación, vaporización

Verdampfungsrückstand
E residue on evaporating
F résidus de vaporisation
S residuo de evaporación

Verdampfungswärme
E heat of evaporation
F chaleur d'évaporation
S calor de evaporación

Verderb
E deterioration
F détérioration, altération
S deterioro

verderben
E deteriorate, to
F se détériorer, s'abîmer
S deteriorar, deteriorarse

verdichten
E compress, to; concentrate, to
F comprimer, concentrer
S concentrar, comprimir

Verdichtung
E compression, concentration
F compression, concentration
S concentración, compresión

verdicken
E concentrate, to; thicken, to
F épaissir
S espesar

Verdickungsmittel
E thickener, thickening agent
F épaississant
S espesante

verdrahten
E wire, to
F enclencher, brancher, connecter
S conectar, conmutar

Verdrillung
E torsion
F torsion
S torsión

Verdunkelung
E darken
F obscurcissement
S oscurecimiento

verdünnen
E dilute, to
F diluer
S diluir

verdünnt
E dilute
F dilué
S diluido

Verdünnung
E dilution
F dilution
S dilución

Verdünnungsmittel
E diluent
F diluant
S diluyente

Verdünnungsreihe
E dilution series
F séries de dilution
S serie de dilución

verdunsten
E evaporate, to
F évaporer, faire évaporer
S evaporar, evaporarse

Verdunstung
E evaporation
F évaporation
S evaporación, vaporización

Verdunstungsverlust
E evaporative loss
F perte due à l'évaporisation
S pérdida de evaporación

Vereinbarung
E agreement
F accord, convention
S acuerdo, convenio

English German French Spanish

English German French Spanish

Verengung
E constriction
F constriction
S constricción, estrechamiento

Veresterung
E esterification
F estérification
S esterificación

Verfahren
E procedure
F procédé
S procedimiento

Verfahrensänderung
E procedural change
F modification d'un procédé
S modificación del procedimiento

Verfahrensentwicklung
E process development
F développement d'un procédé
S desarrollo de un procedimiento

Verfahrensqualifizierung
E performance qualification
F qualification des performances (d'un procédé)
S cualificación de un procedimiento

Verfahrenstechnik
E process technology
F technique des procédés
S técnica del procedimiento

verfallen
E expire, to
F expirer
S caducar, expirar

Verfallsdatum
E expiration date, expiry date
F date d'expiration
S fecha de caducidad, fecha de expiración

verfälschen
E falsify, to
F falsifier
S falsificar

Verfälschung
E falsification
F falsification
S falsificación

Verfärbung
E discoloration
F décoloration
S decoloración

verflüchtigen, sich
E volatilise, to
F volatiliser
S volatilizarse

Verflüchtigung
E volatilisation
F volatilisation
S volatilización

verflüssigen
E fluidise, to; liquify, to
F liquéfier
S licuar, licuefacer

verflüssigte Gase
E liquified gases
F gaz liquéfiés
S gases licuados

Verformfolie
E forming foil
F feuille thermoformée
S lámina termoformada

Verformung
E deformation
F déformation
S deformación

verfügbar
E available
F disponible
S disponible

vergällt
E denatured
F dénaturé
S desnaturalizado

Vergällungsmittel
E denaturing agent
F agent dénaturant
S agente desnaturalizante

Vergleichslösung
E reference solution
F solution de référence
S solución de referencia

Vergrößerung
E enlargement, magnification
F agrandissement
S agrandamiento, aumento

Vergütung
E remuneration
F rémunération
S remuneración

Verhalten
E behaviour
F comportement
S comportamiento

thermisches Verhalten
E thermal behaviour
F comportement thermique
S comportamiento térmico

Verhältnis
E ratio
F rapport, taux
S proporción

verhindern
E prevent, to
F empêcher, éviter
S evitar, impedir

Verifizierung
E verification
F vérification
S verificación

verjüngt
E tapered, conical
F conique
S disminuido, estrechado, cónico

Verjüngung
E conicalness, conicity
F amincissement
S disminución, estrechamiento, conicidad

Verkabelung
E wiring
F câblage
S cables

verkanten
E cant, to
F mettre sur l'arête
S ladear

verkapseln
E encapsulate, to
F encapsuler
S capsular

Verkauf
E sales
F ventes
S ventas, volumen de ventas

Verkaufscharge
E approved batch
F lot de production
S lote de venta

verkleidet
E covered
F revêtu, recouvert
S recubierto, revestido

Verkleidung (von Rohrleitungen)
E cover, cladding (of piping)
F revêtement (de tuyauteries)
S cubierta, revestimiento, recubrimiento (de conducciones)

Verkleidungsblech
E cover, casing
F couvercle, capuchon
S chapa de revestimiento

Verkürzung
E abridgement
F raccourci
S acortamiento, abreviación, abreviatura

English German French Spanish

verlagern
E transfer, to; relocate, to
F transférer, déplacer
S desplazar, transferir, trasladar

verlängern
E extend, to; prolong, to
F prolonger, rallonger
S alargar, prolongar

verlängerte Wirkstoff-Freigabe
E extended release
F libération prolongée
S liberación prolongada de sustancia activa

Verlängerungskabel
E extension cable
F câble de rallonge
S alargadera, cable de prolongación

verläßlich
E reliable
F fiable
S digno de confianza

Verläßlichkeit
E reliability
F fiabilité
S fiabilidad

Verletzung
E infringement
F contrefaire un brevet
S lesión (herida), infracción

Verletzungsgefahr
E risk of injury
F risque de blessures
S riesgo de lesión

Verlust
E loss
F perte
S pérdida

Vermahlung
E grinding
F moulage
S molienda, molturado

vermeiden
E avoid, to
F éviter
S eludir, evitar

Vermeidung
E prevention
F prévention
S evitación

vermindern
E diminish, to
F diminuer
S disminuir, reducir

Vermischung
E mix in, mix
F mélange
S entremezcla

vernebeln
E nebulise, to
F nébuliser
S nebulizar

Vernebler
E nebuliser
F nébuliseur
S nebulizador

vernetzt
E reticular
F réticulaire
S integrado en una red, reticular

vernichten
E destroy, to
F détruire
S destruir

Vernichtung
E destruction
F destruction
S destrucción

Veröffentlichung
E publication
F publication
S publicación

Verordnung (rechtlich)
E regulation
F décret
S decreto, prescripción

Verordnung, ärztliche
E medical prescription
F ordonnance, prescription
S prescripción médica

verpacken
E pack, to; package, to
F emballer
S embalar, empaquetar, envasar

Verpackung (als Vorgang)
E packaging
F conditionnement, emballage
S embalaje, empaquetado, envasado

Verpackung, kindersichere
E child-proof packaging
F emballage de sécurité pour enfants
S embalaje a prueba de niños

Verpackung, luftdichte
E air-tight pack
F emballage étanche à l'air
S embalaje impermeable al aire

Verpackungsanweisung
E packaging instruction
F instruction d'emballage
S instrucción de embalaje

Verpackungsauftrag
E packaging order
F commande de conditionnement
S encargo de embalaje

Verpackungsdesign
E package design
F design du conditionnement
S diseño de un envase

Verpackungsfehler
E packaging defect
F défaut de conditionnement
S defecto de embalaje

Verpackungslinie
E packaging line
F chaîne de conditionnement, rampe de conditionnement
S cadena de empaquetado

Verpackungsmaschine
E packaging machine
F conditionneuse
S empaquetadora

Verpackungsmaterial
E packaging material
F matériel d'emballage
S material de embalaje

Verpackungsprotokoll
E batch packaging record
F compte rendu de conditionnement
S protocolo de embalaje

verpflichtend
E compulsory
F obligatoire
S obligatorio

verplombt
E sealed
F fermé hermétiquement
S precintado

verputzt
E plastered
F crépi
S enlucido, revocado

verputzte Wand
E plastered wall
F mur revêtu d'un crépi
S pared revocada

Verrohrung
E plumbing
F plomberie
S instalación de conducciones

versagen
E fail, to
F faillir à sa tâche
S fracasar

English German French Spanish

Versand
E dispatch, shipment, shipping
F expédition, envoi
S envío, expedición

Versandeinheit
E dispatch unit
F unité d'expédition
S unidad de envío

Versandkarton
E shipping carton
F conteneur
S cartón de envío

Verschleiß
E wear and tear
F usure
S desgaste

Verschleißerscheinung
E wear and tear
F usure
S manifestación de desgaste

Verschleißteil
E part subject to wear
F pièce sujette à l'usure
S pieza desgastable

Verschleißwiderstand
E resistance to wear
F résistance à l'usure
S resistencia al desgaste

verschließen
E seal, to
F sceller, clore, fermer
S cerrar

Verschließmaschine
E capping machine
F capsuleuse
S máquina de cierre

Verschluß
E closure, seal, cap
F bouchon, capuchon, couvercle
S cierre

hermetischer Verschluß
E hermetic seal
F fermeture hermétique
S cierre hermético

kindersicherer Verschluß
E child-resistant closure
F fermeture de sécurité pour enfants
S cierre a prueba de niños

mechanischer Verschluß
E mechanical seal
F fermeture mécanique
S cierre mecánico

Tubenverschluß
E tube closure
F bouchon de tube
S cierre de un tubo

unter Verschluß
E locked location
F enfermé
S cerrado

Verschluß mit Tropfer
E dropper applicator
F applicateur compte-gouttes
S cierre con cuentagotas

Verschlußklappe
E lid flap
F clapet de fermeture
S válvula de cierre

Verschlußmaterial
E closure material
F matériau de fermeture
S material de cierre

Verschlußstation
E sealing station
F station de scellage
S estación de cierre

verschmutzen
E contaminate, to
F contaminer
S contaminar, ensuciar

Verschraubung
E screw fitting
F connexion à filetage
S atornilladura

Verschreibung
E prescription
F ordonnance
S prescripción, receta

verschreibungspflichtig
E prescription
F vendu sur ordonnance
S de receta obligatoria

nicht verschreibungspflichtig
E non-prescription
F vendu sans ordonnance
S de venta libre

verschütten
E spill, to
F renverser, répandre
S derramar, verter

verschweißt
E welded
F soudé
S soldado

versehentlicher Gebrauch
E inadvertent use
F utilisation par inadvertance
S uso por inadvertencia

verseifen
E saponify, to
F saponifier
S saponificar

Verseifung
E saponification
F saponification
S saponificación

Verseifungszahl
E saponification value
F indice de saponification
S índice de saponificación

versenden
E dispatch, to; ship, to
F expédier
S enviar, expedir

versiegeln
E seal, to
F sceller, clore, fermer hermétiquement
S sellar

Versiegelung
E seal
F joint, fermeture
S sellado

Versiegelungsverpackung
E sealed packaging
F emballage hermétique
S embalaje sellado

Version
E edition, version, issue
F édition, version
S edición, versión

Versionsnummer
E version number
F numéro de version
S número de versión

versorgen mit
E supply, to
F fournir, livrer
S abastecer, proveer, suministrar

Versorgung
E supply
F alimentation
S abastecimiento, suministro

Versorgungsanschluß
E supply connection, supply input
F connection de charge
S conexión de abastecimiento

Versorgungsstrom
E power supply
F courant d'alimentation
S corriente de alimentación

English German French Spanish

verständlich
E comprehensible
F compréhensible
S comprensible

Verstärker
E amplifier
F amplificateur
S amplificador

verstärkt
E reinforced
F renforcé
S intensificado, reforzado

Verstärkung
E amplification
F amplification
S amplificación, intensificación, refuerzo

verstopft
E clogged, blocked
F obstrué, bouché
S obstruido

Versuch
E trial, experiment
F essai, expérience
S ensayo, experimento, prueba

Versuchsanlage
E pilot plant
F usine pilote
S instalación piloto

Versuchsanordnung
E trial design
F design d'un essai clinique
S disposición del ensayo

Versuchsbedingungen
E experimental conditions
F conditions expérimentales
S condiciones experimentales

Versuchscharge
E pilot batch, trial batch
F lot pilote
S lote piloto

Versuchsmaßstab
E pilot scale
F échelle pilote
S escala piloto

Verteiler
E dispenser
F distributeur
S distribuidor

Verteilerkasten
E junction box
F boîte de distribution
S caja de distribución

Verteilung (einer Flüssigkeit)
E distribution, dispensing (of a liquid)
F distribution, délivrance (d'un liquide)
S distribución (de un líquido)

Verteilungsvolumen
E dispensing volume
F volume de délivrance
S volumen de distribución

Vertiefung
E recess, cavity, well
F cavité, puits
S cavidad, depresión

Vertikalautoklav
E vertical autoclave
F autoclave vertical
S autoclave vertical

Vertikalelektrophorese
E vertical electrophoresis
F électrophorèse verticale
S electroforesis vertical

Vertikalgranulator
E vertical granulator
F granulateur vertical
S granulador vertical

Vertrag
E contract
F contrat
S contrato

Verträglichkeit
E compatibility
F compatibilité
S compatibilidad

Vertrauensbereich
E confidence area
F plage de confiance
S área de confianza, intervalo de confianza

Vertrauensgrenzen
E confidence limits
F limites de confiance
S límites de confianza

Vertrauensintervall
E confidence interval
F intervalle de confiance
S intervalo de confianza

Vertrauensniveau
E confidence level
F niveau de confiance
S nivel de confianza

Vertraulichkeit
E confidentiality
F confidentialité
S confidencialidad

Vertrieb
E sales
F ventes
S distribución, venta

Vertriebsleiter
E sales manager
F directeur des ventes
S director de ventas

Vertriebsweg
E sales channel
F canal de distribution
S canal de distribución

Verunreinigung
E impurity, contamination
F impureté, contamination
S contaminación, impureza

reduzierende Verunreinigung
E reducing impurity
F pollution réductrice
S impureza reductora

Verunreinigung in Spuren
E trace impurity
F impureté à l'état de traces
S impureza vestigial

Verunreinigungsprofil
E impurity profile
F profil d'impuretés
S perfil de impurezas

verursachen
E cause, to
F provoquer
S causar, provocar

Verwaltung
E administration
F administration
S administración

Verwaltungsverfahren
E method of administration
F méthode d'administration
S procedimiento administrativo

verwandte Substanz
E related substance
F substance apparentée
S sustancia emparentada

Verwarnung (der FDA)
E warning letter (from FDA)
F lettre d'avertissement (de la FDA)
S carta de aviso (de la FDA)

Verwechslung
E confusion, misidentification
F méprise, erreur
S confusión

Verweilzeit
E residence time
F temps de résidence
S tiempo de permanencia

mittlere Verweilzeit
E mean residence time (MRT)
F temps de résidence moyen
S tiempo promedio de permanencia

Verweis auf
E reference to
F référence à
S referencia a

verweisen auf
E refer to, to
F faire référence à
S referir a

verworfenes Produkt
E rejected product
F produit rejeté
S producto desechado

Verzeichnis
E index, contents, list
F répertoire, registre
S índice

verzinkt
E galvanised
F galvanisé au zinc
S galvanizado con zinc

verzögert
E delayed
F retardé
S retardado, retrasado

Verzögerung
E delay
F retard
S retardo, retraso

Verzögerungszeit
E delay time
F retard
S tiempo de retraso

Verzweigung
E branching
F ramification
S ramificación

VE-Wasser
E demineralised water
F eau déminéralisée
S agua completamente desmineralizada

Vibration
E vibration
F vibration
S oscilación, vibración

Vielfachkanalpipettiersystem
E multi-channel pipetting system
F système de pipettage à canaux multiples
S sistema de pipeteo con canales múltiples

virales Agens
E viral agent
F agent viral
S agente viral

Viren
E viruses
F virus
S virus

Virologie
E virology
F virologie
S virología

Virusabreicherung
E removal of viruses
F élimination des virus
S eliminación de virus

Virusentfernung
E virus removal
F élimination des virus
S eliminación de virus

Virusimpfstoff
E viral vaccine
F vaccin viral
S vacuna viral

viskos
E viscous
F visqueux
S viscoso

viskoses Lösungsmittel
E viscous solvent
F solvant visqueux
S solvente viscoso

Viskosität
E viscosity
F viscosité
S viscosidad

Viskositätsmessung
E viscometry
F viscosimétrie
S medida de la viscosiad

visuelle Überwachung
E visual observation
F contrôle visuel
S control visual

Vlies
E fleece
F toison
S vellocino

vollautomatisch
E fully automatic
F entièrement automatique
S completamente automático

vollentsalzt
E demineralised
F complètement désalinisé
S completamente desmineralizado

Vollpipette
E calibrated pipette
F pipette calibrée
S pipeta calibrada

Volumenstromregler, variabler
E variable flowmeter
F régulateur de flux
S regulador variable de flujo

Volumetrie
E volumetry
F volumétrie
S volumetría

volumetrisch
E volumetric
F volumétrique
S volumétrico

volumetrische Analyse
E volumetric analysis
F analyse volumétrique
S análisis volumétrico

voluminös
E voluminous
F volumineux
S voluminoso

von Hand
E hand-operated, manual
F manuel
S manual

vor Ort
E on-site
F sur site
S en el lugar

Vorabnahme (beim Hersteller)
E pre-delivery check, factory acceptance test
F contrôle avant livraison
S control antes de entrega

Vorarbeiter
E foreman
F contremaître
S capataz

Vorauskosten
E up-front costs
F coûts préalables
S costes preliminares

Vorauswahl
E pre-selection
F pré-sélection
S preselección

vorbedruckt
E pre-printed
F imprimé à l'avance
S preimpreso

Vorbehandlung
E pre-treatment
F traitement préalable
S pretratamiento

vorbeugende Wartung
E preventive maintenance
F entretien préventif
S mantenimiento preventivo

Vorcharge
E preliminary batch
F lot préliminaire
S carga previa

Vordruck
E pre-printed form
F formulaire
S formulario

Vordruckrolle (Tablettenpresse)
E pre-pressing roller
F rouleau presseur
S rollo de prensado previo (comprimidos)

Voreinschub
E pre-insertion
F pré-insertion
S preinserción

Voreinstellung
E pre-setting
F pré-réglage
S prerreglaje

Vorfall
E incident
F incident
S incidente

Vorfilter
E pre-filter
F filtre préalable
S filtro previo

Vorgang
E operation
F processus
S proceso

nicht unter Beobachtung stehender Vorgang
E unattended operation
F processus non soumis à un contrôle
S proceso no observado

Vorgänger
E predecessor
F prédécesseur
S predecesor

vorgefaltete Packungsbeilage
E pre-folded package insert
F notice explicative dépliante
S prospecto informativo del medicamento previamente plegado

vorgemischt
E pre-mixed
F mélangé à l'avance
S mezclado previamente

vorläufig
E temporary
F temporaire
S provisional, temporal, transitorio

vormischen
E pre-blend, to; pre-mix, to
F mélanger à l'avance
S mezclar previamente

Vormischung
E pre-mix
F pré-mélange
S mezcla previa

Vormontage
E pre-assembly
F pré-assemblé
S montaje previo

Vorpreßkraft
E pre-compression force
F force de compression préalable
S fuerza de compresión previa

Vorprodukt
E semi-finished product
F produit semi-fini
S producto semiterminado

Vorratsgefäß
E reservoir
F réservoir
S recipiente de depósito

Vorratstank
E storage vessel, reservoir
F récipient de stockage
S tanque de depósito

Vorrichtung
E device
F appareillage, dispositif
S dispositivo

Vorsäule
E pre-column
F colonne préalable
S columna previa

Vorschrift
E instruction, specification
F instruction, spécification
S prescripción

vorschriftsmäßig
E complying with specification
F en conformité avec les spécifications
S conforme a las prescripciones

Vorsichtsmaßnahme
E precaution
F précaution
S medida precautoria

Vorsichtsmaßnahmen bei der Lagerung
E storage precautions
F précautions de stockage
S medida precautoria al almacenar

Vorstand
E board of directors, director
F comité de direction
S junta directiva

Vorstandsmitglied
E director
F directeur
S miembro de la junta directiva

Vorverstärkung
E pre-amplification
F préamplification
S preamplificación

Waage
E balance
F balance
S balanza

oberschalige Waage
E top-loading balance
F balance à plat en haut
S balanza de carga superior

waagerecht
E horizontal
F horizontal
S horizontal

Waagschale
E weighing pan, weighing scale
F plateau de balance
S platillo de balanza

Wachs
E wax
F cire
S cera

Wachstum, mikrobielles
E microbial growth
F croissance microbienne
S crecimiento microbiano

Wachstumsdefekt
E growth defect
F défaut de croissance
S defecto de crecimiento

Wachstumsfaktoren
E growth factors
F facteurs de croissance
S factores de crecimiento

Wachstumsförderung
E growth promotion
F promotion de la croissance
S estimulación del crecimiento

Wägekabine
E weighing cubicle
F cabine de pesée
S cabina de pesado

wahre Dichte
E true density
F densité réelle
S densidad real

Walze
E roller, drum
F rouleau, cylindre, tambour
S cilindro, rodillo

walzen
E roll, to
F passer au rouleau
S allanar, aplanar, cilindrar

Walzenbürste
E revolving brush
F brosse rotative
S cepillo rotatorio

Walzenmühle
E roll mill
F broyeur à cylindres
S molino de cilindros

Walzentrockner
E drum dryer
F séchoir à cylindres
S secador de cilindros

Wand, verputzte
E plastered wall
F mur revêtu d'un crépi
S pared revocada

Wandanschluß
E wall connection
F connexion murale
S conexión de pared

Wandbelag
E deposit
F dépôt
S recubrimiento de la pared, depósito

Wanddicke
E wall thickness
F épaisseur d'un mur
S espesor de tabique

Wanddurchführung
E wall opening, duct
F ouverture dans le mur, conduite
S pasamuros

Wanderung
E migration
F migration
S migración

Wandsockel
E wall skirting
F bordure d'un mur
S zócalo de la pared

Wandung
E wall
F paroi
S pared

Warenannahme, zentrale
E central receiving
F réception de marchandises
S recepción central de mercancías

Wareneingang
E receipt (of goods)
F entrée des marchandises
S entrada de mercancías

Wareneingangsbuch
E receiving log book
F livre d'entrées de marchandises
S libro de entrada de mercancías

Wareneingangscode
E receiving code
F code d'entrée de marchandises
S código de entrada de mercancías

Wareneingangsprüfung
E inspection of incoming goods
F contrôle des livraisons de marchandises
S control de entrada de mercancías

Warenlager
E warehouse
F entrepôt
S almacén de mercancías

Warenzeichen
E trade mark
F marque déposée
S marca (de fábrica)

Wärme
E heat
F chaleur
S calor

Wärmeausdehnung
E thermal expansion
F thermodilatation
S termodilatación

Wärmebehandlung
E heat treatment
F traitement thermique
S tratamiento térmico

Wärmeflußkalorimeter
E heat flow calorimeter
F calorimètre à flux de chaleur
S calorímetro de flujo de calor

Wärmefühler
E temperature sensor
F sonde thermique
S sensor térmico

Wärmeisolierung
E heat insulation
F isolation thermique
S aislamiento térmico

Wärmeleitfähigkeit
E thermal conductivity
F conductivité thermique
S conductividad térmica

Wärmeleitfähigkeitsdetektor
E conductivity detector
F conductimètre
S detector de conductividad térmica

Wärmeleitung
E conductive heat
F conduction thermique
S conducción térmica

Wärmerückgewinnung
E heat recovery
F récupération de la chaleur
S recuperación de calor

Wärmeschock
E thermal shock
F choc thermique
S choque térmico

Wärmeschrank
E oven, incubator
F incubateur
S incubadora

Wärmestrahlung
E convective heat
F rayonnement thermique
S radiación térmica

Wärmetauscher
E heat exchanger
F échangeur de chaleur
S intercambiador de calor

Wärmeübergang, gleichmäßiger
E uniform heat transfer
F transition thermique uniforme
S transición térmica uniforme

wärmeübertragendes Öl
E heat-transmitting oil
F huile conductrice de chaleur
S aceite transmisor de calor

Wärmeübertragung
E heat transfer
F transfert de chaleur
S transferencia térmica

Wärmeverlust
E heat loss
F déperdition de chaleur
S pérdida calórica

Wärmeverteilung
E heat distribution
F distribution de chaleur
S distribución de calor

Warngrenze
E alert limit
F limite d'alerte
S límite de alerta

Warnhinweis
E warning
F avertissement
S aviso de alarma

Warnsignal
E alarm
F alarme
S señal de alarma

Wartung
E maintenance
F entretien, maintenance
S entretenimiento, mantenimiento

vorbeugende Wartung
E preventive maintenance
F entretien préventif
S mantenimiento preventivo

Wartung der Ausrüstung
E equipment maintenance
F entretien de l'équipement
S mantenimiento del equipo

Waschbecken
E wash basin
F évier
S lavabo

Waschdüse
E cleaning nozzle
F buse de nettoyage
S aplicador de lavado

Waschflasche
E wash bottle
F flacon laveur
S frasco de lavado

Wasser
E water
F eau
S agua

Wasser für Injektionszwecke
E water for injection (WFI)
F eau PPI
S agua para inyección

Wasser, demineralisiertes
E demineralised water
F eau déminéralisée
S agua desmineralizada

Wasser, destilliertes
E distilled water
F eau distillée
S agua destilada

Wasser, durch Umkehrosmose entsalztes
E reverse osmosis water
F eau désalinisée par osmose inverse
S agua desalinizada mediante ósmosis inversa

Wasser, entionisiertes
E deionised water
F eau déionisée
S agua desionizada

Wasser, entmineralisiertes
E demineralised water
F eau déminéralisée
S agua desmineralizada

Wasser, gereinigtes
E purified water
F eau purifiée
S agua purificada

Wasser, hochreines
E ultrapure water
F eau ultra pure
S agua ultrapurificada

Wasser, nukleasefreies
E nuclease-free water
F eau dénuée de nucléase
S agua sin nucleasas

Wasserabscheider
E water separator
F séparateur d'eau
S separador de agua

wasserabweisend
E hydrophobic, water-repellent
F hydrophobe
S hidrófobo, hidrófugo

wasseranziehend
E hygroscopic
F hygroscopique
S hidrófilo

Wasseraufbereitung
E water purification
F traitement des eaux usées
S purificación de agua

Wasseraufbereitungsanlage
E water treatment system
F système de traitement de l'eau
S sistema de tratamiento de agua

Wasseraufnahmevermögen
E water absorption capacity
F capacité d'absorption d'eau
S capacidad de absorción de agua

Wasserbad
E water bath
F bain-marie
S baño de agua

Wasserbestimmung
E water determination
F détermination de la teneur en eau
S determinación del contenido en agua

Wasserdampf, gesättigter
E saturated steam
F vapeur d'eau saturée
S vapor de agua saturado

Wasserdampf, gespannter
E super-heated steam
F vapeur surchauffée
S vapor de agua sobrecalentado

Wasserdampfdurchlässigkeit
E water vapour permeability
F perméabilité à la vapeur d'eau
S permeabilidad al vapor de agua

wasserdicht
E water-tight, waterproof
F imperméable à l'eau
S impermeable al agua

wasserdichter Anzug
E waterproof jump-suit
F combinaison imperméable à l'eau
S traje impermeable al agua

Wasserenthärter
E water-softener
F adoucisseur d'eau
S reblandecedor del agua

Wasserenthärtung
E water softening
F adoucissage de l'eau
S reblandecimiento del agua

wasserfrei
E anhydrous
F anhydre
S anhidro

Wassergehalt
E water content
F teneur en eau
S contenido en agua

Wasserhärte
E water hardness
F dureté de l'eau
S dureza del agua

Wasser-in-Öl-Emulsion
E water/oil emulsion
F émulsion d'eau dans l'huile
S emulsión de agua en aceite

Wasserleitung
E water piping
F conduite d'eau
S conducción de agua

Wassermantel
E water jacket
F chemise d'eau
S camisa de agua

Wasserringpumpe
E water-ring pump
F pompe à anneau d'eau
S bomba de anillo de agua

Wassersäule
E water column
F colonne d'eau
S columna de agua

Wasserstoff
E hydrogen
F hydrogène
S hidrógeno

Wasserstoffbrückenbindung
E hydrogen bond
F liaison hydrogène
S puente de hidrógeno

Wasserstoffperoxid
E hydrogen peroxide
F eau oxygénée, peroxide d'hydrogène
S peróxido de hidrógeno

Wasserstrahlpumpe
E water jet pump
F pompe d'une trompe à eau
S bomba de chorro de agua

Wasserversorgung
E water supply
F alimentation en eau
S suministro de agua

wäßrig
E aqueous
F aqueux
S acuoso

wäßrige Phase
E aqueous phase
F phase aqueuse
S fase acuosa

wäßriges Polymer
E aqueous polymer
F polymère aqueux
S polímero acuoso

Watte
E cotton wool
F ouate
S algodón

Wattebausch
E cotton plug
F tampon d'ouate
S torunda de algodón

Wechsel
E change
F changement
S cambio

Wechselstrom
E alternating current (AC)
F courant alternatif
S corriente alterna

Wechselwirkung
E interaction
F interaction, action réciproque
S acción recíproca, interacción

Wegwerfpackung
E disposable packaging
F conditionnement à usage unique
S embalaje de uso único

Weichgelatinekapsel
E soft gelatine capsule
F gélule molle
S cápsula de gelatina blanda

Weichmacher
E softening agent, plasticiser
F plastifiant
S plastificante

Weite
E width
F largeur, étendue
S anchura, amplitud, extensión

Weithalsflasche
E wide-necked bottle
F bouteille à col large
S botella de cuello ancho

Weithalsgefäß
E jar, wide-necked vessel
F fiole, jarre
S recipiente de cuello ancho

Welle (techn.)
E shaft
F arbre, essieu, tige
S árbol, asta, eje

Wellenlänge
E wavelength
F longueur d'onde
S longitud de onda

Wellenlängengenauigkeit
E wavelength accuracy
F exactitude de longueur d'onde
S exactitud de la longitud de onda

Wellenlängenprogrammierung
E wavelength programming
F programmation de la longueur d'onde
S programación de la longitud de onda

Wellenlängenumschaltung
E wavelength switching
F changement de longueur d'onde
S conmutación de la longitud de onda

Wellpappe
E corrugated cardboard (carton)
F carton ondulé
S cartón ondulado

Weltgesundheitsorganisation
E World Health Organisation (WHO)
F organisation mondiale de la santé (OMS)
S Organización Mundial de la Salud (OMS)

Werkbank
E work bench
F établi
S banco de trabajo

reine Werkbank
E clean bench
F paillasse sous flux laminaire
S banco de trabajo estéril

Werksabnahme
E factory acceptance test (FAT)
F réception en usine
S test de aceptación en fábrica

Werksleiter
E plant manager
F directeur d'usine
S director de taller

Werkstatt
E workshop
F atelier
S taller

Werkstoff
E material
F matériau
S material

Werkzeug
E tool
F outil
S instrumento

Wertigkeit
E valency
F valence
S valencia

Widerstand, elektrischer
E electrical resistance
F résistance électrique
S resistencia eléctrica

widerstandsfähig
E resistant
F résistant
S resistente, tenaz

Widerstandsspule
E resistance coil
F bobine de résistance
S bobina de resistencia

wiederaufbereitetes Produkt
E reprocessed product
F produit recyclé
S producto reciclado

Wiederaufbereitung
E reprocessing
F retraitement
S reprocesado

wiedereinschleusen
E reintroduce, to
F réintroduire
S reintroducir

Wiederfindungsrate
E recovery rate
F taux de récupération,
taux de rendement
S tasa de recuperación

wiedergewinnen
E recover, to
F récupérer
S recuperar

Wiedergewinnung
E recovery
F récupération, rendement
S recuperación

Wiederherstellung
E reconstitution
F rétablissement, reconstitution
S reconstitución, restablecimiento

Wiederholbarkeit
E repeatability
F répétitivité
S repetitividad

Wiederholbarkeit der Präzision
E precision repeatability
F répétitivité de la précision
S repetitividad de la precisión

Wiederholung
E repetition
F répétition
S repetición

Wiederholungsanalyse
E replicate analysis
F analyse répétée
S análisis de repetición

Wiederholungsprüfung
E re-test
F essai répété
S ensayo de repetición

Wiederverpackung
E re-packaging
F action de réemballer
S reembalaje

wiederverwendbar
E re-usable
F réutilisable
S reutilizable

Wiederverwendung
E re-use
F réutilisation
S reutilización

Wiederverwertung
E re-cycling
F recyclage
S reciclaje

Wiederzusammenbau
E re-assembly
F réassemblage
S reensamblaje

Wiegeanlage
E weighing facility
F installation de pesage
S instalación de pesado

Wiegebalken
E weighing beam
F fléau de balance
S ástil, cruz de la balanza

Winkel
E angle
F angle
S ángulo

Wirbelschicht
E fluid bed
F lit fluidisé
S lecho fluidificado

Wirbelschichtgranulator
E fluid bed spray granulator
F granulateur en lit fluidisé
S granulador de lecho fluidificado

Wirbelschichttrockner
E fluid bed dryer
F sécheur en lit fluidisé
S secador de lecho fluidificado

Wirbelschichtverfahren
E fluidisation
F fluidisation
S procedimiento de lecho fluidificado

wirksam
E effective, potent
F efficace
S activo, eficaz

wirksamer Bestandteil
E active substance, active ingredient
F composant actif
S componente activo

Wirksamkeit
E efficacy
F efficacité
S eficacia

Wirkstoff (als Rohstoff)
E bulk pharmaceutical chemical (BPC)
F matière première en vrac
S sustancia activa (materia prima)

Wirkstoff (im Arzneimittel)
E active substance, active pharmaceutical ingredient (API)
F principe actif (d'un médicament)
S principio activo (medicamento)

Wirkstoffe, natürlich vorkommende
E natural active substances
F principes actifs naturels
S sustancias activas naturales

Wirkstoff-Freigabe
E active substance release
F libération d'un principe actif
S liberación del principio activo

verlängerte Wirkstoff-Freigabe
E extended release
F libération prolongée d'un principe actif
S liberación prolongada del principio activo (de sustancia activa)

verzögerte Wirkstoff-Freigabe
E delayed release
F libération retardée d'un principe actif
S liberación retardada del principio activo

Wirkstoffscreening
E active substance screening
F screening de principes actifs
S detección de sustancias activas

Wirkungsmechanismus
E drug mechanism
F mécanisme d'action
S mecanismo de acción

Wischblatt (z. B. im Mischbehälter)
E wiper paddle (e. g. of a mixing vessel)
F lame d'essuyage (dans la cuve de mélange)
S goma limpia cristales (p. ej. en mezclador)

Wischtest
E wipe test, swab test
F essai de prélèvement par tampon d'ouate
S prueba de prelavado con torunda de algodón

Wolframbogenlampe
E tungsten arc lamp
F lampe à arc de tungstène
S lámpara de arco de tungsteno

Wundauflage
E wound dressing
F pansement
S compresa, vendaje de una herida

X-Achse
E X-axis
F axe des abscisses
S eje X

Y-Achse
E Y-axis
F axe des ordonnées
S eje Y

zäh
E tough
F visqueux, épais
S resistente, tenaz

zähflüssig
E viscous
F visqueux
S espeso, viscoso

Zähigkeit
E toughness
F viscosité
S resistencia, tenacidad, viscosidad

Zahl der theoretischen Böden
E number of theoretical plates
F nombre de plateaux théoriques
S número de placas teóricas

Zählbrett (für Tabletten)
E tablet counter
F compteur de comprimés
S contador de comprimidos

Zähler
E counter
F compteur
S contador

Zählung lebensfähiger Partikel
E viable particle count
F comptage de particules viables
S recuento de partículas viables

Zange
E tongs
F pince, tenailles
S pinza

Zäpfchen gießen
E mould, to (suppositories)
F mouler des suppositoires
S moldear supositorios

Zäpfchengießmaschine
E suppository machine
F machine à mouler des suppositoires
S máquina de moldear supositorios

Zeichenerklärung
E legend
F légende
S leyenda

Zeichnung
E drawing
F dessin, figure, schéma
S dibujo

technische Zeichnung
E engineering drawing
F dessin technique
S dibujo técnico

Zeiger
E pointer
F aiguille, indicateur
S indicador

Zeitaufwand
E time required
F temps requis
S tiempo invertido

Zeitersparnis
E time-saving
F économie de temps
S ahorro de tiempo

Zeitgeber
E timer
F minuterie
S sincronizador del tiempo

Zeitkonstante
E time constant
F constante de temps
S constante de tiempo

zeitlich gesteuerte Freigabe
E timed release
F libération contrôlée
S liberación temporalmente controlada

Zeitplan
E schedule
F plan, programme
S horario, calendario

Zeitverzögerung
E time lag
F retard
S retraso

Zelldichte
E cell density
F densité de cellules
S densidad de células

Zelle
E cell
F cellule
S célula

Zellernte
E cell harvesting
F récolte de cellules
S recolección de células

Zellkultur
E cell culture
F culture de cellules
S cultivo celular

diploide Zellkultur
E diploid cell culture
F culture de cellules diploides
S cultivo de células diploides

heteroploide Zellkultur
E heteroploid cell culture
F culture de cellules hétéroploïde
S cultivo celular heteroploide

Zellpopulation
E cell population
F population de cellules
S población celular

Zellstoff
E cellulose
F cellulose
S celulosa

Zelltrennung, magnetische
E magnetic cell separation
F clivage cellulaire magnétique
S separación magnética de células

zelluläre Anomalie
E cellular anomaly
F anomalie cellulaire
S anomalía celular

Zellvermehrung
E cell proliferation
F prolifération de cellules
S proliferación celular

Zellwachstum
E cell growth
F croissance de cellules
S crecimiento celular

Zellwand
E cell wall
F membrane cellulaire
S pared celular

Zellzähler
E cell counter
F compteur de cellules
S contador de células

Zementestrich
E cement flooring
F chape de ciment
S suelo de cemento

zensiert
E censored
F censuré
S censado

zentrale Einwaage
E central weighing area
F aire centrale de pesage
S área central de pesado

zentrieren
E centre, to
F centrer
S centrar

Zentrifugalkraft
E centrifugal force
F force de centrifugation
S fuerza centrífuga

Zentrifugalventilator
E centrifugal fan
F ventilateur centrifuge
S ventilador centrífugo

Zentrifugation
E centrifugation
F centrifugation
S centrifugación

Zentrifuge
E centrifuge
F centrifugeuse
S centrífuga

zentrifugieren
E centrifuge, to
F centrifuger
S centrifugar

Zerbeißkapsel
E biting capsule
F capsule à croquer
S cápsula mordible

zerbrechlich
E fragile
F fragile
S frágil

Zerfall
E disintegration
F désintégration
S desintegración

zerfallen
E disintegrate, to
F se désintégrer, se désagréger
S desintegrar(se)

Zerfallsprodukt
E degradation product
F produit de dégradation
S producto de desintegración

Zerfallsprüfung
E disintegration test
F essai de désintégration
S ensayo de desintegración

Zerfallszeit
E disintegration time
F temps de désintégration
S tiempo de desintegración

Zerhacker
E chopper
F hachoir, couperet
S troceadora

Zerhackergeschwindigkeit
E chopper speed
F vitesse de hachoir
S velocidad de troceo

Zerkleinerer
E homogeniser, shredder
F hachoir
S trituradora

zerkleinern
E homogenise, to; shred, to
F hacher
S triturar

Zerlegung
E dismantling, disassembly
F démontage
S desmontaje

Zerreißfestigkeit
E tensile strength
F résistance au déchirement
S resistencia al desgarro

Zersetzung
E decomposition
F décomposition
S degradación, descomposición

Zersetzungsprodukt
E decomposition product
F produit de décomposition
S producto de degradación

zerstäuben
E atomise, to; vaporise, to
F atomiser, pulvériser
S atomizar, pulverizar

Zerstäuber
E atomiser
F atomiseur, pulvérisateur
S atomizador, pulverizador

Zerstäuberluft
E atomising air
F air d'atomiseur
S aire de atomizador

zerstoßen
E crush, to; grind, to; mill, to
F broyer, concasser, piler
S machacar, pulverizar, triturar

Zertifikat
E certificate
F certificat
S certificado

zertifizieren
E certificate, to
F certifier
S certificar

Zertifizierung
E certification
F certification
S certificación

Zonenkonzept
E zonal concept
F concept de zones
S concepción por zonas

Zubehör
E accessory
F accessoire
S accesorios

Zubereitung
E preparation, formulation
F préparation, formulation
S formulación, preparación

Zuckerdragee
E sugar-coated tablet
F comprimé dragéifié, dragée
S gragea azucarada, gragea

Zufallsgenerator
E random number generator
F générateur de hasard
S generador aleatorio

Zufallsverteilung
E random distribution
F distribution randomisée
S distribución aleatoria

Zufuhr
E feed
F alimentation, charge
S alimentación, suministro

Zufuhr durch Gefälle
E gravity feed
F alimentation par gravité
S alimentación por gravedad

Zufuhrrinne
E feed chute
F rigole d'alimentation, conduit d'alimentation
S canal de alimentación

Zuführtisch
E feed table
F table de chargement, table d'alimentation
S mesa de abastecimiento

Zug
E tension
F tension, traction
S tensión, tracción

Zug- und Druckfestigekit
E traction-compression resistance
F résistance à la traction et à la compression
S resistencia a la tracción y a la presión

Zugabe
E addition
F adjonction
S adición, suplemento

Zugang
E access
F accès
S acceso

autorisierter Zugang
E authorised access
F droit d'accès
S acceso autorizado

eingeschränkter Zugang
E limited access, restricted access
F accès limité
S acceso limitado

kontrollierter Zugang
E controlled access
F accès contrôlé
S acceso controlado

Zugang zum System
E system access
F accès au système
S acceso al sistema

Zugänglichkeit
E accessibility
F accessibilité
S accesibilidad

schwer zugängliche Stellen
E poorly accessible points
F endroits difficilement accessibles
S lugares de dificil acceso

Zugangsberechtigung
E authorised access
F autorisation d'accès
S derecho de acceso

zugeben
E add, to
F ajouter
S añadir

Zugkraft
E tensile force
F force de traction
S fuerza de tracción

zulässig
E permissible
F permis
S permitido

Zulassung
E marketing authorisation/approval
F autorisation de mise sur le marché (A.M.M.)
S autorización de (para) venta en el mercado

Zulassung als Generikum
E generic marketing authorisation
F autorisation de mise sur le marché comme médicament générique
S autorización como genérico

Zulassungsabteilung
E regulatory affairs department
F département des affaires réglementaires
S departamento de registros y licencias sanitarias

Zulassungsantrag
E application for marketing authorisation
F demande d'autorisation de mise sur le marché
S solicitud de autorización

Zulassungsbehörde
E regulatory authorities
F autorités compétentes responsables des autorisations de mise sur le marché
S agencia de autorización de licencias sanitarias

Zulassungsdossier
E submission file for marketing authorisation
F dossier de demande d'autorisation de mise sur le marché
S dosier de solicitud de autorización

Zuleitung
E feed
F tuyauterie d'alimentation
S alimentación, tubería de alimentación

Zuluft
E inlet air
F entrée d'air
S entrada de aire

Zuluftklappe
E air inlet cover
F couvercle d'entrée d'air
S válvula de entrada de aire

Zündquelle
E ignition source
F source d'inflammation
S fuente de ignición

Zündung
E ignition
F inflammation
S encendido, ignición

piezoelektrische Zündung
E piezo ignition
F allumage piezoélectrique
S encendido piezoeléctrico

zurückgegebene Ware
E returned goods
F marchandise retournée
S mercancía devuelta

zurückgewiesene Materialien
E rejected materials
F matériaux rejetés, matériaux refusés
S materiales rechazados

zurückhaltend
E retentive
F réservé, effacé, réticent
S reservado

zurückweisen
E reject, to
F rejeter
S rechazar

Zurückweisung
E rejection
F rejet
S rechazo

Zusammenbacken (z. B. von Kristallen)
E baking (e. g. of crystals)
F agglomération (par ex. de cristaux)
S cocción (p. ej. de cristales)

Zusammenbau
E assembly, set-up
F assemblage, montage
S ensamblaje, montaje

Zusammenfassung der Produktmerkmale
E summary of product characteristics (SPC)
F résumé des caractéristiques du produit
S resumen de características del producto

Zusammenschluß von Firmen
E merger, fusion
F fusion (d'entreprises)
S fusión de empresas

zusammensetzen
E assemble, to
F assembler
S ensamblar, montar

Zusammensetzung
E composition
F composition
S composición

Zusatzstoff
E additive
F additif, adjuvant
S aditivo

English German French Spanish

zuschmelzen (Ampullen)
E flame-seal, to (ampoules)
F obturer par vitrification (ampoules)
S obturar por vitrificación, cerrar ampollas a la llama

Zutritt
E access
F accès
S acceso

zuverlässig
E reliable
F fiable
S fiable, confiable

Zuverlässigkeit
E reliability
F fiabilité
S fiabilidad, confiabilidad

Zuverlässigkeit der Dosierung
E dose reliability
F fiabilité d'une dose
S fiabilidad de la dosificación

Zwangsmischer
E forced-circulation mixer, high shear mixer
F mélangeur à circulation forcée
S mezclador de circulación forzada

Zweikomponenten-Reagenz
E dual-component reagent
F réactifs à deux composants
S reactivo de doble componente

Zweischichtverpressung
E double-layer compression
F compression à double couche
S compresión de doble capa

Zweistoffdüse
E binary nozzle
F buse binaire
S aplicador binario

Zwischendecke
E intermediate ceiling, suspended ceiling
F faux plafond
S techo intermedio

Zwischenfall
E incident
F incident
S incidente

Zwischengeschoß
E mezzanine
F étage intermédiaire
S piso intermedio

Zwischenkontrolle
E intermediate control
F contrôle intermédiaire
S control intermediario

Zwischenlagerung
E interim storage
F stockage intermédiaire
S almacenaje intermediario

Zwischenprodukt
E intermediate product
F produit intermédiaire
S producto intermediario

Zwischenraum
E space
F espace
S espacio (intermedio)

Zwischenstufe
E intermediate stage
F état intermédiaire
S nivel intermediario

Zwischenwand
E partition (wall), baffle
F mur de séparation
S tabique

Zyklonabscheidung
E cyclone separation
F séparateur à cyclone
S separación por centrifugación

French A – Z

English

German

French

Indications pour l'emploi du dictionnaire:
p. 12–13

Spanish

Zyklus
E cycle
F cycle
S ciclo

Zyklussequenz
E cycle sequence
F séquence de cycles
S secuencia de ciclos

zylindrisch
E cylindrical
F cylindrique
S cilíndrico

Zytostatica
E cytostatics
F cytostatiques
S citostáticos, agentes citostáticos

abaissement du point de congélation
E depression of freezing point
G Gefrierpunktserniedrigung
S reducción del punto de congelación

abaisser
E lower, to; reduce, to
G senken
S bajar, reducir

abîmer, s'
E deteriorate, to
G verderben
S deteriorar, deteriorarse

abrasion
E friability, abrasion
G Abrieb, Abtrag
S abrasión

absence
E absence
G Abwesenheit
S ausencia

absolu
E absolute
G absolut
S absoluto, absolutamente

absorbant
E absorbent
G Absorbens, Absorptionsmittel
S medio de absorción

absorber
E absorb, to
G absorbieren
S absorber

absorbeur d'énergie
E power absorber
G Kraftaufnehmer
S absorbedor de fuerza

absorption
E absorption, absorbance
G Absorption, Extinktion
S absorción, extinción

absorption d'humidité
E moisture uptake
G Feuchtigkeitsaufnahme
S absorción de humedad

absorption UV
E UV absorption
G UV-Absorption
S absorción UV

abus
E abuse
G Mißbrauch
S abuso

accélérateur
E accelerator
G Beschleuniger
S acelerador

accélérateur de faisceau d'électrons
E electron beam accelerator
G Elektronenstrahlbeschleuniger
S acelerador de haz de electrones

accélérer
E accelerate, to
G beschleunigen
S acelerar

acceptance
E acceptance
G Annahme
S aceptación

acceptation
E acceptance
G Annahme
S aceptación

accès
E access
G Zugang, Zutritt
S acceso

droit d'accès
E authorised access
G autorisierter Zugang
S acceso autorizado

English German French Spanish

accès au système
E system access
G Zugang zum System
S acceso al sistema

accès contrôlé
E controlled access
G kontrollierter Zugang
S acceso controlado

accès limité
E limited access, restricted access
G eingeschränkter Zugang
S acceso limitado

accès restrictif
E limited access, restricted access
G beschränkter Zugang, eingeschränkter Zugang
S acceso limitado

accessibilité
E accessibility
G Zugänglichkeit
S accesibilidad

accessible
E accessible, walk-in
G begehbar
S practicable, viable

accessoire
E accessory
G Ausrüstungsteil, Zubehör
S accesorio

accessoires d'un équipement
E instrument accessories
G Gerätezubehör
S accesorios del aparato

accident
E accident
G Unfall
S accidente

accord
E agreement
G Vereinbarung
S acuerdo, convenio

accord de confidentialité
E secrecy agreement
G Geheimhaltungsvertrag
S contrato de confidencialidad

accoupler
E couple, to
G ankuppeln
S acoplar

accoutumance
E addiction
G Sucht
S adicción

accréditer
E accredit, to
G akkreditieren
S acreditar

accrocher
E couple, to
G ankuppeln
S acoplar

accumulation
E accumulation
G Anhäufung
S acumulación

accumulation de particules
E accumulation of particles
G Partikelansammlung
S acumulación de partículas

achats
E procurement
G Beschaffung
S adquisición

acheter
E purchase, to
G kaufen
S comprar

achèvement
E completion
G Beendigung
S conclusión, terminación

acide
E acid
G sauer, Säure
S ácido

acide aminé
E amino acid
G Aminosäure
S aminoácido

acide aminé essentiel
E essential amino acid
G essentielle Aminosäure
S aminoácido esencial

acide carboxylique
E carboxylic acid
G Carbonsäure
S ácido carbónico

acide chlorhydrique
E hydrochloric acid
G Salzsäure
S ácido clorhídrico

acide concentré
E concentrated acid
G starke Säure
S ácido concentrado

acide faible
E weak acid
G schwache Säure
S ácido débil

acide fumant
E fuming acid
G rauchende Säure
S ácido fumante

acide gras
E fatty acid
G Fettsäure
S ácido graso

acide nitrique
E nitric acid
G Salpetersäure
S ácido nítrico

acide nucléique
E nucleic acid
G Nukleinsäure
S ácido nucleico

acide silicique
E silicic acid
G Kieselsäure
S ácido silícico

acide sulfurique
E sulphuric acid
G Schwefelsäure
S ácido sulfúrico

acide sulfurique chromique
E chromosulphuric acid
G Chromschwefelsäure
S ácido sulfúrico crómico

acidifier
E acidify, to
G ansäuern
S acidificar

acidité
E acidity
G Azidität
S acidez

acier
E steel
G Stahl
S acero

acier inoxydable, inox
E stainless steel
G Edelstahl
S acero inoxidable

acier au carbone
E carbon steel
G Karbonstahl
S acero al carbono

acier chromé
E chrome steel
G Chromstahl
S acero cromado

English German French Spanish

acier chromé et nickelé
E nichrome steel
G Chromnickelstahl
S acero cromado y niquelado

acquérir
E acquire, to; purchase, to
G kaufen, aufkaufen
S adquirir, comprar

acte du personnel
E personnel file
G Personalakte
S acta personal

action corrective
E corrective action
G Korrekturmaßnahme
S acción correctora

action de corriger
E trouble-shooting, failure rectification
G Fehlerbehebung
S corrección de errores

action de dépoussiérer
E dedusting
G Entstaubung
S desempolvamiento

action de réemballer
E re-packaging
G Wiederverpackung
S reembalaje

action de tuer
E killing
G Abtötung
S destrucción

action de vider un flacon
E vessel emptying
G Gefäßentleerung
S vaciamiento de un recipiente

action de vider un récipient
E vessel emptying
G Gefäßentleerung
S vaciamiento de un recipiente

action réciproque
E interaction
G Wechselwirkung
S acción recíproca, interacción

activation
E actuation, activation
G Aktivierung
S activación

activité de surface
E surface activity
G Oberflächenaktivität
S actividad de superficie

activité pharmacologique
E pharmacological activity
G pharmakologische Aktivität
S actividad farmacológica

actualiser
E update, to
G aktualisieren
S actualizar

adapté à l'utilisateur
E user-friendly
G bedienerfreundlich
S confortable para el usuario

additif
E additive
G Zusatzstoff
S aditivo

additif alimentaire
E food additive
G Nahrungsergänzungsmittel
S aditivo alimentario

addition en bout de chaîne
E tailings
G Nachlauf
S adición al final de la cadena

adéquat
E suitable, appropriate, adequate
G angemessen, geeignet
S adecuado, apropiado

adhérence
E adherence
G Adhärenz
S adherencia

adhérer
E adhere, to; stick, to (tablets)
G kleben (bei Tabletten)
S adherir (comprimidos)

adhésif pour feuilles
E film laminating adhesive
G Folienverbundkleber
S adhesivo para láminas

adhésif thermofusible
E heat-sealing adhesive
G Heißsiegelkleber
S adhesivo termofusible

adhésion
E adhesion
G Haftung (physikalisch)
S adhesión (física)

adjonction
E addition
G Zugabe
S adición, suplemento

adjuvant
E additive, excipient, adjuvant
G Zusatzstoff, Hilfsstoff
S aditivo, excipiente, sustancia auxiliar

administration
E administration
G Verabreichung, Verwaltung
S administración

administration (d'un médicament)
E administration (of a drug)
G Darreichung (eines Medikaments)
S administración (de un medicamento)

administration orale
E oral administration
G perorale Darreichung
S administración peroral

administration orale, pour
E for oral use
G zum Einnehmen
S para uso oral

adoucir (eau)
E soften, to (water)
G enthärten (Wasser)
S ablandar (agua)

adoucissage de l'eau
E water softening
G Wasserenthärtung
S reblandecimiento del agua

adoucisseur d'eau
E water-softener
G Wasserenthärter
S reblandecedor del agua

adsorbant
E adsorbent
G Adsorptionsmittel
S medio de adsorción

adsorption
E adsorption
G Adsorption
S adsorción

adsorption d'un principe actif
E absorption of medicinal substance
G Arzneistoffaufnahme
S absorción del principio activo

aération du réservoir
E tank aspiration
G Tankbelüftung
S ventilación del tanque

aérer
E vent, to; ventilate, to
G belüften
S airear, ventilar

aérobie
E aerobic
G aerob
S aerobio

aéroporté
E airborne
G aerogen
S aerógeno

aérosol pour mousse
E foam spray
G Schaumspray
S aerosol de espuma

aérosol sublingual
E sub-lingual spray
G Sublingualspray
S spray sublingual

affichage à cristaux liquides
E liquid crystal display (LCD)
G Flüssigkristallanzeige
S pantalla de cristal líquido

affichage d'une erreur
E fault (failure) display
G Störanzeige
S pantalla de aviso de avería

affichage électroluminescent
E LED readout
G LED-Anzeige
S pantalla electroluminiscente

affichage numérique
E analogue display
G Analoganzeige
S pantalla análoga

affiche avec consignes de sécurité
E safety poster
G Plakat mit Sicherheitshinweisen
S cartel con avisos de seguridad

afficher
E display, to; indicate, to
G anzeigen
S indicar, mostrar

affinité
E affinity
G Affinität
S afinidad

agar
E agar
G Agar
S agar

agar oblique
E sloping agar
G Schrägagar
S agar oblicuo

agar-agar
E agar
G Agar
S agar

agence pour la protection de l'environnement
E environmental protection agency (EPA)
G Umweltschutzbehörde
S autoridades de protección del medio ambiente

agent antimousse
E anti-foaming agent
G Antischaummittel
S agente antiespumante

agent antistatique
E anti-static agent
G Antistatikum
S antiestático

agent aromatique
E flavouring agent, flavour
G Geschmackstoff
S agente saporífero

agent chélatant
E chelating agent
G Komplexiermittel
S agente quelante

agent chimique
E chemical agent
G chemisches Mittel
S agente químico

agent de dessication
E drying agent
G Trockenmittel
S agente desecante

agent de dispersion
E dispersion agent
G Dispersionsmittel
S agente dispersor

agent de nettoyage
E cleansing agent, detergent
G Reinigungsmittel
S detergente, producto de limpieza

agent de précipitation
E precipitation agent
G Ausfällungsmittel, Fällungsmittel
S agente precipitador, agente de precipitación

agent de résorption
E resorption agent
G Resorptionsvermittler
S agente de resorción

agent délitant
E disintegrant, tablet disintegrant
G Sprengmittel
S desintegrante

agent dénaturant
E denaturing agent
G Denaturierungsmittel, Vergällungsmittel
S agente desnaturalizante

agent d'inactivation
E inactivation agent
G Inaktivierungsmittel
S agente inactivador

agent filmogène
E film-forming agent
G Filmbildner
S agente formador de películas

agent nocif
E harmful agent
G schädliches Mittel
S agente nocivo

agent pathogène atténué
E attenuated pathogen
G abgeschwächter Erreger
S agente patógeno atenuado

agent stabilisant
E stabilising agent
G Stabilisator
S estabilizador

agent thérapeutique
E therapeutic agent
G Heilmittel
S agente terapéutico

agent viral
E viral agent
G virales Agens
S agente viral

agents chimiques
E chemical agents
G chemische Agenzien
S agentes químicos

agglomérat
E agglomerate
G Agglomerat
S aglomerado

agglomération (par ex. de cristaux)
E baking (e. g. of crystals)
G Zusammenbacken (z. B. von Kristallen)
S cocción (p. ej. de cristales)

agglomérer
E agglomerate, to
G agglomerieren
S aglomerar

agglutination
E agglutination
G Agglutination
S aglutinación

agglutiner (colonne)
E bake off, to (column)
G verbacken (Säule)
S preparar (columna)

agitateur
E stirrer, agitator
G Rührer, Rührwerk
S agitador

agitateur à ancre
E anchor stirrer
G Ankerrührer
S agitador de ancla

agitateur à pales
E blade stirrer
G Flügelrührer
S agitador de aletas

agitateur magnétique
E magnetic stirrer, magnetic stirring bar
G Magnetrührer, Rührfisch
S agitador magnético

agitation vigoureuse
E vigorous stirring
G kräftiges Rühren
S agitación intensa

agiter
E stir, to
G rühren
S agitar

agrandissement
E enlargement, magnification
G Vergrößerung
S agrandamiento, aumento

agrandissement d'une installation
E plant expansion
G Betriebserweiterung
S ampliación de la empresa

agrégat
E aggregate
G Aggregat
S agregado

aide temporaire
E temporary help
G Aushilfe
S ayuda temporal

aides au fonctionnement
E operative aids
G Bedienhilfen
S ayudas de funcionamiento

aiguille
E pointer
G Zeiger
S indicador

dans le sens des aiguilles d'une montre
E clockwise
G im Urzeigersinn
S sentido horario

aiguille de remplissage
E filling needle
G Abfüllnadel
S aguja de envasado

aiguille d'injection
E filling nozzle
G Düsennadel
S aguja de inyección

aiguille pour injection
E injection needle
G Injektionsnadel
S aguja de inyección

aiguisé
E sharp
G scharf
S afilado, agudo, cortante

ailette
E fan wheel, blade, vane, rotor, impeller
G Laufrad, Flügelrad
S rueda de aletas, rueda de paletas, rueda portante

air comprimé
E compressed air
G Druckluft, Preßluft
S aire comprimido

air conditionné
E air-conditioned
G klimatisiert
S climatizado

air d'atomiseur
E atomising air
G Zerstäuberluft
S aire de atomizador

air de recirculation
E recirculating air
G Umluft
S aire circulante

air d'échappement
E exhaust air, outlet air
G Abluft
S aire de escape

air d'évacuation
E exhaust air, outlet air
G Abluft
S aire de escape

air filtré
E clean air
G Reinluft
S aire limpio

air frais
E outside air, external air
G Außenluft
S aire fresco, aire libre

air libre
E outside air, external air
G Außenluft
S aire fresco, aire libre

aire
E surface
G Oberfläche
S superficie

aire spécifique
E specific surface area
G spezifische Oberfläche
S superficie específica

aire centrale de pesage
E central weighing area
G zentrale Einwaage
S área central de pesado

aire de collage
E splice point
G Klebestelle
S zona de adherencia

aire de fermentation
E fermentation room
G Fermentationsraum
S área de fermentación

aire de pulvérisation
E spray area
G Sprühbereich
S área de pulverización

aire de stockage
E warehouse, storage area
G Lager(bereich)
S almacén

aire d'encartonnage
E cartoning section
G Kartonierteil
S área de encartonamiento

aire d'entreposage
E warehouse, storage area
G Lager(bereich)
S almacén

aire totale
E total area
G Gesamtfläche
S superficie total

ajout
E spike
G Spike
S punta

ajouter
E add, to
G zugeben
S añadir

ajustable
E controllable, adjustable
G einstellbar, regelbar, regulierbar
S ajustable, regulable

ajustage de la matrice
E die alignment
G Matrizenausrichtung
S disposición de matrices

ajustement
E adjustment, setting
G Einstellung, Regulierung
S ajuste, regulación

ajustement de fonctionnement
E operational adjustment, process adjustment
G betriebliche Anpassung, Prozeßanpassung
S ajuste del funcionamiento, ajuste de un proceso

ajustement de la vitesse
E speed adjustment
G Geschwindigkeitseinstellung
S ajuste de la velocidad

ajustement du pH
E pH adjustment
G pH-Wert-Einstellung
S ajuste del pH

ajustement d'un procédé
E operational adjustment, process adjustment
G betriebliche Anpassung, Prozeßanpassung
S ajuste del funcionamiento, ajuste de un proceso

ajuster
E adjust, to; align, to
G einstellen, ausrichten
S ajustar, alinear, orientar, regular

alarme
E alarm
G Warnsignal
S señal de alarma

alarme de mauvais fonctionnement
E malfunction indication, malfunction alarm, failure alarm
G Störungsmeldung
S aviso de avería

alarme d'incendie
E fire alarm
G Feuermelder
S alarma de incendio

alcalin
E alkaline, basic
G alkalisch, basisch
S alcalino, básico

alcaliniser
E deacidify, to
G entsäuern
S alcalinizar, desacidificar

alcalinité
E alkalinity
G Alkalinität
S alcalinidad, basicidad

alcoolate
E alcoholate
G Alkoholauszug
S extracto alcohólico

aldéhyde
E aldehyde
G Aldehyd
S aldehído

aligner
E align, to
G ausrichten
S ajustar, alinear, orientar

aliment
E food
G Lebensmittel
S alimento

alimentation
E supply
G Versorgung
S abastecimiento, suministro

alimentation du vide
E vacuum feed
G Vakuumbeschickung
S alimentación de vacío

alimentation en air
E air supply
G Luftversorgung
S abastecimiento de aire

alimentation en courant électrique
E power supply
G Netzgerät, Stromversorgung
S alimentador a la red, suministro eléctrico

alimentation en eau
E water supply
G Wasserversorgung
S suministro de agua

alimentation en feuilles
E film supply
G Folienbeschickung
S abastecimiento de láminas

alimentation en gaz
E gas supply
G Gaszufuhr
S alimentación de gas

alimentation en produit
E product feed
G Produktzufuhr
S suministro de un producto

alimentation par gravité
E gravity feed
G Zufuhr durch Gefälle
S alimentación por gravedad

alimenter
E fill, to; charge, to
G einfüllen
S envasar, llenar

aliquoter
E aliquot, to
G aliquotieren
S alicuotar

alkylation
E alkylation
G Alkylierung
S alquilación

allergène
E allergen
G Allergen
S alergeno

allergisant
E sensitising
G allergisierend
S alergizante

alliage
E alloy
G Legierung
S aleación

allumage piezoélectrique
E piezo ignition
G piezoelektrische Zündung
S encendido piezoeléctrico

allumer
E switch on, to
G einschalten
S conectar, encender

altération
E deterioration
G Verderb
S deterioro

alupalette
E aluminium pallet
G Alupalette
S paleta de aluminio

amélioration de la qualité
E quality improvement
G Qualitätsverbesserung
S mejora de la calidad

améliorer
E improve, to
G verbessern
S mejorar

amendement
E amendment
G Änderungsanzeige
S anuncio de enmienda

amer
E bitter
G bitter
S amargo

amiante
E asbestos
G Asbest
S asbesto

amidon
E starch
G Stärke
S almidón

amidon du maïs
E corn starch
G Maisstärke
S almidón de maíz

amincissement
E conicalness, conicity
G Verjüngung, Konizität
S disminución, estrechamiento, conicidad

amines
E amines
G Amine
S aminas

amines aromatiques
E aromatic amines
G aromatische Amine
S aminas aromáticas

amines primaires
E primary amines
G primäre Amine
S aminas primarias

amines secondaires
E secondary amines
G sekundäre Amine
S aminas secundarias

amines tertiaires
E tertiary amines
G tertiäre Amine
S aminas terciarias

amorcer
E prime, to
G grundieren
S enderezar, dar la primera capa

amorphe
E amorphous
G amorph
S amorfo

amortisseur de son
E silencer, attenuator
G Schalldämpfer
S silenciador

amovible
E detachable, removable
G entfernbar, abnehmbar
S desmontable

ampérage
E amperage
G Stromstärke
S amperaje, intensidad de corriente

ampèremètre
E ammeter
G Amperemeter, Strommesser
S amperímetro

amplificateur
E amplifier
G Verstärker
S amplificador

amplificateur de signal
E signal amplifier
G Signalverstärker
S amplificador de señal

amplification
E amplification
G Verstärkung
S amplificación, intensificación, refuerzo

amplitude
E amplitude
G Amplitude
S amplitud

ampoule
E ampoule
G Ampulle
S ampolla

ampoule autocassable
E one-point cut (OPC) ampoule
G Brechampulle
S ampolla de apertura manual

ampoule buvable
E oral ampoule
G Trinkampulle
S ampolla bebible

ampoule de verre
E glass ampoule
G Spießampulle
S ampolla de vidrio

ampoule en plastique
E plastic ampoule
G Kunststoffampulle
S ampolla de plástico

anaérobe
E anaerobic
G anaerob
S anaerobio

analyse
E analysis, control test
G Analyse, Prüfung
S análisis, examen, ensayo, prueba, test

analyse à poids sec
E dry weight analysis
G Trockengewichtanalyse
S análisis de peso seco

analyse coulométrique
E coulometric analysis
G coulometrische Analyse
S análisis coulométrico

analyse de données matricielles
E matrix data analysis
G Matrixdatenanalyse
S análisis de datos en matriz

analyse de la demande biologique d'oxygène (DBO)
E biochemical oxygen demand (bod) analysis
G biochemischer Sauerstoffbedarf (BSB)
S necesidades bioquímicas de oxígeno

analyse de la teneur totale du pétrole en hydrocarbures
E total petroleum hydrocarbon (tph) analysis
G Analyse auf Gesamt-(Petroleum)-Kohlenwasserstoffe
S análisis de hidrocarburos totales (de petróleo)

analyse de l'environnement
E environmental analysis
G Umweltanalyse
S análisis del medio ambiente

analyse de libération
E release analysis
G Freigabeuntersuchung
S análisis de autorización

analyse de modes et effets des pannes (FMEA)
E failure mode and effect analysis (FMEA)
G Fehlermöglichkeits- und Einflußanalyse (FMEA)
S análisis de influencia y posibilidad de defectos

analyse de traces
E trace analysis
G Spurenanalyse
S análisis de vestigios

analyse d'échantillon
E sample assay, sample analysis
G Probenanalyse
S análisis de muestras

analyse des risques
E risk analysis
G Risikoanalyse
S análisis del riesgo

English
German
French
Spanish

analyse des selles
E faeces test
G Stuhluntersuchung
S examen de heces

analyse des tendances
E trend analysis
G Trendermittlung
S análisis de tendencias

analyse du poids
E gravimetric analysis
G Gewichtsanalyse
S análisis del peso

analyse d'un produit
E product assay, product analysis
G Produktanalyse
S análisis del producto

analyse élémentaire
E elementary analysis
G Elementaranalyse
S análisis elemental

analyse par activation neutronique
E neutron activation analysis
G Neutronenaktivierungsanalyse
S análisis de activación de neutrones

analyse répétée
E replicate analysis
G Wiederholungsanalyse
S análisis de repetición

analyse structurelle
E structural analysis
G Strukturaufklärung
S análisis estructural

analyse volumétrique
E volumetric analysis
G volumetrische Analyse
S análisis volumétrico

analyseur à balayage
E see-through scanner
G Durchlichtkontrolleinrichtung
S dispositivo de control por transiluminación

analyseur robot
E robotic system
G Robotersystem
S sistema robot

analyte
E analyte
G Analyt
S sustancia a analizar

analytique
E analytical
G analytisch
S analítico

anémomètre à ailettes
E fan wheel anemometer
G Flügelradanemometer
S anemómetro de rueda de aletas

anémomètre à moulinet
E fan wheel anemometer
G Flügelradanemometer
S anemómetro de rueda de aletas

anémomètre à résistance électrique
E hot-wire anemometer
G Hitzedrahtanemometer
S anemómetro de resistencia eléctrica

angle
E angle
G Winkel
S ángulo

angle de pente
E angle of slope, angle of gradient
G Neigungswinkel, Böschungswinkel
S ángulo de inclinación, ángulo de la pendiente

angle de réflexion
E angle of reflection
G Reflektionswinkel
S ángulo de reflexión

angle de réfraction
E angle of refraction
G Brechungswinkel
S ángulo de refracción

angle d'incidence
E angle of incidence
G Einfallswinkel
S ángulo de incidencia

angles, à
E angled, angular
G abgewinkelt
S angulado, doblado, escuadrado

angulaire
E angled, angular
G abgewinkelt
S angulado, doblado, escuadrado

anhydre
E anhydrous
G wasserfrei
S anhidro

anneau
E collar
G Manschette
S manguito

anneau de support
E retaining ring
G Haltering
S anillo de soporte

annexe
E insert, enclosure, appendix
G Beilage, Anlage (zur Dokumentation)
S anexo, apéndice (de un documento)

anomalie cellulaire
E cellular anomaly
G zelluläre Anomalie
S anomalía celular

anorganique
E inorganic
G anorganisch
S anorgánico

antibiotique
E antibiotic
G Antibioticum
S antibiótico

anticorps
E antibody
G Antikörper
S anticuerpo

anticorps monoclonal
E monoclonal antibody
G monoklonaler Antikörper
S anticuerpo monoclonal

anti-déflagrant
E explosion-proof
G explosionssicher
S a prueba de explosión

anti-dérapant
E slip-proof, non-slip
G rutschsicher
S antideslizante

antidote
E antidote
G Gegengift
S antídoto

antifongique
E anti-fungal
G pilzabtötend
S antifúngico, fungicida

antimousse
E anti-foaming agent, defoamer
G Entschäumer
S agente antiespumante

antioxydant
E anti-oxidant
G Antioxidans
S antioxidante

antipodes optiques
E optical antipodes
G optische Antipoden
S antípodas ópticos

apathogène
E apathogenic
G apathogen
S apatógeno

aplati
E flattened
G abgeflacht
S aplanado

aplatissement
E flattening
G Abflachung
S aplanamiento

appareil à corbeille
E basket apparatus
G Korbgerät
S aparato de cesto

appareil à teindre
E stainer
G Färbegerät
S teñidor

appareil d'analyses
E analytical apparatus
G Analysengerät
S aparato de análisis

appareil de chauffage
E heating aggregate
G Heizaggregat
S aparato de calefacción

appareil de climatisation
E air conditioner
G Klimaanlage
S aire acondicionado

appareil de contrôle
E monitoring device
G Überwachungseinrichtung
S dispositivo de vigilancia

appareil de distillation
E still
G Destille
S alambique

appareil de distillation à colonnes multiples
E pressure column distillation plant
G Druckkolonnendestillationsanlage
S aparato de destilación a columna de presión

appareil de mesure des particules
E particle measuring instrument
G Partikelmeßgerät
S aparato de medición de partículas

appareil de surveillance
E monitoring device
G Überwachungseinrichtung
S dispositivo de vigilancia

appareil d'éclairage
E light, light fittings
G Beleuchtungskörper
S aparato de iluminación

appareil doseur
E metering device, dosing device
G Dosiereinrichtung
S dispositivo dosificante

appareillage
E device
G Vorrichtung
S dispositivo

appareillage compact
E compact line
G Kompaktanlage
S instalación compacta

appareillage d'alimentation
E filling device, charging device
G Einfüllvorrichtung
S dispositivo de relleno

appareillage élévateur
E lifting device
G Hubvorrichtung
S dispositivo elevador

appareillage expérimental
E apparatus, equipment
G Geräte
S aparatos

appareils périphériques
E peripheral instrumentation
G periphere Geräte
S aparatos periféricos

apparence
E appearance
G äußere Beschaffenheit
S aspecto externo

apparence générale
E general appearance
G allgemeines Aussehen
S aspecto general

appel d'offres
E tender
G Ausschreibung
S anuncio, concurso, convocatoria

appellation
E designation
G Bezeichnung
S denominación, marcado, rotulación

appendice
E enclosure, appendix
G Anlage (zur Dokumentation), Anhang
S anexo, apéndice (de un documento)

applicabilité
E applicability
G Anwendbarkeit
S aplicabilidad

applicateur
E applicator
G Applikator
S aplicador

applicateur compte-gouttes
E dropper applicator
G Verschluß mit Tropfer
S cierre con cuentagotas

applicateur nasal
E nasal applicator
G Nasenolive
S aplicador nasal

application
E application
G Anwendung
S aplicación

pour application externe
E for external application
G zur äußerlichen Anwendung
S para aplicación externa

application d'échantillons (sur plaque de CCM)
E sample spotting (on TLC plate)
G Probenauftrag (als Fleck auf DC-Platte)
S depósito de muestras (como mancha sobre la placa de cromatografía en capa fina)

applications potentielles
E potential applications
G potentielle Anwendungen
S aplicaciones potenciales

appliquer (un échantillon)
E apply, to (sample)
G aufgeben (Probe), aufbringen, auftragen
S aplicar (una muestra), extender, untar

apposer
E apply, to; attach, to
G anbringen
S instalar, montar

apprenti
E apprentice
G Auszubildender, Lehrling
S aprendiz

apprentissage
E apprenticeship
G Lehre
S aprendizaje, enseñanza

approbation
E approval
G Billigung
S aprobación

approprié
E suitable, appropriate, adequate, relevant, pertinent
G angemessen, geeignet, relevant
S adecuado, apropiado, relevante

approuver
E approve, to
G billigen
S aprobar

approvisionnement en dépliants
E leaflet feed
G Prospektzuführung
S suministro de prospectos

approvisionnement public en eau
E public water supply
G öffentliche Wasserversorgung
S abastecimiento público de agua

apte à l'emmagasinage
E suitable for storage
G lagerfähig
S adecuado para almacenaje

aptitude à être étendu
E spreadability
G Streichfähigkeit
S untabilidad

aptitude à être stérilisé
E sterilisability
G Sterilisierbarkeit
S esterilizabilidad

aqueux
E aqueous
G wäßrig
S acuoso

arbre
E shaft
G Schaft, Welle
S árbol, asta, eje

arbre à cames
E camshaft
G Nockenwelle
S árbol de levas

arbre de transmission
E drive shaft
G Antriebswelle
S árbol motor

archivage
E archiving, retention, storage,
G Archivierung, Aufbewahrung
S archivado, conservación, almacenaje

archives
E archive
G Archiv
S archivo

arête
E edge
G Rand
S arista, borde

arête d'un comprimé
E rim, bur of a tablet
G Grat einer Tablette
S borde de un comprimido

armoire électrique
E switch box, control box, wiring box
G Schaltkasten
S caja de distribución

arrêt (par ex. d'une machine)
E shut down (e. g. of a machine)
G Abschaltung (z. B. einer Maschine)
S desconexión (p. ej. de una máquina)

à l'arrêt
E at rest
G im Ruhezustand
S parado

arrêt de machine
E machine stoppage
G Maschinenstillstand
S detención de la máquina

arrêt d'urgence
E emergency off
G Not-Aus
S interruptor de emergencia

arrêter
E switch off, to
G abschalten
S desconectar

arrière-goût
E after-taste
G Nachgeschmack
S regusto

arrivée d'air frais
E fresh air inlet
G Frischluftzufuhr
S entrada de aire fresco

arrivée d'eau potable
E tap water feed
G Trinkwasserzufuhr
S abastecimiento de agua potable

arrondi au chiffre inférieur
E rounded off
G abgerundet
S redondeado a la cifra inferior

arrondir
E round off, to
G abrunden
S redondear a la cifra inferior

artisan
E workman, tradesman
G Handwerker
S artesano, trabajador manual

ascenseur
E lift, elevator
G Aufzug
S ascensor

aseptique
E aseptic
G aseptisch
S aséptico

aspect
E appearance
G äußere Beschaffenheit
S aspecto externo

aspersion d'eau chaude
E hot water spraying
G Heißwasserberieselung
S rociado con agua caliente

aspirer
E aspirate, to
G ansaugen, absaugen
S aspirar, succionar

assainissement
E reorganisation, restructuring
G Sanierung
S saneamiento

assemblage
E assembly, mounting, set-up
G Montage, Zusammenbau
S ensamblaje, montaje

assembler
E assemble, to
G zusammensetzen
S ensamblar, montar

assise
E bearing (mach.)
G Lager (Maschinenteil)
S asiento, cojinete, soporte

assistant de laboratoire
E laboratory assistant
G Laborant
S asistente de laboratorio

assisté par ordinateur
E computerised, computer-assisted
G computergestützt
S asistido por ordenador

association professionelle
E trade association
G Berufsgenossenschaft
S asociación profesional

assurance de conformité
E conformity assurance
G Konformitätssicherung
S aseguramiento de conformidad

assurance-qualité
E quality assurance (QA)
G Qualitätssicherung (QS)
S aseguramiento de la calidad

assurer
E guarantee, to; secure, to; ensure, to
G sicherstellen
S asegurar, garantizar

atelier
E workshop
G Werkstatt
S taller

atomiser
E atomise, to; vaporise, to; spray, to
G zerstäuben, aufsprühen
S atomizar, pulverizar

atomiseur
E atomiser
G Zerstäuber, Nebelgenerator
S atomizador, pulverizador

attache
E tab, tongue
G Einstecklasche
S cubrejunta de pestaña

atteinte à l'environnement
E environmental damage
G Umweltschaden
S daño ecológico

atténuation (d'un signal)
E attenuation (of a signal)
G Abschwächung (eines Signals)
S atenuación (de una señal)

audit
E audit
G Audit
S auditoría

audit d'un fabricant
E manufacturer audit
G Herstelleraudit
S inspección de un fabricante

audit d'une installation
E plant audit
G Betriebsprüfung
S auditoría de empresa

audit interne
E internal audit
G internes Audit
S auditoría interna

augmentation de pression
E pressure increase
G Druckanstieg
S aumento de presión

augmentation de température
E temperature increase
G Temperaturerhöhung
S aumento de temperatura

augmentation du rendement
E yield enhancement
G Ausbeutesteigerung
S aumento del rendimiento

auto-adhésif
E self-adhesive
G selbstklebend
S autoadhesivo

autoclavable
E autoclavable
G autoklavierbar
S esterilizable en autoclave

autoclave
E autoclave, steriliser
G Autoklav, Sterilisator
S autoclave, esterilizador

autoclave vertical
E vertical autoclave
G Vertikalautoklav
S autoclave vertical

autoclaver
E autoclave, to
G autoklavieren
S esterilizar en autoclave

autographe
E signature
G eigenhändige Unterschrift
S firma autógrafa

auto-inspection
E self-check, self-inspection
G Selbstüberprüfung, Selbstinspektion
S autocomprobación, autoinspección

automate programmable industriel
E programmable logic control (PLC)
G speicherprogrammierbare Steuerung (SPS)
S control programable mediante memoria

automatisation
E automation
G Automation
S automa(tiza)ción

automatisation d'un procédé
E process automation
G Prozeßautomatisierung
S automa(tiza)ción de un proceso

automatiser
E automate, to
G automatisieren
S automatizar

automédication
E self-medication
G Selbstmedikation
S automedicación

autorisation
E authorisation, approval, authority
G Genehmigung, Befugnis
S autorización, competencia

autorisation d'accès
E authorised access
G Zugangsberechtigung
S derecho de acceso

autorisation de fabrication
E manufacturing authorisation
G Herstellerlaubnis
S permiso de fabricación

autorisation de mise sur le marché (A.M.M.)
E marketing authorisation
G Zulassung, Marktzulassung
S autorización de (para) venta en el mercado

autorisation de mise sur le marché comme médicament générique
E generic marketing authorisation
G Zulassung als Generikum
S autorización como genérico

autorisation de production
E production licence
G Produktionsgenehmigung
S permiso de producción

autorisation d'imprimer
E print release
G Druckfreigabe
S autorización para imprimir

autorisation d'une autorité réglementaire
E licence, approval, authorisation
G behördliche Genehmigung
S autorización oficial

autorisation électronique
E electronic approval
G elektronische Genehmigung
S autorización electrónica

autoriser
E authorise, to; approve, to
G genehmigen
S autorizar

autorité réglementaire
E authorities
G Behörde
S autoridades, organismos oficiales

autorités compétentes responsables des autorisations de mise sur le marché
E regulatory authorities
G Zulassungsbehörde
S agencia de autorización de licencias sanitarias

auxiliaires de conditionnement
E packaging aids
G Packhilfsmittel
S materiales auxilares para envasado

avertissement
E warning
G Warnhinweis
S aviso de alarma

avis d'expert
E expertise
G Gutachten
S dictamen

axe de rotation
E axis of rotation
G Drehachse
S eje de rotación

axe des abscisses
E X-axis
G X-Achse
S eje X

axe des ordonnées
E Y-axis
G Y-Achse
S eje Y

axe longitudinal
E longitudinal axis
G Längsachse
S eje longitudinal

azote
E nitrogen
G Stickstoff
S nitrógeno

bac
E bin, container, vessel
G Behälter
S recipiente

backup d'une base de données
E data base backup
G Datenbanksicherheitskopie
S copia de seguridad de un banco de datos

bactéricide
E bactericidal
G bakterizid
S bactericida

bactérie
E bacteria
G Bakterien
S bacterias

bague
E collar
G Manschette
S manguito

baguette de verre
E glass rod
G Glasstab
S barra de vidrio, bastón de vidrio

bain à ultra-sons
E ultrasonic bath
G Ultraschallbad
S baño ultrasónico

bain de bouche
E mouthwash
G Mundwasser
S enjuague bucal

bain d'huile
E oil bath
G Ölbad
S baño de aceite

bain d'immersion
E immersion bath
G Tauchbad
S baño de sumersión

bain-marie
E water bath
G Wasserbad
S baño de agua

baisse de qualité
E loss of quality
G Güteminderung
S pérdida de calidad

baisse de température
E temperature decrease
G Temperaturabfall
S descenso de temperatura

baisser
E lower, to; reduce, to
G senken
S bajar, reducir

balance
E balance
G Waage
S balanza

balance à plat en haut
E top-loading balance
G oberschalige Waage
S balanza de carga superior

balance à ressort
E spring balance
G Federwaage
S balanza de resorte

balance d'analyse
E analytical balance
G Analysenwaage
S báscula de análisis

balance de contrôle
E control balance
G Kontrollwaage
S báscula de control

balance de convoyeur
E band balance, conveyor balance
G Bandwaage
S báscula de cinta

balance de précision
E precision balance
G Feinwaage, Präzisionswaage
S balanza de precisión

balance de torsion
E torsion balance
G Torsionswaage
S balanza de torsión

ballon
E flask
G Kolben (Glasgefäß)
S alambique, matraz, retorta

ballon à fond rond
E round-bottomed flask
G Rundkolben
S matraz esférico

ballon conique
E conical flask
G Spitzkolben
S matraz cónico

ballon de verre
E glass balloon
G Glasballon
S balón de vidrio

ballon gradué
E volumetric flask
G Meßkolben
S matraz graduado

ballon rodé
E ground-joint flask
G Schliffkolben
S matraz esmerilado

bandage
E bandage
G Verband
S vendaje

bandage d'occlusion
E occlusive dressing
G Okklusivverband
S vendaje oclusivo

bande (par ex. d'étoffe)
E sheet (e. g. of foil)
G Bahn (z. B. Folien-)
S rollo, tira (p. ej. de una lámina)

bande adhésive
E adhesive tape
G Klebeband
S cinta adhesiva

English German French Spanish

bande continue
E continuous band
G Endlosbahn
S cinta sin fin

bande de gaze
E gauze bandage
G Mullbinde
S venda de gasa

bande de papier d'enregistreur
E recorder chart
G Schreiberstreifen
S registro de diagramas

bande de spores
E spore strip
G Sporenstreifen
S banda de esporas

bande de triage
E sorting belt
G Sortierband
S cinta clasificadora

bande d'étoffe
E sheet of film
G Folienbahn
S banda de láminas

bande magnétique
E magnetic tape
G Magnetband
S cinta magnética

banderole
E band, banderole, tape
G Banderole
S precinto

bandes d'interférence
E interfering bands
G Störbanden, interferierende Banden
S bandas de interferencia

banque de cellules souches
E stem cell bank
G Stammzellbank
S banco de células germinales

banque du sang
E blood bank, blood donor service
G Blutbank, Blutspendewesen
S banco de sangre, servicio de donantes de sangre

barreau aimanté
E magnetic stirring bar
G Rührfisch
S agitador magnético

barrière fluidique
E barrier fluid
G Sperrflüssigkeit
S barrera líquida

barrière optique
E optical barrier, light barrier
G Lichtschranke
S barrera luminosa, barrera óptica

bas de la colonne de distillation
E distillation bottom
G Destillationsboden
S fondo de destilación

basculer
E tilt, to
G kippen
S verter, volcar

base
E base, basis
G Base, Basis
S base

base d'absorption
E absorption base (for ointments)
G Absorptionsgrundlage (für Salben)
S base de absorción (para pomadas)

base organique
E organic base
G organische Base
S base orgánica

base perforée
E perforated base
G Lochboden
S suelo perforado

basicité
E basicity
G Basizität
S basicidad, alcalinidad

basique, alcalin
E basic, alkaline
G basisch
S básico, alcalino

bassin de descente
E catch basin, drain
G Sinkkasten
S fuente (descendente) de recogida

bâtiment
E building
G Gebäude
S edificio

bâtonnet de test
E test strip
G Teststäbchen
S bastoncillos de prueba

beaume
E embrocation, liniment
G Einreibemittel
S bálsamo, linimento

bec de Bunsen
E Bunsen burner
G Bunsenbrenner
S mechero Bunsen

bec de gaz
E Bunsen burner
G Bunsenbrenner
S mechero Bunsen

bécher
E beaker
G Becherglas
S probeta

biais
E slope
G Schräge
S inclinación, oblicuidad

biberon
E aspirator bottle
G Saugflasche
S biberón

bidon d'aérosol
E aerosol can
G Aerosoldose
S tubo aerosol

bilan
E reconciliation
G Bilanzierung
S hacer balance

bilan d'étiquettes
E label reconciliation
G Etikettenbilanzierung
S balance de etiquetas

bimétal
E bimetal
G Bimetall
S bimetal

biocompatible
E biocompatible
G biokompatibel
S biocompatible

biodégradable
E biodegradable
G biologisch abbaubar
S degradable biológicamente

biodégradation
E biodegradation
G biologischer Abbau
S degradación biológica

biodisponibilité
E bioavailability
G Bioverfügbarkeit
S biodisponibilidad

bioéquivalence
E bioequivalence
G Bioäquivalenz
S bioequivalencia

biogène
E biogenic
G biogen
S biógeno

biogénérateur
E biogenerator
G Biogenerator
S biogenerador

biogenèse
E biogenesis
G Biogenese
S biogénesis

biologie moléculaire
E molecular biology
G Molekularbiologie
S biología molecular

bioluminescence
E bioluminescence
G Biolumineszenz
S bioluminiscencia

biomasse
E biomass
G Biomasse
S biomasa

bio-sécurité
E biosafety
G biologische Sicherheit
S seguridad biológica

biosynthèse
E biosynthesis
G Biosynthese
S biosíntesis

biotechnologie
E biotechnology
G Biotechnologie
S biotecnología

biseau
E bevel
G Abschrägung, Facette
S bisel, faceta

biseau (d'un poinçon à comprimés)
E punch chamfer (of tablet punch)
G Fase (am Tablettenstempel)
S bisel (del troquel de comprimidos)

biseau, en
E sloping
G abgeschrägt
S biselado

biseauté
E sloping
G abgeschrägt
S biselado

blister
E blister, well, cup (of blister)
G Blister, Napf (beim Blister)
S blister, pocillo del blíster

bloc de moulage
E die block
G Formblock
S bloque de moldeo

bloc d'injection
E injection block
G Einspritzblock
S bloque de inyección

blocage
E blockage
G Blockierung
S bloqueo

bloquer
E block, to; jam, to
G blockieren
S bloquear

blouse
E lab coat, gown, smock
G Kittel, Kurzkittel
S bata, blusa

blouse de laboratoire
E lab coat, gown
G Laborkittel
S bata de laboratorio

bobine de résistance
E resistance coil
G Widerstandsspule
S bobina de resistencia

boîte
E box, carton, outer carton
G Schachtel, Umkarton
S caja, carton

boîte d'ampoules
E ampoule box
G Ampullenschachtel
S caja de ampollas

boîte de bornes
E terminal box
G Klemmkasten
S caja de terminales

boîte de distribution
E junction box
G Verteilerkasten
S caja de distribución

boîte de fusibles
E fuse box
G Sicherungskasten
S caja de fusibles

boîte de Petri
E Petri dish
G Petrischale
S placa de Petri

boîte de stockage
E stacking box
G Stapelkasten
S caja de apilamiento

boîte pliante
E folding carton
G Faltschachtel
S caja plegable

boîtier
E housing
G Gehäuse
S caja, estuche

boîtier de filtre
E filter housing
G Filtergehäuse
S armazón del filtro

bombe aérosol
E aerosol can
G Aerosoldose
S tubo aerosol

bonnes pratiques cliniques (GCP)
E Good Clinical Practice (GCP)
G Gute Klinische Praxis
S Prácticas Clínicas Correctas (GCP)

bonnes pratiques de fabrication (GMP)
E Good Manufacturing Practice (GMP)
G Gute Herstellungspraxis (GMP)
S Prácticas Correctas de Fabricación (GMP)

bonnes pratiques de laboratoire (GLP)
E Good Laboratory Practice (GLP)
G Gute Laborpraxis (GLP)
S Prácticas Correctas de Laboratorio (GLP)

bonnet
E head covering, headgear, cap
G Kopfbedeckung, Kopfhaube
S sombrero, capucha, cofia

bord
E edge
G Rand
S arista, borde

bordereau de livraison
E delivery note
G Lieferschein
S talón de entrega

bordure d'un mur
E wall skirting
G Wandsockel
S zócalo de la pared

bordure triangulaire
E triangular skirting
G Dreikantsockel
S zócalo triangular

borne
E socket, terminal
G Buchse, Klemme
S casquillo, hembrilla, manguito, borne, pinza, terminal,

bouche
E duct
G Schacht
S conducto, pozo

bouché
E clogged, blocked
G verstopft
S obstruido

bouche d'égout
E floor drain
G Fußbodenabfluß
S sumidero

boucher
E tighten, to; seal, to
G abdichten
S cerrar herméticamente

boucheuse
E capper, crimping machine
G Bördelmaschine
S máquina de rebordeo

bouchon
E closure, seal, cap, plug, stopper
G Verschluß, Stopfen
S cierre, tapón

bouchon à compte-gouttes
E dropper insert
G Tropfeinsatz
S tapón cuentagotas

bouchon à vis
E screw cap
G Schraubkappe
S cierre de rosca

bouchon de tube
E tube closure
G Tubenverschluß
S cierre de un tubo

bouchon en caoutchouc
E rubber stopper
G Gummistopfen
S tapón de goma

bouchon en caoutchouc butyle
E butyl rubber stoppers
G Stopfen aus Butylgummi
S tapón de caucho butílico

bouchon graisseur
E lubricating nipple
G Schmiernippel
S boquilla lubri(fi)cante

bouchon rodé
E ground stopper
G Schliffstopfen
S tapón esmerilado

boucle d'asservissement
E control loop
G Regelkreis
S circuito regulador

boucle de dosage
E dosing loop
G Dosierschleife
S bucle de dosificación

boucle de recirculation
E main ring
G Ringleitung
S cañería en anillo, red anular

boucle de test
E test loop
G Testschleife
S bucle de pruebas

boucle d'eau de refroidissement
E cooling water loop
G Kühlwasserschleife
S serpentín para el agua de refrigeración

boucle d'échantillon
E sample loop
G Probenschleife
S bucle para toma de muestras

bouillir
E boil, to
G aufkochen, sieden
S hervir

bouilloire
E vessel, boiler
G Kessel
S caldera, marmita

bouillon de culture
E culture broth
G Kulturbouillon, Nährbouillon, Nährlösung
S caldo de cultivo, solución de cultivo, solución nutritiva

boulette
E pellet, compressed core
G Preßling
S masa comprimida

boulon
E bolt
G Bolzen
S clavija, perno

bourre
E floc
G Flocke
S copo, flóculo

bourrelet
E bead
G Bördelrand
S burlete rebordeado, canto rebordeado

bout
E stub
G Stichleitung
S adaptador de guiaondas

bouteille
E bottle
G Flasche
S botella

bouteille à col large
E wide-necked bottle
G Weithalsflasche
S botella de cuello ancho

bouteille d'aluminium
E aluminium bottle
G Aluminiumflasche
S botella de aluminio

bouteille de gaz
E gas cylinder
G Gasflasche, Druckgasflasche
S botella de gas, botella de gas a presión

bouteille en plastique
E plastic bottle
G Kunststoff-Flasche
S botella de plástico

bouteille munie d'un bouchon à vis
E screw-cap bottle
G Flasche mit Schraubverschluß
S botella con cierre de rosca

bouteille perforable
E perforable bottle
G Durchstechflasche
S botella perforable

bouton d'ajustement
E adjusting knob
G Einstellknopf
S botón de ajuste

bouton de contrôle
E control knob
G Bedienungselement
S elemento de manejo

bouton marche/arrêt
E on/off switch
G Abschalter, Ausschalter
S interruptor (de desconexión)

brancher
E wire, to
G schalten, verdrahten
S conectar, conmutar

bras de levier
E yoke
G Gabelarm, Joch
S brazo de horquilla

bras d'un robot
E robotic arm
G Roboterarm
S brazo de robot

bras pivotant
E swivel arm
G Schwenkarm
S brazo giratorio

brevet
E patent
G Patent
S patente

approbation de brevet
E patent approval
G Erteilung eines Patentes
S aprobación de patente

violation de brevet
E infringement of a patent
G Verletzung eines Patentes
S violación de patente

breveté
E patented
G patentiert
S patentado

bride
E flange
G Flansch
S brida, collar

brider
E flange, to
G flanschen
S bridar

brillance
E gloss
G Glanz
S brillo, lustre

brillant
E glossy
G glänzend
S brillante, lustrado

brillant comme de la soie
E silk glossy
G seidenglänzend
S brillante como seda

broche
E pin
G Stift (technisch)
S clavija, perno, pivote

brochure d'information pour patient
E patient information leaflet
G Patientenbroschüre
S folleto de información del paciente

bromage
E bromination
G Bromierung
S bromado

brosse
E brush
G Bürste
S cepillo

brosse de laminage
E revolving brush
G Bürstenwalze
S cepillo rotativo, cilindro cepillador

brosse rotative
E revolving brush
G Walzenbürste
S cepillo rotatorio

brouillard
E fog
G Nebel
S niebla

broyage humide
E wet grinding
G Naßvermahlung
S molido húmedo

English German French Spanish

broyer
E mill, to; crush, to; grind, to
G mahlen
S moler

broyeur
E mill
G Mühle
S molino

broyeur à boulets
E ball mill, pebble mill
G Kugelmühle
S molinillo a bolas

broyeur à broches
E pin mill
G Stiftmühle
S molino de clavija

broyeur à cylindres
E roll mill
G Walzenmühle
S molino de cilindros

broyeur à marteau
E hammer mill
G Hammermühle
S molino triturador

broyeur à pommade
E ointment mill
G Salbenmühle
S molino de pomada

brucelles
E tweezers
G Pinzette
S pinzas

bruit
E noise
G Rauschen
S ruido (de fondo)

bruit de fond d'une ligne de base
E baseline noise
G Basislinienrauschen
S ruido (de fondo) en la línea de base

brut
E coarse
G grob
S grosero, grueso

bulle
E bubble, blister
G Blase
S ampolla, burbuja, vejiga

bulle d'air piégée
E entrapped air bubble
G eingeschlossene Luftblase
S burbuja de aire capturada

bulle de gaz
E gas bubble
G Gasblase
S burbuja de gas

burette
E burette
G Bürette
S bureta

buse
E nozzle, nozzle head
G Düse, Sprühkopf
S aplicador, inyector, tobera, cabeza del inyector

buse à billes
E ball nozzle
G Kugeldüse
S aplicador de bola

buse binaire
E binary nozzle
G Zweistoffdüse
S aplicador binario

buse de nettoyage
E cleaning nozzle
G Waschdüse
S aplicador de lavado

buse de remplissage
E filling nozzle
G Füllventil
S válvula de relleno

buse d'injection
E injection port
G Einspritzdüse
S inyector

cabine de pesée
E weighing cubicle
G Wägekabine
S cabina de pesado

câblage
E wiring
G Verkabelung
S cables

câble
E cable
G Kabel
S cable

câble de rallonge
E extension cable
G Verlängerungskabel
S alargadera, cable de prolongación

câbles électriques
E electrical cables
G elektrische Zuleitungen
S cables de conducción eléctrica

cachet
E cachet, capsule
G Oblate, Oblatenkapsel
S oblea, gragea, cápsula amilácea

cadence
E cycle number
G Taktzahl
S número de ciclos

cadre
E stand, frame
G Gestell
S armazón, bastidor, soporte

cadre dirigeant
E executive
G Führungskraft
S directivo, ejecutivo

cahier de laboratoire
E laboratory notebook, log book
G Laborjournal
S diario de laboratorio

cahier de route
E log book
G Logbuch
S cuaderno de bitácora

cahier des charges
E user requirements, user specifications
G Lastenheft
S requerimientos del usuario

caisse en bois
E wooden case
G Holzkiste
S caja de madera

calciner, se
E ignite, to
G ausglühen
S calcinar

calcul
E calculation
G Berechnung
S cálculo

calcul du rendement
E yield calculation
G Ausbeuteberechnung
S cálculo del rendimiento

calculation
E calculation
G Rechnung
S cálculo

calculer
E calculate, to
G berechnen
S calcular

calibration
E calibration
G Kalibrierung, Eichung
S calibración

calibration par points de mesure multiples
E multiple point calibration
G Kalibrierung anhand mehrerer Meßpunkte
S calibración por varios puntos

calibration par un point de mesure
E single point calibration
G Ein-Punkt-Kalibrierung
S calibración por punto único

calibration de l'équipement
E instrument calibration
G Gerätekalibrierung
S calibración de aparatos

calibrer
E calibrate, to
G kalibrieren, eichen
S calibrar

calmant
E sedative
G Beruhigungsmittel
S sedante, tranquilizante

calorimètre
E calorimeter
G Kalorimeter
S calorímetro

calorimètre à flux de chaleur
E heat flow calorimeter
G Wärmeflußkalorimeter
S calorímetro de flujo de calor

came
E cam
G Nocke
S leva

came (de poinçon) ascendante
E lifting cam (of upper punch)
G Aufzugsschiene (des Oberstempels)
S carril de ascenso (del troquel superior)

came de poinçon descendante
E pull-down cam
G Niederzugsschiene
S carril de tracción inferior, corredera de tracción inferior

came de remplissage
E filling cam (tablet press)
G Füllkurve (bei der Tablettenpresse)
S curva de relleno (prensa de comprimidos)

came d'éjection
E ejector cam
G Auswerfkurve, Auswurfkurve (bei der Tablettenpresse)
S curva de expulsión (de prensa de comprimidos)

campagne
E campaign
G Kampagne
S campaña

canal
E duct, channel
G Kanal
S canal, tubo, conducto

canal de câbles
E cable duct
G Kabelkanal
S canal de cables

canal de distribution
E sales channel
G Vertriebsweg
S canal de distribución

canal de purge anti-déflagrant
E ex-duct, explosion vent
G Ex-Kanal
S orificio (válvula) de seguridad (antideflagrante)

canal d'évacuation de l'air
E exhaust air duct
G Abluftkanal
S canal del aire de escape

English German French Spanish

English German French Spanish

canalisation
E pipe(work), pipeline
G Rohrleitung
S canalización

canalisation d'aération
E venting line
G Entlüftungsleitung
S conducción de ventilación

canalisation d'air
E air duct, air shaft
G Luftschacht
S canalización de aire

canalisation de décompression
E pressure relief duct
G Druckentlastungskanal
S canal de descompresión

canalisation de ventilation
E venting line
G Entlüftungsleitung
S conducción de ventilación

canalisation d'élimination des déchets
E waste duct
G Ablaufrinne
S canal de salida

cancérogène
E carcinogenic
G karzinogen, cancerogen, krebserregend
S cancerógeno

canne
E can, tin
G Dose
S bote, caja, lata

cannelé
E corrugated
G geriffelt
S acanalado, estriado

canneler
E corrugate, to
G riffeln
S acanalar, estriar

cannelure
E groove
G Nut, Rille
S acanaladura, estría, muesca, ranura

cannelure pour joint
E gasket channel
G Dichtungsführung
S guía para la junta

cantine
E canteen
G Kantine
S cantina

canule
E cannula, injection needle
G Kanüle
S cánula

caoutchouc
E rubber
G Gummi
S goma

caoutchouc durci
E hard rubber, vulcanite
G Hartgummi
S ebonita

capable d'écoulement
E capable of flowing, flowable
G rieselfähig
S capaz de fluir

capacité
E capacity, throughput
G Kapazität, Durchsatz
S capacidad, rendimiento

capacité
E capacity, volume
G Fassungsvermögen
S capacidad

capacité d'absorption
E absorptivity, absorption capacity, absorptive capacity, absorbing power, absorbing capacity
G Absorptionsfähigkeit, Absorptionsvermögen
S capacidad de absorción

capacité d'absorption d'eau
E water absorption capacity
G Wasseraufnahmevermögen
S capacidad de absorción de agua

capacité d'adsorption
E adsorptivity, adsorption capacity
G Adsorptionsfähigkeit
S capacidad de adsorción

capacité d'analyse d'échantillons
E sample throughput
G Probendurchsatz
S rendimiento en muestras

capacité de chargement
E load capacity
G Belastbarkeit
S capacidad de carga

capacité de coloration
E colour capacity
G Färbevermögen
S capacidad colorante

capacité de fixation
E binding capacity
G Bindungsvermögen
S capacidad de enlace, capacidad de fijación

capacité de gonflement
E swelling capacity
G Quellfähigkeit
S capacidad de hinchamiento

capacité de récupération
E recovery capability
G Erholungsfähigkeit
S capacidad de recuperación

capacité de séparation
E separation capacity
G Trennungskapazität
S capacidad de separación

capacité d'un tampon
E buffering capacity
G Pufferkapazität
S capacidad de tamponamiento

capillaire
E capillary
G Kapillare
S capilar

capillaire d'ébullition
E boiling capillary
G Siedekapillare
S capilar de ebullición

capsule
E capsule, cachet
G Kapsel, Oblate
S cápsula, oblea, gragea

capsule à bouteilles
E bottle cap
G Flaschenverschluß
S cierre de botella, tapa de botella

capsule à croquer
E biting capsule
G Zerbeißkapsel
S cápsula mordible

capsule de gélatine
E gelatine capsule
G Gelatinekapsel
S cápsula de gelatina

capsule d'évaporation
E evaporating dish
G Abdampfschale
S cápsula de evaporación

capsuler (comprimés)
E cap, to; crimp, to (tablets)
G deckeln, verbördeln (bei Tabletten)
S cubrir, recubrir, rebordear cantos (comprimidos)

capsuleuse
E capping machine
G Verschließmaschine
S máquina de cierre

capter
E collect, to; entrap, to
G auffangen
S captar, colectar, recoger

English
German
French
Spanish

capteur
E sensor, transducer
G Fühler, Meßwertaufnehmer
S sensor, registrador de valores medidos, transductor

capteur de conductivité
E conductivity sensor
G Leitfähigkeitsmesser
S sensor de conductividad

capteur de fibres
E fibre catcher
G Faserfänger
S captador de fibras

capuchon
E closure, seal, cap, cover, hood, casing
G Verschluß, Haube, Abdeckung, Verkleidungsblech
S cierre, casquete, cubierta, sombrerete, chapa de revestimiento

capuchon à usage unique
E disposable cover
G Einmalabdeckung
S cubierta de uso único

caractérisation (d'un composé organique)
E characterisation (of a compound)
G Charakterisierung (einer Verbindung)
S caracterización (de un compuesto)

caractérisation d'un produit
E product description
G Produktbeschreibung
S descripción de un producto

caractéristique
E feature, curve, property
G Merkmal, Kennlinie, Eigenschaft
S característica, propiedad

caracteristique de qualité
E quality attribute
G Qualitätsmerkmal
S característica de calidad

caractéristique de sécurité
E safety feature
G Sicherheitsmerkmal
S característica de seguridad

caractéristique du défaut
E defect characteristic
G Fehlermerkmal
S característica de defecto

caractéristique individuelle
E individual characteristic
G Einzelmerkmal
S característica individual

caractéristique physique
E physical characteristic
G physikalische Eigenschaft
S propiedad física

caractéristiques de compression
E compression characteristics
G Preßeigenschaften
S características de compresión

caractéristiques physico-chimiques
E physical-chemical characteristics
G physikalisch-chemische Eigenschaften
S propiedades fisicoquímicas

caractéristiques physiques
E physical characteristics
G physikalische Eigenschaften
S propiedades físicas

carbone
E carbon
G Kohle
S carbón

carcinogène
E carcinogenic
G karzinogen, krebserregend
S carcinógeno

carence
E deficiency
G Mangel
S carencia, defecto, deficiencia, insuficiencia

carreau
E tile
G Fliese
S baldosa

carte de contrôle de qualité
E quality control card
G Qualitätsregelkarte
S ficha de control de calidad

carter à huile
E sump
G Ölwanne
S cárter

carter d'un moteur
E motor housing
G Motorgehäuse
S cárter del motor

carton
E box, carton, outer carton, pasteboard, cardboard
G Karton, Pappe, Pappschachtel, Umkarton
S caja, cartón, caja de cartón

carton à fibres
E fibre cardboard
G Fiberkarton
S cartón de fibra

carton d'expédition
E outer carton
G Umkarton
S cartón externo

carton ondulé
E corrugated cardboard (carton)
G Wellpappe
S cartón ondulado

cartonner
E carton, to
G kartonieren
S encartonar

cartouche
E cartridge
G Kartusche, Patrone
S cartucho

cartouche de filtre
E filter cartridge
G Filterpatrone
S cartucho de filtro

casque de protection
E safety helmet, hard hat
G Schutzhelm
S casco protector

cassant
E brittle
G brüchig, spröde
S frágil, quebradizo

casser
E bend, to; buckle, to
G knicken
S doblar, quebrar

casser une ampoule
E break an ampoule, to; snap, to (an ampoule)
G Ampulle aufbrechen, abknicken
S romper, romper por el cuello (una ampolla)

catalyseur
E catalyst
G Katalysator
S catalizador

cataplasme
E poultice
G Umschlagpaste
S cataplasma

catégorie du comprimé
E tablet category
G Tablettenkategorie
S categoría de comprimido

cathéter
E catheter
G Katheter
S catéter

cathode
E cathode
G Kathode
S cátodo

English German French Spanish

cation
E cation
G Kation
S catión

cause du défaut
E cause of failure
G Fehlerursache
S causa de error

caustique
E caustic
G ätzend
S cáustico

cavité
E cavity, hollow space, recess, well
G Hohlraum
S cavidad, espacio hueco

cavité de matrice
E die bore
G Matrizenöffnung
S abertura de matriz

cellule
E cell
G Zelle
S célula

cellule de détection
E detector cell
G Detektorzelle
S célula de detección

cellule de mesure de conductivité
E conductivity cell
G Leitfähigkeitsmeßzelle
S célula de medida de la conductividad

cellule de mesure du débit
E flow-through cell, flow cell
G Durchflußzelle
S célula de fluxometría

cellule photoélectrique
E photo cell, photoelectric cell
G Photozelle
S célula fotoeléctrica

cellulose
E cellulose
G Zellstoff
S celulosa

cendre
E ash
G Asche
S ceniza

cendre sulfatée
E sulphate ash
G Sulfatasche
S ceniza sulfatada

cendres résiduelles
E residue on ignition
G Verbrennungsrückstand
S cenizas residuales

censuré
E censored
G zensiert
S censado

centrale énergétique
E power station
G Kraftwerk
S central energética

centre de gravité
E centre of gravity
G Schwerpunkt
S baricentro, centro de gravedad

centrer
E centre, to
G zentrieren
S centrar

centrifugation
E centrifugation
G Zentrifugation
S centrifugación

centrifuger
E centrifuge, to
G zentrifugieren
S centrifugar

centrifugeuse
E centrifuge
G Zentrifuge
S centrífuga

certificat
E certificate
G Urkunde, Zertifikat
S documento, certificado

certificat d'analyse
E certificate of analysis, test certificate
G Analysenzertifikat, Prüfzertifikat
S certificado de análisis, certificado de prueba

certificat de calibration
E calibration certificate
G Eichschein, Kalibrierschein
S certificado de calibración

certificat de conformité
E certificate of conformity
G Konformitätszertifikat
S certificado de conformidad

certification
E certification
G Zertifizierung
S certificación

certifié ISO
E ISO-certificated
G ISO-zertifiziert
S ISO-certificado

certifier
E certificate, to
G zertifizieren
S certificar

chaîne carbonée
E carbon chain
G Kohlenstoffkette
S cadena carbonada

chaîne de conditionnement
E packaging line
G Verpackungslinie
S cadena de empaquetado

chaîne de production
E production line
G Produktionslinie
S cadena de producción

chaîne de réfrigération
E refrigerating chain
G Kühlkette
S cadena de refrigeración

chaîne de remplissage
E filling line, bottling line
G Abfüllstraße
S cadena de envasado

chaîne longue, à
E long-chained
G langkettig
S de cadena larga

chaleur
E heat
G Wärme
S calor

chaleur d'évaporation
E heat of evaporation
G Verdampfungswärme
S calor de evaporación

chaleur due à la réaction
E heat of reaction
G Reaktionswärme
S calor de reacción

chaleur perdue
E waste heat
G Abwärme
S calor de escape, pérdida calórica

chaleur spécifique
E specific heat
G spezifische Wärme
S calor específico

chambre
E chamber
G Kammer
S cámara

chambre d'autoclave
E autoclave (sterilisation) chamber
G Sterilisierkammer
S cámara de esterilización

chambre de climatisation
E climatic chamber
G Klimaprüfkammer
S cámara de aclimat(iz)ación

chambre de compression
E compression chamber
G Preßkammer
S cámara de compresión

chambre de développement (chromatographie)
E developing chamber (chromatography)
G Chromatographiekammer
S cámara cromatográfica

chambre de développement pour chromatographie sur couche mince
E thin layer chromatography developing chamber
G Dünnschichtchromatographiekammer
S cámara de cromatografía en capa fina

chambre de dosage
E metering chamber, dosing chamber
G Dosierkammer
S cámara de dosificación

chambre d'incubation
E incubation room
G Inkubationsraum
S cámara de incubación

chambre froide
E cold room
G Kühlraum
S cámara frigorífica

chambre tropicale
E tropical chamber
G Tropenkammer
S cámara tropical

champ d'application
E area of application, scope, validity
G Anwendungsgebiet, Geltungsbereich
S campo de aplicación

champignon
E fungus, mould
G Schimmelpilz
S moho

champignons
E fungi, moulds
G Pilze
S hongos

chandelle filtrante
E filter cartridge
G Filterkerze
S candela filtrante

changement
E change, variation
G Änderung, Wechsel
S cambio, modificación, variación

changement de bobine
E reel changes
G Rollenwechsel
S cambio de bobina

changement de couleur
E colour change
G Farbumschlag
S cambio de color

changement de longueur d'onde
E wavelength switching
G Wellenlängenumschaltung
S conmutación de la longitud de onda

changer l'emballage
E re-pack, to
G umpacken
S envasar de nuevo

chape de ciment
E cement flooring
G Zementestrich
S suelo de cemento

chape de compensation
E screed, floor leveller
G Ausgleichsestrich
S pavimento compensador

chape inclinée
E sloping flooring, screed
G Gefälleestrich
S pavimento inclinado

charbon actif
E activated charcoal
G Aktivkohle
S carbón activado

charge
E load, feed
G Beschickung, Ladung, Zufuhr
S carga, suministro

charge (électricité)
E charge (electricity)
G Ladung (Elektrizität)
S carga (electricidad)

charge de pression
E pressure loading
G Druckbelastung
S carga de presión

charge dynamique
E dynamic load
G dynamische Belastung
S carga dinámica

charge électrique
E electrical charge
G elektrische Ladung
S carga eléctrica

charge électrostatique
E electrostatic charge
G elektrostatische Aufladung
S carga electrostática

charge maximale
E maximum load
G Höchstlast
S carga máxima

charge statique
E static charge, static load
G statische Aufladung, statische Belastung
S carga estática

charge thermique
E thermal load
G thermische Belastung
S carga térmica

chargement
E loading
G Belastung
S carga

charger
E fill, to; charge, to; load, to
G einfüllen, beladen
S envasar, llenar, carga

chariot de montage
E mounting trolley
G Montagewagen
S carro de montaje

chariot de transport
E transport cart
G Transportwagen
S carro de transporte

chariot dévidoir
E tube carriage
G Schlauchwagen
S transportador de tubos

chariot élévateur
E fork-lift truck, lifting truck, stacker
G Gabelstapler, Hubwagen, Stapler
S carretilla elevadora de horquilla, carro elevador, apilador

chassis mobile
E trolley
G Fahrgestell
S bastidor, chasis

chaudière
E vessel, boiler
G Kessel
S caldera, marmita

English German French Spanish

chauffage avec apport de vapeur externe
E external steam heating
G Beheizung mit externer Dampfzufuhr
S calefacción con suministro de vapor externo

chauffé à la vapeur
E steam-heated
G dampfbeheizt
S calentado al vapor

chauffe-liquide
E immersion heater
G Tauchsieder
S calentador de inmersión

chauffer
E heat, to
G beheizen
S caldear

chaussures de laboratoire
E laboratory shoes
G Laborschuhe
S calzado de laboratorio

chef de département
E head of department, group manager
G Abteilungsleiter, Gruppenleiter
S director de departamento, director de grupo

chef de service
E head of department
G Abteilungsleiter
S director de departamento

chélate
E chelate, chelate complex
G Chelatkomplex
S complejo de quelatos

chemin de dégradation
E degradation path, metabolic path
G Abbauweg
S vía de degradación

chemin de remplissage
E filling section
G Abfüllstrecke
S sección de llenado

chemise de refroidissement
E cooling jacket
G Mantelkühlung
S camisa de refrigeración

chemise d'eau
E water jacket
G Wassermantel
S camisa de agua

chevauchement
E overlap
G Überschneidung
S entrecruzamiento, interferencia

cheville
E bolt
G Bolzen
S clavija, perno

chewing-gum médicamenté
E medicated chewing gum
G medizinisches Kaugummi
S goma de mascar medicamentosa

chicane
E baffle
G Schikane, Ablenkplatte
S vejación, placa de desviación

chicane de déviation
E baffle
G Umlenkblech
S chapa desviadora

chiffon
E cleaning cloth, cleaning tissue
G Reinigungstuch
S paño de limpieza

chiffre d'affaires
E turnover, sales
G Umsatz
S movimiento, volumen de negocios

chimie analytique
E analytical chemistry
G analytische Chemie
S química analítica

chimie humide
E wet chemistry
G Naßchemie
S química húmeda

chimiluminescence, chimioluminescence
E chemiluminescence
G Chemilumineszenz
S quimioluminiscencia

chimique humide
E wet chemical
G naßchemisch
S químicamente húmedo

chimiquement pur
E chemically pure
G chemisch rein
S químicamente puro

chiralité
E chirality
G Chiralität
S quiralidad

chlor
E chlorine
G Chlor
S cloro

chlorure de polyvinyl (PVC)
E polyvinyl chloride (PVC)
G Polyvinylchlorid (PVC)
S cloruro de polivinilo

chlorurer
E chlorinate, to
G chlorieren
S clorar

choc
E impact
G Stoß
S choque, golpe, impacto

choc thermique
E thermal shock
G Wärmeschock
S choque térmico

chromatogramme
E chromatogram
G Chromatogramm
S cromatograma

chromatographie
E chromatography
G Chromatographie
S cromatografía

chromatographie ascendante
E ascending chromatography
G aufsteigende Chromatographie
S cromatografía ascendente

chromatographie d'adsorption
E adsorption chromatography
G Adsorptionschromatographie
S cromatografía de adsorción

chromatographie d'affinité
E affinity chromatography
G Affinitätschromatographie
S cromatografía de afinidad

chromatographie d'échange de ligands optiquement actifs
E chiral ligand exchange chromatography
G chirale Ligandenaustausch-chromatographie
S cromatografía de intercambio de ligandos ópticamente activos

chromatographie descendante
E descending chromatography
G absteigende Chromatographie
S cromatografía descendente

chromatographie d'exclusion ionique
E ion exclusion chromatography
G Ionenausschlußchromatographie
S cromatografía de exclusión iónica

English German French Spanish

chromatographie en phase gazeuse
E gas chromatography
G Gaschromatographie
S cromatografía de gases

chromatographie en phase inverse
E reverse-phase chromatography
G Umkehrphasenchromatographie
S cromatografía en fase inversa

chromatographie liquide sous haute pression
E high pressure liquid chromatography (HPLC)
G Hochdruckflüssigkeitschromatographie
S cromatografía líquida a alta presión

chromatographie par échange de ligands optiquement actifs
E chiral ligand exchange chromatography
G Ligandenaustauschchromatographie, chirale
S cromatografía de intercambio de ligandos ópticamente activos

chromatographie par échange d'ions
E ion exchange chromatography
G Ionenaustauschchromatographie
S cromatografía de intercambio iónico

chromatographie par limite d'exclusion
E size exclusion chromatography
G Ausschlußchromatographie
S cromatografía de exclusión

chromatographie par paires d'ions
E ion pair chromatography
G Ionenpaarchromatographie
S cromatografía de pares de iones

chromatographie sur couche mince
E thin layer chromatography (TLC)
G Dünnschichtchromatographie (DC)
S cromatografía en capa fina

chromatographie sur gel
E gel chromatography
G Gelchromatographie
S cromatografía sobre gel

chromatographie sur résine échangeuse de cations
E cation chromatography
G Kationenchromatographie
S cromatografía de cationes

chromé
E chromium plated
G verchromt
S cromado

chute de pression
E pressure drop
G Druckabfall
S descenso de presión

cinétique
E kinetics
G Kinetik
S cinética

circonférence
E circumference
G Umfang
S circunferencia, perímetro, extensión

circuit
E circuit (electrical), loop
G Stromkreis, Schaltung (elektrisch)
S circuito eléctrico, conexión (eléctrica)

circuit de visite
E visitor tour
G Besuchergang
S recorrido de visita

circuit principal
E main circuit
G Hauptstromkreis
S circuito eléctrico principal

circulation d'air
E air flow
G Luftströmung
S flujo de aire

circulation fermée
E closed loop
G geschlossener Kreislauf
S circulación cerrada

cire
E wax
G Wachs
S cera

cire à cacheter
E sealing wax
G Siegellack
S lacre

clair
E distinct, clear, unambiguous
G deutlich, eindeutig
S claro, distinto, inequívoco, unívoco

clapet
E flap
G Klappe
S tapa, válvula

clapet à billes
E ball valve
G Kugelventil
S válvula esférica

clapet anti-déflagrant
E explosion panel
G Ex-Klappen
S válvula antideflagrante

clapet antirefouleur
E back flow preventer,
back flow flap
G Rückstauklappe
S válvula de retención

clapet anti-retour
E flap trap
G Rückschlagklappe
S válvula de retención

clapet de fermeture
E lid flap, shut-off flap
G Absperrklappe, Verschlußklappe
S válvula de cierre

clapet de réglage
E control flap, control valve
G Regelklappe
S válvula reguladora

clapet de ventilation
E vent flap
G Entlüftungsklappe
S válvula de ventilación

clapet d'évacuation d'air
E exhaust valve
G Abluftregelklappe
S válvula de evacuación de aire

clareté
E clarity
G Klarheit
S claridad

classe de dangers
E hazard class
G Gefahrenklasse
S clase de peligro

classe d'environnement
E cleanliness class,
cleanliness grade
G Reinheitsklasse
S nivel de pureza

classe d'inflammables
E inflammability class
G Brandklasse
S clase inflamable

classification
E grade
G Einstufung
S clasificación

classifier
E classify, to; grade, to
G sichten, klassieren
S clasificar, ordenar

clavette (de poinçon)
E key (of punch)
G Paßfeder, Schlüssel (des Stempels)
S llave (de troquel)

English German French Spanish

clavier
E key board
G Tastatur(feld)
S teclado

clavier à effleurement
E membrane key pad
G Folientastatur
S teclado de membrana plástica

clé BTR
E Allen key
G Inbusschlüssel
S llave hexagonal

clé en main
E turnkey
G schlüsselfertig
S llave en mano

clef de serrage
E wrench
G Schraubenschlüssel
S cierre de tornillo

cliché
E printing block
G Klischee
S cliché

client
E contract provider, principal, client, contract acceptor, customer
G Auftraggeber, Abnehmer, Kunde, Auftragnehmer
S cliente, comitente, comisionista

clientèle de référence
E reference customers
G Referenzkunden
S clientes de referencia

climatisation
E air-conditioning
G Klimatisierung
S climatizador

clivage cellulaire magnétique
E magnetic cell separation
G magnetische Zelltrennung
S separación magnética de células

clonage
E cloning
G Klonierung
S clonación

clore (comprimés)
E seal, to (tablets)
G verschließen, siegeln, einsiegeln (Tabletten)
S precintar, sellar, cellar, cerrar, estampar (comprimidos)

coagulation
E coagulation
G Gerinnung, Koagulation
S coagulación

coaguler
E coagulate, to
G gerinnen
S coagular

codage de couleurs
E colour code
G Farbcodierung
S codificación de colores

codage de la date d'expiration
E expiration coding
G Codierung des Verfalldatums
S codificación de la fecha de caducidad

codage d'un lot
E batch code
G Chargencode
S código de un lote

code à barres
E code bars
G Codestriche
S barras de código

code d'entrée de marchandises
E receiving code
G Wareneingangscode
S código de entrada de mercancías

code numérique non équivoque
E unequivocal code number
G eindeutige Codenummer
S número codificador inequívoco

code régional
E local code
G regionales Regelwerk
S código regional

coefficient d'absorption
E absorption coefficient, coefficient of absorbance
G Absorptionskoeffizient, Extinktionskoeffizient
S coeficiente de absorción, coeficiente de extinción

coefficient de friction
E coefficient of friction
G Reibungskoeffizient
S coeficiente de fricción

coefficient de frottement
E coefficient of friction
G Reibungskoeffizient
S coeficiente de fricción

coefficient de variation
E coefficient of variation
G Variationskoeffizient
S coeficiente de validación

coefficient d'expansion
E coefficient of expansion
G Dehnungskoeffizient
S coeficiente de dilatación

coefficient d'extinction UV
E UV coefficient of absorbance
G UV-Extinktionskoeffizient
S coeficiente de extinción UV

coenzyme
E coenzyme
G Koenzym
S coenzima

cohérent
E coherent
G kohärent
S coherente

cohésion
E cohesion
G Kohäsion
S cohesión

coin
E corner
G Ecke
S esquina

col de bouteille
E bottle neck
G Flaschenhals
S cuello de botella, gollete

col d'une ampoule
E ampoule neck
G Ampullenhals
S cuello de ampolla

colis
E itemised goods
G Stückgut
S bultos sueltos

collant
E sticky, tacky
G klebrig
S pegajoso

collation de données
E collation of data
G Datenüberprüfung
S comprobación de datos

colle
E adhesive, glue
G Kleber, Leim
S cola, sustancia adhesiva

collecte de gouttelettes
E drop-collection
G Tröpfchenabscheidung
S separación de gotitas

collecteur
E reservoir, collector
G Sammelbehälter
S depósito (colector)

collecteur de fractions
E fraction collector
G Fraktionssammler
S colector de fracciones

English German French Spanish

collecteur de solvant
E solvent collector
G Lösungsmittelauffangbehälter
S colector de solvente

coller
E glue, to
G kleben, leimen
S encolar, pegar

collerette
E flange
G Flansch
S brida, collar

collet
E bush, bushing (mach.)
G Muffe
S manguito

collet du poinçon
E punch neck
G Stempelhals
S cuello de troquel

collet d'une bouteille
E shoulder section (of a bottle)
G Schulter (einer Flasche)
S ensanchamiento de una botella

collier
E collar, clip
G Manschette, Schelle
S abrazadera, collar, manguito

collodion
E film-forming liquid, collodion
G filmbildende Flüssigkeit
S colodión

colmatant (une fissure)
E crack-filling
G rißüberbrückend
S rellenante de una fisura

colmater
E tighten, to; seal, to
G abdichten
S cerrar herméticamente

colonne analytique
E analytical column
G analytische Säule
S columna analítica

colonne d'ascension
E dip tube
G Steigrohr
S tubo ascensional, tubo montante

colonne d'eau
E water column
G Wassersäule
S columna de agua

colonne d'immersion
E dip tube
G Tauchrohr
S tubo de inmersión

colonne préalable
E pre-column
G Vorsäule
S columna previa

colonne sous pression
E pressure column
G Druckkolonne
S columna a presión

colorant
E colouring agent, dye, stain
G Färbemittel, Farbstoff
S colorante, pigmento, tintura

coloration
E colouration
G Färbung
S coloración

colorer
E stain, to
G färben
S colorear, teñir

combinaison à usage unique
E disposable jump-suit
G Einmalanzug
S ropa de uso único

combinaison imperméable à l'eau
E waterproof jump-suit
G wasserdichter Anzug
S traje impermeable al agua

combustibilité
E flammability
G Brennbarkeit
S combustibilidad, inflamabilidad

combustible
E combustible, flammable
G brennbar
S combustible, inflamable

combustion
E combustion, incineration
G Verbrennung, Veraschung
S combustión, incineración

comité de direction
E board of directors, director
G Vorstand
S junta directiva

comité directeur de validation
E validation review committee
G Steuerungsausschuß zur Validierung
S comisión fiscal de validación

commande
E order
G Bestellung
S pedido

commande de conditionnement
E packaging order
G Verpackungsauftrag
S encargo de embalaje

commande de fabrication
E manufacturing order
G Herstellungsauftrag
S encargo de producción

commande de fabrication par sous-traitance
E contract manufacturer order
G Lohnherstellungsauftrag
S encargo de fabricación por comisión

commandé par menu
E menu-controlled
G menügesteuert
S dirigido por minuta

commercial
E sales representative
G Außendienstmitarbeiter
S agente externo de ventas

commettant
E contract provider, principal, client
G Auftraggeber
S cliente, comitente

commission d'éthique
E ethics committee
G Ethikkomission
S comisión ética

compacteur
E compactor
G Kompaktierer
S compactador

compagnie
E company, concern
G Gesellschaft, Konzern
S sociedad, consorcio

compatibilité
E compatibility
G Verträglichkeit, Kompatibilität
S compatibilidad

compatibilité des matériaux
E material compatibility
G Materialverträglichkeit
S compatibilidad de materiales

compatible
E compatible
G kompatibel
S compatible

compensation de pression
E pressure equilibrium
G Druckausgleich
S equilibrio de presión

English German French Spanish

compensation de température
E temperature equalisation
G Temperaturausgleich
S compensación de temperatura

compétiteur
E competitor
G Mitbewerber
S competidor

compilation (de documents)
E compilation (of documents)
G Erstellung (von Dokumenten)
S redacción (de documentos)

compiler
E compile, to
G erstellen
S elaborar, producir, redactar

complément
E supplementation
G Ergänzung
S complemento, suplemento

complètement désalinisé
E demineralised
G vollentsalzt
S completamente desmineralizado

complexe de chélation
E chelate, chelate complex
G Chelatkomplex
S complejo de quelatos

comportement
E behaviour
G Verhalten
S comportamiento

comportement de dissolution
E dissolution behaviour
G Auflösungsverhalten
S comportamiento en disolución

comportement de libération
E release behaviour
G Freisetzungsverhalten
S comportamiento de liberación

comportement thermique
E thermal behaviour
G thermisches Verhalten
S comportamiento térmico

composant
E component, constituent, ingredient
G Bestandteil
S componente, ingrediente

composant (d'une presse à comprimés)
E component (of a tablet press)
G Formatteil (bei einer Tablettenpresse)
S componente formador (de una prensa de comprimidos)

composant actif
E active substance, active ingredient
G wirksamer Bestandteil
S componente activo

composant amer
E bitter component
G Bitterstoff
S sustancia amarga

composant clé
E key component
G Schlüsselkomponente
S componente clave

composant de base d'un suppositoire
E suppository base
G Suppositoriengrundlage
S excipiente de un supositorio

composant moulé par injection
E injection-moulded component
G Spritzgußteil
S componente moldeado por inyección

composants
E components
G Einzelteile
S componentes

composé comprimable
E compression material, moulding compound
G Preßmasse
S masa comprimible

composé hydrocarboné
E hydrocarbon
G Kohlenwasserstoff
S hidrocarburo

composé organique chélaté
E chelated compound
G Chelatverbindung
S compuesto quelado

composé organo-métallique
E organo-metallic compound
G metallorganische Verbindung
S compuesto organometálico

composition
E composition
G Zusammensetzung
S composición

compréhensible
E comprehensible
G verständlich
S comprensible

compresse
E compress
G Kompresse
S compresa

compression
E compression, concentration
G Verdichtung
S concentración, compresión

compression à double couche
E double-layer compression
G Zweischichtverpressung
S compresión de doble capa

compression directe
E direct tablet compression
G Direkttablettierung
S compresión directa

comprimé
E tablet
G Tablette
S comprimido

apparence d'un comprimé
E tablet appearance
G Aussehen der Tablette
S aspecto de un comprimido

hétérogénéité des comprimés
E tablet inconsistency
G Uneinheitlichkeit von Tabletten
S heterogeneidad de los comprimidos

résistance à la rupture d'un comprimé
E tablet crushing strength
G Bruchfestigkeit einer Tablette
S resistencia a la ruptura de un comprimido

uniformité de la couleur d'un comprimé
E tablet colour uniformity
G Einheitlichkeit der Tablettenfarbe
S uniformidad del color de los comprimidos

comprimé à libération retardée
E retard tablet, delayed action tablet
G Retardtablette
S comprimido retard

comprimé à mâcher
E chewing tablet
G Kautablette
S comprimidos masticables

comprimé allongé
E oblong tablet
G längliche Tablette
S comprimido elongado

comprimé dragéifié
E sugar-coated tablet
G Dragee, Zuckerdragee
S gragea, gragea azucarada

English German French Spanish

comprimé effervescent
E effervescent tablet
G Brausetablette
S comprimido efervescente

comprimé multicouche
E laminated tablet
G Manteltablette
S comprimido de cubierta estratificada

comprimé oblong
E oblong tablet
G Oblongtablette
S comprimido oblongo

comprimé pelliculé
E coated tablet
G Filmtablette
S gragea

comprimé rond
E round tablet
G Rundtablette
S comprimido redondo

comprimé vaginal
E vaginal tablet
G Vaginaltablette
S comprimido vaginal

comprimer
E compress, to; concentrate, to
G verdichten
S concentrar, comprimir

comprimés défectueux
E faulty tablets
G fehlerhafte Tabletten
S comprimidos defectuosos

compromettre (la qualité)
E endanger, to (quality)
G gefährden (Qualität)
S arriesgar, poner en peligro (la calidad)

comptage de particules viables
E viable particle count
G Zählung lebensfähiger Partikel
S recuento de partículas viables

comptage d'étiquettes
E label count
G Etikettenzählung
S recuento de etiquetas

compte rendu de conditionnement
E batch packaging record
G Verpackungsprotokoll
S protocolo de embalaje

compte rendu d'un lot
E batch record
G Chargenprotokoll
S protocolo de lotes

compte-gouttes
E drop counter
G Tropfenzähler
S cuentagotas

compte-rendu de réclamation
E complaint report
G Beanstandungsbericht
S informe de reclamaciones

compte-rendu des insuffisances
E deficiency report
G Mängelrüge
S reclamación por vicios

compte-tours
E revolution counter, tachymeter
G Drehzahlmesser
S contador de revoluciones, taquímetro

compteur
E counter
G Zähler
S contador

compteur de cellules
E cell counter
G Zellzähler
S contador de células

compteur de comprimés
E tablet counter
G Zählbrett (für Tabletten)
S contador de comprimidos

compteur de particules
E particle counter
G Partikelzähler
S contador de partículas

compteur d'étiquettes
E label counter
G Etikettenzähler
S contador de etiquetas

compteur d'heures de mise en service
E running time meter
G Betriebsstundenzähler
S contador de horas de funcionamiento

concasser
E crush, to; grind, to; mill, to
G zerstoßen
S machacar, pulverizar, triturar

concave
E concave
G nach innen gewölbt, konkav
S cóncavo

concentration
E compression, concentration, enrichment
G Konzentration, Verdichtung, Anreicherung
S concentración, compresión, enriquecimiento

concentration critique de micelles
E critical micelle concentration
G kritische Micellkonzentration
S concentración crítica de micelas

concentration d'un colorant
E dye concentration
G Farbstoffkonzentration
S concentración de colorante

concentration en poussière
E dust concentration
G Staubanteil
S proporción de polvo

concentration maximale de postes de travail
E maximum allowable concentration (MAC)
G maximale Arbeitsplatzkonzentration (MAK)
S concentración máxima de puestos de trabajo

concentré
E concentrate
G Dickextrakt
S extracto concentrado

concentré sec
E dried concentrate
G Trockenextrakt
S concentrado seco

concentrer
E concentrate, to; enrich, to; compress, to
G anreichern, verdichten, einengen
S concentrar, enriquecer, espesar

concept de zones
E zonal concept
G Zonenkonzept
S concepción por zonas

condensat
E condensate
G Kondensat
S condensado

condensation
E condensation
G Kondensation
S condensación

condenseur
E condenser
G Kondensator
S condensador

condition de test simulée
E simulated test condition
G simulierte Testbedingung
S condiciones simuladas de ensayo

English German French Spanish

condition d'exploitation, à
E in process
G im Betriebszustand
S funcionando

conditionnement
E package, pack, container, packaging
G Packung, Gebinde, Verpacken, Konfektionierung
S embalaje, envase, envoltura, contenedor, envasado, empaquetado

conditionnement à bulles
E blister pack
G Blisterverpackung
S embalado en blísters

conditionnement à usage unique
E disposable packaging
G Einwegverpackung, Wegwerfpackung
S embalaje de uso único

conditionnement blister
E blister pack
G Blisterverpackung
S embalado en blísters

conditionnement de sécurité pour enfants
E child-resistant pack
G kindergesicherte Verpackung
S envase a prueba de niños

conditionnement d'origine
E original package
G Orginalpackung
S envase original

conditionnement d'une colonne
E column conditioning
G Säulenkonditionierung
S acondicionamiento de la columna

conditionnement en plusieurs phases
E portioned packaging
G portionierte Abpackung
S envase porcionado

conditionnement final
E final container
G Endbehältnis
S recipiente final

conditionnement multi-doses
E multiple-dose container
G Mehrdosenbehältnis
S recipiente de dosis múltiple

conditionnement non-imprimé
E unprinted packaging material
G unbedrucktes Packmittel
S medio de envasado no impreso

conditionnement pour hôpitaux
E hospital pack
G Klinikpackung
S embalaje para clínica

conditionnement primaire
E packaging material, primary
G primäres Packmittel
S medio de envasado primario

conditionnement secondaire
E packaging material, secondary
G sekundäres Packmittel
S medio de envasado secundario

conditionnement sous blister
E blister pack
G Tiefziehverpackung
S envase blíster

conditionnement thermoformé
E blister pack
G Tiefziehverpackung
S envase termoformado

conditionneuse
E packaging machine
G Verpackungsmaschine
S empaquetadora

conditions
E conditions
G Bedingungen
S condiciones

conditions de l'environnement
E environmental conditions
G Umgebungsbedingungen
S condiciones ambientales

conditions de production
E manufacturing conditions
G Herstellungsbedingungen
S condiciones de producción

conditions de réaction
E reaction conditions
G Reaktionsbedingungen
S condiciones de reacción

conditions de réaction adiabatiques
E adiabatic reaction conditions
G adiabatische Reaktionsbedingungen
S condiciones adiabáticas de reacción

conditions de service
E operating conditions
G Betriebsbedingungen
S condiciones de funcionamiento

conditions de stockage
E storage conditions
G Lagerungsbedingungen
S condiciones de almacenamiento

conditions expérimentales
E experimental conditions
G Versuchsbedingungen
S condiciones experimentales

conditions préalables uniformes
E uniform preconditions
G einheitliche Voraussetzungen
S presupuestos uniformes

conducteur
E conductive
G leitfähig
S conductor

conductimètre
E conductivity meter, conductivity detector
G Leitfähigkeitsmesser, Wärmeleitfähigkeitsdetektor
S conductímetro, detector de conductividad térmica

conduction thermique
E conductive heat
G Wärmeleitung
S conducción térmica

conductivité
E conductivity
G Leitfähigkeit
S conductibilidad

conductivité électrique
E conductivity
G elektrische Leitfähigkeit
S conductividad eléctrica

conductivité thermique
E thermal conductivity
G Wärmeleitfähigkeit
S conductividad térmica

conduit d'alimentation
E feed chute
G Zufuhrrinne
S canal de alimentación

conduit d'écoulement
E drain
G Abguß
S decantación, vaciado

conduite
E wall opening, duct
G Wanddurchführung, Schacht
S pasamuros, conducto, pozo

conduite (de gaz, d'eau)
E piping (gas, water)
G Leitung (Gas, Wasser)
S conducción, tubería (gas, agua)

conduite d'alimentation
E filling tube, charging tube, charge tube
G Einfüllrohr, Befüllrohr
S tubo de relleno, conducto de carga, conducto de alimentación

conduite de charge
E charge tube
G Befüllrohr
S conducto de carga, conducto de alimentación

conduite de remplissage
E filling hose, filling pipe
G Abfüllrohr
S conducto de envasado

conduite de vapeur
E steam line
G Dampfleitung
S conducción de vapor

conduite d'eau
E water piping
G Wasserleitung
S conducción de agua

conduite destinée aux déchets
E waste output
G Entsorgungsanschluß
S empalme de eliminación

conduite destinée aux eaux résiduelles
E waste water line
G Abwasserleitung
S conducción de aguas residuales

conduite d'évacuation
E exhaust line
G Abluftleitung
S conducto de evacuación de aire

conduite d'évacuation d'air
E exhaust pipe
G Abluftrohr
S tubo de evacuación de aire

cône
E cone
G Kegel, Konus
S cono

confidentialité
E confidentiality
G Vertraulichkeit
S confidencialidad

configuration de l'instrument
E instrument configuration
G Gerätekonfiguration
S configuración de aparatos

configuration stérique
E sterical arrangement
G sterische Anordnung
S configuración estérica

conforme aux bonnes pratiques de fabrication
E GMP-conform
G GMP-gerecht
S conforme a GMP

conformité
E compliance, conformity
G Einhaltung, Konformität, Übereinstimmung
S cumplimiento, observancia, conformidad, concordancia, coincidencia

conformité aux bonnes pratiques de fabrication
E GMP compliance
G GMP-Entsprechung
S conformidad con GMP

congédier
E make redundant, to
G entlassen
S despedir

congélateur
E freezer
G Gefrierschrank
S congelador

congelé
E deep-frozen
G tiefgefroren
S congelado

congeler
E deep-freeze, to
G tieffrieren
S congelar

conique
E tapered, conical
G verjüngt, konisch, kegelförmig
S disminuido, estrechado, cónico

connecté
E connected
G angeschlossen
S conectado

faussement connecté
E wrongly connected
G falsch angeschlossen
S mal conectado

connecter
E connect, to; wire, to
G anschließen, schalten, verdrahten
S conectar, conmutar

connection de charge
E supply connection, supply input
G Versorgungsanschluß
S conexión de abastecimiento

connection parallèle
E parallel connection
G Parallelschaltung
S conexión paralela

connections sanitaires
E sanitary fittings
G Sanitäranschlüsse
S conexiones sanitarias

connexion
E connection
G Anschluß, Verbindung
S conexión, compuesto

connexion (électrique)
E circuit (electrical)
G Schaltung (elektrisch)
S conexión (eléctrica)

connexion à collerette instantanée
E quick-flange connection
G Schnellverschluß
S cierre rápido

connexion à fiche(s)
E plug connection
G Steckkupplung
S conexión de enchufe

connexion à filetage
E screw fitting
G Verschraubung
S atornilladura

connexion de conduite à vapeur
E steam connection
G Dampfleitungsverbindung
S conexión de conducción de vapor

connexion étanche
E bulkhead connection
G Schottverschraubung
S atornillado hermético

connexion instantanée
E quick coupling, instant coupling
G Schnellkupplung
S conexión rápida

connexion latérale
E cross-linking
G Quervernetzung
S conexión lateral

connexion murale
E wall connection
G Wandanschluß
S conexión de pared

conscience de l'environnement
E environmental awareness
G Umweltbewußtsein
S conciencia del medio ambiente

conservateur
E preservative, anti-microbial agent
G Konservierungsmittel
S medio de conservación

conservation
E retention, storage, archiving, preservation
G Aufbewahrung, Konservierung
S conservación, almacenaje

conservé
E preserved
G konserviert
S conservado

conserver
E preserve, to; retain, to; store, to; retain, to; store, to
G konservieren, aufbewahren
S conservar, guardar

consignes de sécurité
E safety requirements
G Sicherheitsanforderungen
S requisito de seguridad

consistance
E uniformity, consistency
G Gleichförmigkeit, Konsistenz
S homogeneidad, uniformidad

consistance d'un lot
E batch consistency
G Chargenkonsistenz
S consistencia de un lote

consommables
E consumables
G Verbrauchsmaterial
S material consumible

consommateur
E consumer
G Verbraucher
S consumidor

consommation
E consumption
G Verbrauch
S consumo

consommation de vapeur
E steam consumption
G Dampfverbrauch
S consumo de vapor

consommation d'électricité
E power consumption, power consumption
G Stromaufnahme, Energieverbrauch
S consumo de electricidad

consommation d'énergie
E energy consumption, power consumption
G Energieverbrauch, Leistungsverbrauch
S consumo energético, consumo de energía

consortium
E company, concern
G Konzern
S consorcio

constance d'un poids
E constant weight
G Gewichtskonstanz
S constancia del peso

constante de temps
E time constant
G Zeitkonstante
S constante de tiempo

constituant
E component, constituent, ingredient
G Bestandteil
S componente, ingrediente

constituants d'un emballage
E packaging components
G Bestandteile der Packung
S componentes del envase

constriction
E constriction
G Verengung
S constricción, estrechamiento

construction de soutien
E supporting construction
G Stützkonstruktion
S construcción de sostén

construit pour
E designed for
G ausgelegt für
S construido para, diseñado para

container
E container, reaction vessel
G Behältnis, Ansatzbehälter
S recipiente, contenedor

container final
E final container
G Endbehältnis
S recipiente final

contaminants
E contaminants
G kontaminierende Stoffe
S sustancias contaminantes

contaminants microbiens
E microbial contaminants
G mikrobielle Kontaminanten
S contaminantes microbianos

contamination
E impurity, contamination
G Verunreinigung
S contaminación, impureza

contamination aéroportée
E airborne contamination
G aus der Luft stammende Kontamination
S contaminación procedente del aire

contamination croisée
E cross-contamination
G Kreuzkontamination
S contaminación cruzada

contamination d'un produit
E product contamination
G Produktverunreinigung
S contaminación de un producto

contamination primaire
E primary contamination
G Primärkontamination
S contaminación primaria

contamination secondaire
E secondary contamination
G Sekundärkontamination
S contaminación secundaria

contamination transportée par l'air
E airborne contamination
G aus der Luft stammende Kontamination
S contaminación procedente del aire

contaminé
E contaminated
G kontaminiert
S contaminado

contaminer
E contaminate, to
G kontaminieren, verschmutzen
S contaminar, ensuciar

contenance
E capacity, volume
G Fassungsvermögen
S capacidad

conteneur
E shipping carton
G Versandkarton
S cartón de envío

conteneur final
E final container
G Endbehältnis
S recipiente final

contenu
E content
G Gehalt, Inhalt
S contenido

contenu minimal
E minimum contents
G Mindestinhalt
S contenido mínimo

continu
E continuous
G stufenlos
S continuo

English German French Spanish

English German French Spanish

contrainte de cisaillement
E shear stress
G Scherspannung
S tensión de cizallamiento

contrainte de poussée
E shear stress
G Schubspannung
S tensión de empuje

contrat
E contract
G Vertrag
S contrato

contrat de fabrication
E manufacturing contract
G Lohnauftrag
S negocio de comisión

contrat de licence
E licensing agreement
G Lizenzabkommen
S acuerdo de licencia

contre le sens des aiguilles d'une montre
E anticlockwise
G gegen Uhrzeigersinn
S sentido antihorario

contre-bride
E counter-flange
G Gegenflansch
S contrabrida

contrefaire un brevet
E infringement
G Verletzung
S lesión (herida), infracción

contre-indication
E contraindication
G Kontraindikation, Gegenanzeige
S contraindicación

contre-indiqué
E contraindicated
G kontraindiziert
S contraindicado

contre-ion
E counter-ion
G Gegenion
S contraión, ion complementario

contremaître
E foreman
G Vorarbeiter
S capataz

contrepoids
E counter-weight
G Gegengewicht
S contrapeso

contre-pression
E back pressure, support pressure
G Gegendruck (in der Chromatographie), Stützdruck
S contrapresión (en cromatografía)

contrôle
E control, check, monitoring
G Kontrolle, Steuerung, Überwachung
S control, supervisión, vigilancia

contrôlé
E checked, inspected
G geprüft
S comprobado

contrôle avant livraison
E pre-delivery check, factory acceptance test
G Vorabnahme (beim Hersteller)
S control antes de entrega

contrôle continu
E continuous monitoring
G ständige Überwachung
S vigilancia continua

contrôle de la poussière
E dust control
G Staubkontrolle
S control de polvo

contrôle de la pression
E pressure control (excess pressure)
G Druckkontrolle (bei Überdruck)
S control de presión (en caso de sobrepresión)

contrôle de la qualité
E quality control (QC)
G Qualitätskontrolle (QK)
S control de calidad

contrôle de la quantité de remplissage
E quantity control
G Füllmengenkontrolle
S control de la cantidad de relleno

contrôle de l'éjection
E ejection control
G Auswurfgegenkontrolle
S control de la expulsión

contrôle de l'environnement
E environmental monitoring, environmental control
G Umgebungskontrolle, Umweltkontrolle
S control del entorno, control ecológico

contrôle de l'impression
E print control (printed matter)
G Druckkontrolle (von Aufdruckdaten)
S control de impresos

contrôle des changements
E change control, change management
G Änderungskontrolle
S control de modificaciones

contrôle des déchirures de feuilles
E film tear sensor
G Folienrißkontrolle
S control de desgarro de láminas

contrôle des fragments
E fragment control
G Bruchstückkontrolle
S control de fragmentos

contrôle des livraisons de marchandises
E inspection of incoming goods
G Wareneingangsprüfung
S control de entrada de mercancías

contrôle des lots
E batch control
G Chargenkontrolle
S control de lotes

contrôle des modifications
E change control, change management
G Änderungskontrolle
S control de modificaciones

contrôle des particules
E particle monitoring
G Partikelmonitoring
S control de partículas

contrôle du contenu
E content control
G Füllgutkontrolle
S control del contenido

contrôle du poids
E weight control
G Gewichtskontrolle
S control del peso

contrôle d'un comprimé
E tablet checking
G Tablettenkontrolle
S control de comprimidos

contrôle d'un procédé
E process control
G Prozeßsteuerung
S control de un proceso

contrôle d'un programme
E programme control
G Programmsteuerung
S control del programa

contrôle intermédiaire
E intermediate control
G Zwischenkontrolle
S control intermediario

contrôle lors de la fabrication
E in-process control (IPC)
G In-Prozeß-Kontrolle
S control durante el proceso

contrôle microbien
E microbial control
G mikrobielle Kontrolle
S control microbiano

contrôlé par ordinateur
E computer-controlled
G computergesteuert
S controlado por ordenador

contrôlé par placebo
E placebo-controlled
G placebokontrolliert
S controlado por placebo

contrôle visuel
E visual control, visual observation
G optische Kontrolle, Sichtkontrolle, visuelle Überwachung
S control óptico, control visual

contrôle-qualité
E quality control (QC)
G Qualitätskontrolle (QK)
S control de calidad

contrôler
E monitor, to; supervise, to; control, to; check, to
G überwachen, überprüfen
S supervisar, vigilar, comprobar

convection de l'air
E air convection
G Luftkonvektion
S convección de aire

convenable
E suitable
G passend
S adecuado, conveniente

convention
E agreement
G Vereinbarung
S acuerdo, convenio

conversion
E conversion
G Umrechnung
S conversión

conversion thermique
E thermal conversion
G thermische Umwandlung
S conversión térmica

convertibilité (d'une substance en une réaction)
E convertibility (of a substance in a reaction)
G Umwandlungsfähigkeit (einer Substanz in einer Reaktion)
S convertibilidad (de una sustancia en una reacción)

convertisseur
E converter, measurement converter
G Umwandler, Meßumformer
S transformador, convertidor de mediciones

convexe
E convex
G nach außen gewölbt, konvex
S convexo

convivial pour l'utilisateur
E user-friendly
G bedienerfreundlich
S confortable para el usuario

convoyeur
E conveyor, conveyor belt
G Bandzufuhr, Bandförderer
S transportador, transportador de cinta, suministro por cinta

convoyeur à bande
E conveyor belt
G Fließband, Förderband, Transportband
S cinta transportadora

convoyeur à vis doseuse
E dosing screw conveyor
G Schneckendosiermaschine
S máquina dosificadora de tornillo sin fin

copie de sauvegarde
E back-up file
G Sicherheitskopie
S copia de seguridad

corbeille
E retaining basket
G Fangkorb
S cesto colector

corbeille d'autoclave
E autoclave basket
G Korbeinsatz für Autoklaven
S cesto para autoclave

corbeille rotative
E rotary basket
G Drehkörbchen
S cesto rotatorio

corps creux
E hollow article, hollow body
G Hohlkörper
S cuerpo hueco

corps étranger
E foreign body
G Fremdkörper
S cuerpo extraño

correction
E correction
G Berichtigung, Korrektur
S corrección, enmienda, rectificación

correspondre (à)
E correspond, to
G entsprechen
S corresponder

différent de
E not corresponding to
G nicht entsprechen
S no corresponder

corridor
E corridor
G Flur
S corredor

corridor de service
E service corridor
G Technikgang
S corredor de servicio

corroder
E corrode, to; etch, to
G korrodieren, einätzen
S corroer, grabar (al aguafuerte)

corrosif
E corrosive
G korrodierend
S corroyente

corrosion
E corrosion
G Korrosion
S corrosión

cosmétiques
E cosmetics
G Kosmetika
S cosméticos

cosse de câble
E cable lug
G Kabelschuh
S terminal de cable

côté supérieur
E upper side, top side
G Oberseite
S lado superior

coton
E cotton
G Baumwolle
S algodón

couche
E coat, coating, film, layer
G Beschichtung, Überzug, Lage, Schicht
S estrato, cubierta, revestimiento

couche aqueuse pelliculaire
E aqueous film coating
G wäßrige Filmbeschichtung
S película acuosa de revestimiento

couche de barrage
E barrier layer
G Sperrschicht
S estrato barrera

English German French Spanish

English German French Spanish

couche de résine synthétique
E synthetic resin screed
G Kunstharzestrich
S pavimento de resina sintética

couche d'isolation
E insulating layer
G Isolierschicht
S capa aislante

coude d'un tuyau
E tube kink
G Schlauchknick
S acodadura de un tubo

couder
E bend, to; buckle, to
G knicken
S doblar, quebrar

coulage de plaques (microbiologie)
E plate method (in microbiology)
G Plattengußverfahren (Mikrobiologie)
S método de placas (microbiología)

couler
E run off, to, slip, to
G auslaufen, gleiten
S escaparse, salirse, deslizar, resbalar

couleur de fabrication de comprimés
E tablet dye
G Tablettierfarbe
S color de fabricación de comprimidos

couleur d'imprimante
E printer ink
G Druckerfarbe
S impresora a color

coup
E impact
G Schlag, Stoß
S choque, golpe, impacto

coupant
E sharp
G scharf
S afilado, agudo, cortante

coupe
E cup
G Meßbecher
S vaso graduado

coupe transversale
E cross-section
G Querschnitt
S sección transversal

couper
E switch off, to
G abschalten
S desconectar

couperet
E chopper
G Zerhacker
S troceadora

couplage
E coupling
G Kupplung
S acoplamiento, embrague

couplage de colonnes
E column coupling
G Säulenverbindung
S acople de columna

couple
E torque
G Drehmoment
S momento de torsión, par, par motor

coupure de courant
E power failure
G Stromausfall
S corte de corriente

coupure de courant intermittente
E intermittent power interruption
G zeitweiser Stromausfall
S corte intermitente de corriente, corte transitorio de corriente

courant
E current
G laufend
S corriente

courant (électr.)
E current, electricity
G Strom
S corriente eléctrica

courant alternatif
E alternating current (AC)
G Wechselstrom
S corriente alterna

courant continu
E direct current
G Gleichstrom
S corriente continua

courant d'alimentation
E power supply
G Versorgungsstrom
S corriente de alimentación

courant de cheminement
E leakage current
G Kriechstrom
S corriente de fuga

courant de coupure
E breaking current
G Ausschaltstrom
S corriente de desconexión

courant triphasé
E three-phase current
G Drehstrom
S corriente trifásica

courbe ascendante
E ascending curve
G Aufwärtskurve
S curva ascendente

courbe d'acceptance
E acceptance graph
G Annahmekennlinie
S característica de aceptación

courbe de calibration
E calibration curve
G Kalibrierkurve
S curva de calibración

courbe de dosage
E titration curve
G Titrationskurve
S curva de titulación

courbe de titrage
E titration curve
G Titrationskurve
S curva de titulación

courbure
E bend, flexure
G Biegung
S flexión, curvatura

courroie excentrique
E eccentric band
G Exzenterband
S cinta excéntrica

courroie trapézoïdale
E fan belt
G Keilriemen
S correa trapezoidal

course de piston
E stroke
G Hub, Kolbenweg
S carrera del émbolo

court-circuit
E short circuit
G Kurzschluß
S cortocircuito

coussinet
E sheath, bush, sleeve, bearing
G Hülle, Hülse, Peilung
S envoltura, cápsula, cáscara, sondeo

coûts de fonctionnement
E operational costs
G Betriebskosten
S costes de funcionamiento

coûts d'exploitation
E current cost
G laufende Kosten
S costes de explotación

coûts d'investissements
E investment costs
G Investitionskosten
S costes de inversión

coûts du personnel
E personnel cost
G Personalkosten
S costes del personal

coûts d'une installation
E installation costs
G Installationskosten
S costes de instalación

coûts préalables
E up-front costs
G Vorauskosten
S costes preliminares

couture
E seam
G Naht
S costura

couture de pliage
E lock seam
G Falznaht
S soldadura del encaje

couvercle
E lid, cover, hood, casing
G Deckel, Abdeckhaube, Haube, Abdeckung, Verkleidungsblech
S tapa, tapadera, casquete, cubierta, sombrerete, chapa de revestimiento

couvercle à enclenchement
E snap cap, snap lid
G Schnappdeckel
S tapa de cierre de golpe

couvercle à usage unique
E disposable cover
G Einmalabdeckung
S cubierta de uso único

couvercle anti-éclaboussures
E spray protection
G Spritzschutz
S protección frente al salpicado

couvercle de canalisation anti-déflagrant
E explosion relief duct cover
G Ex-Kanalabdeckung
S cubierta del orificio de seguridad

couvercle de machine
E machine cover
G Maschinenabdeckung
S cubierta de la máquina

couvercle d'entrée d'air
E air inlet cover
G Zuluftklappe
S válvula de entrada de aire

couvercle pivotant (par ex. d'un autoclave)
E swivel lid (e. g. of autoclave)
G Drehdeckel (z. B. eines Autoklaven)
S tapa de rosca (p. ej. de autoclave)

couvert d'écailles
E scaly
G schuppig
S escamoso

couverture en polyéthylène
E polyethylene coating
G Polyethylenbeschichtung
S cubierta de polietileno

couvre-chaussure
E overshoe
G Überschuhe
S chanclos

covalent
E covalent
G kovalent
S covalente

crachat
E sputum
G Sputum
S esputo

crémage (d'une émulsion)
E creaming (of emulsions)
G Aufrahmung (bei Emulsionen)
S cremado (de emulsiones)

crémaillère pour filtre
E filter suspension rack
G Filteraufhängevorrichtung
S dispositivo de suspensión de filtros

crème
E cream
G Creme
S crema

crème auriculaire
E ear cream
G Ohrencreme
S crema auricular

crème évanescente
E water-soluble cream
G abwaschbare Salbe
S pomada evanescente

crème nasale
E nasal cream
G Nasencreme
S crema nasal

crème ophtalmique
E eye cream
G Augencreme
S crema oftálmica

crème rectale
E rectal cream
G Rektalcreme
S crema rectal

crème vaginale
E vaginal cream
G Vaginalcreme
S crema vaginal

crépi
E plastered
G verputzt
S enlucido, revocado

creuset
E crucible
G Tiegel
S crisol

creux
E hollow
G hohl
S hueco

crevasse
E slit, cleft
G Spalte
S fisura

crible bas
E bottom screen
G Bodensieb
S tamiz base

cristallin
E crystalline
G kristallin
S cristalino

cristallisation
E crystallisation
G Kristallisierung, Auskristallisierung
S cristalización

cristallisation occlusive
E inclusion crystallisation
G Einschlußkristallisation
S cristalización de inclusión

cristalliser
E crystallise, to
G kristallisieren
S cristalizar

cristalliser complètement, se
E crystallise out, to
G auskristallisieren
S cristalizar completamente

English German French Spanish

English German French Spanish

cristaux secondaires
E secondary crystals
G Sekundärkristalle
S cristales secundarios

critère
E criterion
G Kriterium
S criterio

selon des critères sévères (par ex. un test)
E according to stringent criteria (e. g. testing)
G gemäß strengen Kriterien (z. B. Test)
S siguiendo criterios estrictos (p. ej. test)

critère d'acceptation
E acceptance criterion
G Akzeptanzkriterium
S criterio de aceptación

critère de dosage
E dose criterion
G Dosiskriterium
S criterio de dosificación

croissance de cellules
E cell growth
G Zellwachstum
S crecimiento celular

croissance microbienne
E microbial growth
G mikrobielles Wachstum
S crecimiento microbiano

croquis de section
E sectional drawing
G Querschnittszeichnung
S croquis transversal

cuillère-mesure
E measuring spoon
G Meßlöffel
S cuchara de medida

cuivre
E copper
G Kupfer
S cobre

culture de cellules
E cell culture
G Zellkultur
S cultivo celular

culture de cellules de mammifère
E mammalian cell culture
G Säugetierzellkultur
S cultivo de células de mamífero

culture de cellules diploides
E diploid cell culture
G diploide Zellkultur
S cultivo de células diploides

culture de cellules hétéroploïde
E heteroploid cell culture
G heteroploide Zellkultur
S cultivo celular heteroploide

culture de cellules tissulaires
E tissue cell culture
G Gewebezellkultur
S cultivo de células tisulares

culture en continu
E continuous culture
G kontinuierliche Kultur
S cultivo continuo

culture mère
E stock culture
G Stammkultur (von Organismen)
S cultivo madre (de organismos)

culture repiquée
E sub-culture
G Subkultur
S subcultivo

curseur
E cursor
G Schieber
S compuerta, corredera, cursor

cuve
E bin, container, vessel
G Behälter
S recipiente

cuve mobile, cuve sur roues
E mobile vessel, mobile container
G fahrbarer Behälter, fahrbarer Ansatzbehälter
S contenedor portátil, recipiente portátil

cuve à réaction sous pression
E pressurised reaction vessel
G Druckreaktionskessel
S caldera presurizada de reacción

cuve de collecte
E collection vessel
G Auffanggefäß
S recipiente colector

cuve de fermentation
E fermentation vessel
G Fermentationskessel
S caldera de fermentación

cuve de stockage
E holding tank, storage vessel
G Lagertank
S tanque depósito

cuvette
E cuvette, cell
G Küvette
S cubeta

cuvette en verre
E glass cuvette
G Glasküvette
S cubeta de vidrio

cycle
E cycle, run
G Zyklus, Lauf
S ciclo, marcha, recorrido

cycle de fonctionnement
E operational cycle
G Arbeitsablauf
S ciclo de funcionamiento

cycle de mélange
E blending cycle
G Mischzyklus
S ciclo de mezcla

cycle de pulvérisation
E spray cycle
G Sprühzyklus
S ciclo de pulverización

cycle de séchage
E drying cycle
G Trocknungszyklus
S ciclo de desecación

cycle de validation
E validation run
G Validierungslauf
S ciclo de validación

cycle de vie
E life cycle
G Lebenszyklus
S ciclo vital

cylindre
E roller, drum
G Walze
S cilindro, rodillo

cylindre à imprimer
E printing roller
G Druckwalze
S rodillo de imprenta

cylindre de compression
E compressed air cylinder, compression roll, compaction roll (tablet press)
G Druckluftzylinder, Druckrolle (an der Tablettenpresse)
S cilindro de aire comprimido, cilindro compresor (en la prensa de comprimidos)

cylindre de seringue
E syringe cylinder
G Spritzenzylinder
S cilindro de jeringa

cylindrique
E cylindrical
G zylindrisch
S cilíndrico

cytométrie à débit liquide
E flow cytometry
G Durchflußzytometrie
S citometría de flujo

cytostatiques
E cytostatics
G Zytostatica
S citostáticos, agentes citostáticos

dalle (de sol)
E bottom plate
G Bodenplatte
S placa del suelo

danger
E safety risk
G Sicherheitsrisiko
S riesgo para la seguridad

danger biologique
E biohazard
G Biogefahr, Gefahr durch biologische Agenzien
S peligro biológico

danger d'explosion
E explosion hazard
G Explosionsgefahr
S peligro de explosión

dangereux
E hazardous, dangerous, harmful
G gefährlich, gesundheitsschädlich
S peligroso, perjudicial

dangereux pour la santé lors d'un contact cutané
E harmful in contact with skin
G gesundheitsschädlich bei Hautkontakt
S perjudicial para la salud si entra en contacto con la piel

dangereux pour la santé si ingéré
E harmful if swallowed
G gesundheitsschädlich beim Verschlucken
S perjudicial para la salud si se ingiere

dangereux pour la santé si inhalé
E harmful by inhalation
G gesundheitsschädlich bei Inhalation
S perjudicial para la salud si se inhala

date de libération
E release date
G Freigabedatum
S fecha de liberación

date de livraison
E due date, delivery date
G Lieferdatum
S fecha de entrega

date d'expiration
E expiration date, expiry date
G Verfallsdatum
S fecha de caducidad, fecha de expiración

débimètre
E flowmeter
G Durchflußmesser
S fluxómetro

débit
E flow, flow rate
G Durchfluß, Durchflußgeschwindigkeit, Fließgeschwindigkeit, Strömungsgeschwindigkeit
S paso (de un líquido), flujo, velocidad de flujo

débit de diffusion
E diffusion flow
G Diffusionsfluß
S flujo de difusión

débit de gaz
E gas flow
G Gasstrom
S corriente gaseosa

débit de production de comprimés
E tablet output
G Tablettenausstoß, Tablettierausstoß
S rendimiento en comprimidos, rendimiento de la máquina de comprimidos

débit d'écoulement d'air
E air throughput
G Luftdurchsatz
S rendimiento de aire

débit horaire
E output per hour
G Stundenleistung
S rendimiento horario

débitmètre
E flow meter
G Strömungswächter
S fluxómetro

débordement
E overflow
G Überlauf
S desbordamiento, rebosadero

débris
E debris
G Bruch, Trümmer
S despojos, restos, escombros

débris de verre
E breakage of glassware
G Glasbruch
S ruptura de vidrio

décalage
E slippage
G Durchschlupf
S postigo, puerta falsa

décanter
E decant, to
G abgießen, dekantieren
S decantar, verter

décapé
E pickled
G gebeizt
S decapado, macerado

décaper
E corrode, to; etch, to
G korrodieren, einätzen
S corroer, grabar (al aguafuerte)

décharge
E relief
G Entlastung
S alivio, descarga

décharge d'explosion
E explosion relief
G Explosionsentlastung
S descarga de explosión

décharger
E discharge, to
G entladen
S descargar

décharger (la pommade du conteneur)
E discharge, to (ointment from container)
G austragen (Salbe aus Container)
S descargar (pomada del contenedor)

déchets
E rubbish, waste, waste material
G Müll, Abfall, Abfallprodukt, Ausschuß
S basura, desechos, producto de desecho, residuos

déchiffreur électronique de codage
E electronic code reader
G elektronisches Codelesegerät
S lector electrónico de códigos

déchirure
E crack, tear
G Riß
S desgarro, fisura

décoction
E decoction
G Abkochung, Decoct
S decocción

décodeur
E decoder
G Entschlüssler
S descodificador

English German French Spanish

English
German
French
Spanish

décoloration
E discoloration
G Verfärbung
S decoloración

décomposition
E decomposition
G Zersetzung
S degradación, descomposición

décontamination
E decontamination
G Dekontamination
S descontaminar

découper à l'emporte-pièce
E die-cut, to; punch, to; stamp, to
G ausstanzen
S estampar, perforar, punzonar

décret
E regulation
G Verordnung
S decreto, prescripción

décret concernant les matières dangereuses
E regulations for hazardous goods, toxic chemical ordinance
G Gefahrstoffverordnung
S decreto sobre sustancias peligrosas

décret concernant les narcotiques
E narcotics regulation
G Betäubungsmittelgesetz
S decreto sobre narcóticos

défaillance (machine)
E breakdown, downtime (machine), failure
G Ausfall
S avería, desperfecto, fallo

défaut
E defect, error, failure, fault, mistake
G Fehler
S error

défaut de conditionnement
E packaging defect
G Verpackungsfehler
S defecto de embalaje

défaut de croissance
E growth defect
G Wachstumsdefekt
S defecto de crecimiento

défaut de qualité
E defect, shortcoming
G Qualitätsmangel
S defecto de calidad

défaut de registre
E register defect
G Passerfehler
S defecto de registro

défectueux
E defective, damaged, faulty
G beschädigt, fehlerhaft
S dañado, estropeado, perjudicado, defectuoso

déficience
E deficiency
G Mangel
S carencia, defecto, deficiencia, insuficiencia

déflecteur
E baffle, deflector
G Leitblech
S deflector, disruptor

déformation
E deformation
G Verformung
S deformación

défraîchir, se
E fade, to
G verblassen
S empalidecer

dégasification à vide
E vacuum degasification
G Vakuumentgaser
S desgasificador de vacío

dégâts
E damage
G Beschädigung
S daño, perjuicio

dégâts dûs au transport
E transport damage
G Transportschaden
S daños de transporte

dégazage
E degassing, deaeration (of liquids)
G Entgasung (von Flüssigkeiten)
S desgasificación (de líquidos)

dégazer
E degas, to; deaerate, to
G entgasen
S desgasificar

dégeler
E defrost, to; thaw, to
G auftauen
S descongelar

dégradable
E degradable
G abbaubar
S degradable

dégradation
E degradation
G Abbau
S degradación

dégraisser
E degrease, to
G entfetten
S desengrasar

degré de liberté
E degree of freedom
G Freiheitsgrad
S grado de libertad

degré de lustre
E grade of gloss, grade of lustre
G Glanzgrad
S grado de brillantez

degré de qualité
E quality grade
G Güteklasse
S grado de calidad

degré d'innovation (par ex. d'un produit)
E novelty (e. g. of a product)
G Neuheitsgrad (z. B. eines Produktes)
S grado de novedad (p. ej. de un producto)

degré hydrolytique
E hydrolytic grade
G hydrolytischer Grad
S grado hidrolítico

déhydratation
E dehydration
G Dehydratisierung
S deshidratación

délai
E time limit, deadline
G Frist
S plazo

délivrance
E dispensing (of a liquid)
G Verteilung (einer Flüssigkeit)
S distribución (de un líquido)

demande
E application
G Antrag
S solicitud, instancia

demande d'autorisation d'un médicament auprès de la FDA
E New Drug Application (NDA)
G Antrag auf Produktzulassung bei der FDA
S solicitud de aprobación de un producto por la FDA

English German French Spanish

demande d'autorisation de mise sur le marché (AMM)
E Medicines Marketing Authorisation Application (MAA), Product License Application (PLA), Application for Marketing Approval/Authorisation
G Antrag auf Zulassung zum Inverkehrbringen von Arzneimitteln in der EU, Antrag auf Vertriebsgenehmigung eines Arzneimittels bei der FDA (USA), Zulassungsantrag, Produktzulassungsantrag
S solicitud de autorización de venta de medicamentos en la UE, solicitud de permiso a la FDA (EE.UU.) para poner a la venta un medicamento, solicitud de autorización, solicitud de autorización de un producto (para la venta)

demande d'autorisation d'étude clinique d'un nouveau médicament (IND) auprès de la FDA
E Investigational New Drug Application (IND)
G Antrag an die FDA (USA) zur klinischen Prüfung eines Arzneimittels
S solicitud a la FDA (EE.UU.) para investigar clínicamente un nuevo medicamento

demande de brevet
E patent application
G Patentbeantragung
S solicitud de patente

demande de modification
E change request
G Änderungsantrag
S solicitud de cambio

démarrage d'un essai clinique
E start of study, start of trial
G Studienstart
S comienzo del estudio

démarrer
E start, to; start-up, to
G anfahren
S poner en marcha

démarrer (un procédé)
E start, to (a process)
G starten (Ablauf)
S comenzar (un proceso)

déménagement
E change of site, change of location
G Standortwechsel
S cambio de emplazamiento

déminéraliser
E deionise, to
G entmineralisieren
S desmineralizar

demi-vie
E half-life
G Halbwertszeit
S tiempo de vida media

démixtion
E demixing, separation
G Entmischung
S separación

démontable
E detachable, removable
G entfernbar, abnehmbar
S desmontable

démontage
E removal, disassembly, dismantling
G Ausbau, Demontage, Zerlegung
S desmontaje

démontage de filtre
E filter removal
G Filterausbau
S desmontaje de un filtro

dénaturation
E denaturing
G Denaturierung
S desnaturalización

dénaturé
E denatured
G denaturiert, vergällt
S desnaturalizado

densité
E density
G Dichte
S densidad

densité absolue
E absolute density
G absolute Dichte
S densidad absoluta

densité apparente
E bulk density
G Schüttdichte
S densidad aparente

densité de cellules
E cell density
G Zelldichte
S densidad de células

densité de package
E tapped density, packed density
G Stampfdichte
S densidad de compresión

densité de tassement
E packed density, tapped density
G Stampfdichte
S densidad de apisonamiento

densité d'une poudre
E powder density
G Pulverdichte
S densidad del polvo

densité réelle
E true density
G wahre Dichte
S densidad real

densité relative
E relative density
G relative Dichte
S densidad relativa

dépannage
E trouble-shooting, failure rectification
G Fehlerbehebung
S corrección de errores

département
E department, division
G Abteilung, Sparte
S departamento, especialidad, rama, sector

département de développement galénique
E galenical development department
G Galenikabteilung
S departamento de farmacia galénica

département des affaires réglementaires
E regulatory affairs department
G Zulassungsabteilung
S departamento de registros y licencias sanitarias

département des ressources humaines
E personnel department
G Personalabteilung
S departamento de personal

dépenser
E dispense, to
G ausgeben
S distribuir, gastar

déperdition de chaleur
E heat loss
G Wärmeverlust
S pérdida calórica

dépistage
E screening
G Erkennung
S detección

English
German
French
Spanish

déplacer
E transfer, to; relocate, to
G verlagern
S desplazar, transferir, trasladar

déposition (d'une demande d'autorisation de mise sur le marché)
E submission (of an application for marketing approval)
G Einreichung (eines Zulassungsantrags)
S presentación (de una solicitud de autorización)

dépôt
E deposit, sediment
G Wandbelag, Ablagerung
S recubrimiento de la pared, depósito, sedimento

dépôt de demande de brevet
E patent filing
G Patentanmeldung, Patenteinreichung
S solicitud de patente

dépôt de palettes
E pallet store
G Palettenstellplatz
S almacén para paletas

dépourvu de joint
E seamless
G nahtlos
S sin sutura

dépourvu de pores
E pore-free
G porenfrei
S sin poros

dépourvu de pyrogènes
E pyrogen-free
G pyrogenfrei
S sin pirógenos

dépourvu de rouille
E rust-free
G rostfrei
S sin orín

dépourvu de volume mort
E dead volume-free
G totraumfrei
S sin espacios muertos

dépoussiérage
E dedusting
G Entstaubung
S desempolvamiento

dépoussiéreur
E deduster
G Entstauber
S desempolvante

depression
E negative pressure
G Unterdruck
S depresión, hipotensión

dépression atmosphérique
E sub-atmospheric pressure
G Atmosphärenunterdruck
S presión atmosférica baja

dépressurisation
E pressure drop
G Druckabfall
S descenso de presión

déprotonation
E deprotonation
G Deprotonierung
S desprotonización

dépyrogénation
E depyrogenation
G Entpyrogenisierung
S despirogenación, eliminación de pirógenos

dépyrogéner
E depyrogenate, to
G entpyrogenisieren
S despirogenar, eliminar pirógenos

dérangement
E malfunction, interference
G Störung
S avería, fallo

dérivé
E derivative
G Abkömmling, Derivat
S derivado

dérivé d'acide aminé
E amino acid derivative
G Aminosäurederivat
S derivado de aminoácido

dérive de la ligne de base
E baseline drift
G Basisliniendrift
S desviación de la línea de base

dérive du point zero
E zero drift
G Nullpunktabweichung
S desviación del punto cero

dernier cri de la technique
E state-of-the-art
G Stand der Technik
S estado (actual) de la técnica

déroulement d'un procédé
E sequence of operation
G Ablauf (eines Prozesses)
S secuencia (de un proceso)

déroulement d'une réaction
E course of a reaction
G Reaktionsverlauf
S transcurso de la reacción

désaérer
E degas, to; deaerate, to; ventilate, to; vent, to
G entgasen, entlüften
S desgasificar, airear, ventilar

désagréger, se
E disintegrate, to
G zerfallen
S desintegrar(se)

description
E description
G Beschreibung
S descripción

description d'un emploi
E job description
G Stellenbeschreibung
S descripción de un puesto de trabajo

déshuileur
E oil separator, oil trap
G Ölabscheider
S separador de aceite

déshydratant
E desiccant
G Trocknungsmittel
S desecante, deshidratante

design
E design
G Bauart
S tipo de construcción

design du conditionnement
E package design
G Verpackungsdesign
S diseño de un envase

design d'un essai clinique
E study design, trial design
G Studiendesign, Versuchsanordnung
S diseño de un estudio (clínico), disposición del ensayo

design modulaire
E modular design
G Baukastenprinzip, Modularbauweise
S principio de unidades de montaje, diseño modular

désignation
E designation
G Bezeichnung
S denominación, marcado, rotulación

désigné (pour)
E designated (for)
G bestimmt (für)
S designado (para)

désinfectable
E disinfectable
G desinfizierbar
S desinfectable

English German French Spanish

English German French Spanish

désinfectant
E disinfectant
G Desinfektionsmittel
S agente desinfectante

désinfectants autorisés
E approved disinfectants
G zugelassene Desinfektionsmittel
S desinfectantes autorizados

désinfecter
E disinfect, to
G desinfizieren, entkeimen
S desinfectar

désinfection
E disinfection
G Desinfektion
S desinfección

désinfection de locaux
E room disinfection
G Raumdesinfektion
S desinfección de la sala

désinfection des instruments
E instrument disinfection
G Gerätedesinfektion
S desinfección de instrumentos

désinfection des mains
E hand disinfection
G Händedesinfektion
S desinfección de manos

désintégrant
E disintegrant, tablet disintegrant
G Sprengmittel
S desintegrante

désintégration
E disintegration
G Zerfall
S desintegración

désintégration radioactive
E radioactive decay
G radioaktiver Zerfall
S desintegración radiactiva

désintégrer, se
E disintegrate, to
G zerfallen
S desintegrar(se)

dessaler
E desalt, to
G entsalzen
S desalinizar

desséchant
E desiccant
G Trocknungsmittel
S desecante, deshidratante

dessicateur
E desiccator
G Exsiccator
S desecante, exicante

dessicateur à claies
E tray dryer
G Hordentrockenschrank
S armario de secado en bandeja

dessicateur à plateaux
E tray dryer
G Hordentrockenschrank
S armario de secado en bandeja

dessication sous vide
E vacuum drying
G Vakuumtrocknung
S secado al vacío

dessication sur claies
E tray drying
G Hordentrocknung
S secado en bandeja

dessin
E drawing
G Zeichnung
S dibujo

dessin technique
E engineering drawing
G technische Zeichnung
S dibujo técnico

dessiquer
E dry out, to; desiccate, to
G austrocknen, eintrocknen
S desecar, secar

destruction
E destruction
G Vernichtung
S destrucción

détachable
E detachable, removable
G abnehmbar
S desmontable

détaché
E separated, segregated
G abgetrennt
S aislado, separado

détartrant
E decalcifier
G Entkalker
S agente descalcificante

détartrer
E decalcify, to
G entkalken
S descalcificar

détectable
E detectable
G nachweisbar, detektierbar
S detectable

indétectable
E undetectable
G nicht nachweisbar
S no detectable

détecteur à capture électronique
E electron capture detector (ECD)
G Elektroneneinfangdetektor
S detector de captura electrónica

détecteur à ionisation de flamme
E flame ionisation detector (FID)
G Flammenionisationsdetektor (FID)
S detector de ionización de llama

détecteur ampérométrique
E amperometric detection
G amperometrische Detektion
S detección amperométrica

détecteur d'azote phosphorisé
E nitrogen-phosphorous detector (NPD)
G Stickstoff-Phosphor-Detektor
S detector de nitrógeno fosforado

détecteur de fumée
E smoke detector
G Rauchmelder
S detector de humo

détecteur de lumière diffuse
E light-scattering detector
G Streulicht-Detektor
S detector de luz dispersa

détecteur de métaux
E metal detector
G Metallsuchgerät
S detector de metales

détecteur de niveau
E level detector, level sensor
G Füllstandsmelder, Pegelmesser
S detector de nivel de relleno, sensor de nivel

détecteur de pression atmosphérique
E air pressure sensor
G Luftdruckfühler
S sensor de presión atmosférica

détecteur d'humidité
E humidity detector
G Feuchtesensor
S detector de humedad

détecteur UV/VIS
E UV/VIS detector
G UV/VIS-Detektor
S detector UV/VIS

détection
E detection, evidence, proof
G Nachweis
S demostración, prueba

détérioration
E deterioration
G Verderb
S deterioro

détériorer, se
E deteriorate, to
G verderben
S deteriorar, deteriorarse

déterminant la qualité
E quality-determining
G qualitätsbestimmend
S determinante de la calidad

détermination
E determination
G Bestimmung
S análisis, determinación

détermination de la teneur en eau
E water determination
G Wasserbestimmung
S determinación del contenido en agua

détermination du contenu
E determination of content
G Gehaltsbestimmung
S determinación del contenido

détermination du nombre de micro-organismes
E microbial count determination
G Keimzahlbestimmung
S recuento de gérmenes

déterminer
E determine, to
G bestimmen, ermitteln
S averigar, determinar

détruire
E destroy, to; kill, to
G vernichten, abtöten
S destruir, matar

développement
E development
G Entwicklung
S desarrollo, evolución

développement analytique
E analytical development
G Entwicklungsanalytik
S analítica de desarrollo

développement d'un nouveau produit
E new product development
G Entwicklung eines neuen Produktes
S desarrollo de un producto nuevo

développement d'un procédé
E process development
G Verfahrensentwicklung
S desarrollo de un procedimiento

développement d'un produit
E product development
G Produktentwicklung
S desarrollo de un producto

développement d'une résistance
E development of resistance
G Resistenzentwicklung
S desarrollo de resistencia

déverrouiller
E unlock, to
G entriegeln
S desbloquear

déversoir pour comprimés
E tablet gate
G Tablettenablaufweichen
S lámina divisoria para comprimidos

déviation
E deviation
G Abweichung
S desviación

déviation (d'une aiguille)
E deflection (of pointer)
G Ausschlag (eines Zeigers)
S desviación (de una aguja indicadora)

déviation de température
E temperature deviation
G Temperaturabweichung
S desviación de temperatura

déviation standard
E standard deviation
G Standardabweichung
S desviación estándar

déviation standard maximum permise
E maximum permitted standard deviation
G maximal zulässige Standardabweichung
S desviación estándar máxima permitida

dévier
E deflect, to
G ablenken
S desviar

dévisser
E screw on, to
G aufschrauben
S atornillar

dextrogyre
E dextro-rotatory
G rechtsdrehend
S dextrógiro

diagnose
E diagnosis, report, finding
G Befund
S diagnóstico

diagnostic in-vitro
E in-vitro diagnosis
G In-vitro-Diagnose
S diagnóstico in vitro

diagnostiques
E diagnostics
G Diagnostica
S agentes diagnósticos

diagramme
E diagram
G Diagramm
S diagrama

diagramme à secteurs
E pie chart
G Kreisdiagramm
S diagrama circular

diagramme arborescent
E tree diagram
G Baumdiagramm
S diagrama en árbol

diagramme d'affinité
E affinity diagram
G Affinitätsdiagramm
S diagrama de afinidad

diagramme de phases
E phase diagram
G Phasendiagramm
S diagrama de fases

diagramme des connexions
E wiring diagram
G Schaltdiagramm
S diagrama de circuito

diagramme matriciel
E matrix diagram
G Matrixdiagramm
S diagrama en matriz

diamètre
E diameter
G Durchmesser
S diámetro

diamètre de bobine
E reel diameter
G Rollendurchmesser
S diámetro de bobina

diamètre de colonne
E column diameter
G Säulendurchmesser
S diámetro de la columna

diamètre du plateau d'une matrice
E die plate diameter
G Matrizenscheibendurchmesser
S diámetro del disco matriz

diamètre d'un comprimé
E tablet diameter
G Tablettendurchmesser
S diámetro del comprimido

diamètre d'un pore
E pore diameter
G Porendurchmesser
S diámetro de poro

diamètre d'une surface
E surface diameter
G Oberflächendurchmesser
S diámetro de una superficie

diamètre interne
E internal diameter
G lichter Durchmesser
S diámetro interno

diaphragme
E aperture, diaphragm
G Lochblende
S diafragma

différence de pression
E pressure differential
G Druckdifferenz
S diferencia de presión

différence de registre
E register difference
G Passerdifferenz
S diferencia de registro

différentiation microbienne
E microbial differentiation
G Keimdifferenzierung
S diferenciación de gérmenes

difficulté de glissement d'un poinçon
E punch sticking
G Stempelschwergängigkeit
S dificultad de deslizamiento del troquel

diffraction de la lumière
E diffraction
G Lichtbeugung
S difracción luminosa

diffusion
E diffusion
G Diffusion
S difusión

diffusion (de valeurs)
E spread, distribution (of values)
G Streuung (von Werten)
S dispersión (de valores)

diluant
E diluent
G Verdünnungsmittel
S diluyente

dilué
E dilute
G verdünnt
S diluido

diluer
E dilute, to
G verdünnen
S diluir

dilution
E dilution
G Verdünnung
S dilución

dilution maximale autorisée
E maximum valid dilution (MVD)
G maximal zulässige Verdünnung (MZV)
S dilución máxima permitida

dimension interne
E internal dimension
G Innenmaß
S dimensión interna

dimensions
E dimensions
G Abmessungen, Ausmaß
S dimensiónes, medidas, cuantía

dimensions d'un comprimé
E tablet dimensions
G Tablettenabmessungen
S dimensiones del comprimido

dimensions externes
E external dimensions
G Außenmaße
S dimensiones externas

dimensions totales
E overall dimensions
G Gesamtabmessungen
S dimensiones totales

diminuer
E diminish, to
G vermindern
S disminuir, reducir

dioxyde de carbone
E carbon dioxide
G Kohlendioxyd
S anhídrido carbónico

directeur
E director, head (person), executive
G Direktor, Leiter (als Person), Vorstandsmitglied
S director, miembro de la junta directiva

directeur de production
E head of production
G Herstellungsleiter
S director de producción

directeur des ventes
E sales manager
G Vertriebsleiter
S director de ventas

directeur du département d'ingénierie
E head of engineering department
G Technischer Leiter
S director del departamento técnico

directeur d'usine
E plant manager
G Werksleiter
S director de taller

directeur technique
E Plant Manager
G Betriebsleiter
S director técnico de la empresa

direction de l'écoulement d'air
E air flow direction
G Luftströmungsrichtung
S dirección del flujo aéreo

direction de rotation
E direction of rotation
G Drehrichtung
S sentido de la rotación

direction d'une société
E company management
G Geschäftsleitung
S gerencia

directive
E directive, policy, guideline
G Richtlinie, Leitlinie
S directiva, directriz

directives GMP de la CE
E EC-GMP Guideline
G EG-GMP-Leitfaden
S Líneas directrices de la EC sobre GMP

diriger
E guide, to
G leiten
S conducir, dirigir

disparité
E discrepancy
G Diskrepanz
S discrepancia

disperser
E disperse, to
G dispergieren
S dispersar

dispersion
E dispersion, stray range, spread, distribution
G Dispersion, Streubreite
S dispersión

dispersion colloïdale
E colloidal dispersion
G Kolloiddispersion
S dispersión coloidal

dispersion de la couleur
E colour dispersion
G Farbdispersion
S dispersión cromática

dispersion de la lumière
E light scattering, stray light
G Lichtstreuung
S dispersión luminosa

dispersion refractive
E refractive dispersion
G Brechungsdispersion
S dispersión refringente

disponible
E available
G verfügbar
S disponible

disponible seulement sur ordonnance
E prescription only
G rezeptpflichtig
S con receta médica

dispositif
E device
G Vorrichtung
S dispositivo

dispositif adaptable
E attachment, module
G Anbauteil
S pieza de montaje

dispositif d'aide au dosage
E metering aid, dosing aid
G Dosierhilfe
S dispositivo para dosificar

dispositif d'alimentation
E filling device, charging device
G Einfüllvorrichtung
S dispositivo de relleno

dispositif de basculement
E tilting device
G Kippvorrichtung
S dispositivo basculante

dispositif de guidage
E guide, guiding device, guiding mechanism
G Führungsvorrichtung
S dispositivo de guía, guía

dispositif de levage
E lifting device
G Hebevorrichtung
S dispositivo elevador

dispositif de mesure d'un niveau
E level-measuring device
G Füllstandsmesser
S sistema de medida del nivel de relleno

dispositif de nettoyage de filtre
E filter cleaning device
G Filterabreinigungsvorrichtung
S dispositivo de limpieza de filtros

dispositif de refroidissement
E cooling device
G Abkühlvorrichtung
S dispositivo de enfriamiento

dispositif de sécurité
E safety device
G Sicherheitsvorrichtung
S dispositivo de seguridad

dispositif de serrage rapide
E fast-clamping device
G Schnellspannvorrichtung
S dispositivo tensor rápido

dispositif de stockage
E stacking device
G Stapelvorrichtung
S dispositivo de apilamiento

dispositif d'échantillonnage
E powder sampler, sampling device, sampling pipette
G Stechheber
S pipeta (de toma de muestras)

dispositif d'orientation
E swing-out device, swivelling device
G Ausschwenkvorrichtung
S dispositivo giratorio

dispositions (légales) concernant les déchets
E waste regulations
G Abfallbestimmungen
S prescripciones sobre desechos

disque de rupture
E bursting disk, rupture disk
G Berstscheibe
S disco de ruptura

dissémination de (poussière)
E dissemination of (dust)
G Verbreitung von (Staub)
S diseminación de (polvo)

dissociation
E dissociation
G Dissoziation
S disociación

dissolution
E dissolution
G Auflösung
S dilución, disolución

dissoudre
E dissolve, to
G auflösen, lösen
S diluir, disolver

distance entre plateaux
E plate spacing
G Plattenabstand
S distancia entre placas

distillat
E distillate
G Destillat
S destilado

distillation sous vide
E vacuum distillation
G Vakuumdestillation
S destilación en vacío

distiller
E distil, to; distil off, to
G destillieren, abdestillieren
S destilar

distinct
E distinct, clear
G deutlich
S claro, distinto

distribuer
E dispense, to
G ausgeben
S distribuir, gastar

distributeur
E dispenser
G Spender,
Verteiler
S distribuidor

distribution
E distribution
G Verteilung
S distribución

distribution de chaleur
E heat distribution
G Wärmeverteilung,
Hitzeverteilung
S distribución de calor

distribution de fréquences
E frequency distribution
G Häufigkeitsverteilung
S distribución de
frecuencias

distribution de la taille des particules
E particle size distribution
G Korngrößenverteilung
S distribución del tamaño
de los granos

distribution de phases
E phase distribution
G Phasenverteilung
S distribución de fases

distribution des particules
E particle distribution
G Partikelverteilung
S distribución de partículas

distribution des sommes
E sum distribution
G Summenverteilung
S distribución de sumas

distribution du matériel d'emballage
E packaging material dispensary
G Packmittelausgabe
S distribución de material de embalaje

distribution randomisée
E random distribution
G Zufallsverteilung
S distribución aleatoria

division pharmaceutique
E pharmaceutical division
G Pharma-Sparte
S sector farmacéutico

documentation
E documentation
G Dokumentation
S documentación

documentation d'un procédé
E process documentation
G Prozeßdokumentation
S documentación de un proceso

documentation électronique
E electronic batch recording
G elektronische Chargendokumentation
S documentación electrónica de lotes

documenter
E document, to; protocol, to; record, to
G dokumentieren, protokollieren
S documentar, levantar acta, protocolar

domaine d'application
E area of application, scope, validity
G Anwendungsgebiet, Geltungsbereich
S campo de aplicación

dommage
E damage, impairment
G Beschädigung, Beeinträchtigung
S daño, perjuicio, merma

données
E data
G Daten
S datos

données
E data, specifications
G Angaben
S datos, especificaciones

données brutes
E raw data
G Rohdaten
S datos brutos

données de production
E production data
G Produktionsdaten
S datos de producción

données de validation
E validation data
G Validierungsdaten
S datos de validación

données génomiques
E genomic data
G Genomdaten
S datos genómicos

donneur (personne)
E donor (person)
G Spender (als Person)
S donante

donneur d'ordre
E contract provider, principal, client
G Auftraggeber
S cliente, comitente

dosage de précipitation
E precipitation titration
G Fällungstitration
S volumetría de precipitación

dose
E dose
G Dosis
S dosis

dose de maintien
E maintenance dosage
G Erhaltungsdosis
S dosis de mantenimiento

dose faible
E low dosage
G niedrige Dosis
S dosis baja

dose faible, à
E low-dosed
G niedrig dosiert
S dosis reducida

dose journalière
E daily dosage
G Tagesdosis
S dosis diaria

dose liminaire
E threshold dosage
G Schwellendosis
S dosis liminar, dosis umbral

dose maximale
E maximum dosage
G Höchstdosis
S dosis máxima

dose mortelle
E fatal dose
G tödliche Dosis
S dosis mortal

dose unique
E single dose
G Einzeldosis
S dosis única

dose unitaire
E dosage unit
G Dosierungseinheit
S unidad de dosificación

doser
E meter, to; dose, to
G abmessen, dosieren
S medir, dosificar, calibrar

dossier de demande d'autorisation de mise sur le marché
E submission file for marketing authorisation
G Zulassungsdossier
S dosier de solicitud de autorización

double aveugle, en
E double-blind
G doppelblind
S doble ciego

double faisceau
E double beam
G Doppelstrahl
S haz doble, rayo doble

double manchon
E double jacket
G Doppelmantel
S cubierta doble

double manteau
E double jacket
G Doppelmantel
S cubierta doble

douche de rinçage pour les yeux
E eye wash equipment
G Augendusche
S equipo de lavado oftálmico

douille
E sheath, bush, sleeve
G Hülle, Hülse
S envoltura, cápsula, cáscara

douille de connexion
E connection port, connection nipple
G Anschlußstutzen
S empalme de conexión

dragée
E sugar-coated tablet
G Dragee, Zuckerdragee
S gragea, gragea azucarada

dragéification (à la turbine)
E coating pan
G Dragierkessel
S caldera para gragear

English German French Spanish

dragéifier
E pan-coat, to
G dragieren (mit Zuckerüberzug)
S preparar grageas (con cubierta de azúcar), gragear

drain
E drain
G Abguß, Abfluß
S decantación, vaciado, desagüe

dresser (un carton)
E set up, to (a folding carton)
G aufrichten (eine Faltschachtel)
S montar (una caja plegable)

droit
E right-handed
G rechtsgängig
S de paso derecho

droit d'accès
E authorised access
G autorisierter Zugang
S acceso autorizado

droits liés à un brevet
E patent claim
G Patentanspruch
S reclamación de patente

duplicata
E duplicate
G Duplikat
S duplicado

durable
E durable, stable
G dauerhaft
S duradero

durcissage
E hardening
G Härten
S endurecimiento

durée
E duration
G Dauer
S duración

durée de conservation
E shelf-life
G Haltbarkeitsdauer
S duración de conservación

durée de résidence gastrique
E gastric duration, gastric residence
G Aufenthalt im Magen
S permanencia en el estómago

durée de stérilisation
E duration of sterilisation
G Sterilisationszeit
S tiempo de esterilización

durée de stockage
E shelf-life
G Haltbarkeitsdauer
S duración de conservación

durée de validité
E period of validity
G Gültigkeitsdauer
S período de validez

durée de validité d'un brevet
E patent duration, patent life
G Patentgültigkeitsdauer
S duración de la validez de una patente

durée d'exposition à l'irradiation
E duration of exposure to radiation
G Bestrahlungsdauer
S duración de la irradiación

durée d'opération
E running time
G Laufzeit
S tiempo de funcionamiento

durée d'un cycle
E running time
G Laufzeit
S tiempo de funcionamiento

durée d'un essai
E duration of trial
G Studiendauer
S duración de prueba

dureté
E hardness
G Härte
S dureza

dureté (par ex. d'un comprimé)
E strength (e. g. of a tablet)
G Stärke (z. B. einer Tablette)
S fuerza (p. ej. de un comprimido)

dureté à la bille
E ball hardness
G Kugeldruckhärte
S dureza de la bola

dureté de l'eau
E water hardness
G Wasserhärte
S dureza del agua

dureté d'un comprimé
E tablet hardness
G Tablettenhärte
S dureza del comprimido

dureté permamente (de l'eau)
E permanent hardness (of water)
G permanente Härte (von Wasser)
S dureza permanente (del agua)

dureté résiduelle (par ex. de l'eau)
E residual hardness (e. g. of water)
G Resthärte (z. B. von Wasser)
S dureza residual (p. ej. del agua)

dureté Rockwell (outils)
E Rockwell hardness (of tools)
G Rockwell-Härte (von Werkzeug)
S dureza rockwell (de herramientas)

dureté temporaire (de l'eau)
E temporary hardness (of water)
G temporäre Härte (von Wasser)
S dureza temporal (del agua)

dysfonctionnement
E malfunction
G Funktionsstörung
S disfunción

eau
E water
G Wasser
S agua

eau chlorée
E chlorinated water
G Chlorwasser
S agua clorada

eau condensée
E condense water
G Kondenswasser
S agua condensada

eau d'alimentation
E feed water
G Speisewasser
S agua de alimentación

eau de cristallisation
E water of crystallisation
G Kristallwasser
S agua de cristalización

eau de haute pureté
E high purity water
G Reinstwasser
S agua ultrapurificada

eau de refroidissement
E cooling water
G Kühlwasser
S agua de refrigeración

eau de rinçage
E rinsing water
G Spülwasser
S agua de lavado

eau de ruissellement
E splash water
G Spritzwasser
S agua de inyección, agua de rociado

eau déionisée
E deionised water
G entionisiertes Wasser
S agua desionizada

English German French Spanish

eau déminéralisée
E demineralised water
G demineralisiertes Wasser, entmineralisiertes Wasser, VE-Wasser
S agua desmineralizada, agua completamente desmineralizada

eau dénuée de nucléase
E nuclease-free water
G nukleasefreies Wasser
S agua sin nucleasas

eau désalinisée par osmose inverse
E reverse osmosis water
G durch Umkehrosmose entsalztes Wasser
S agua desalinizada mediante ósmosis inversa

eau distillée
E distilled water
G destilliertes Wasser, Aqua dest.
S agua destilada

eau du robinet
E tap water
G Leitungswasser
S agua corriente

eau glacée
E ice water
G Eiswasser
S agua helada

eau médicinale
E medicinal water
G Heilwasser
S agua medicinal

eau mère
E mother liquor
G Mutterlauge
S lejía madre

eau oxygénée
E hydrogen peroxide
G Wasserstoffperoxid
S peróxido de hidrógeno

eau pharmaceutique
E pharmaceutical water
G Pharma-Wasser
S agua farmacéutica

eau potable
E drinking water, potable water
G Trinkwasser
S agua potable, agua corriente potable

eau pour opérations
E process water
G Prozeßwasser
S agua de procesado

eau pour préparation injectable (eau PPI)
E water for injection (WFI), pure water, redistilled water, double-distilled water
G Wasser für Injektionszwecke, Reinstwasser, Aqua bidest.
S agua para inyección, agua purificada, agua bidestilada

eau purifiée
E purified water
G gereinigtes Wasser, Aqua purificata
S agua purificada

eau ultra pure
E ultrapure water
G hochreines Wasser
S agua ultrapurificada

eaux d'égouts
E waste water
G Abwasser
S aguas residuales

eaux résiduelles
E waste water
G Abwasser
S aguas residuales

eaux usées
E waste water
G Abwasser
S aguas residuales

ébarbage
E deburring
G Entgratung
S desbarbado

ébarber
E deburr, to
G entgraten
S desbarbar

ébarbeur
E deburrer
G Entgrater
S desbarbador, desbastador

ébauche
E draft, blank
G Entwurf, Rohling
S bosquejo, diseño, esbozo, proyecto, pieza bruta

ébonite
E hard rubber, vulcanite
G Hartgummi
S ebonita

écart
E deviation, discrepancy
G Abweichung, Diskrepanz
S desviación, discrepancia

écart entre les poids d'un cachet
E tablet weight variation
G Schwankung des Tablettengewichts
S fluctuación del peso de los comprimidos

écart entre les poids d'un comprimé
E tablet weight variation
G Schwankung des Tablettengewichts
S fluctuación del peso de los comprimidos

écart-type relatif
E relative standard deviation
G relative Standardabweichung
S desviación estándar relativa

échafaudage
E supporting structure
G Gerüst
S andamio, armazón, esqueleto

échancrure
E recess
G Aussparung
S hueco, vacío

échange d'halogène
E halogen exchange
G Halogenaustausch
S intercambio de halógenos

échange d'ions
E ion exchange
G Ionenaustausch
S intercambio de iones

échange d'ions sur lit mixte
E mixed bed ion exchange
G Gemischtbett-Ionenaustauscher
S intercambiador de iones de lecho mixto

échangeur de cations
E cation exchanger
G Kationentauscher
S intercambiador de cationes

échangeur de chaleur
E heat exchanger
G Wärmetauscher
S intercambiador de calor

échangeur de chaleur à faisceaux tubulaires
E tube bundle heat exchanger
G Rohrbündelwärmetauscher
S intercambiador de calor de haces tubulares

échangeur de cuvette
E cell changer
G Küvettenwechsler
S intercambiador de cubetas

échangeur d'ions
E ion exchanger
G Ionenaustauscher
S intercambiador de iones

échangeur d'ions à lit mixte
E mixed bed ion exchanger
G Mischbettionentauscher, Gemischtbett-Ionenaustauscher
S intercambiador de iones de lecho mixto

échangeur d'ions anioniques
E anion exchanger
G Anionenaustauscher
S intercambiador de aniones

échantillon
E sample, test sample, specimen
G Probe, Prüfmuster, Muster, unverkäufliches Muster
S muestra, muestra de prueba, espécimen, muestra gratuita

échantillon clinique
E clinical trial sample
G klinisches Prüfmuster
S muestra para ensayos clínicos

échantillon de référence
E retained sample, reference sample
G Rückstellmuster
S muestra de referencia

échantillon du mélange
E composite sample
G Mischprobe
S muestra mixta

échantillon fortuit du fournisseur
E supplier's random sample
G Lieferantenstichprobe
S muestra al azar del abastecedor

échantillon mixte
E composite sample
G Mischmuster
S muestra mixta

échantillon pharmaceutique
E pharmaceutical sample
G Ärztemuster
S muestra farmacéutica

échantillon prélevé au hasard
E random sample
G Stichprobe
S muestra al azar

échantillon soumis à un effort
E stressed sample
G beanspruchte Probe
S muestra sometida a carga

échantillonnage
E sampling
G Probenahme, Musterziehung
S toma de muestra

critères d'échantillonnage
E sampling criteria
G Schärfe der Stichprobenanweisung
S rigor de las instrucciones para tomar muestras

échantillonneur d'air
E microbial collector
G Luftkeimsammler
S colector de gérmenes del aire

échantillonneuse
E sampler
G Probengeber
S aparato de toma de muestras

échelle
E scale, standard, range
G Skala, Maßstab, Bandbreite
S escala, estándar, patrón, anchura de banda, gama, márgenes

à l'échelle
E true to scale
G maßstabgerecht
S a escala

échelle de laboratoire
E laboratory scale
G Labormaßstab
S escala de laboratorio

échelle de mesure
E measuring scale
G Meßskala
S escala de medida

dans l'échelle de mesure
E on-scale
G innerhalb des Anzeigebereichs
S dentro de la escala de medida

en dehors de l'échelle de mesure
E off-scale
G außerhalb des Anzeigebereichs
S fuera de la escala de medida

échelle de production
E production scale
G Produktionsmaßstab
S escala de producción

échelle pilote
E pilot scale
G Versuchsmaßstab
S escala piloto

échelonné
E stepwise
G stufenweise
S gradualmente

éclaboussures
E splashes
G Spritzer
S inyección, rociado, salpicadura

éclairage
E lighting, illumination
G Beleuchtung
S iluminación

éclairage par l'arrière
E back illumination
G Beleuchtung von hinten
S iluminación desde atrás

éclairage plafonnier
E ceiling lighting
G Deckenbeleuchtung
S alumbrado de techo

éclater
E burst, to
G bersten
S estallar, reventar

éclats de verre
E glass splinters
G Glassplitter
S añicos de vidrio

écologique
E environmentally friendly, non-polluting
G umweltfreundlich
S ecológico

écologiste
E environmentalist, ecologist
G Umweltschützer
S ecologista

économie de temps
E time-saving
G Zeitersparnis
S ahorro de tiempo

économique
E cost-efficient
G kosteneffizient
S económico

écoulant librement, s'
E free flowing
G freifließend
S fluyendo libremente

écoulement d'air
E air current
G Luftstrom
S corriente de aire

écran
E screen
G Bildschirm
S pantalla

écran de protection
E protective screen
G Schutzschirm
S pantalla protectora

écran de protection constitué de verre de sécurité
E safety glass screen
G Schutzschirm aus Sicherheitsglas
S pantalla protectora de vidrio de seguridad

English German French Spanish

écraser
E pinch, to; squeeze, to
G quetschen
S aplastar

écrou
E nut
G Mutter, Schraubenmutter
S tuerca

écrou moleté
E knurled nut
G Rändelmutter
S tuerca moleteada

édifice
E building
G Gebäude
S edificio

édition
E edition, version, issue
G Ausgabe, Version
S edición, versión

édition numérique
E digital read out
G digitale Ausgabe
S edición digital

éducation
E education, training
G Ausbildung, Schulung
S educación, formación, adiestramiento, instrucción

édulcorant
E sweetener
G Süßstoff
S edulcorante

effacé
E retentive
G zurückhaltend
S reservado

effervescent
E effervescent
G schäumend
S espumante

effet
E effect
G Einwirkung
S efecto

effet adverse
E adverse reaction
G unerwünschte Reaktion
S reacción indeseable

effet secondaires
E side effect
G Nebenwirkung
S efecto colateral, efecto secundario

efficace
E effective, potent
G wirksam
S activo, eficaz

efficacité
E efficacy, efficiency
G Wirksamkeit, Effizienz
S eficacia, eficiencia

efficacité de la désinfection
E disinfecting effectiveness
G desinfizierende Wirksamkeit
S eficacia desinfectante

efficacité de rétention (pour un filtre)
E retention efficiency (in filters)
G Rückhaltevermögen (bei Filtern)
S capacidad de retención (de un filtro)

effluent
E effluvium
G Ausdünstung
S evaporación, transpiración

effluent aqueux
E aqueous waste
G Flüssigabfall
S desecho fluido

effluent de filtration
E filtrate waste
G Filtrationsabfall
S desecho de filtración

efflux
E effluvium
G Ausdünstung
S evaporación, transpiración

égoût
E floor drain
G Gulli, Bodenabfluß
S sumidero

éjecter
E eject, to
G ausstoßen
S emitir, expeler, expulsar

éjection
E ejection
G Auswurf, Auswurf
S eyección

éjection automatique
E automatic ejection
G automatischer Auswurf
S expulsión automática

éjection d'un comprimé
E tablet ejection
G Tablettenauswurf
S eyección de comprimidos

élasticité
E elasticity
G Elastizität
S elasticidad

élastique
E elastic
G elastisch
S elástico

électricité
E current, electricity
G Strom
S corriente eléctrica

électrode
E electrode
G Elektrode
S electrodo

électrode de verre
E glass electrode
G Glaselektrode
S electrodo de vidrio

électrolyse
E electrolysis
G Elektrolyse
S electrólisis

électrolyte
E electrolyte
G Elektrolyt
S electrólito

électrophorèse capillaire
E capillary electrophoresis
G Kapillarelektrophorese
S electroforesis capilar

électrophorèse horizontale
E horizontal electrophoresis
G Horizontalelektrophorese
S electroforesis horizontal

électrophorèse verticale
E vertical electrophoresis
G Vertikalelektrophorese
S electroforesis vertical

électro-poli
E electro-polished
G elektropoliert
S pulido eléctricamente

électrotechnique et techniques de mesure et de réglage
E measuring and control technology
G Elektro-, Meß- und Regeltechnik (EMR)
S electrotécnica y técnicas de medida y regulación

élément chauffant
E heating element
G Heizelement
S elemento calefactor

élément commutateur
E switch module
G Schaltelement
S elemento interruptor

English
German
French
Spanish

English German French Spanish

élimination
E disposal, remova, deconcentration
G Beseitigung, Abreicherung, Entfernung, Entsorgung
S eliminación, reducción, desecho

élimination de déchets
E waste disposal
G Abfallbeseitigung
S eliminación de desechos

élimination des résidus
E waste disposal
G Abfallentsorgung
S eliminación de desechos

élimination des virus
E removal of viruses, virus removal
G Virusabreicherung, Virusentfernung
S eliminación de virus

élimination d'un principe actif
E excretion of medicinal substance
G Arzneistoffausscheidung
S eliminación del principio activo

éliminer (par ex. des virus)
E deplete, to; reduce, to (e. g. viruses)
G abreichern (z. B. Viren)
S eliminar (p. ej. virus)

éliminer une erreur
E eliminate a failure (fault), to
G Fehler beseitigen
S eliminar errores

éluant
E eluant
G Elutionsmittel
S agente levigante

éluat
E eluate
G Eluat
S levigado, eluado

élucider (une structure)
E elucidate, to (a structure)
G aufklären (Struktur)
S aclarar, esclarecer (una estructura)

émail
E enamel
G Email
S esmalte

émaillé
E enamelled
G emailliert
S esmaltado

emballage
E package, pack, packaging
G Packung, Verpacken
S embalaje, envase, envoltura, envasado, empaquetado

emballage à bulles
E blister, well, cup (of blister)
G Blister, Napf (beim Blister)
S blister, pocillo del blíster

emballage à l'export
E export package
G Exportverpackung
S embalaje de exportación

emballage avec gaz inerte
E inert gas packaging
G Schutzgasverpackung
S embalaje con gas inerte

emballage de sécurité pour enfants
E child-proof packaging
G kindersichere Verpackung
S embalaje a prueba de niños

emballage entamé
E open case, open package
G Anbruch
S envase abierto

emballage étanche à l'air
E air-tight pack
G luftdichte Verpackung
S embalaje impermeable al aire

emballage externe
E outer packaging
G Umverpackung
S embalaje externo

emballage fini
E finished pack
G Fertigpackung
S envase terminado

emballage hermétique
E sealed packaging
G Versiegelungsverpackung
S embalaje sellado

emballage manuel
E manual packaging
G Handverpackung
S empaquetado manual

emballage ouvert
E open case, open package
G Anbruch
S envase abierto

emballage plastique
E plastic packaging
G Kunststoffverpackung
S embalaje de plástico

emballage pour hôpitaux
E hospital pack
G Anstaltspackung
S envase clínico

emballage sous film rétractable
E shrink-pack
G eingeschrumpftes Gebinde
S haz contraído, haz comprimido

emballer
E pack, to; package, to
G einpacken, verpacken, konfektionieren
S embalar, empaquetar, envasar

emballer en sachets
E package in bags, to
G in Beutel verpacken
S empaquetar en sobres

embout
E mouthpiece, support
G Mundstück, Stutzen
S boquilla, embocadura, empalme, tubuladura

emboutir
E deep draw, to
G tiefziehen
S embutir a profundidad

emboutissage
E thermoforming
G Thermoverformung
S deformación térmica

emboutisseuse
E thermoforming machine
G Thermoformmaschine
S máquina de deformación térmica

embrayage magnétique
E magnetic clutch
G Magnetkupplung
S acoplamiento magnético

embrocation
E embrocation
G Einreibung
S fricción, frotamiento

émission
E emission
G Emission
S emisión

émissions sonores
E noise development
G Geräuschentwicklung
S producción de ruido

empaquetage par sous-traitance
E contract packaging
G Lohnverpackung
S embalaje por comisión

empaqueter
E package, to
G verpacken
S empaquetar

empaqueteur
E contract packager
G Lohnabpacker
S empaquetador comisionado

empêcher
E prevent, to
G verhindern
S evitar, impedir

empilage
E stacking
G Stapelung
S apilamiento

empilage de conditionnement
E package stacking
G Packungsstapelung
S apilamiento de envases

empilement de réserve
E back-up stack
G Nachlegestapel
S montón de reserva

empiler
E stack, to
G stapeln
S almacenar, amontonar, apilar

empirique
E empirical
G empirisch
S empírico

emplacement
E site, location
G Standort
S emplazamiento, ubicación

emplacement de l'éjection
E reject position
G Auswurfstelle
S zona de expulsión

emplacement des essais cliniques
E clinical trial location
G klinische Prüfeinrichtung
S centro de investigación clínica

emploi
E employment, job
G Arbeitsstelle
S puesto de trabajo

employé
E employee
G Angestellter
S empleado

employé à mi-temps
E part-time employee
G Teilzeitkraft
S empleado a tiempo parcial

empreindre
E emboss, to; imprint, to
G einprägen, aufprägen
S estampar, imprimir

empreinte digitale IR
E IR fingerprint
G IR-Fingerabdruck
S huella dactilar IR

émulseur
E emulsifier
G Emulgiergerät
S emulsor

émulsifiant
E emulsifier, emulsifying agent
G Emulgator
S emulsivo

émulsion
E emulsion
G Emulsion
S emulsión

émulsion de silicone
E silicone emulsion
G Silikonemulsion
S emulsión de silicona

émulsion d'eau dans l'huile
E water/oil emulsion
G Wasser-in-Öl Emulsion
S emulsión de agua en aceite

émulsion d'huile dans l'eau
E oil/water emulsion
G Öl-in-Wasser Emulsion
S emulsión de aceite en agua

émulsionner
E emulsify, to
G emulgieren
S emulsionar

énantiomère
E enantiomer
G Enantiomere
S enantiómero

encapsuler
E encapsulate, to
G verkapseln
S capsular

encapsuleur
E capping machine
G Deckelverschließmaschine
S máquina para cerrar cápsulas

encapsuleuse
E capsule filling machine, encapsulator
G Kapselfüllmaschine, Kapselmaschine
S máquina de relleno de cápsulas, máquina encapsuladora

encastré
E fitted
G eingebaut
S incorporado, instalado, montado

enceinte de risques biologiques
E biohazard cabinet
G Biosicherheitskabinett
S gabinete de seguridad biológica

enchâssé
E encased
G eingeschlossen, umgeben von
S rodeado de

enclencher
E wire, to
G schalten, verdrahten
S conectar, conmutar

encoche de rupture
E break notch, breaking notch, break score
G Bruchrille, Kreuzbruchkerbe
S ranura de ruptura, surco de ruptura, muesca de ruptura

encre
E ink
G Tinte
S tinta

endommagé
E defective, damaged
G beschädigt
S dañado, estropeado, perjudicado

endotoxine
E endotoxin
G Endotoxin
S endotoxina

endotoxine bactérienne
E bacterial endotoxin
G Bakterienendotoxin
S endotoxina bacteriana

endroit
E location
G Lage, Ort
S lugar, situación

endroits difficilement accessibles
E poorly accessible points
G schwer zugängliche Stellen
S lugares de difícil acceso

endroits inaccessibles
E inaccessible points
G unzugängliche Stellen
S lugares inaccesibles

enduction
E coat, coating, film, layer
G Beschichtung, Überzug, Lage, Schicht
S estrato, cubierta, revestimiento

enduire
E coat, to; laminate, to
G beschichten
S laminar, recubrir

enduire à la brosse
E brush coat, to
G einstreichen (mit einer Bürste)
S untar con cepillo

enduit
E coated (tablets)
G überzogen (Tabletten)
S recubierto (comprimidos)

énergie d'activation
E activation energy
G Aktivierungsenergie
S energía de activación

enfermé
E locked location
G unter Verschluß
S cerrado

engendrement
E generation (of)
G Erzeugung
S generación, producción

engrais
E fertiliser
G Düngemittel
S abono, fertilizante

engrenage
E transmission, drive
G Getriebe
S engranaje, transmisión

engrenage à vis sans fin
E worm gear box
G Schneckengetriebe
S engranaje de tornillo si fin

enregistrement
E recording, record, log, registration
G Aufnahme, Aufzeichnung, Registrierung, Protokoll
S toma, registro, protocolo

enregistrement de données
E data recording
G Datenaufnahme
S registro de datos

enregistrement d'un lot
E batch record
G Chargenprotokoll
S protocolo de lotes

enregistrer
E protocol, to; record, to; document, to; enter, to
G protokollieren, eintragen
S levantar acta, protocolar, inscribir, registrar

enregistrer des données
E log, to; record, to; register, to (data)
G aufzeichnen, erfassen (Daten)
S registrar (datos)

enregistreur
E recorder, chart recorder
G Schreiber
S registradora

enregistreur à canaux multiples
E multi-channel recorder
G Mehrkanalschreiber
S registradora de canales múltiples

enregistreur de température
E temperature recorder
G Temperaturschreiber
S registrador de temperatura

enregistreur graphique
E chart recorder
G Diagrammschreiber
S registrador gráfico

enregistreur par ligne pointillée
E dotted-line recorder
G Punktschreiber
S registradora de línea de puntos

enrobage entérique, à
E enteric-coated
G magensaftresistent überzogen
S con cubierta resistente al jugo gástrico

enrober (comprimés)
E coat, to (tablets)
G überziehen (Tabletten)
S recubrir (comprimidos)

ensemencement
E smear
G Ausstrich
S extensión, frotis

ensemencer (colonies microbiol.)
E smear, to (microbiological colonies); inoculate, to
G ausstreichen (mikrobiol. Kolonien), beimpfen (mit Keimen)
S sembrar (colonias microbiológicas), inocular

entaille de rupture
E break notch, break score
G Bruchrille, Bruchkerbe
S ranura de ruptura, surco de ruptura, muesca de ruptura

entéro-soluble
E entero-soluble
G dünndarmlöslich
S soluble en el intestino delgado

entièrement automatique
E fully automatic
G vollautomatisch
S completamente automático

entonnoir
E funnel, hopper
G Trichter
S embudo, tolva

entonnoir d'alimentation
E hopper, funnel
G Schütttrichter
S tolva

entonnoir de Büchner
E Buchner funnel
G Nutsche
S embudo de Buechner

entonnoir séparateur
E separating funnel
G Scheidetrichter
S embudo de separación

entraînement
E training, drive
G Schulung, Antrieb
S adiestramiento, instrucción, impulso, propulsión, tracción

entraînement par chaînes
E chain drive
G Kettenantrieb
S propulsión por cadena

entraînement par courroie
E belt drive
G Riemenantrieb
S propulsión por correa

entraînement par courroie trapézoïdale
E belt drive
G Keilriemenantrieb
S propulsión por correa trapezoidal

entraînement par piston
E piston drive
G Kolbenantrieb
S propulsión por émbolo

entrée d'air
E inlet air
G Zuluft
S entrada de aire

entrée de détecteur
E detector inlet
G Detektoreinlaß
S entrada al detector

entrée des marchandises
E receipt (of goods)
G Wareneingang
S entrada de mercancías

entrée d'une commande
E command, entry
G Befehlseingabe
S entrada de un comando

entrée d'une pompe
E pump inlet
G Pumpeneinlaß
S entrada de una bomba

entreposage non ordonné
E random location storage system
G Lagerhaltung, chaotische
S gestión de stocks caótica

entrepôt
E warehouse, storage room
G Lagerraum, Warenlager
S almacén, almacén de mercancías, depósito

entreprise de nettoyage
E contract cleaner
G Reinigungsfirma
S empresa de limpieza

entreprise de traitement des résidus
E waste disposal company
G Abfallentsorgungsfirma
S empresa de eliminación de desechos

entreprise d'élimination des résidus
E waste disposal company
G Abfallentsorgungsfirma
S empresa de eliminación de desechos

entretien
E maintenance
G Instandhaltung, Wartung
S mantenimiento, entretenimiento

entretien de l'équipement
E equipment maintenance
G Wartung der Ausrüstung
S mantenimiento del equipo

entretien préventif
E preventive maintenance
G vorbeugende Wartung
S mantenimiento preventivo

enveloppe
E jacket, mantle
G Ummantelung
S revestimiento

environnement
E environment
G Umgebung, Umwelt
S entorno, medio ambiente

environnement d'un procédé
E process environment
G Prozeßumgebung
S entorno de un proceso

environnement non controlé
E uncontrolled environment
G nicht kontrollierte Umgebung
S entorno no controlado

envoi
E dispatch, shipment, shipping
G Versand
S envío, expedición

enzyme
E enzyme
G Enzym
S enzima

enzyme de modification de l'ADN
E DNA-modifying enzyme
G DNA-modifizierendes Enzym
S enzima modificador del ADN

enzyme de restriction
E restriction enzyme
G Restriktionsenzym
S enzima restrictivo

épais
E thick, tough
G dick, zäh
S compacto, espeso, grueso, macizo, resistente, tenaz

épaisseur
E thickness
G Dicke
S espesor, grosor

épaisseur de feuille
E film thickness
G Foliendicke
S espesor de lámina

épaisseur de la couche
E coating thickness
G Auftragsdicke
S espesor de la capa

épaisseur de l'enduit
E coating thickness
G Auftragsdicke
S espesor de la capa

épaisseur d'un comprimé
E tablet thickness
G Tablettendicke
S espesor del comprimido

épaisseur d'un mur
E wall thickness
G Wanddicke
S espesor de tabique

épaissir
E concentrate, to; thicken, to
G eindicken, verdicken
S concentrar, condensar, espesar

épaississant
E thickener, thickening agent
G Verdickungsmittel
S espesante

épaulement de pic
E peak shoulder
G Peakschulter
S hombro del pico

épimérisation
E eperimisation
G Epimerisierung
S epimerización

épitaxie d'une couche d'atomes
E atomic layer epitaxy (ALE)
G Atomschichtepitaxie
S epitaxia de un estrato atómico

éponge
E sponge
G Schwamm
S esponja

épreuve du feu, à l'
E fire-proof
G feuergeschützt
S protegido frente al fuego

éprouvette graduée
E graduated measuring cylinder
G graduierter Meßzylinder
S probeta graduada

équation
E equation
G Gleichung (mathematisch)
S ecuación (matemática)

équilibre
E equilibrium
G Gleichgewicht
S equilibrio

rééquilibre
E re-equilibrium
G erneutes Gleichgewicht
S reequilibrio

équipe (de travail)
E shift (working)
G Schicht, Arbeits-
S turno de trabajo

équipement
E equipment
G Ausrüstung
S equipamiento

équipement dédié
E dedicated equipment
G Ausrüstung nur für ein Produkt
S equipamiento sólo para un producto

équipement multi-usage
E multipurpose equipment
G Ausrüstung für verschiedene Produkte
S equipamiento para diferentes productos

équipement de calibration
E calibrating equipment
G Prüfmittel (zur Kalibrierung)
S sistema de prueba (para calibrar)

équipement de nettoyage
E cleaning equipment
G Reinigungsgerät
S aparato de limpieza

équipement d'un procédé de fabrication
E process equipment
G Produktionsanlagen
S equipo de instrumentos para el proceso de producción

équipement pour le prélèvement d'un échantillon
E sampling equipment, sampler
G Probenahmegerät
S aparato de toma de muestras

équiper
E provide with, to; equip, to
G ausrüsten
S equipar

équivalence
E equivalency
G Äquivalenz
S equivalencia

équivalent
E equivalent
G äquivalent
S equivalente

Erlenmeyer
E Erlenmeyer flask
G Erlenmeyerkolben
S matraz de Erlenmeyer

erreur
E defect, error, failure, fault, mistake, confusion, misidentification
G Fehler, Verwechslung
S error, confusión

erreur aléatoire
E random error
G zufälliger Fehler
S error casual

erreur de calcul
E calculation error
G Rechenfehler
S error de cálculo

erreur de mesure
E measuring error
G Meßfehler
S error de medición

erreur de transfer
E transfer error
G Übertragungsfehler
S error de transferencia

erreur humaine
E human error
G menschlicher Fehler
S error humano

escaliers
E stairs
G Treppenhaus
S escalera de la casa

escarpé
E steep
G steil
S empinado, escarpado

espace
E space
G Zwischenraum
S espacio (intermedio)

espace creux
E cavity, hollow space
G Hohlraum, Vertiefung
S cavidad, depresión, espacio hueco

espace de stockage
E storage space
G Lagerplatz
S lugar de almacenamiento

espace de tête
E head space
G Kopfraum, Gasraum
S espacio para la cabeza

espace libre
E clearance
G Freiraum
S espacio libre

espace mort
E dead space
G Totraum
S espacio muerto

espèce
E species
G Art, Gattung, Spezies
S especie, género

espèce d'origine
E origin of species
G Ursprungsart
S especie de origen

essai
E trial, experiment
G Versuch
S ensayo, experimento, prueba

essai clinique
E clinical trial, clinical study
G klinische Prüfung, klinische Studie
S ensayo clínico

réservé aux essais cliniques
E for clinical trial use
G zur klinischen Prüfung bestimmt
S reservado para ensayos clínicos

essai d'aptitude d'un système
E system suitability test
G Systemeignungstest
S ensayo de adecuación de un sistema

essai de compression
E moulding trial
G Preßversuch
S ensayo de compresión

essai de désintégration
E disintegration test
G Zerfallsprüfung
S ensayo de desintegración

essai de dissolution
E dissolution study
G Auflösungsstudie
S estudio de dilución

essai de fonctionnement
E trial run, test run
G Probelauf
S marcha de ensayo

essai de fuite
E leak-test
G Dichtigkeitsprüfung
S prueba de estanqueidad

essai de pénétration thermique
E heat penetration test
G Hitzedurchdringungstest
S prueba de penetración térmica

essai de perte
E leak-test
G Dichtigkeitsprüfung
S prueba de estanqueidad

essai de point de bulle
E bubble point test
G Blasendrucktest
S prueba de presión de vejiga, cistometría

essai de prélèvement par tampon d'ouate
E wipe test, swab test
G Wischtest
S prueba de prelavado con torunda de algodón

essai d'étanchéité
E leak test
G Lecktest, Dichtigkeitsprüfung
S prueba de escape, prueba de estanqueidad

essai en double aveugle
E double-blind study
G Doppelblindversuch
S ensayo de doble ciego

essai répété
E re-test
G Wiederholungsprüfung
S ensayo de repetición

English German French Spanish

essieu
E shaft
G Schaft, Welle
S árbol, asta, eje

estampage
E embossment
G Prägung
S acuñado, estampado, troquelado

estampé
E embossed
G geprägt
S acuñado, estampado

estamper
E punch, to; emboss, to; stamp, to
G einstanzen, stanzen, prägen
S estampar, troquelar, acuñar, punzonar

estérification
E esterification
G Veresterung
S esterificación

établi
E bench, work bench
G Arbeitstisch, Werkbank
S mesa de trabajo, banco de trabajo

établir
E implement, to
G implementieren
S establecer, realizar

établissement industriel
E facility, plant (machines)
G Anlage (Maschine)
S equipo, instalación (máquina)

étage du service technique
E technical floor
G Technikgeschoß
S piso de servicio técnico

étage intermédiaire
E mezzanine
G Zwischengeschoß
S piso intermedio

étagère
E shelf
G Regal
S estante

étagère de stockage
E high-bay storage, shelf
G Hochregallager, Lagerregal
S almacén de estanterías altas, estante de almacén

étagère d'entreposage
E shelf
G Lagerregal
S estante de almacén

étalement de pic
E peak spreading
G Peakverbreiterung
S ensanchamiento del pico

étalon interne
E internal standard
G interner Standard
S estándar interno

étalonnement
E alignment, adjustment
G Justierung
S ajuste

étalonner
E adjust, to
G justieren
S ajustar

étanche
E leak-tight, impervious to moisture
G dicht, feuchtigkeitsundurchlässig
S hermético, impermeable a la humedad

non étanche
E leaky
G undicht
S permeable

étanche à la poussière
E dust-tight
G staubdicht
S hermético para el polvo

étanche à l'air
E air-tight
G luftdicht
S hermético, impermeable al aire

étanche au gaz
E gas-tight
G gasdicht
S impermeable al gas

étanchéifier
E tighten, to; seal, to
G abdichten
S cerrar herméticamente

étanchéité
E tightness
G Dichtigkeit
S estanqueidad, hermeticidad

étanchéité d'un poinçon
E punch tightness
G Stempeldichtigkeit
S estanqueidad del troquel

étanchement d'un filtre
E filter seal
G Filterabdichtung
S cierre hermético de un filtro

étape critique d'un procédé
E critical processing step
G kritischer Prozeßschritt
S etapa crítica de un proceso

étape de fabrication
E manufacturing step
G Herstellungsstufe
S etapa de producción

étape de permutation
E switching stage
G Schaltstufe
S etapa de conmutación

étapes, par
E stepwise
G stufenweise, schrittweise
S gradualmente, paso a paso

état de développement
E development status
G Entwicklungsstatus
S status de desarrollo

état intermédiaire
E intermediate stage
G Zwischenstufe
S nivel intermediario

état membre
E member state
G Mitgliedstaat
S estado miembro

éteindre
E blow out, to
G ausblasen
S apagar soplando

étendre
E apply, to
G aufbringen, auftragen
S aplicar, extender, untar

étendue
E circumference, width
G Umfang, Weite
S circunferencia, perímetro, anchura, amplitud, extensión

étendue d'un brevet
E patent scope
G Patentumfang
S extensión de una patente

éthique
E ethical
G ethisch
S ético

étincelles
E sparks
G Funken
S chispas

étiquetage
E labelling, lettering
G Etikettierung, Beschriftung, Kennzeichnung
S etiquetado, marcado, rotulado

étiqueter
E mark, to; label, to; designate, to
G kennzeichnen, bezeichnen
S etiquetar, marcar, denominar, rotular

étiquette
E label
G Eitkett
S etiqueta

étiquettes autoadhésives
E self-adhesive labels
G selbstklebende Etiketten, Haftetiketten
S etiquetas autoadhesivas

étiquettes en rouleaux
E roll-fed labels
G Etiketten auf Rollen
S etiquetas en rollo

étiquettes prédécoupées
E loose labels, cut labels, transferable labels
G lose Etiketten, Abziehetiketten
S etiquetas sueltas, etiquetas separables

être chargé (d'une affaire)
E be in charge of, to
G beauftragt sein mit
S estar encargado de

être en conformité avec
E conform with, to
G übereinstimmen mit
S coincidir con

étude de stabilité
E stability study
G Stabilitätsuntersuchung
S ensayo de estabilidad

étude de stabilité à court terme
E short-term stability
G Kurzzeitstabilität
S estabilidad a corto plazo

étude de stabilité à long terme
E long-term stability
G Langzeitstabilität
S estabilidad a largo plazo

étude toxicologique
E toxicological testing
G toxikologische Prüfung
S prueba toxicológica

étui du capteur
E sensor housing
G Sensorgehäuse
S caja del sensor

étuve
E dry heat oven
G Trockenofen
S estufa de secado, horno de secado

eutectique
E eutectic
G eutektisch
S eutéctico

évacuer
E empty, to; evacuate, to
G entleeren
S vaciar

évaluation
E interpretation, evaluation, determination
G Auswertung, Bestimmung
S evaluación, interpretación, análisis, determinación

évaluation (de données)
E evaluation, assessment (of data)
G Bewertung (von Daten)
S evaluación (de datos)

évaluer
E evaluate, to; assess, to; determine, to
G bewerten, ermitteln, bestimmen
S evaluar, averiguar, determinar

évaporateur
E evaporator
G Verdampfer
S evaporador

évaporateur Kestner
E rising film evaporator
G Kletterverdampfer
S evaporador Kestner

English German French Spanish

évaporateur rotatif
E rotatory evaporator
G Rotationsverdampfer
S evaporador rotatorio

évaporateur sous vide
E vacuum evaporation
G Vakuumverdampfer
S evaporador de vacío

évaporation
E evaporation
G Verdunstung
S evaporación, vaporización

évaporation du solvant
E solvent evaporation
G Verdampfen des Lösungsmittels
S evaporación del solvente

évaporer
E evaporate, to
G eindampfen, verdunsten, abdampfen
S evaporar, evaporarse, volatilizar

évaporisation
E vaporisation
G Verdampfung
S evaporación, vaporización

évidure
E recess
G Aussparung
S hueco, vacío

évier
E sink, wash basin
G Ausguß, Waschbecken
S descarga, orificio de descarga, lavabo

éviter
E prevent, to; avoid, to
G verhindern, vermeiden
S evitar, impedir, eludir

évolution de la teneur en oxygène
E oxygen release
G Sauerstoffentwicklung
S liberación de oxígeno

exactitude
E accuracy
G Richtigkeit (einer Prüfmethode)
S corrección, exactitud (de un método de prueba)

exactitude de contrôle
E control accuracy
G Regelgenauigkeit
S exactitud de la regulación

exactitude de dosage
E metering accuracy
G Dosiergenauigkeit
S exactitud de la dosificación

exactitude de longueur d'onde
E wavelength accuracy
G Wellenlängengenauigkeit
S exactitud de la longitud de onda

exactitude de réglage
E control accuracy
G Regelgenauigkeit
S exactitud de la regulación

exactitude d'un poids
E weight accuracy
G Gewichtsgenauigkeit
S exactitud del peso

examen d'entrée
E examination on receipt
G Eingangsprüfung
S examen inicial

examen médical
E medical examination
G ärztliche Untersuchung
S exploración médica

examen médical suite à une embauche
E medical examination on starting a new job
G Einstellungsuntersuchung
S exploración médica al ser empleado

examen physiologique
E physiological testing
G physiologische Prüfung
S prueba fisiológica

examen supplétif
E subsequent test
G Nachuntersuchung
S examen adicional

examen visuel
E visual examination
G Sichtprüfung
S inspección visual

examens biologiques
E biological testing
G biologische Prüfung
S prueba biológica

excédent de poids
E excess weight
G Mehrgewicht
S excedente de peso

excéder une limite
E exceed, to (a limit)
G überschreiten
S exceder

excès
E excess
G Überschuß
S excedente, sobrante

excipient
E excipient, adjuvant
G Hilfsstoff
S excipiente, sustancia auxiliar

excrétion
E excretion
G Exkretion
S excreción

exécutant
E operator
G Durchführender
S ejecutante,operador

exécuter
E carry out, to; execute, to
G durchführen
S ejecutar, llevar a cabo, realizar

exempt de vibration
E vibration-free
G erschütterungsfrei
S sin vibración

exigé
E required
G gefordert
S exigido, reclamado

exigence
E requirement
G Anforderung, Erfordernis
S exigencia, requerimiento, necesidad

exigence légale
E legal requirement
G gesetzliche Anforderung
S requerimiento legal

exiger
E require, to; demand, to
G erfordern, fordern
S exigir, necesitar, requerir

expansion
E expansion
G Ausdehnung
S ampliación, dilatación, expansión, extensión

expédier
E dispatch, to; ship, to
G versenden
S enviar, expedir

expédition
E dispatch, shipment, shipping
G Versand
S envío, expedición

expérience
E trial, experiment, run
G Versuch, Lauf
S ensayo, experimento, prueba, ciclo, marcha, recorrido

expériences réalisées sur animaux
E animal experiment
G Tierversuch
S experimento con animales

expert
E expert, qualified person, assessor
G Begutachter, Sachkundiger, Sachverständiger
S asesor, experto, perito

expertise
E expertise
G Gutachten
S dictamen

expiration d'un brevet
E patent expiry
G Auslaufen des Patentes
S expiración de una patente

expirer
E expire, to
G verfallen
S caducar, expirar

explication
E rationale, reasoning
G Begründung
S argumentación, razonamiento

explosivité
E explosiveness
G Explosivität
S explosividad

exposé des motifs
E rationale, reasoning
G Begründung
S argumentación, razonamiento

expulser
E eject, to
G ausstoßen
S emitir, expeler, expulsar

extension longitudinale
E linear extension
G Längenausdehnung
S expansión longitudinal

externe
E external
G äußerlich
S externo

extincteur
E fire extinguisher
G Feuerlöscher
S extintor (de incendios)

extraction
E extraction
G Extraktion
S extracción

extraction en phase solide
E solid phase extraction
G Festphasenextraktion
S extracción en fase sólida

extraction liquide-liquide
E liquid-liquid extraction
G flüssig-flüssig-Extraktion
S extracción líquido-líquido

extrahir par percolation
E percolate, to
G perkolieren
S percolar

extraire
E extract, to
G extrahieren
S extraer

extrait
E extract
G Extrakt, Auszug
S extracto

extrait liquide
E liquid extract
G Flüssigextrakt
S extracto líquido

extrait sec
E dry extract
G Trockenextrakt
S extracto seco

extrait solide
E solid extract
G Dickextrakt
S extracto sólido

English German French Spanish

extrapolation (d'un procédé)
E scale-up (of a procedure)
G Maßstabsvergößerung (eines Verfahrens)
S aumento a escala (de un proceso)

extrémités
E dead spots
G tote Enden
S extremos de desecho

extruder
E extrude, to
G extrudieren
S extrudir

extrudeuse
E extruder
G Extruder, Strangpresse
S extrusor, prensa extrusora

extrusion
E extrusion
G Extrusion
S extrusión

fabricant
E manufacturer
G Hersteller
S fabricante

fabricant de cuves
E vessel manufacturer
G Behälterbauer
S fabricante de recipientes

fabricant de matériel d'emballage
E packaging material manufacturer
G Packmittelhersteller
S fabricante de material de embalaje

fabricant d'équipement
E equipment manufacturer
G Gerätehersteller
S fabricante de aparatos

fabrication
E manufacture, production, processing
G Herstellung, Bearbeitung, Verarbeitung
S fabricación, elaboración, transformación

fabrication à l'échelle industrielle
E industrial scale manufacture
G Herstellung im industriellen Maßstab
S fabricación a escala industrial

fabrication aseptique
E aseptic processing
G aseptische Herstellung
S fabricación aséptica

fabrication de comprimés
E tabletting, compression, compaction
G Tablettierung
S fabricación de comprimidos

fabrication de comprimés informatisée
E computer-integrated tabletting (CIT)
G computerintegrierte Tablettierung
S fabricación informatizada de comprimidos

fabrication en continu
E continuous operation
G Dauerbetrieb
S funcionamiento continuo

fabrication en sous-traitance
E contract manufacture
G Herstellung im Lohnauftrag
S fabricación por comisión

fabrication informatisée
E computer-integrated manufacturing (CIM)
G computerintegrierte Herstellung
S fabricación informatizada

fabrication par sous-traitance
E contract manufacture
G Lohnherstellung
S fabricación por comisión

fabrication standard
E standard construction
G Grundausführung
S versión básica

face inférieure
E base
G Unterseite
S lado inferior

face supérieure
E upper side, top side
G Oberseite
S lado superior

facilité de glissement d'un poinçon
E easy punch sliding
G Stempelleichtgängigkeit
S facilidad de deslizamiento del troquel

façonnage de feuilles
E film forming
G Folienverformung
S deformación de láminas

facteur de rétention
E retention factor
G Retentionsfaktor
S factor de retención

facteur de standardisation
E standardisation factor
G Standardfaktor
S factor estándar

facteurs de croissance
E growth factors
G Wachstumsfaktoren
S factores de crecimiento

fade
E tasteless, flavourless
G geschmacklos
S insípido

faillir à sa tâche
E fail, to
G versagen
S fracasar

faire couler
E drain, to; discharge, to (liquids)
G ablassen (Flüssigkeiten)
S dar salida, dejar escapar

faire fermenter
E ferment, to
G fermentieren
S fermentar

faire fondre
E melt, to; fuse, to
G einschmelzen
S fundir

faire référence à
E refer to, to
G verweisen auf
S referir a

faire rougir
E ignite, to
G ausglühen
S calcinar

faire saillir
E project, to; protrude, to
G überhängen, überstehen
S pender sobre, sobresalir, resaltar

faisceau de référence
E reference beam
G Referenzstrahl
S rayo de referencia

falsification
E falsification
G Fälschung, Verfälschung
S falsificación

falsifier
E falsify, to
G verfälschen
S falsificar

fatigue du matériel
E material fatigue
G Materialermüdung
S fatiga del material

English German French Spanish

faux plafond
E intermediate ceiling, suspended ceiling
G Zwischendecke, abgehängte Decke
S techo intermedio, techo suspendido

fécondité
E non-sterility
G Unsterilität
S fertilidad, fecundidad

fêlé
E cracked (glass)
G gesprungen (Glas)
S quebrado (vidrio)

fenêtre de visée
E observation window
G Sichtfenster
S ventana visual

fenêtre d'observation
E observation window, observation port
G Schauglas, Beobachtungsfenster
S ventana de observación

fente
E slit, cleft, notch
G Spalte, Spalt, Schlitz, Kerbe
S fisura, hendidura, raja, muesca

fermé hermétiquement
E sealed
G verplombt
S precintado

fermentation
E fermentation
G Fermentation, Gärung
S fermentación

fermenteur
E fermenter
G Fermenter
S fermentador

fermer
E seal, to; close off, to
G verschließen, absperren
S cerrar, cortar

fermer à clef
E lock, to
G arretieren
S fijar, parar, retener

fermer une ampoule
E seal an ampoule, to
G Ampulle verschließen
S cerrar una ampolla

fermeture
E seal
G Versiegelung
S sellado

fermeture à baïonnette
E bayonet connection
G Bajonettverschluß
S conexión de bayoneta

fermeture à vis
E screw connection
G Schraubverschluß
S cierre de rosca

fermeture de sécurité pour enfants
E child-resistant closure
G Verschluß, kindersicherer
S cierre a prueba de niños

fermeture hermétique
E hermetic seal
G hermetischer Verschluß
S cierre hermético

fermeture mécanique
E mechanical seal
G Verschluß, mechanischer
S cierre mecánico

fermeture pour gel
E gel seal
G Gelverschluß
S cierre por gel

feuille
E foil, film
G Folie
S hoja, lámina

feuille continue
E continuous foil, continuous film
G endlose Folie
S lámina continua

feuille d'aluminium
E aluminium foil
G Aluminiumfolie
S hoja de aluminio

feuille de données de sécurité
E material safety data sheet (MSDS)
G Sicherheitsdatenblatt
S hoja de datos de seguridad, pliego de datos de seguridad

feuille de protection
E cover foil
G Deckfolie
S hoja de recubrimiento

feuille en gaine
E tubular film, film tube
G Schlauchfolie
S película tubular

feuille enduite
E coated foil, coated film
G beschichtete Folie
S lámina recubierta

feuille estampée
E embossed film
G Prägefolie
S lámina de estampado

feuille rétractable
E shrink foil, shrink film
G Schrumpffolie
S lámina retraíble

feuille stratifiée
E laminated foil, composite foil
G Verbundfolie
S hoja laminada, lámina estratificada

feuille thermoformée
E forming foil, thermoforming foil
G Verformfolie, Tiefziehfolie
S lámina termoformada

feuille transparente
E transparent foil
G Klarsichtfolie
S lámina transparente, película transparente

feuillet de données sur la sécurité
E safety data sheet
G Sicherheitsdatenblatt
S pliego de datos de seguridad, hoja de datos de seguridad

feux clignotant
E flash light
G Blinklicht
S luz intermitente

fiabilité
E reliability
G Zuverlässigkeit, Verläßlichkeit
S fiabilidad, confiabilidad

fiabilité d'une dose
E dose reliability
G Zuverlässigkeit der Dosierung
S fiabilidad de la dosificación

fiable
E reliable
G zuverlässig, verläßlich
S fiable, confiable

fibre
E fibre
G Faser
S fibra

fibre artificielle
E artificial fibre
G Kunstfaser
S fibra artificial

fibre de verre
E fibreglass
G Glasfaser
S fibra de vidrio

figure
E drawing
G Zeichnung
S dibujo

fil
E thread
G Faden
S hilo

fil métallique
E wire
G Draht
S alambre

filetage
E thread, screw thread
G Gewinde, Schraubgewinde
S filete, rosca, filete de tornillo, rosca de tornillo

à droite
E right-handed
G rechtsgängig
S de paso derecho

à gauche
E left-handed
G linksgängig
S de paso izquierdo

filets du tube
E tube thread
G Tubengewinde
S rosca de tubo

filiale (société)
E subsidiary company
G Tochterfirma
S empresa filial, empresa subsidiaria

film adhésif
E adhesive film
G Klebefolie
S película adhesiva

film aqueux
E aqueous film coating
G wäßrige Filmbeschichtung
S película acuosa de revestimiento

film de revêtement
E coating
G Filmüberzug
S película de revestimiento

film plastique
E plastic film
G Plastikfolie
S lámina de plástico

film rétractable
E shrink foil, shrink film
G Schrumpffolie
S lámina retraíble

filtrat
E filtrate
G Filtrat
S filtrado

filtration
E filtration
G Filtration
S filtración

filtration par membrane
E membrane filtration
G Membranfiltration
S filtración por membrana

filtration stérile
E sterile filtration
G Sterilfiltration
S filtración estéril

filtration sur gel
E gel filtration
G Gelfiltration
S filtración por gel

filtre
E filter
G Filter
S filtro

filtre à air
E air filter
G Luftfilter
S filtro de aire

filtre à air d'évacuation
E exhaust air filter
G Abluftfilter
S filtro del aire de escape

filtre à membrane
E membrane filter
G Membranfilter
S filtro de membrana

filtre à particules
E particle filter
G Partikelfilter
S filtro de partículas

filtre à poches
E filter bag
G Filtersack
S bolsa filtro

filtre à poussières fines
E fine dust filter
G Feinstaubfilter
S filtro de polvo fino

filtre antipoussières à haute performance
E high efficiency particulate air (HEPA) filter
G Hochleistungsschwebstoffilter
S filtro antipolvo de gran rendimiento

filtre au carbone
E carbon filter
G Kohlefilter
S filtro de carbón

filtre biologique
E biological filter
G Biofilter
S filtro biológico

filtre cannelé
E fluted filter
G Faltenfilter
S filtro acanalado

filtre coalescent
E coalescing filter
G Koaleszenzfilter
S filtro de coalescencia

filtre d'admission
E inlet filter
G Eingangsfilter, Einlaßfilter
S filtro de entrada

filtre de graviers
E gravel filter
G Kiesbettfilter
S filtro de grava

filtre de retenue d'huile
E oil-separating filter
G Ölabscheidefilter
S filtro de separación de aceite

filtre de sortie
E outlet filter
G Auslaßfilter
S filtro de descarga, filtro de salida

filtre de ventilation
E vent filter
G Belüftungsfilter
S filtro de ventilación

filtre d'entrée
E inlet filter
G Eingangsfilter, Einlaßfilter
S filtro de entrada

filtre en amiante
E asbestos filter
G Asbestfilter
S filtro de asbesto

filtre microporeux
E membrane filter
G Membranfilter
S filtro de membrana

filtre nervuré
E fluted filter
G Faltenfilter
S filtro acanalado

filtre préalable
E pre-filter
G Vorfilter
S filtro previo

filtre profondeur
E depth filter
G Tiefenfilter
S filtro de profundidad

filtre renforcé à la fibre de verre
E fibreglass-reinforced filter
G glasfaserverstärkter Filter
S filtro reforzado con fibra de vidrio

filtre stérile terminal
E terminal sterile filter
G Sterilfilter, endständiger
S filtro estéril terminal

filtre terminal
E terminal filter
G endständiger Filter
S filtro terminal

filtrer
E filter, to
G filtrieren, abnutschen, kolieren
S filtrar

filtres HEPA
E HEPA (high efficiency particulate air) filters
G HEPA-Filter
S filtro HEPA

fin d'un essai clinique
E end of study, end of trial
G Studienende
S fin del estudio

fiole
E jar, wide-necked vessel, vial
G Weithalsgefäß, Gläschen
S recipiente de cuello ancho, vial

fiole en verre
E glass vial
G Glasfläschchen
S vial de vidrio

fiole Eppendorf
E Eppendorf reaction vessel
G Eppendorf-Reaktionsgefäß
S tubo de ensayo Eppendorf

fissure
E crack, tear, slit, cleft
G Riß, Schlitz, Spalt, Spalte
S desgarro, fisura, hendidura, raja

fissure capillaire
E hairline crack
G Haarriß
S fisura capilar

fixation
E fixing, attachment
G Befestigung
S fijación

flacon
E flask, vial
G Kolben, Gläschen, Fläschchen
S alambique, matraz, retorta, botellín, frasco, vial

flacon à fond plat
E Erlenmeyer flask
G Erlenmeyerkolben
S matraz de Erlenmeyer

flacon compte-gouttes
E dropping bottle
G Tropfflasche
S frasco cuentagotas

flacon de pipette
E pipette bottle
G Pipettenflasche
S frasco de pipeteo

flacon d'échantillon
E sample vial
G Probenfläschchen
S vial de muestras

flacon d'injection
E injection vial
G Injektionsflasche
S vial de inyección

flacon d'iode
E iodine flask
G Iodzahlkolben
S matraz de índice de iodo

flacon doseur
E dropping bottle
G Tropfflasche
S frasco cuentagotas

flacon en verre
E glass vial
G Glasfläschchen
S vial de vidrio

flacon laveur
E wash bottle
G Waschflasche, Spritzflasche
S frasco de lavado, matraz de lavado

flacon saupoudreur
E sprinkler can
G Streudose
S frasco espolvoreador

flacon souple doseur
E squeeze bottle
G Quetschflasche
S recipiente flexible

flamme ouverte
E naked flame
G offene Flamme
S llama abierta

fléau de balance
E weighing beam
G Wiegebalken
S ástil, cruz de la balanza

fleur
E blossom
G Blüte
S flor

flexible
E flexible, pliable
G biegsam
S flexible, maleable, plegable

floconneux
E flaky
G flockig
S flocular

floculation
E flocculation
G Flockung
S floculación

floculer
E flocculate, to; flake, to
G ausflocken
S flocular

fluctuation de pression
E pressure fluctuation
G Druckschwankung
S fluctuación de presión

fluctuer
E vary, to; fluctuate, to
G schwanken
S fluctuar, variar

fluide
E non-viscous, thin, thin-bodied, free flowing
G dünnflüssig, freifließend
S fluido, fluyendo libremente

fluidifiant
E flow promoter (in tabletting)
G Fließmittel (in der Tablettierung)
S fluidificante (fabricación de comprimidos)

fluidisation
E fluidisation
G Wirbelschichtverfahren
S procedimiento de lecho fluidificado

fluidité
E flowability
G Fließfähigkeit
S fluidez

fluorescence
E fluorescence
G Fluoreszenz
S fluorescencia

fluorescent
E fluorescent
G fluoreszierend
S fluorescente

fluorométrie
E fluorometry
G Fluorometrie
S fluorometría

fluoruration
E fluorination
G Fluorierung
S fluoración

fluorure de polyvinylidène (PVDF)
E polyvinylidene fluoride (PVDF)
G Polyvinylidenfluorid
S fluoruro de polivinilideno

flux d'air laminaire
E laminar air flow
G Laminarströmung
S corriente laminar

flux des matériaux
E material flow
G Materialfluß
S flujo de material

flux du personnel
E personnel flow
G Personalfluß
S flujo de personal

flux laminaire
E laminar flow
G Laminarfluß, laminare Strömung
S flujo laminar

flux turbulent
E turbulent flow
G turbulente Strömung
S flujo turbulento

fonction d'audit
E audit function
G Auditfunktion
S función de la auditoría

fonction d'écrasement
E overwrite function
G Überschreibfunktion
S función sobreescribir

fonctionnalité
E operability, functionality
G Funktionsfähigkeit
S capacidad funcional

fonctionnement automatique
E automatic operation, unmanned operation
G automatischer Betrieb
S funcionamiento automático

fondé de pouvoirs
E executive with power of procuration
G Prokurist
S apoderado general

fondre
E melt, to; fuse, to
G schmelzen, einschmelzen
S fundir

fongicide
E fungicide, fungicidal
G Fungizid, fungizid
S fungicida

forage
E bore
G Bohrung
S perforación

force
E force
G Kraft
S fuerza

force d'adhérence
E adhesive strength
G Klebekraft
S fuerza adhesiva

force d'adhésion
E adhesive force, adhesive power
G Bindekraft, Haftkraft
S fuerza adhesiva

force d'attraction
E force of attraction
G Anziehungskraft
S fuerza de atracción

force de centrifugation
E centrifugal force
G Zentrifugalkraft, Fliehkraft
S fuerza centrífuga

force de cisaillement
E shear strength
G Scherkraft
S fuerza de cizallamiento

force de cohésion
E cohesive power
G Kohäsionskraft
S fuerza de cohesión

force de compression
E compaction force
G Preßkraft
S fuerza de compresión

force de compression préalable
E pre-compression force
G Vorpreßkraft
S fuerza de compresión previa

force de frappe
E impact force
G Schlagkraft
S fuerza impactante,
fuerza de percusión

force de friction
E frictional force
G Reibungskraft
S fuerza de fricción

force de frottement
E frictional force
G Reibungskraft
S fuerza de fricción

force de gravité
E gravity
G Schwerkraft
S fuerza de gravedad

force de torsion
E torsion force
G Drehkraft
S fuerza de rotación

force de traction
E tensile force
G Zugkraft
S fuerza de tracción

force de vente
E field force, sales force
G Außendienst
S servicio externo de ventas

force d'éjection
E ejection force
G Ausstoßkraft
S fuerza de eyección

force d'impact
E impact force
G Schlagkraft
S fuerza impactante,
fuerza de percusión

force portante
E loading capacity
G Tragfähigkeit
S capacidad de carga

format
E format, size
G Format
S formato, tamaño

format de compression
E compression format
G Preßformat
S formato de compresión

formation de chélate
E chelate formation
G Chelatbildung
S formación de quelatos

formation de complexes
E complex formation
G Komplexbildung
S secuestración

formation de gel
E gel formation
G Gelbildung
S gelación

formation de moisissure
E mould growth
G Schimmelbefall
S crecimiento de moho

formation de mousse
E foam formation, foaming
G Schaumbildung
S formación de espuma

formation de plis
E wrinkling
G Faltenbildung
S formación de arrugas, formación de pliegues

formation de rides
E wrinkling
G Faltenbildung
S formación de arrugas, formación de pliegues

formation de sels
E salt formation
G Salzbildung
S salificación

formation du personnel
E personnel training
G Personalschulung
S formación del personal

formation d'un front (HPLC)
E fronting (in HPLC)
G Frontbildung (HPLC)
S formación de frente (HPLC)

formation d'un granulome
E granuloma formation
G Bildung eines Granuloms
S formación de un granuloma

formation professionnelle
E vocational training
G Berufsausbildung
S formación profesional

forme (de particules)
E shape (of particles)
G Form (z. B. von Partikeln)
S forma (por ejemplo de partículas)

forme de dosage solide
E solid dosage forms
G feste Formen
S formas sólidas de dosificación

forme d'hélice, en
E spiral
G spiralförmig
S espiraliforme

forme du dosage
E dosage form, administration form
G Darreichungsform
S forma de administración

forme d'un poinçon
E punch shape, punch form
G Stempelform
S forma del troquel

forme d'une particule
E particle form, particle shape
G Partikelform, Teilchenform
S forma de la partícula, forma de las partículas

forme d'une unité de prise
E single dose unit
G einzeldosierte Arzneiform
S forma farmacéutica de dosis única

forme liquide (spécialités pharmaceutiques)
E liquid form
G flüssige Form
S forma líquida de administración

forme ovale
E ovality
G Ovalität
S ovalidad

forme pharmaceutique
E dosage form
G Arzneiform
S forma farmacéutica

forme pharmaceutique monolithique
E single dose form
G monolithische Arzneiform
S formulación monolítica

forme stérile
E sterile form
G sterile Zubereitung
S forma estéril, preparación estéril

formulaire
E form, pre-printed form
G Formular, Vordruck
S formulario

formulation
E preparation, formulation
G Zubereitung, Rezeptur, Formgebung, Galenik
S formulación, preparación, fórmula galénica

formulation avec libération contrôlée
E controlled release formulation
G Formulierung mit kontrollierter Freisetzung
S formulación con liberación controlada

formulation de base
E basic formulation
G Basisformulierung
S formulación básica, formulación de base

formulation primaire
E primary formulation
G Primärformulierung
S formulación primaria

formule
E formula
G Formel
S fórmula

formule brute
E molecular formula
G Molekularformel
S fórmula molecular

formule développée
E structural formula
G Strukturformel
S fórmula estructural

formule empirique
E empirical formula
G empirische Formel
S fórmula empírica

forure d'une matrice
E pitch die
G Matrizenbohrung
S orificio de matriz

four
E furnace
G Schmelzofen
S horno fundidor

four à air chaud
E hot air oven
G Heißluftofen
S horno de aire caliente

four à moufle
E muffle furnace
G Muffelofen
S horno de manguito

four pour colonne
E column oven
G Säulenofen
S horno de columna

fournir
E supply, to
G liefern, versorgen mit
S abastecer, proveer, suministrar

fournisseur
E supplier, vendor
G Lieferant
S abastecedor, proveedor

fraction
E fraction
G Fraktion
S fracción

fraction de poudre
E powder fraction
G Pulverfraktion
S fracción de polvo

fraction de tamisage
E sieve fraction
G Siebfraktion
S fracción de tamizado

fractionner
E fractionate, to
G fraktionieren
S fraccionar

fracture du métal
E metal fracture
G Metallbruch
S fractura de un metal

fragile
E fragile
G zerbrechlich
S frágil

fragilité
E brittleness
G Brüchigkeit
S fragilidad, friabilidad

fragment
E fragment, piece, fraction
G Bruchstück
S fragmento

frais d'achat
E purchase price
G Anschaffungskosten
S costes de adquisición

frein à disques multiples
E multiple disk brake
G Lamellenbremse
S freno de discos múltiples

fréquence
E frequency
G Häufigkeit
S frecuencia

friction
E friction
G Reibung
S fricción, frotamiento

fritte de verre
E glass sinter
G Glassinter
S sínter de vidrio

fritter
E sinter, to
G sintern
S aglomerar, sinterizar

front de migration du solvant
E solvent front
G Fließmittelfront
S frente de migración del solvente

fuire
E drop, to
G tropfen
S gotear

fuite
E leak, leakage
G Leck, Undichtigkeit
S escape, permeabilidad

fumigant
E fumigant
G Begasungsmittel
S fumigante

fumigation
E fumigation, flushing, purging
G Begasung, Raumbegasung
S fumigación

fusible
E fuse
G Sicherung (elektrisch)
S cortacircuito, fusible

fusible à action instantanée
E fast fuse
G flinke Sicherung
S fusible rápido

fusible à action retardée
E slow fuse
G träge Sicherung
S fusible lento

fusion
E melt
G Schmelze
S fundición, fusión

fusion (d'entreprises)
E merger, fusion
G Zusammenschluß von Firmen
S fusión de empresas

gaine
E jacket, mantle
G Ummantelung
S revestimiento

galet de guidage
E casters
G Laufrollen, Lenkrollen
S polea, roldana

galvanisé au zinc
E galvanised
G verzinkt
S galvanizado con zinc

gamme
E range
G Bandbreite
S anchura de banda, gama, márgenes

gamme de couleurs
E colour scale
G Farbskala
S escala cromática

gamme de mesure
E measuring range
G Meßbereich
S zona de medición

gants
E gloves
G Handschuhe
S guante

gants à usage unique
E disposable gloves
G Einmalhandschuhe
S guantes de uso único

gants protecteurs
E protective gloves
G Schutzhandschuhe
S guantes protectores

garantie
E guarantee, warranty
G Garantie
S garantía

garantie de stérilité
E sterility assurance
G Sterilisationssicherheit
S garantía de esterilización

garantir
E guarantee, to; secure, to; ensure, to
G sicherstellen
S asegurar, garantizar

garnissage (de récipients)
E lining (of containers)
G Auskleidung (von Behältern)
S revestimiento (de recipientes)

garniture
E fitting
G Armatur
S armadura, accesorios

garniture de couvercle
E cover fitting
G Haubenhalterung
S soporte del casquete

garniture d'un gicleur
E nozzle insert
G Düseneinsatz
S inserción de la tobera

gas de purge
E purge gas
G Spülgas
S gas purgante

gaspillage
E material wastage
G Materialverschwendung
S derroche de material

gaz
E gas
G Gas
S gas

gaz dissous sous pression
E pressure-dissolved gases
G unter Druck gelöste Gase
S gas diluido a presión

gaz comprimés
E compressed gases
G komprimierte Gase
S gases comprimidos

gaz d'échappement
E exhaust gas, waste gas
G Abgas
S gas de escape

gaz d'évacuation
E exhaust gas, waste gas
G Abgas
S gas de escape

gaz inerte
E inert gas, rare gas
G Edelgas, Schutzgas
S gas noble, gas inerte

gaz liquéfiés
E liquified gases
G verflüssigte Gase
S gases licuados

gaz liquide
E liquid gas
G Flüssiggas
S gas líquido

gaz porteur
E carrier gas
G Trägergas
S gas portador

gaz propulseur
E propellant (gas)
G Treibgas
S propelente

gaz rare
E inert gas, rare gas
G Edelgas
S gas noble

gaze
E swab, gauze, pad
G Mull, Tupfer
S gasa, torunda

gazeux
E gaseous
G gasförmig
S gaseoso

gel
E gel
G Gel
S gel

gel auriculaire
E ear gel
G Ohrengel
S gel auricular

gel bleu
E blue silica gel
G Blaugel
S gel azul de sílice

gel de silice
E silica gel
G Kieselgel, Silicagel
S gel de sílice

gel nasal
E nasal gel
G Nasengel
S gel nasal

gel pour administration orale
E oral gel
G Gel zum Einnehmen
S gel oral

gel pour œil
E eye gel
G Augengel
S gel oftálmico

gel pour utilisation endo-cervicale
E endocervical gel
G Gel zur endozervikalen Anwendung
S gel de uso endocervical

gel rectal
E rectal gel
G Rektalgel
S gel rectal

gel vaginal
E vaginal gel
G Vaginalgel
S gel vaginal

geler
E gel, to
G gelieren
S gelar

gélifiant
E gelling agent, gel-forming agent, gellant
G Geliermittel, Gelbildner
S gelificante

gélose chocolat
E chocolate agar
G Schokoladenagar
S agar chocolate

gélule
E hard gelatine capsule, hard capsule
G Hartgelatinekapsel, Steckkapsel
S cápsula de gelatina dura, cápsula gelatinosa dura

gélule molle
E soft gelatine capsule
G Weichgelatinekapsel
S cápsula de gelatina blanda

générateur
E generator
G Generator
S generador

générateur de courant d'urgence
E emergency power supply
G Notstromaggregat
S generador eléctrico de emergencia

générateur de fumée
E smoke generator
G Raucherzeuger
S generador de humo

générateur de hasard
E random number generator
G Zufallsgenerator
S generador aleatorio

générateur de vapeur pure
E pure steam generator
G Reindampferzeuger
S generador de vapor puro

générateur d'impulsions
E pulse generator
G Impulsgeber
S generador de impulsos

génération de particules
E particle generation
G Partikelerzeugung
S producción de partículas

générique
E generic
G Genericum
S genérico

génie génétique
E gene technology
G Gentechnologie
S tecnología genética

génomique
E genomics
G Genomlehre
S teoría del genoma

germe
E organism
G Keim
S germen

germe cristallin
E seed crystal
G Impfkristall
S cristal de sembrado

germination
E germination
G Auskeimung (von Sporen)
S germinación (de esporas)

gestion de la qualité
E quality management (QM)
G Qualitätsmanagement (QM)
S gestión de la calidad

gestion absolue de la qualité
E total quality management (TQM)
G umfassendes Qualitätsmanagement
S gestión de la calidad absoluta

gestion de l'environnement
E environmental management
G Umweltschutzmanagement
S gestión ecológica

gicleur
E nozzle, nozzle head
G Düse, Sprühkopf
S aplicador, inyector, tobera, cabeza del inyector

glissement d'une feuille
E film slippage
G Folienschlupf
S deslizamiento de una lámina

glisser
E slip, to
G gleiten
S deslizar, resbalar

glissoir de charge
E charge chute
G Befüllrutsche
S tobogán de carga

globule sanguin
E blood corpuscle
G Blutkörperchen
S eritrocito

gluant
E sticky, tacky
G klebrig
S pegajoso

glucides
E carbohydrates
G Kohlenhydrate
S hidratos de carbono

gobelet
E graduated beaker
G Meßbecher, Becherglas
S vaso graduado, probeta

gommer
E gum, to
G gummieren
S engomar, impermeabilizar

gonflable
E inflatable
G aufblasbar
S hinchable

gonfler
E swell, to
G quellen
S brotar, hincharse

gorge
E notch
G Kerbe
S muesca

goulot
E bottle neck
G Flaschenhals
S cuello de botella, gollete

goupille
E pin
G Stift (technisch)
S clavija, perno, pivote

gousse d'une capsule
E capsule shell
G Kapselhülse
S cubierta de una cápsula

goût
E taste, flavour
G Geschmack
S gusto

gouttelettes
E droplet
G Tröpfchen
S gotita

gouttes antitussives
E cough drops
G Hustentropfen
S gotas antitusivas

gouttes auriculaires
E ear drops
G Ohrentropfen
S gotas auriculares

gouttes nasales
E nose drops
G Nasentropfen
S gotas nasales

gouttes ophtalmiques
E eye drops
G Augentropfen
S gotas oftálmicas

gouttes pour voie orale
E oral drops
G Tropfen zum Einnehmen
S gotas orales

gouttière
E gutter
G Rinne
S canal, reguera, surco

gouvernement régional
E regional government
G Regierungspräsidium
S gobierno civil

gradation de couleurs
E colour scale
G Farbabstufung
S gradación de colores

gradient
E slope, gradient
G Neigung, Gradient
S inclinación, pendiente, gradiente

gradient de température
E temperature gradient
G Temperaturgefälle
S gradiente de temperatura

gradient d'écoulement
E flow gradient
G Fließgradient
S gradiente de flujo

graduation
E scale, graduation
G Gradeinteilung, Skaleneinteilung
S graduación,
graduación de una escala

gradué
E graduated
G graduiert
S graduado

grain fin, à
E fine-grained
G feinkörnig
S de grano fino

graisse
E grease
G Schmierfett
S grasa lubri(fi)cante

graisser
E grease, to; lubricate, to
G schmieren, einfetten
S engrasar, lubri(fi)car

Gram-négatif
E Gram-negative
G Gram-negativ
S Gram negativo

Gram-positif
E Gram-positive
G Gram-positiv
S Gram positivo

granulaire
E granular
G körnig
S granular

granulateur en lit fluidisé
E fluid bed spray granulator
G Wirbelschichtgranulator
S granulador de lecho fluidificado

granulateur vertical
E vertical granulator
G Vertikalgranulator
S granulador vertical

granulation
E grain
G Körnung
S granulación

granulation fine
E fine particles, fine grain
G feine Körnung
S granulación fina

granulation (par voie) humide
E wet granulation
G Feuchtgranulierung
S granulación húmeda

granulation de dégradation
E degradation granulation
G Abbaugranulierung
S granulación de degradación

granulation hors taille
E synthetic granulation
G Aufbaugranulierung
S granulación sintética

granulation par séchage
E dry granulation
G Trockengranulierung
S granulación en seco

granule
E granule
G Granulatkorn
S gránulo

granulé
E granulate
G Granulat
S granulado

granule moulée
E moulding granulate
G Preßgranulat
S granulado de compresión

granuler
E granulate, to
G granulieren
S granular

granules à libération retardée
E prolonged release granules
G Retardgranulat
S granulado retard

granules gastro-résistantes
E gastro-resistant granules
G magensaftresistentes Granulat
S granulado resistente al jugo gástrico

granulés grossiers
E coarse granules
G Grobgranulat
S granulado grueso

granulométrie
E sieve analysis
G Siebanalyse
S granulometría

graphe
E graph
G grafische Darstellung
S representación gráfica

graver
E engrave, to
G eingravieren
S grabar

grille
E net, grid, grating
G Netz, Gitter, Gitterrost
S red, retícula

grossier
E coarse, rough
G grob, rauh
S grosero, grueso, áspero

grossièrement cristallin
E course-grained
G grobkristallin
S groseramente cristalino

grossièreté
E roughness
G Rauhigkeit
S aspereza

groupe de travail
E working group, task force
G Arbeitsgruppe
S grupo de trabajo

guidage de clapet
E flap control
G Klappensteuerung
S control de las válvulas

guidage d'un poinçon
E punch guide
G Stempelführung
S guía del troquel

guide
E guide, guiding device, guiding mechanism
G Führungsvorrichtung
S dispositivo de guía, guía

hacher
E homogenise, to; shred, to
G zerkleinern
S triturar

hachoir
E homogeniser, shredder, chopper
G Zerkleinerer, Zerhacker
S trituradora, troceadora

halogénation
E halogenation
G Halogenierung
S halogenación

haute dose, à
E highly dosed
G hoch dosiert
S altamente dosificado

haute performance
E high performance
G Hochleistungs-
S gran rendimiento

haute-résolution
E high-resolution
G hochauflösend
S de alta resolución

hauteur
E height
G Höhe
S altura

hauteur ajustable, à
E height-adjustable
G höhenverstellbar
S de altura regulable

hauteur de bande
E band height (of tablets)
G Steghöhe (bei Tabletten)
S altura de banda (de comprimidos)

hauteur de bande d'un comprimé
E tablet web height
G Tablettensteghöhe
S altura de banda de un comprimido

hauteur de chargement (p. ex. d'un autoclave)
E loading height (e. g. of autoclave)
G Beladungshöhe (z. B. eines Autoklaven)
S altura de carga (p. ej. de autoclave)

hauteur de chute
E drop height
G Fallhöhe
S altura de caída

hauteur de pic
E peak height
G Peakhöhe
S altura del pico

hauteur de remplissage
E filling depth
G Fülltiefe
S altura del relleno

hauteur du plateau d'une matrice
E die plate height
G Matrizentischhöhe
S altura de la mesa para matriz

English German French Spanish

hauteur totale
E overall height
G Gesamthöhe
S altura total

hélice alpha (structure des protéines)
E alpha helix (e. g. of protein)
G Alpha-Helix (z. B. eines Proteins)
S hélice alfa (p. ej. de proteína)

herbicide
E herbicide
G Unkrautvernichtungsmittel
S herbicida

hermétiquement fermé
E tightly closed
G dicht verschlossen
S herméticamente cerrado

hétérocyclique
E heterocyclic
G heterozyklisch
S heterocíclico

hétérogénéité des comprimés
E tablet inconsistency
G Uneinheitlichkeit von Tabletten
S heterogeneidad de comprimidos

homogène
E homogeneous
G homogen
S homogéneo

homogénéiser
E homogenise, to
G homogenisieren
S homogenizar

homogénéiseur
E homogeniser
G Homogenisator
S homogenizador

homogénéité
E homogeneity
G Homogenität
S homogeneidad

homologue
E homologous
G homolog
S homólogo

horizontal
E horizontal
G waagerecht
S horizontal

hotte à flux laminaire
E ventilated hood, fume cupboard
G Abzug
S escape, campana de extracción de gases

hotte chimique
E ventilated hood, fume cupboard
G Abzug
S escape, campana de extracción de gases

huile conductrice de chaleur
E heat-transmitting oil
G wärmeübertragendes Öl
S aceite transmisor de calor

huile essentielle
E essential oil
G ätherisches Öl
S aceite etérico

huileux
E oily
G ölig
S oleaginoso, oleoso

humide
E moist
G feucht
S húmedo

humidificateur
E humidifier
G Befeuchter, Luftbefeuchter
S humidificador de aire

humidification
E humidification
G Befeuchtung
S humectación, humidificación

humidifier
E humidise, to; wet, to; moisten, to
G anfeuchten, befeuchten, benetzen
S humectar, humedecer, mojar, rociar

humidité
E humidity, moisture
G Feuchtigkeit, Luftfeuchtigkeit
S humedad, humedad del aire

humidité adhérente
E bound moisture
G gebundene Feuchtigkeit
S humedad adherente

humidité non liée
E unbound moisture
G nicht gebundene Feuchtigkeit
S humedad no adherente

humidité relative
E relative humidity
G relative Luftfeuchtigkeit
S humedad atmosférica relativa

humidité résiduelle
E residual moisture
G Restfeuchte
S humedad residual

hydrate
E hydrate
G Hydrat
S hidrato

hydrates de carbone
E carbohydrates
G Kohlenhydrate
S hidratos de carbono

hydrocarbures polyaromatiques
E polyaromatic hydrocarbons (PAH)
G polyaromatische Kohlenwasserstoffe (PAK)
S hidrocarburos poliaromáticos

hydrogénation
E hydrogenation
G Hydrogenierung
S hidrogenación

hydrogène
E hydrogen
G Wasserstoff
S hidrógeno

hydrolyse
E hydrolysis
G Hydrolyse
S hidrólisis

hydrolyse partielle
E partial hydrolysis
G Hydrolyse, partielle
S hidrólisis parcial

hydrophile
E hydrophilic
G hydrophil
S hidrófilo

hydrophobe
E hydrophobic, water-repellent
G hydrophob, wasserabweisend
S hidrófobo, hidrófugo

hygiène des installations
E plant hygiene, plant sanitation
G Betriebshygiene
S higiene de la empresa

hygiène du personnel
E personnel hygiene
G Personalhygiene
S higiene personal

hygromètre
E hygrometer
G Hygrometer, Feuchtigkeitsmesser, Feuchtemesser
S higrómetro

hygromètre à cheveux
E hair hygrometer
G Haarhygrometer
S higrómetro capilar

hygroscopie
E hygroscopicity
G Hygroskopizität
S higroscopicidad

hygroscopique
E hygroscopic
G hygroskopisch, wasseranziehend
S higroscópico, hidrófilo

hypertonique
E hypertonic
G hypertonisch
S hipertónico

hypo-dose
E sub-strength
G Unterdosierung
S infradosificación

hypotonique
E hypotonic
G hypotonisch
S hipotónico

identification
E identification
G Identifikation
S identificación

identification de l'aire de collage
E splice recognition
G Klebestellenerkennung
S reconocimiento de la zona de adherencia

identification de l'impression
E print recognition
G Druckerkennung
S identificación del impreso

identification électronique
E electronic identification (EID)
G elektronische Identifikation (EID)
S identificación electrónica

identifier une erreur
E locate a failure (fault), to
G Fehler finden
S encontrar errores

identité
E identity
G Identität
S identidad

ignifugation (d'un instrument)
E flame protector (of instrument)
G Brandschutz (eines Gerätes)
S protección frente al fuego (de un aparato)

ignifugé
E fire-proof
G feuergeschützt
S protegido frente al fuego

ignifugeage (d'un instrument)
E flame protector (of instrument)
G Brandschutz (eines Gerätes)
S protección frente al fuego (de un aparato)

immerger
E immerse, to; dip, to; submerge, to
G eintauchen, untertauchen
S sumergir, sumergirse

immobilisé
E at rest
G im Ruhezustand
S parado

immunoélectrophorèse
E immune electrophoresis
G Immunelektrophorese
S inmunoelectroforesis

immunologique
E immunological
G immunologisch
S inmunológico

impact
E impact
G Schlag, Stoß
S choque, golpe, impacto

imperméabilité
E impermeability, imperviousness
G Undurchlässigkeit
S impermeabilidad

imperméabilité à l'air
E air impermeability, air tightness
G Luftundurchlässigkeit, Luftdichtheit
S impermeabilidad al aire, hermeticidad para el aire

imperméable
E impermeable, impervious
G undurchlässig
S impermeable

imperméable à la poussière
E dustproof
G staubgeschützt
S protegido frente al polvo

imperméable à l'air
E impermeable to air
G luftundurchlässig
S impermeable al aire

imperméable à l'eau
E water-tight, waterproof
G wasserdicht
S impermeable al agua

implant
E implant, pellet, compressed core
G Implantat, Preßling
S implantado, masa comprimida

implémenter
E implement, to
G implementieren
S establecer, realizar

imprécision inhérente (par ex. d'une technologie)
E inherent uncertainty (e. g. of a technique)
G inhärente Ungenauigkeit (z. B. einer Technik)
S inexactitud inherente (p. ej. de una técnica)

imprégner
E soak, to; impregnate, to
G tränken, imprägnieren
S embeber, empapar, impregnar

impression
E imprint
G Aufdruck
S impresión

impression de feuilles
E film printing
G Folienbedruckung
S impresión de láminas

imprimante
E printer
G Drucker
S impresora

imprimante à jet d'encre
E ink jet printer
G Tintenstrahldrucker
S impresora de chorro de tinta

imprimante à laser
E laser printer
G Laserdrucker
S impresora de láser

imprimé
E printout
G Ausdruck, Schreiberausdruck
S impreso

imprimé à l'avance
E pre-printed
G vorbedruckt
S preimpreso

imprimé sur papier
E paper printout, hard copy
G Papierausdruck
S impreso en papel, impreso sobre papel

imprimer
E emboss, to; imprint, to; print, to
G einprägen, aufprägen, aufdrucken, bedrucken
S estampar, imprimir

impureté
E impurity, contamination
G Verunreinigung
S contaminación, impureza

impureté à l'état de traces
E trace impurity
G Verunreinigung in Spuren
S impureza vestigial

in situ
E in-situ
G in-situ
S in situ

English German French Spanish

inaccessible
E inaccessible
G unzugänglich
S inaccesible

inaccessible aux enfants
E child-proof
G kindersicher
S inaccesible para niños

inactivation
E inactivation, deactivation
G Inaktivierung
S inactivación

inactivées
E inactivated
G inaktiviert
S inactivado

incassable
E unbreakable, shatter-proof
G unzerbrechlich, bruchfest
S irrompible

incertitude
E uncertainty
G Unsicherheit
S inseguridad

incertitude analytique
E analytical uncertainty
G analytische Unsicherheit
S inseguridad analítica

incident
E incident, fault, failure, accident
G Vorfall, Zwischenfall, Störfall
S incidente, avería, fallo

incinérateur
E incinerator
G Verbrennungsanlage
S crematorio

incinération
E combustion, incineration, ashing
G Verbrennung
S combustión, incineración

incinération des déchets
E rubbish incineration
G Müllverbrennung
S incineración de desechos

inclinaison
E gradient, slope
G Gefälle
S declive, gradiente, inclinación, pendiente

incliné
E sloped, sloping
G schräg, geneigt, mit Gefälle
S inclinado, oblicuo, con inclinación, con pendiente

inclure
E embed, to
G einbetten
S incluir

inclusion
E inclusion
G Einschluß
S inclusión

inclusion d'air
E air entrapment
G Lufteinschluß
S inclusión de aire

incolore
E colourless
G farblos
S incoloro

incompatibilité
E incompatibility
G Inkompatibilität, Unverträglichkeit
S incompatibilidad, intolerancia

incompatible
E incompatible
G inkompatibel
S incompatible

incomplet
E incomplete
G unvollständig
S incompleto

incubateur
E oven, incubator
G Wärmeschrank, Brutschrank
S incubadora

incuber
E incubate, to
G inkubieren, bebrüten
S incubar

indélébile
E indelible
G unauslöschbar
S indeleble

index de peroxyde
E peroxide number, peroxide index
G Peroxydzahl
S índice de peróxido

index de réfraction
E refractive index
G Brechungsindex, Brechungszahl
S índice de refracción

indicateur
E indicator, pointer, display
G Indikator, Zeiger, Anzeige
S indicador, indicación, pantalla

indicateur biologique
E bioindicator
G Bioindikator
S bioindicador

indicateur de pression différentielle
E pressure differential indicator
G Differenzdruckanzeiger
S indicador de presión diferencial

indicateur du niveau de liquide
E liquid level indicator
G Flüssigkeitsstandsanzeige
S indicador de nivel de líquido

indicateur intégré
E integrated display
G integrierte Anzeige
S pantalla integrada

indicateur optique
E visual display
G optische Anzeige
S pantalla óptica

indication visuelle
E display
G optische Anzeige
S señal óptica

indice d'acceptance
E acceptance number
G Annahmezahl
S número de aceptación

indice d'acide
E acid value
G Säurezahl
S índice de ácido

indice de fusion
E melting index
G Schmelzindex
S índice de fusión

indice de saponification
E saponification value
G Verseifungszahl
S índice de saponificación

indice de saturation
E saturation index
G Sättigungsindex
S índice de saturación

indice d'hydroxyle
E hydroxyl number
G Hydroxylzahl
S índice hidroxílico

indice d'iode
E iodine number
G Iodzahl
S índice de iodo

indiquer
E display, to; indicate, to
G anzeigen
S indicar, mostrar

industriel de la pharmacie
E pharmaceutical manufacturer
G pharmazeutischer Unternehmer
S fabricante farmacéutico

inerte
E inert, poorly reactive
G inert, reaktionsträge
S inerte

infectieux
E infectious
G infektiös
S infeccioso

inflammable
E flammable, ignitable
G entflammbar, entzündbar, feuergefährlich
S inflamable

facilement inflammable
E highly flammable
G leicht entflammbar
S fácilmente inflamable

in-inflammable
E fire-resistant, non-flammable
G feuerfest, nicht brennbar
S ignífugo, resistente al fuego, no combustible, no inflamable

inflammation
E ignition
G Zündung
S encendido, ignición

influence de l'environnement
E environmental influence
G Umwelteinfluß
S influencia del medio ambiente

information technique
E technical information
G Fachinformation
S ficha técnica (de un medicamento)

informatique
E EDP (Electronic Data Processing)
G EDV (Elektronische Datenverarbeitung)
S proceso electrónico de datos

infusion
E infusion
G Infus, Aufguß
S infusión

ingénierie
E engineering
G Technik (als Abteilung)
S departamento técnico

ingénierie des zones d'atmosphère contrôlée
E clean room engineering
G Reinraumtechnik
S técnica para el área estéril

ingénieur
E engineer
G Ingenieur
S ingeniero

ingénieurie
E engineering
G Ingenieurwesen
S ingeniería

ingrédient
E component, constituent, ingredient
G Bestandteil
S componente, ingrediente

ingrédient de base d'une pommade
E ointment base
G Salbengrundlage
S excipiente de una pomada

inhalateur doseur
E metered dose inhaler
G Dosieraerosol
S aerosol dosificante

inhalation
E inhalation
G Inhalation
S inhalación

inhibiteur
E inhibitor
G Hemmstoff
S inhibidor

inhibition
E inhibition
G Hemmung
S inhibición

in-inflammable
E fire-resistant
G feuerfest
S ignífugo, resistente al fuego

initiales
E initials
G Namenszeichen
S iniciales

initiation (d'une réaction)
E initiation (of a reaction)
G Initiierung (einer Reaktion)
S iniciación (de una reacción)

injectable
E injectible
G injizierbar
S inyectable

injecter
E inject, to
G injizieren
S inyectar

injecteur à aiguille
E filling nozzle
G Düsennadel
S aguja de inyección

injecteur automatique
E injector, automatic
G Injektor, automatischer
S inyector automático

injecteur d'implant
E implanter
G Implantatinjektor
S inyector de implantados

injection
E injection
G Einspritzung
S inyección

injection d'échantillon
E sample injection
G Probeneinspritzung
S inyección de muestras

innovant
E innovative
G innovativ
S innovador

inoccupé
E unmanned
G mannlos
S desocupado

inoculation
E inoculation
G Inokulation, Beimpfung
S inoculación, siembra

inoculation directe
E direct inoculation (for microbial count determination)
G Direktbeschickung (zur Keimzahlbestimmung)
S inoculación directa (para recuento microbiano)

inoculer
E inoculate, to
G beimpfen
S inocular, sembrar

insaturé
E unsaturated
G ungesättigt
S insaturado

English German French Spanish

inscrire
E enter, to
G eintragen
S inscribir, registrar

insecticide
E insecticide
G Insektizid, insektizid
S insecticida

insert en polystyrène
E polystyrene insert
G Polystyrol-Einsatz
S inserción de poliestirol

insipide
E tasteless, flavourless
G geschmacklos
S insípido

insoluble
E insoluble
G unlöslich
S insoluble

insonorisation du bruit
E noise insulation
G Geräuschisolierung
S aislamiento sonoro

insonorisé
E noise-proof
G geräuschdämmend
S insonorizado

inspecté
E checked, inspected
G geprüft
S comprobado

inspecter
E investigate, to
G untersuchen
S examinar, explorar, investigar

inspection
E inspection, investigation, audit
G Inspektion, Untersuchung, Audit
S inspección, examen, exploración, investigación, autitoría

inspection (entité admin.)
E inspectorate
G Inspektorat
S inspectoría

inspection physique
E physical inspection, physical examination
G körperliche Untersuchung
S exploración física

inspection visuelle
E visual inspection
G Durchsichtkontrolle
S inspección visual

installation
E installation, mounting, facility, plant (machines)
G Installation, Einbau, Anlage (Maschine)
S instalación, montaje, equipo, instalación (máquina)

installation de pesage
E weighing facility
G Wiegeanlage
S instalación de pesado

installation d'un filtre
E filter installation
G Filtereinbau
S instalación de un filtro

installation industrielle
E facility, plant
G Einrichtung (in Gebäuden)
S instalación (en edificios)

installation industrielle dédiée
E dedicated plant
G Einrichtung für einen bestimmten Zweck
S instalación para un fin determinado

installation pour processus
E processing facility, processing plant
G Prozeßanlage
S instalación para proceso

installation servant à la production d'air comprimé
E compressed air plant
G Druckluftanlage
S instalación de aire comprimido

installation sur site
E on-site installation
G Installation vor Ort
S instalación in situ

installation technique multi-usages
E multi-purpose equipment
G Mehrzweckanlage
S instalación de uso múltiple

installations
E plant, factory, facility
G Betriebsstätte
S plantas empresariales

installé de manière permanente
E permanently installed
G fest installiert
S instalado fijamente

installer
E fit, to; install, to
G einbauen
S instalar, montar

instruction
E instruction, specification
G Anweisung, Vorschrift
S instrucción, prescripción

instruction d'emballage
E packaging instruction
G Verpackungsanweisung
S instrucción de embalaje

instructions de fabrication
E master formula, manufacturing instructions
G Herstellungsanweisung, Herstellungsvorschrift
S instrucción de fabricación, prescripciones de fabricación

instructions de sécurité
E safety instructions
G Sicherheitshinweis
S aviso de seguridad

instructions de service
E operating manual, operating instructions
G Betriebsanleitung
S instrucciones de funcionamiento

instructions d'échantillonnage
E sampling instructions
G Stichprobenanweisung
S instrucciones para tomar muestras

instructions d'un test
E test instructions, testing procedure
G Prüfanweisung, Prüfvorschrift
S instrucciones de prueba, prescripción de prueba

instructions opératoires
E operating instructions
G Bedienungsanleitung
S instrucción de manejo, instrucción de servicio

instructions pour le traitement
E processing instructions
G Verarbeitungsanweisung
S instrucción de procesado

instructions pour l'utilisation
E instructions for use, operating instructions
G Gebrauchsanweisung
S instrucción de uso

instructions vestimentaires
E gowning procedure
G Bekleidungsvorschrift
S prescripción de vestuario

instrument de fabrication de comprimés
E compaction device
G Tablettierwerkzeug
S instrumentos para fabricar comprimidos

instrument de mesure
E measuring instrument, measuring device
G Meßmittel, Meßgerät
S dispositivo de medición, aparato de medición

English German French Spanish

instruments de contrôle
E control instrumentation
G Kontrollinstrumentierung
S instrumentos de control

insuffisance
E deficiency
G Mangel
S carencia, defecto, deficiencia, insuficiencia

insuffisance de poids
E short weight, underweight
G Untergewicht
S falta de peso

intact
E intact, sound, undamaged
G intakt, unbeschädigt
S intacto, indemne

intégrité
E integrity
G Integrität, Unversehrtheit
S integridad

intégrité d'un conditionnement
E package integrity
G Unversehrtheit der Verpackung
S integridad de un embalaje

intégrité d'un filtre
E filter integrity
G Filterintegrität
S integridad del filtro

intensité de cisaillement
E shear intensity
G Scherintensität
S intensidad de cizallamiento

interaction
E interaction
G Wechselwirkung
S acción recíproca, interacción

interaction dipolaire
E dipole-dipole interaction
G Dipol-Dipol-Wechselwirkung
S interacción entre dipolos

interchangeable
E interchangeable, exchangeable
G austauschbar, auswechselbar
S intercambiable

interface
E interface
G Grenzfläche
S interfase, superficie limitante

interface série
E serial interface
G serielle Schnittstelle
S interfase seriada

interférence
E interference
G Interferenz
S interferencia

interférence électrique
E electrical interference
G elektrische Störung
S avería eléctrica

interférence électromagnétique
E electromagnetic interference
G elektromagnetische Interferenz
S interferencia electromagnética

interlocuteur
E contact person
G Ansprechpartner
S interlocutor

interprétation
E interpretation, evaluation
G Auswertung
S evaluación, interpretación

interrupteur
E switch, on/off switch
G Schalter, Abschalter, Ausschalter
S conmutador, interruptor (de desconexión)

interrupteur de courant
E power switch, main switch
G Netzschalter
S interruptor a la red

interrupteur principal
E main switch, power switch
G Hauptschalter
S interruptor principal

interrupteurs à bascule
E lever switch controls
G Kippschalter-Kontrollen
S controles de interruptor unipolar

interruption
E interruption
G Unterbrechung
S interrupción

interruption d'une réaction
E cessation (of a reaction)
G Unterbrechung (einer Reaktion)
S interrupción (de una reacción)

intervalle
E range
G Bereich, Bandbreite
S zona, márgenes, anchura de banda, gama

intervalle autorisé
E acceptable range
G zulässiger Bereich
S zona permitida, márgenes permitidos

intervalle de calibration
E calibration interval
G Kalibrierintervall
S intervalo de calibración

intervalle de confiance
E confidence interval
G Vertrauensintervall
S intervalo de confianza

intervalle de distillation
E distillation range
G Destillationsbereich
S intervalo de destilación

intervalle de tolérance
E tolerance range
G Toleranzbereich
S intervalo de tolerancia

intervalle linéaire
E linear range
G Linearbereich
S área lineal

intervention
E intervention
G Eingriff
S intervención

introduction sur le marché
E placing on the market, launch
G Markteinführung, Inverkehrbringen
S introducción en el mercado

invasion d'insectes
E insect infestation
G Insektenbefall
S infestación con insectos

inventaire
E inventory, stock
G Lagerbestand
S existencias en almacén, stocks

investigation des sources d'une erreur
E error (failure) investigation
G Fehleruntersuchung
S investigación de errores

ion chargé
E charged ion
G geladenes Ion
S ion cargado

ion complémentaire
E counter-ion
G Gegenion
S contraión, ion complementario

ionisation
E ionisation
G Ionisierung
S ionización

irradiation
E irradiation, radiation
G Bestrahlung
S irradiación

English German French Spanish

irradier avec
E irradiate, to (with)
G bestrahlen mit
S irradiar con

irréprochable
E faultless
G einwandfrei
S intacto

irritant pour la peau
E irritating to skin
G hautreizend
S irritante cutáneo

irritant pour le système respiratoire
E irritating to respiratory system
G reizt die Atemwege
S irrita las vías respiratorias

irritant pour les yeux
E irritating to eyes
G reizt die Augen
S irrita los ojos

irritation (chimique)
E irritation (chem.)
G Reizung (chemisch)
S irritación (química)

isocratique
E isocratic
G isokratisch
S isocrático

isolateur
E glove box, isolator
G Isolator
S aislante

isolation
E insulation
G Isolierung
S aislamiento

isolation thermique
E heat insulation
G Wärmeisolierung
S aislamiento térmico

isolé
E separated, segregated
G abgetrennt
S aislado, separado

isomères de conformation
E conformation isomers
G Konformationsisomere
S isómeros de conformación

isotonique
E isotonic
G isoton
S isotónico

jarre
E jar, wide-necked vessel
G Weithalsgefäß
S recipiente de cuello ancho

jauge
E gauge
G Meßlehre
S galga, gálibo, calibre

jauge de contrainte
E wire strain gauge
G Dehnungsmeßstreifen
S extensímetro de resistencia

jauge d'épaisseur
E thickness gauge
G Dickenmeßgerät
S calibre de grosores

jet d'air
E air jet
G Luftstrahl
S chorro de aire

jetable
E disposable
G Einweg-
S uso único, de

joint
E joint, seam, weld, seal, gasket
G Fuge, Naht, Trennfuge, Versiegelung, Dichtung
S junta, soldadura, sutura, sellado

dépourvu de joint
E seamless
G fugenlos
S sin juntas

joint (d'un tube)
E crimp, seam (of a tube)
G Falz (einer Tube)
S encaje, juntura (de un tubo)

joint (rondelle)
E washer, gasket
G Dichtungsscheibe
S disco para cierre hermético

joint à rotule
E ball + socket joint
G Kugelgelenk
S articulación de rótula, unión esférica

joint de cartouche
E cartridge gasket
G Patronendichtung
S junta de cartucho

joint de compensation
E expansion joint
G Dehnungsfuge
S junta de dilatación

joint de construction
E construction joint
G Arbeitsfuge
S junta de construcción

joint de dilatation
E settling joint
G Bewegungsfuge
S junta de movimiento

joint de porte
E door seal
G Türdichtung
S junta de una puerta

joint de silicone gonflable
E inflatable silicone seal
G aufblasbare Silikondichtung
S cierre inflable de silicona

joint d'étanchéité
E sealing ring
G Dichtring
S anillo hermético, arandela hermética

joint dilatable
E expansion joint
G Dehnungsfuge
S junta de dilatación

joint en caoutchouc
E rubber gasket
G Gummidichtung
S junta de goma

joint gonflable
E inflatable gasket
G aufblasbare Dichtung
S junta hinchable

joint sanitaire
E sanitary joint
G Sanitärverbindung
S conexión sanitaria

joint torique
E O-ring
G O-Ring
S anillo tórico

joint torique en forme de rondelle
E gasket ring
G Dichtungsring
S arandela para junta hermética

journalier
E daily
G täglich
S diario

jus
E juice
G Saft
S jugo (animal), zumo (vegetal)

English German French Spanish

kit
E kit
G Bausatz
S kit

laborantin
E laboratory assistant
G Laborant
S asistente de laboratorio

laboratoire
E laboratory, lab
G Labor
S laboratorio

laboratoire conforme aux GMP
E GMP-controlled laboratory
G GMP-Labor
S laboratorio controlado para GMP

laboratoire de fermentation
E fermentation laboratory
G Fermentationslabor
S laboratorio de fermentación

laboratoire de risques biologiques
E biohazard laboratory, biosafety laboratory
G Biosicherheitslabor
S laboratorio de seguridad biológica

laboratoire d'étalonnage homologué
E accredited calibration laboratory
G akkreditiertes Kalibrierlabor
S laboratorio acreditado de calibración

laboratoire sous-traitant
E contract laboratory
G Auftragslabor
S laboratorio comisionado

lactone
E lactone
G Lacton
S lactona

lactose
E lactose
G Lactose
S lactosa

laisser se déposer
E allow to stand, to
G absetzen lassen
S dejar precipitar, dejar sedimentar

laisser s'écouler
E drain, to; discharge, to (liquids)
G ablassen (Flüssigkeiten)
S dar salida, dejar escapar

laisser sédimenter
E allow to stand, to
G absetzen lassen
S dejar precipitar, dejar sedimentar

lame
E cover glass
G Abdeckplatte
S cubreobjetos

lame de protection
E cover glass, cover slip (microscopy)
G Deckglas (Mikroskopie)
S cubreobjetos (microscopio)

lame d'essuyage (dans la cuve de mélange)
E wiper paddle (e. g. of a mixing vessel)
G Wischblatt (z. B. im Mischbehälter)
S goma limpia cristales (p. ej. en mezclador)

lame d'immersion
E immersion sword
G Tauchschwert
S lámina de inmersión

lamelle
E lamella
G Lamelle
S arandela, disco, laminilla

lampe à arc de tungstène
E tungsten arc lamp
G Wolframbogenlampe
S lámpara de arco de tungsteno

lampe de contrôle
E control lamp
G Signallampe
S lámpara de señales

lampe UV
E UV lamp
G UV-Lampe
S lámpara UV

lancement d'un produit
E product launch
G Produkteinführung
S introducción de un producto (en el mercado)

languette
E tab, tear-off tab, tongue
G Einstecklasche, Aufreißlasche
S cubrejunta de pestaña, lengüeta arrancable

laquage superficiel
E surface lacquer
G Oberflächenlackierung
S barnizado de superficies

laque
E lacquer
G Lack
S barniz, laca

laque extérieure
E outer lacquer
G Außenlack
S barniz externo

laque interne
E internal lacquer
G Innenlack
S barniz interno

laque interne de protection
E internal protective lacquer
G Innenschutzlack
S barniz protector interno

laque par immersion
E immersion lacquer
G Tauchlack
S barniz de inmersión

laque thermofusible
E heat-sealing lacquer
G Heißsiegellack
S laca termofusible

laquer
E lacquer, to
G lackieren
S barnizar, lacar

largeur
E width
G Breite, Weite
S anchura, amplitud, extensión

largeur de pic
E peak width
G Peakbreite
S anchura del pico

largeur d'une fente
E slit width
G Spaltbreite
S anchura de la fisura

largeur d'une fissure
E slit width
G Spaltbreite
S anchura de la fisura

largeur nominale
E nominal width
G Nennweite
S anchura nominal

largeur totale
E overall width
G Gesamtbreite
S anchura total

lavement
E enema
G Klistier
S enema, lavativa

lavement intestinal
E enema
G Darmspülung
S enema, lavativa

leader d'opinion
E opinion leader
G Meinungsbildner
S líder de opinión

lecteur (d'un ordinateur)
E disk drive (computer)
G Laufwerk (Computer)
S unidad (de un ordenador)

lecteur de codage de couleurs
E colour ring code reader
G Farbringleser
S lector de anillo cromático

lecture du codage
E code reading
G Codelesung
S lectura de códigos

légende
E legend
G Zeichenerklärung
S leyenda

législation
E legislation
G Gesetzgebung
S legislación

législation allemande sur les substances dangereuses
E German Hazardous Substance Act
G Deutsches Gefahrstoffgesetz
S Ley Alemana de Sustancias Peligrosas

lentille
E lens
G Linse
S lente

lentille-objet
E object lens
G Objektlinse
S lente del objetivo

lessive-mère
E mother liquor
G Mutterlauge
S lejía madre

lettre d'avertissement (de la FDA)
E warning letter (from FDA)
G Verwarnung (der FDA)
S carta de aviso (de la FDA)

levier
E lever
G Hebel
S palanca

lévogyre
E laevo-rotary
G linksdrehend
S levógiro

levure
E yeast
G Hefe
S levadura

liaison
E bond
G Bindung
S enlace

liaison hydrogène
E hydrogen bond
G Wasserstoffbrückenbindung
S puente de hidrógeno

liaison ionique
E ion bonding
G ionische Bindung
S enlace iónico

liaison superficielle
E surface binding
G Oberflächenbindung
S ligadura de superficie

liant
E binding agent
G Bindemittel
S aglomerante, aglutinante

libération
E release
G Freigabe, Freisetzung
S liberación

libération contrôlée
E controlled release, timed release
G kontrollierte Freisetzung, zeitlich gesteuerte Freigabe
S liberación controlada

libération différée
E delayed release
G verzögerte Freisetzung
S liberación retardada

libération immédiate
E immediate release
G schnelle Freisetzung
S liberación inmediata

libération incomplète
E incomplete release
G unvollständige Freisetzung
S liberación incompleta

libération modifiée
E modified release
G modifizierte Freisetzung
S liberación modificada

libération prolongée
E sustained release, extended release
G verlängerte Freisetzung
S liberación prolongada

libération de produit
E product release, extended release
G Produktfreigabe
S aprobación del producto

libération d'un lot
E batch release
G Chargenfreigabe
S liberación de un lote

libération d'un principe actif
E active substance release, release of medicinal substance
G Wirkstoff-Freigabe, Arzneistoff-Freisetzung
S liberación del principio activo

libération prolongée d'un principe actif
E extended release
G verlängerte Wirkstoff-Freigabe
S liberación prolongada del principio activo

libération retardée d'un principe actif
E delayed release
G verzögerte Wirkstoff-Freigabe
S liberación retardada del principio activo

libération immédiate, à
E immediate release
G schnell freisetzend
S de liberación rápida

libération in-vitro
E in-vitro release
G In-vitro-Freisetzung
S liberación in vitro

libération modifiée de granules
E modified release granules
G Granulat mit veränderter Wirkstoff-Freisetzung
S granulado con liberación modificada de la sustancia activa

libéré
E released
G freigegeben
S liberado

libérer
E release, to
G freigeben
S liberar

libérer des particules
E shed particles, to
G Partikel abgeben
S liberar partículas

libre de particules
E particle-free
G partikelfrei
S sin partículas

licence
E licence
G Lizenz
S licencia

licenciement
E redundancy
G Entlassung
S despido

licencier
E make redundant, to
G entlassen
S despedir

license d'importation
E import licence
G Einfuhrerlaubnis
S licencia de importación

lié
E flush
G bündig
S enrasado

lier ensemble
E bundle, to
G bündeln
S enfardar

lieu
E location
G Lage, Ort
S lugar, situación

lieu de production
E manufacturing location/site
G Produktionsort
S lugar de producción

lieu d'installation
E installation location
G Aufstellungsort
S lugar de instalación

lieuse
E bundling machine
G Bündelpacker
S enfardador

ligne de base
E baseline, zero line
G Basislinie, Nullinie
S línea de base

ligne de dégagement (d'une chaîne de conditionnement)
E line clearance (at a packaging line)
G Linienabnahme (an der Verpackungslinie)
S punto de descarga de la cadena de envasado

ligne de fracture
E rupture line, fracture line
G Bruchlinie
S línea de ruptura, línea de fractura

ligne de remplissage
E filling line, bottling line
G Abfüllinie
S cadena de envasado

ligne de rupture
E rupture line, fracture line
G Bruchlinie
S línea de ruptura, línea de fractura

ligne de zéro
E zero line
G Nullinie
S línea de base

ligne droite
E straight, straight line
G Gerade
S recta (línea)

lignée (microbiol.)
E strain
G Stamm
S cepa

lignée de cellule de mammifère
E mammalian cell line
G Säugetierzellinie
S línea de células de mamífero

lignes directrices générales
E cross-functional guideline
G abteilungsübergreifende Richtlinie
S línea directriz general

lime (pour ampoule)
E ampoule file, ampoule cutter
G Ampullenfeile
S lima de ampolla

limitation
E limitation
G Einschränkung
S limitación, restricción

limite
E limit
G Grenzwert
S valor límite

limite d'action
E action limit
G Aktionsgrenze, Stopgrenze
S límite de acción

limite d'alarme
E alarm limit
G Alarmlimit
S límite de alarma

limite d'alerte
E alert limit
G Warngrenze
S límite de alerta

limite de charge
E loading limit, loading capacity
G Belastungsgrenze, Tragfähigkeit
S límite de carga,
capacidad de carga

limite de détection
E limit of detection (LOD)
G Nachweisgrenze
S límite de detección

limite de quantitation
E limit of quantitation (LOQ)
G Bestimmungsgrenze
S límite de análisis,
límite de determinación

limite inférieure de quantitation
E lower limit of quantitation
G untere Bestimmungsgrenze
S límite inferior de determinación

limite supérieure de quantitation
E upper limit of quantitation
G obere Bestimmungsgrenze
S límite superior de determinación

limite de service
E operating limit
G Betriebsgrenze
S límite de funcionamiento

limite de spécification
E specification limit
G Spezifikationsgrenze
S límite de especificación

limite inférieure de spécification
E lower specification limit
G untere Spezifikationsgrenze
S límite inferior de especificación

limite supérieure de spécification
E upper specification limit
G obere Spezifikationsgrenze
S límite superior de especificación

limites étroites de spécification
E tight specification limits
G enge Spezifikationsgrenzen
S límites estrechos de especificación

limite d'écoulement
E yield point
G Fließgrenze
S límite de migración
(en cromatografía)

limite d'exclusion
E exclusion limit
G Ausschlußgrenze
S límite de exclusión

limite d'utilisation
E operating limit
G Betriebsgrenze
S límite de funcionamiento

limites de confiance
E confidence limits
G Vertrauensgrenzen
S límites de confianza

linéarité
E linearity
G Linearität
S linealidad

liniment
E liniment
G Liniment
S linimento

lipide
E lipid
G Lipid
S lípido

lipophile
E lipophilic
G lipophil
S lipófilo

lipophobe
E lipophobic
G lipophob
S lipófobo

liquéfier
E fluidise, to; liquify, to
G verflüssigen
S licuar, licuefacer

liquide
E liquid
G Flüssigkeit, flüssig
S líquido

liquide de granulation
E granulating fluid
G Granulierflüssigkeit
S líquido de granulación

liquide de refroidissement
E refrigerant, coolant
G Kühlmittel
S medio refrigerante

liquide d'étanchéité
E sealing liquid
G Dichtflüssigkeit
S líquido de cerrado hermético

liquide lacrymal
E lacrimal fluid
G Tränenflüssigkeit
S líquido lacrimal

liquides biologiques
E biological fluids
G biologische Flüssigkeiten
S líquidos biológicos

lire
E read, to; read off, to
G ablesen
S leer

lisible
E legible
G lesbar
S legible

lisse
E smooth
G glatt
S liso, pulido, resbaladizo

liste de pièces de rechange
E spare parts list
G Ersatzteilliste
S lista de piezas de recambio

liste détaillée
E bill of materials, list of items
G Stückliste
S especificación, lista detallada, inventario

liste-inventaire
E bill of materials, list of items
G Stückliste
S especificación, lista detallada, inventario

lit de filtre
E filter bed
G Filterbett
S lecho filtrante

lit de mortier
E mortar bed
G Mörtelbett
S lecho de mortero

lit de poudre
E powder bed
G Pulverbett
S lecho de polvo

lit fluidisé
E fluid bed
G Wirbelschicht
S lecho fluidificado

lit mixe
E mixed bed
G Mischbett
S lecho mixto

livraison
E delivery
G Ausgabe, Auslieferung, Lieferung
S distribución, entrega

livre d'entrées de marchandises
E receiving log book
G Wareneingangsbuch
S libro de entrada de mercancías

livrer
E supply, to
G liefern, versorgen mit
S abastecer, proveer, suministrar

locaux
E premises
G Räumlichkeiten
S locales

logiciel configurable
E configurable software
G konfigurierbare Software
S software configurable

logiciel d'application
E application software
G Anwendungssoftware
S sistema lógico de aplicación, software de aplicación

logistique
E logistics
G Logistik
S logística

logo
E logo
G Firmenzeichen, Logo
S logotipo

loi
E law, statute
G Gesetz
S ley

loi pour la protection contre les radiations
E radiation protection act
G Strahlenschutzgesetz
S ley de protección frente a radiaciones ionizantes

longueur
E length
G Länge
S longitud

longueur de colonne
E column length
G Säulenlänge
S longitud de la columna

longueur de la tête du poinçon
E punch tip length
G Stempelkopflänge
S longitud de la cabeza de troquel

longueur d'onde
E wavelength
G Wellenlänge
S longitud de onda

longueur totale
E overall length
G Gesamtlänge
S longitud total

loquet
E latch, door handle
G Klinke
S picaporte, gatillo, trinquete

English German French Spanish

lot
E batch, lot
G Charge
S lote

sous-lot
E sub-batch, partial batch
G Teilcharge
S lote parcial

lot de production
E production batch, approved batch
G Produktionscharge, Verkaufscharge
S lote de producción, lote de venta

lot défectueux
E defective batch, failed batch
G Fehlcharge
S lote defectuoso

lot partiel
E sub-batch, partial batch
G Teilcharge
S lote parcial

lot pilote
E pilot batch, trial batch
G Versuchscharge
S lote piloto

lot préliminaire
E preliminary batch
G Vorcharge
S carga previa

lotion
E lotion
G Lotion
S loción

lotion capillaire
E medicated hair tonic
G medizinisches Haarwasser
S loción capilar

lotion pour œil
E eye lotion
G Augenbad
S loción oftálmica

louche
E ladle, scoop
G Schöpfkelle
S cazo, vasija

loupe
E magnifying glass
G Lupe
S lupa

lubrifiant
E lubricant
G Gleitmittel, Schmiermittel
S lubri(fi)cante

lubrification d'un instrument
E instrument lubrication
G Geräteschmierung
S lubricación del aparato

lubrifier
E grease, to; lubricate, to
G schmieren
S engrasar, lubri(fi)car

lumière diffuse
E stray light
G Streulicht
S luz difusa

lunettes de protection
E safety spectacles
G Schutzbrille
S gafas protectoras

lunettes de sécurité
E safety spectacles
G Sicherheitsbrille
S gafas de seguridad

lustre
E gloss
G Glanz
S brillo, lustre

lustré
E glossy
G glänzend
S brillante, lustrado

lutte antiparasitaire
E pest control
G Schädlingsbekämpfung
S control de plagas, lucha antiparasitaria

lyophilisat
E lyophilisate
G Lyophilisat
S liofilizado

lyophilisateur
E freeze dryer, lyophiliser
G Gefriertrockner
S liofilizador

lyophilisation
E freeze drying, lyophilisation
G Gefriertrocknung, Lyophilisation
S liofilización

lyophilisé
E freeze-dried, lyophilised
G gefriergetrocknet
S liofilizado

lysat
E lysate
G Lysat
S lisado

macération
E maceration
G Mazeration
S maceración

machine à cartonner
E cartoning machine
G Kartonierer
S máquina encartonadora

machine à laver les bouchons
E stopper washing machine
G Stopfenwaschmaschine
S máquina de lavado de tapones

machine à mouler des suppositoires
E suppository machine
G Zäpfchengießmaschine
S máquina de moldear supositorios

machine à sceller les boîtes pliantes
E folding carton sealing machine
G Faltschachtelverschließmaschine
S máquina de cierre de cajas plegables

machine à serrage de couvercles
E screw-cap closing machine
G Schraubdeckelverschließmaschine
S máquina de cierre de rosca

machine à tester la dureté
E hardness tester
G Härtetester
S máquina de comprobación de dureza

machine de fabrication de comprimés
E tabletting machine
G Tablettiermaschine
S máquina de fabricación de comprimidos

machine de remplissage des bouteilles
E bottling machine
G Flaschenabfüllmaschine
S embotelladora

machine de remplissage pour tubes
E tube-filling machine
G Tubenfüllmaschine
S máquina de llenado por tubos

machine d'empaquetage
E bundling machine
G Bündelmaschine
S máquina de embalaje

machine d'encapsulage
E bottle-closing machine
G Flaschenverschließmaschine
S máquina de cierre de botellas

machine d'enrobage à tambour
E pan coater
G Trommelcoater
S máquina de tambor para gragear

machine excentrique
E eccentric machine
G Exzentermaschine
S máquina excéntrica

machine pour conditionnements thermoformés
E blister (forming) line
G Tiefziehmaschine
S máquina para troquelar en caliente

mâchoire
E jaw (tech.)
G Backe (techn.)
S mandíbula, mordaza

mâchoire chauffante
E heating jaw
G Heizbacke
S mordaza de calefacción

mâchoires de fermeture
E sealer jaws
G Siegelbacken
S mandíbulas de sellado

macro-molécule
E macromolecule
G Makromolekül
S macromolécula

macropores
E macropores
G Makroporen
S macroporos

madré
E mottled
G gesprenkelt
S moteado, salpicado

magasin d'articles de conditionnement
E packaging warehouse
G Packmittel-Lager
S almacén de medios de envasado

maintenance
E maintenance
G Wartung
S entretenimiento, mantenimiento

maintenance d'une installation
E plant maintenance
G Anlagenwartung
S mantenimiento de equipo e instalaciones

maître
E foreman, supervisor
G Meister
S maestro

majoration
E supplement, overage
G Aufschlag
S aumento, suplemento

maladie infectieuse
E infectious disease
G ansteckende Krankheit
S enfermedad contagiosa

malaxer
E knead, to
G kneten
S amasar

malaxeur
E blender, blending apparatus
G Mischer
S mezclador

malaxeur à chute libre
E tumbler mixer
G Freifallmischer
S mezclador por basculado

management d'une installation
E plant management
G Betriebsführung
S gestión empresarial

manchette d'étanchéité
E sealing collar
G Dichtmanschette
S manguito hermético

manchon
E sleeve, sheath, bush, bushing (mach.)
G Muffe, Hülse, Hülle
S manguito, cápsula, cáscara, envoltura

manchon d'aspiration
E aspiration nipple
G Ansaugstutzen
S empalme de aspiración

manchon de connexion
E connection port, connection nipple
G Anschlußstutzen
S empalme de conexión

manchon de drainage
E discharge nipple, drain nipple, outlet nipple
G Ablaßstutzen
S empalme de salida

manchon de purge
E outlet nipple
G Auslaufstutzen
S empalme de salida

manchon d'écoulement
E discharge port, outlet port, discharge nipple, drain nipple, outlet nipple
G Ablaufstutzen, Ablaßstutzen
S empalme de salida

maniement
E handling (of)
G Handhabung, Umgang (mit)
S manejo, tratamiento, trato (con)

manipulation des matériaux
E materials handling, materials management
G Materialwirtschaft
S administración del material

manipulation génétique
E genetic engineering
G Genmanipulation
S manipulación genética

manomètre
E manometer, pressure gauge
G Druckmeßgerät
S manómetro

manomètre de pression
E manometer
G Manometer
S manómetro

manomètre différentiel
E differential manometer
G Differenzdruckmesser
S manómetro diferencial

manteau chauffant
E heating mantle
G Heizpilz
S manguito de caldeo

manteau de refroidissement
E cooling jacket
G Kühlmantel
S camisa refrigerante

manuel
E hand-operated, manual
G von Hand, manuell
S manual

manuel (d'utilisation)
E instruction manual
G Handbuch
S manual de instrucciones

manuel d'instructions
E instrument manual
G Gerätehandbuch
S manual de instrucciones

manufacturé par biotechnologie
E manufactured biotechnologically
G biotechnologisch hergestellt
S fabricado biotecnológicamente

marchandise en vrac
E bulk (material)
G Bulkware
S mercancía a granel

marchandise retournée
E returned goods
G zurückgegebene Ware
S mercancía devuelta

marchandises receptionnées
E incoming goods
G angelieferte Materialien
S materiales suministrados

marge brute
E gross margin
G Bruttomarge
S margen bruto

marge d'erreur
E margin of error
G Fehlergrenze
S límite de error, margen de error

mariner
E marinate, to; pickle, to
G beizen
S adobar, cauterizar, desinfectar

marquage
E labelling, lettering
G Beschriftung, Kennzeichnung
S etiquetado, marcado, rotulado

marquage de l'appareil
E apparatus designation
G Gerätekennzeichnung
S caracterización de aparatos

marquage des tuyaux
E piping designation
G Rohrleitungskennzeichnung
S caracterización de cañerías

marquage isotopique
E radio-label
G radioaktive Markierung
S marcado radiactivo

marque de commerce
E brand name, registered name, trade name
G Handelsmarke
S marca comercial

marque de graduation
E graduation mark
G Strichmarkierung, Teilstrich
S marca de graduación

marque déposée
E trade mark
G Warenzeichen
S marca (de fábrica)

marque inconstante
E marker (on leaflet)
G Flattermarke
S marca inconstante

marquer
E mark, to; label, to
G kennzeichnen
S etiquetar, marcar

marqueur
E marker, tracer
G Leitsubstanz
S marcador

masquage d'une saveur
E taste masking
G Geschmacksüberdeckung
S enmascaramiento del sabor

masque
E mask, masking
G Maske, Maskierung
S máscara, enmascaramiento

masque contre la poussière
E dust mask
G Staubmaske
S máscara contra el polvo

masque de protection facial
E face mask
G Mundschutz
S protección bucal

masque respiratoire de protection
E respiratory protection
G Atemschutz
S protección respiratoria

masquer
E mask, to
G maskieren
S enmascarar

masse de fabrication pour comprimés
E tabletting mass
G Tablettiermasse
S masa para comprimidos

masse thermique
E thermal mass
G thermische Masse
S masa térmica

mat
E mat
G matt
S mate

matériau
E material
G Werkstoff
S material

matériau de fermeture
E closure material
G Verschlußmaterial
S material de cierre

matériau d'étanchéité
E sealant
G Dichtungsmittel
S material de cierre, material de sellado

matériau d'obturation
E sealant
G Dichtungsmittel
S material de cierre, material de sellado

matériau en vrac
E bulk material
G Schüttgut
S carga a granel

matériau libérant des particules
E particle-releasing material
G partikelabgebendes Material
S material que desprende partículas

matériau monolithique
E monolithic material
G monolithisches Material
S material monolítico

matériau pour joint
E jointing material
G Fugenmaterial
S material de junta

matériaux de filtre
E filter materials
G Filtermaterialien
S materiales de filtración

matériaux de réaction
E reaction materials
G Ansatz
S planteamiento, inserción, materiales de reacción

matériaux refusés
E rejected materials
G zurückgewiesene Materialien
S materiales rechazados

matériaux rejetés
E rejected materials
G zurückgewiesene Materialien
S materiales rechazados

matériel dangereux
E hazardous material, dangerous material
G Gefahrstoff
S sustancia peligrosa

matériel de départ
E starting material, raw material
G Ausgangsstoff
S sustancia de partida, sustancia inicial

matériel de laboratoire
E lab ware
G Laborartikel
S artículo de laboratorio

matériel de moulage
E pressing material
G Preßmaterial
S material de prensado

matériel de pressage
E pressing material
G Preßmaterial
S material de prensado

matériel de remplissage d'une colonne
E column filler
G Säulenfüllmaterial
S material de relleno de la columna

English German French Spanish

matériel d'emballage
E packaging material
G Packmaterial, Verpackungsmaterial, Packmittel
S material de embalaje

matériel d'emballage imprimé
E printed packaging material
G bedrucktes Packmaterial
S material impreso de embalaje

matériel d'emballage primaire
E primary packaging material
G Primärpackmittel
S material primario de envase

matériel d'emballage secondaire
E secondary packaging material
G Sekundärpackmittel
S material de envase secundario

matière brute
E raw material
G Rohmaterial, Rohstoff
S materia prima

matière de remplissage
E contents, charge
G Füllgut
S material de relleno

matière hautement infectieuse
E highly infectious material
G hochinfektiöses Material
S material muy infeccioso

matière moulée
E compression material, moulding compound
G Preßmasse
S masa comprimible

matière première
E starting material, raw material
G Ausgangsstoff
S sustancia de partida, sustancia inicial

matière première en vrac
E bulk pharmaceutical chemical (BPC)
G Wirkstoff (als Rohstoff)
S sustancia activa (materia prima)

matière première inactive
E inactive raw material
G inaktiver Rohstoff
S materia prima inactiva

matrice
E stencil, template
G Schablone
S modelo, patrón, plantilla

matrice (d'une presse à comprimés)
E die (of tabletting machine)
G Matrize (an der Tablettenpresse)
S matriz (de una prensa de comprimidos)

matrice pour outil multiple
E multi-bore die
G Matrize für Mehrfachwerkzeug
S matrices para herramientas de uso múltiple

mauvaise qualité, de
E inferior
G minderwertig
S de menor calidad

mécanique
E mechanical
G maschinell
S mecánico

mécanisme d'action
E drug mechanism
G Wirkungsmechanismus
S mecanismo de acción

mécanisme de guidage
E guide, guiding device, guiding mechanism
G Führungsvorrichtung
S dispositivo de guía, guía

mécanisme de réaction
E reaction mechanism
G Reaktionsmechanismus
S mecanismo de reacción

mécanisme de séparation
E separation mechanism
G Trennungsmechanismus
S mecanismo de separación

médecin responsable d'essais cliniques
E trial physician, investigator
G Prüfarzt
S médico investigador

médicament
E medicinal product, drug
G Arzneimittel
S medicamento

médicament à usage vétérinaire
E veterinary medicament
G Tierarzneimittel
S medicamento de uso veterinario

médicament fini
E finished medicinal product
G Fertigarzneimittel
S medicamento manufacturado, especialidad farmacéutica manufacturada

médicament optiquement actif
E chiral medicinal substance
G chiraler Arzneistoff
S sustancia medicamentosa ópticamente activa

médicament pour nourriture animale
E drugs for animal feed
G Fütterungsarzneimittel
S medicamento para el pienso

médicament produit par génie génétique
E genetically manufactured medicinal product
G gentechnologisch hergestelltes Arzneimittel
S medicamento producido mediante tecnología genética

médicament retard
E depot drug
G Depotpräparat
S preparado retard

médication
E medication
G Medikation
S medicación

médication alternative
E alternative medication
G Ausweichmedikation
S medicación alternativa

médium d'archivage
E archiving media
G Archivierungsmedien
S medios de archivado

médium de concentration
E concentration medium, enrichment medium
G Anreicherungsmedium
S medio de concentración, medio de enriquecimiento

médium de culture exempt de sérum
E serum-free media
G serumfreie Nährmedien
S medios de cultivo sin suero

mélange
E blend, mix, mixture, mix in
G Mischung, Gemisch, Untermischung, Vermischung
S mezcla, mixtura, entremezcla

mélangé à l'avance
E pre-mixed
G vorgemischt
S mezclado previamente

mélange comprimable
E compactible mixture
G preßfertige Mischung
S mezcla comprimible

mélange de poudre
E powdered mixture
G Pulvermischung
S mezcla de polvo

mélange homogénéisé
E blending mixture
G Mischgut
S mezcla homogeneizada

mélanger
E blend, to; mix, to
G mischen
S mezclar

English German French Spanish

mélanger à l'avance
E pre-blend, to; pre-mix, to
G vormischen
S mezclar previamente

mélangeur
E blender, blending apparatus
G Mischer
S mezclador

mélangeur à circulation forcée
E forced-circulation mixer
G Zwangsmischer
S mezclador de circulación forzada

mélangeur à forces de cisaillement
E high shear mixer
G Pflugscharmischer
S mezclador de cizallamiento

mélangeur à pales
E propeller mixer
G Propellermischer
S mezclador de hélice

mélangeur à tambour
E drum mixer
G Trommelmischer
S mezclador de tambor

mélangeur avec forces de cisaillements importantes
E high-shear mixer
G Mischer mit hohem Scherkraftanteil
S mezclador intenso de cizallamiento

mélangeur culbuteur
E tumbler mixer, tumble blender
G Freifallmischer, Taumelmischer
S mezclador por basculado, mezclador de volteo

mélangeur en cube
E cube mixer
G Kubusmischer
S mezclador cúbico

mélangeur excentrique
E forced-circulation mixer
G Zwangsmischer
S mezclador de circulación forzada

mélangeur planétaire
E planetary mixer
G Planetenmischer
S mezclador planetario

mélangeur turbulent
E tumble blender
G Taumelmischer
S mezclador de turbulencia

membrane
E membrane, diaphragm
G Membran
S membrana

membrane cellulaire
E cell wall
G Zellwand
S pared celular

membrane de micro-filtration
E micro-filtration membrane
G Mikrofiltrationsmembran
S membrana de microfiltración

membrane perméable
E permeable membrane
G permeable Membran
S membrana permeable

membrane semi-perméable
E semi-permeable membrane
G semipermeable Membran
S membrana semipermeable

mémoire d'un instrument
E instrument memory
G Gerätespeicher
S memoria de un instrumento

mention de venue
E sign-in log
G Ankunftsvermerk
S nota de llegada

mention d'origine
E sign-out log
G Ausgangsvermerk
S mención inicial, nota inicial

méprise
E confusion, misidentification
G Verwechslung
S confusión

mésopores
E mesopores
G Mesoporen
S mesoporos

message d'erreur
E failure message
G Fehlermeldung
S aviso de errores

mesurable
E measurable
G meßbar
S medible, mensurable

mesure
E measure, measurement
G Maßnahme, Messung
S medida, medición

mesure (de la dose) d'un aérosol
E aerosol measurement
G Aerosolmessung
S medida de aerosol

mesurer
E measure, to
G messen
S medir

mesures propres à favoriser un produit
E product promotion
G Produktförderung
S promoción de un producto

métal
E metal
G Metall
S metal

métal lourd
E heavy metal
G Schwermetall
S metal pesado

métal précieux
E precious metal
G Edelmetall
S metal noble

méthode
E method, technique
G Methode, Technik
S método, técnica

méthode analytique
E test method, analytical method
G Prüfmethode
S método de prueba

méthode chromatographique
E chromatographic assay
G chromatographische Methode
S método cromatográfico

méthode d'administration
E method of administration
G Verwaltungsverfahren
S procedimiento administrativo

méthode d'agitation à corbeilles
E basket stirring method
G Drehkörbchenmethode
S método de agitación con cesto rotatorio

méthode de coloration de Gram
E Gram staining
G Gramfärbung
S tinción de Gram

méthode de contrôle
E test method, analytical method
G Prüfmethode
S método de prueba

méthode de filtration
E filtration method
G Filtrationsmethode
S método de filtración

English German French Spanish

méthode de séparation
E separating method
G Trennmethode
S método de separación

mettre à la terre
E ground, to; earth, to
G erden
S conectar a tierra

mettre en danger (la qualité)
E endanger, to (quality)
G gefährden (Qualität)
S arriesgar, poner en peligro (la calidad)

mettre en fonctionnement
E put into operation, to
G in Betrieb setzen
S poner en funcionamiento

mettre en place
E set up, to
G einrichten
S instalar

mettre sur l'arête
E cant, to
G verkanten
S ladear

microbien
E microbial
G mikrobiell
S microbiano

microbiologie
E microbiology
G Mikrobiologie
S microbiología

microbiologique
E microbiological
G mikrobiologisch
S microbiológico

microcospe
E microscope
G Mikroskop
S microscopio

microcristallin
E microcrystalline
G mikrokristallin
S microcristalino

micro-encapsulé
E micro-encapsulated
G mikroverkapselt
S microencapsulado

micro-filtration
E micro-filtration
G Mikrofiltration
S microfiltración

micromètre
E fine adjusting screw, micrometer screw
G Mikrometerschraube
S tornillo micrométrico

micronisation
E micronisation
G Mikronisierung
S micronización

microniseur à jet d'air
E air attrition mill, fluid energy mill
G Luftstrahlmühle
S micronizador del chorro de aire

micro-onde
E microwave
G Mikrowelle
S microonda

micro-organismes
E microorganisms
G Mikroorganismen
S microorganismos

micro-organismes non-pathogènes
E non-pathogenic microorganisms
G apathogene Mikroorganismen
S microorganismos apatógenos

micro-organismes pathogènes
E pathogenic microorganisms
G pathogene Mikroorganismen
S microorganismos patógenos

micro-organismes viables
E viable microorganisms
G lebensfähige Mikroorganismen
S microorganismos viables

micro-pipettage
E micro-pipetting
G Mikropipettierung
S micropipetado

micro-plasma
E micro-plasma
G Mikroplasma
S microplasma

migration
E migration
G Migration, Wanderung
S migración

milieu
E medium
G Medium
S medio

milieu de culture
E culture medium, nutrient medium
G Nährmedium, Nährboden
S medio de cultivo

milieu de culture déhydraté
E dehydrated culture medium
G Trockennährmedium
S medio de cultivo deshidratado

milieu de culture sélectif
E selective culture medium
G Selektivnährmedien
S medios de cultivo selectivos

milieu de dissolution
E dissolution medium
G Lösemedium, Auflösemedium
S disolvente, diluyente, medio de disolución

milieu de rinçage
E rinsing medium
G Spülmedium
S medio de lavado

milieu de séparation
E separating medium, separation media
G Trennmittel, Trennmedium
S medio de separación, medio separador

milieu non aquatique
E non-aqueous environment
G nicht-wäßrige Umgebung
S entorno no acuoso

milieux liquides
E liquid media
G Flüssigmedien
S medios líquidos

minuterie
E timer
G Zeitgeber
S sincronizador del tiempo

minuterie (d'un ordinateur)
E disk drive (computer)
G Laufwerk (Computer)
S unidad (de un ordenador)

minutie
E thoroughness
G Gründlichkeit
S minuciosidad

minutieusement
E thorough
G gründlich
S minucioso, minuciosamente

miscible
E miscible
G mischbar
S miscible

non miscible
E immiscible
G nicht mischbar
S no miscible

mise à la terre
E ground, earth
G Ableitung, Erdung
S derivación, toma de tierra

English German French Spanish

mise à zéro
E zero adjustment
G Nulleinstellung
S posición cero, puesta a cero

mise au point précise
E fine adjustment
G Feineinstellung
S ajuste fino

mise en forme
E processing
G Bearbeitung, Verarbeitung
S elaboración, transformación

mise en garde
E hazard indication
G Gefahrenhinweis
S aviso de peligro

cancéreux si inhalé
E may cause cancer by inhalation
G kann beim Einatmen Krebs erzeugen
S cancerógeno si se inhala

dangereux pour les enfants pendant une grossesse
E may cause harm to unborn child
G gefährdet ungeborene Kinder
S peligroso para el feto

peut altérer la fertilité
E may impair fertility
G kann die Fruchtbarkeit beeinträchtigen
S puede dañar la fertilidad

peut être la cause de dommages génétiques héréditaires
E may cause heritable genetic damage
G kann vererbliche Genschäden verursachen
S puede originar daños genéticos hereditarios

peut irriter le système respiratoire
E irritating to respiratory system
G reizt die Atemwege
S irrita las vías respiratorias

peut provoquer de (sévères) brûlures
E causes (severe) burns
G verursacht (schwere) Verbrennungen
S causa (graves) quemaduras

peut provoquer des irritations aux yeux
E irritating to eyes
G reizt die Augen
S irrita los ojos

peut provoquer un cancer
E may cause cancer
G kann Krebs erzeugen
S puede causar cáncer

toxique au contact de la peau
E toxic in contact with skin
G giftig bei Hautkontakt
S tóxico para la piel

toxique si ingéré
E toxic if swallowed
G giftig beim Verschlucken
S tóxico si se ingiere

toxique si inhalé
E toxic by inhalation
G giftig beim Einatmen
S tóxico si se inhala

mise en service
E start-up
G Inbetriebnahme
S puesta en marcha, puesta en servicio

mise la terre
E grounding, earthing
G Erdung
S toma de tierra

mixture
E blend, mixture
G Mischung
S mezcla, mixtura

mixture devant être agitée
E mixture to be shaken
G Schüttelmixtur
S mezcla a agitar

mm de pression d'eau
E mm water
G mm Wassersäule
S mm de presión de agua

mobile
E mobile
G fahrbar
S móvil, portátil

mode d'emploi
E instruction, operating manual, operating instructions
G Anweisung, Betriebsanleitung, Bedienungsanleitung
S instrucción, instrucciones de funcionamiento, instrucción de manejo, instrucción de servicio

mode d'utilisation
E operating mode
G Bedienungsmodus
S modo de servicio

mode indéréglable
E fail-safe mode
G fehlersicherer Modus
S modo a prueba de errores

mode opératoire
E test instructions
G Prüfanleitung
S instrucciones de prueba

modelage de substance
E substance modelling
G Substanzmodellierung
S modelado de sustancias

modelage moléculaire
E molecular modelling
G Molekularmodellierung
S modelado molecular

modèle d'écoulement d'air
E air flow pattern
G Luftführung
S patrón de conducción de aire

modernisation
E re-equipping
G Umrüstung
S modernización, reorganización

moderniser
E upgrade, to; re-equip, to
G aufrüsten, umrüsten
S modernizar, renovar, reorganizar

modification chimique
E chemical modification
G chemische Modifikation
S modificación química

modification d'un format
E size changeover
G Formatumstellung
S cambio de formato

modification d'un procédé
E procedural change
G Verfahrensänderung
S modificación del procedimiento

modifié
E modified
G modifiziert
S modificado

module
E attachment, module
G Anbauteil, Baustein
S módulo, pieza de montaje, piedra de construcción

moisi
E mouldy, mildewed
G schimmelig
S enmohecido, mohoso

moisissure
E mould
G Schimmel
S moho

molaire
E molar
G molar
S molar

molarité
E molarity
G Molarität
S molaridad

English German French Spanish

mole
E mole
G Mol
S mol

moléculaire
E molecular
G molekular
S molecular

monochromateur
E monochromator
G Monochromator
S monocromador

monochromatique
E monochromatic
G monochrom
S monocromo

monographie de la pharmacopée
E pharmacopoeial monograph
G Arzneibuchmonographie
S monografía de farmacopea

monomère
E monomer
G Monomer
S monómero

monovalent
E monovalent
G einwertig
S monovalente

montage
E installation, mounting, assembly, set-up
G Einbau, Zusammenbau, Montage
S instalación, montaje, ensamblaje

montage des instruments
E instrument set-up
G instrumenteller Aufbau
S montaje de instrumentos

monter (un carton)
E set up, to (a folding carton)
G aufrichten (eine Faltschachtel)
S montar (una caja plegable)

morceau
E fragment, piece, fraction
G Bruchstück
S fragmento

mortier
E mortar
G Mörser, Reibschale
S mortero

mot de passe
E password
G Paßwort
S consigna

moteur de transmission
E drive motor
G Antriebsmotor
S motor de propulsión

moteur électrique triphasé
E three-phase current motor
G Drehstrommotor
S motor de corriente trifásica

moteur propulsif
E drive motor
G Antriebsmotor
S motor de propulsión

mouillant
E wetting agent
G Benetzungsmittel, Feuchthaltemittel, Netzmittel
S humectante

mouiller
E wet, to; moisten, to
G benetzen
S humedecer, mojar, rociar

moulage
E grinding
G Vermahlung
S molienda, molturado

moulage par procédé pressé-soufflé
E blow moulding
G Blasverformung
S moldeo por inyección

mouler des suppositoires
E mould, to (suppositories)
G Zäpfchen gießen
S moldear supositorios

moulu
E moulded, ground
G geformt, gepreßt, geschliffen
S moldeado, comprimido

moulure creuse
E recess
G Hohlkehle
S canal, garganta, media caña

moussage
E foam formation, foaming
G Schaumbildung
S formación de espuma

mousse
E foam
G Schaum
S espuma

mousse en plastique
E foam plastic
G Schaumstoff
S espuma

mousse pour utilisation cutanée
E cutaneous foam
G Schaum zur Anwendung auf der Haut
S espuma cutánea

mousse rectale
E rectal foam
G Rektalschaum
S espuma rectal

mousser
E foam, to
G schäumen
S espumar

mouvement d'agitation
E shaking movement
G Schüttelbewegung
S movimiento de agitación

mouvement des matériaux
E material movement
G Materialbewegung
S movimiento de material

moyen de remplissage
E filler
G Füllmittel
S medio de relleno

moyenne
E average, mean
G Durchschnitt
S media, promedio

moyenne arithmétique
E arithmetic mean
G arithmetisches Mittel
S media aritmética

moyens de production
E utilities
G Medien, Betriebsmittel
S medios de producción

moyens d'exploitation
E utilities
G Betriebsmittel, Medien
S medios de explotación empresarial

moyeu d'agitateur
E stirrer hub
G Rührwerksnabe
S cubo del agitador

mucilage
E mucilage
G Schleim
S mucosidad

mucus
E mucilage
G Schleim
S mucosidad

multicentrique
E multicentric
G multizentrisch
S multicéntrico

muqueuse
E mucous membrane
G Schleimhaut
S mucosa

muqueux
E mucous
G schleimig
S mucoso, mucilaginoso

mur de partage
E partition
G Stellwand
S pantalla protectora

mur de séparation
E partition (wall), baffle
G Trennwand, Zwischenwand
S tabique (de separación)

mur revêtu d'un crépi
E plastered wall
G verputzte Wand
S pared revocada

mutagène
E mutagenic
G mutagen
S mutágeno

narcotique
E narcotic
G Rauschmittel
S narcótico

nature (d'une substance)
E nature (of a substance)
G Beschaffenheit (einer Substanz)
S naturaleza (de una sustancia)

nébuliser
E nebulise, to
G vernebeln
S nebulizar

nébuliseur
E nebuliser
G Vernebler
S nebulizador

nécessaire de transfusion
E transfusion set
G Transfusionsbesteck
S instrumental de transfusión

nécessaire pour infusion
E infusion assembly
G Infusionsbesteck
S instrumental de infusión

nécessiter
E require, to
G erfordern
S exigir, necesitar, requerir

nettoyage
E cleaning, purification
G Reinigung
S limpieza

nettoyage d'échantillons
E sample clean-up
G Probenaufreinigung
S purificación de muestras

nettoyage en place (CIP)
E cleaning in-place (CIP)
G Reinigung (von Anlagen) im geschlossenen System
S limpieza (de instalaciones) en sistema cerrado

niche
E niche, recess
G Nische
S nicho

niveau
E level
G Pegel, Pegelstand, Füllstand
S nivel, nivel de relleno

niveau de bio-sécurité
E biosafety level
G biologische Sicherheitsstufe
S grado de seguridad biológica

niveau de confiance
E confidence level
G Vertrauensniveau
S nivel de confianza

niveau de contamination
E contamination level
G Kontaminationsgrad
S grado de contaminación

niveau de pressurisation
E pressurisation level
G Druckhöhe
S altura de presión

niveau de production
E output
G Ausstoß (Menge)
S volumen de producción

niveau de propreté
E cleanliness grade (e. g. room), purity (product)
G Reinigungsgrad, Reinheitsgrad
S grado de limpieza, grado de pureza

niveau de qualité acceptable
E acceptable quality level (AQL)
G Annehmbare Qualitätsgrenzlage (AQL)
S límite de calidad aceptable

niveau individuel de qualité acceptable
E individual AQL
G Einzel-AQL
S límite individual de calidad aceptable

niveau total de qualité acceptable
E class AQL
G Gesamt-AQL
S límite total de calidad aceptable

niveau de remplissage
E filling level
G Füllhöhe
S nivel de llenado

niveau de rendement
E output
G Ausstoß (Menge)
S volumen de producción

niveau de stérilité
E clean room grade, clean room class
G Reinraumklasse
S nivel de esterilidad

niveau du bruit
E noise level
G Geräuschpegel
S nivel sonoro

niveau du liquide
E liquid level
G Flüssigkeitsstand
S nivel de líquido

nivellement
E levelling
G Nivellierung
S nivelación

nocif
E harmful, hazardous
G schädlich
S dañino, nocivo

nom commercial
E brand name
G Markenname
S nombre comercial

nom de commerce
E commercial name
G Handelsname
S nombre comercial

nombre de micro-organismes
E microbial count
G Keimzahl
S número de gérmenes

nombre de micro-organismes de l'air
E air microbial count
G Luftkeimzahl
S número de gérmenes del aire

nombre de particules
E particle count
G Partikelzahlen
S número de partículas

nombre de pièces
E number of items
G Stückzahl
S número de piezas

nombre de plateaux
E plate number
G Bodenzahl
S número de placa

nombre de plateaux théoriques
E number of theoretical plates
G Zahl der theoretischen Böden
S número de placas teóricas

nombre de rejet
E rejection number
G Rückweisezahl
S número de rechazo

nombre de rotations
E revolutions
G Drehzahl
S número de revoluciones

nombre de tours
E revolutions
G Umdrehungszahl
S número de revoluciones

nombre d'ester
E ester number
G Esterzahl
S número de éster

nombre d'iode
E iodine number
G Iodzahl
S índice de iodo

nombre total de micro-organismes
E total microbial count
G Gesamtkeimzahl
S número total de gérmenes

non aqueux
E non-aqueous
G nicht-wäßrig
S no acuoso

non conformité
E non-compliance
G Nichteinhaltung
S no observancia

non emballé
E unpacked
G unverpackt
S no embalado

non équivoque
E unequivocal
G unzweideutig, eindeutig
S inequívoco

non linéaire
E non-linear
G nichtlinear
S no lineal

non polaire
E non-polar
G unpolar
S no polar

non valable
E invalid
G ungültig
S inválido

non volatile
E non-volatile
G nichtflüchtig
S no volátil

normalité (d'une solution)
E normality (of a solution)
G Normalität (einer Lösung)
S normalidad (de una disolución)

norme
E standard
G Norm
S norma

norme de travail
E working standard
G Arbeitsstandard
S norma de trabajo

normes de sécurité
E safety standards
G Sicherheitsstandards
S estándares de seguridad

notes explicatives
E recommendation
G Empfehlung
S recomendación

notice (d'un emballage)
E package leaflet, package insert
G Beipackzettel
S prospecto acompañante (del medicamento)

notice explicative
E package insert, package leaflet
G Packungsbeilage
S prospecto informativo del medicamento

notice explicative dépliante
E pre-folded package insert
G vorgefaltete Packungsbeilage
S prospecto informativo del medicamento previamente plegado

nourriture
E food
G Lebensmittel
S alimento

nouvelle formulation
E reformulation
G Umformulierung
S nueva formulación, reformulación

noyau
E nucleus
G Kern
S núcleo

noyau d'un comprimé
E tablet core
G Tablettenkern
S núcleo del comprimido

nuance d'une couleur
E colour shade, hue
G Farbton
S matiz del color

numéro de commande
E order number, purchase order number
G Auftragsnummer, Bestellauftragsnummer
S número del encargo, número del encargo de pedido

numéro de lot
E batch number
G Chargennummer
S número de lote

numéro de série
E serial number
G Seriennummer
S número de serie

numéro de version
E version number
G Versionsnummer
S número de versión

numéro d'identification d'un patient
E patient identification number
G Patientennummer
S número de identificación del paciente

nutriment
E nutrient
G Nährstoff
S nutriente, sustancia nutricia

obligatoire
E binding, compulsory
G verbindlich, obligatorisch
S obligatorio

ne comportant aucune obligation
E without obligation
G unverbindlich
S no obligatorio

oblique
E sloping
G schräg
S inclinado, oblicuo

English
German
French
Spanish

obscurcissement
E darken
G Verdunkelung
S oscurecimiento

observation particulière
E observation, special
G Beobachtung, besondere
S observación especial

obsolète
E obsolete
G veraltet
S envejecido, obsoleto

obstrué
E clogged, blocked
G verstopft
S obstruido

obturateur doseur
E drop closure
G Tropfverschluß
S tapón cuentagotas

obturer (des ampoules)
E tip seal, to (ampoules)
G abschmelzen (Ampullen)
S sellar (ampollas)

obturer par vitrification (ampoules)
E flame-seal, to (ampoules)
G zuschmelzen (Ampullen)
S obturar por vitrificación, cerrar ampollas a la llama

obturer une ampoule
E seal an ampoule, to
G Ampulle verschließen
S cerrar una ampolla

occulaire
E ocular
G Okular
S ocular

odeur
E odour, fragrance
G Geruch, Duft
S olor, aroma

sans odeur
E odourless
G geruchlos
S inodoro

œillet
E eye, eyelet
G Öse
S ojal

œillet d'inoculation
E inoculating loop
G Impföse
S ojal de inoculación

office des brevets
E patent office
G Patentamt
S oficina de patentes

oligoélément
E trace elements
G Spurenelemente
S oligoelementos

oligomères
E oligomers
G Oligomere
S oligómero

omission
E omission
G Auslassung
S omisión

onguent
E embrocation, liniment
G Einreibemittel
S bálsamo, linimento

opalescence
E opalescence
G Opaleszenz
S opalescencia

opaque
E opaque
G undurchsichtig, lichtundurchlässig
S opaco

opérateur
E operator
G Durchführender
S ejecutante,operador

opération
E operation, run
G Arbeitsgang, Lauf
S turno de trabajo, ciclo, marcha, recorrido

opération continue
E continuous operation
G Dauerbetrieb, kontinuierlicher Betrieb
S funcionamiento continuo

opération électro-pneumatique
E electro-pneumatic operation
G elektro-pneumatischer Betrieb
S funcionamiento electroneumático

opération en une seule étape
E single step operation
G in einem Arbeitsgang
S operación en etapa única

opérations en zone d'atmosphère contrôlée
E clean room operations
G Arbeitsvorgänge im Reinraum
S procesos de trabajo en área estéril

opinion d'expert
E expert opinion
G Begutachtung
S dictamen, peritaje

optimisation
E optimisation
G Optimierung
S optim(iz)ación

options d'un équipement
E instrument options
G Geräteoptionen
S opciones del aparato

oral
E oral
G oral
S oral

ordonnance
E prescription, medical prescription
G Rezept, Verschreibung, ärztliche Verordnung
S receta, prescripción, prescripción médica

ordre de magnitude
E order of magnitude
G Größenordnung
S orden de magnitud

ordures
E waste
G Abfall
S desecho

organigramme
E organisation chart, organogram
G Organigramm
S organigrama

organisation mondiale de la santé (OMS)
E World Health Organisation (WHO)
G Weltgesundheitsorganisation
S Organización Mundial de la Salud (OMS)

organisme cité
E Notified Body
G Benannte Stelle
S departamento citado

organisme de contrôle
E test organism
G Prüfkeim
S germen de prueba

organisme indicateur
E indicator organism
G Indikatorkeim
S germen indicador

organisme microbien
E organism
G Keim
S germen

English German French Spanish

organismes génétiquement modifiés (OGM)
E genetically modified organisms (GMO)
G genetisch veränderte Organismen
S organismos modificados genéticamente

orifice
E outlet, orifice
G Auslaß, Austritt, Mündung
S descarga, escape, salida, desembocadura, orificio

orifice d'alimentation
E charge port, nipple
G Befüllstutzen
S tubuladura de carga, tubuladura de alimentación

orifice de charge
E charge port, nipple
G Befüllstutzen
S tubuladura de carga, tubuladura de alimentación

orifice de purge
E vent
G Belüftungsloch
S orificio de ventilación

orifice de purge anti-déflagrant
E ex-duct, explosion vent
G Ex-Kanal
S orificio o válvula de seguridad (antideflagrante)

orifice de ventilation
E vent
G Belüftungsloch
S orificio de ventilación

orifice d'entrée de liquide
E inlet
G Einfluß
S orificio de entrada de líquido

origine du produit
E product origin
G Produktherkunft
S procedencia del producto

oscillation
E oscillation
G Oszillation
S oscilación

osmolalité
E osmolality
G Osmolalität
S osmolalidad

osmomètre
E osmometer
G Osmometer
S osmómetro

osmose
E osmosis
G Osmose
S ósmosis

osmose inverse
E reverse osmosis (RO)
G Umkehrosmose
S ósmosis inversa

ouate
E cotton wool
G Watte
S algodón

ouate à pansement
E cotton wool
G Verbandwatte
S algodón de vendaje

ourlet
E seam
G Naht
S costura

outil
E tool
G Werkzeug
S instrumento

outil de compression
E compaction device, compression mould
G Preßwerkzeug
S instrumental de compresión

outil de perforation
E perforation tool
G Perforierwerkzeug
S instrumentos de perforación

outiller
E provide with, to; equip, to
G ausrüsten
S equipar

ouverture
E opening
G Öffnung
S abertura

ouverture dans le mur
E wall opening, duct
G Wanddurchführung
S pasamuros

ouverture de chargement
E filling port
G Einfüllöffnung
S abertura de relleno

ouverture de décompression
E pressure relief opening
G Druckentlastungsöffnung
S orificio de descompresión

ouverture de maille
E mesh size
G Maschenweite
S tamaño del orificio de la malla

ouverture d'un entonnoir
E funnel opening
G Trichteröffnung
S abertura del embudo

ouverture d'un trémie
E funnel opening
G Trichteröffnung
S abertura del embudo

ouverture d'une matrice
E die opening
G Matrizenöffnung
S abertura de matriz

ouvrier
E workman, tradesman
G Handwerker
S artesano, trabajador manual

ouvrier qualifié
E skilled worker
G Facharbeiter
S tabajador cualificado

oximation
E oximation
G Oximierung, Oximbildung
S oximación

oxydable
E oxidisable
G oxydierbar
S oxidable

oxydant
E oxidising agent
G Oxydationsmittel
S oxidante

oxydation
E oxidation
G Oxydierung
S oxidación

oxydé (électrolytiquement)
E anodised
G eloxiert
S oxidado electrolíticamente

oxyde d'aluminium
E alumina, aluminium oxide
G Aluminiumoxid
S óxido de aluminio

oxygénation
E oxygenation
G Oxigenierung
S oxigenación

oxygène
E oxygen
G Sauerstoff
S oxígeno

English German French Spanish

oxygène dissous
E dissolved oxygen (DO)
G gelöster Sauerstoff
S oxígeno disuelto

ozonation
E ozonisation
G Ozonisierung
S ozon(iz)ación

ozone
E ozone
G Ozon
S ozono

ozonisation
E ozonisation
G Ozonisierung
S ozon(iz)ación

package de colonne
E column packing
G Säulenfüllung
S llenado de la columna

paillasse de laboratoire
E bench
G Labortisch
S mesa de laboratorio

paillasse sous flux laminaire
E clean bench
G reine Werkbank
S banco de trabajo estéril

pale
E blade
G Schaufel
S pala

pale d'agitation
E paddle stirrer, stirring blade
G Blattrührerapparatur, Rührflügel
S pala de agitación, aleta de agitación

palette
E pallet
G Palette
S paleta

alupalette, palette en aluminium
E aluminium pallet
G Alupalette
S paleta de aluminio

palette en bois
E wooden pallet
G Holzpalette
S paleta de madera

palette en plastique
E plastic pallet
G Kunststoffpalette
S paleta de plástico

palettiser
E palletise, to
G palettieren
S cargar con paleta

palettiseur
E palletiser
G Palettiermaschine
S máquina de carga con paleta

palmer
E thickness gauge
G Dickenmeßgerät
S calibre de grosores

palpeur de remplissage
E product scanner
G Füllguttaster
S sensor del contenido

panne
E breakdown, downtime (machine), failure, fault, accident
G Störfall, Ausfall, Panne
S avería, incidente, desperfecto, fallo

pansement
E wound dressing, bandage
G Wundauflage, Verband
S compresa, vendaje, vendaje de una herida

pansement transcutané
E transdermal patch
G transdermales Pflaster
S emplasto transdérmico

papier de tournesol
E litmus paper
G Lackmuspapier
S papel de tornasol

papier filtre
E filter paper
G Filtrierpapier
S papel de filtro

papier vernis
E varnished cardboard
G lackierte Pappe
S cartón barnizado

paramètre critique
E critical parameter
G kritischer Parameter
S parámetro crítico

paramètre d'analyse
E testing parameter
G Prüfparameter
S parámetro de prueba

paramètre de service
E operational parameter
G Betriebsparameter
S parámetro de servicio

paroi
E wall
G Wandung
S pared

paroi d'un récipient
E vessel wall
G Gefäßwand
S pared de un recipiente

paroi d'une matrice
E die wall
G Matrizenwand
S pared de matriz

participation
E participation, involvement
G Beteiligung
S participación

particularité
E feature
G Merkmal
S característica

particule
E particle, particulate matter
G Partikel, Teilchen
S partícula

particule de verre
E glass particle
G Glaspartikel
S partícula de vidrio

particule fine
E fine particle
G Feinkorn
S partícula fina

particule grossière
E coarse particle
G Grobkorn
S grano grueso

particules aéroportées
E airborne particles
G aus der Luft stammende Partikel
S partículas procedentes del aire

particules de poussière
E dust particles
G Staubpartikel
S partícula de polvo

particules de verre fritté
E fused glass particles
G Sinterglasteilchen
S partículas de vidrio sinterizado

particules viables
E viable particles
G lebensfähige Partikel
S partículas viables

partie
E part, moiety
G Teil
S parte

pas gauche, à
E left-hand
G linksgängig
S de paso izquierdo

passage
E passage
G Durchlauf
S paso

passage intercalé de conditionnements
E package loading
G Packguteinschub
S inserción de embalajes

passant (tamisage)
E fines (sieve)
G Durchgang (beim Sieben)
S tamizado, paso de tamiz

passer à la vapeur
E strip, to; evaporate, to
G ausdampfen
S evaporar, volatilizar

passer au rouleau
E roll, to
G walzen
S allanar, aplanar, cilindrar

passif (finance)
E liability (financial)
G Verbindlichkeit (finanz.)
S obligación, pasivo (contabilidad)

passivation (par ex. de l'acier inoxydable)
E passivation (e. g. of steel)
G Passivierung (z. B. von Stahl)
S pasivación (p. ej. de acero)

passivé
E passivated
G passiviert
S pasivado

pasteurisation
E pasteurisation
G Pasteurisierung
S paste(u)rización

pastille
E pastille, lozenge, pellet, compressed core
G Pastille, Lutschtablette, Preßling
S pastilla, comprimido para chupar, masa comprimida

pastiller
E pelletise, to
G pelletieren
S transformar en pellets

pastilleuse
E tablet press
G Tablettenpresse
S prensa de comprimidos

pâte
E paste
G Paste
S pasta

pâte pour utilisation cutanée
E cutaneous paste
G Paste zur Anwendung auf der Haut
S pasta cutánea

pâte pour utilisation orale
E oral paste
G Paste zum Einnehmen
S pasta oral

pâteux
E pasty, paste-like, doughy
G pastenartig, pastös, teigartig
S pastoso

pathogène
E pathogen
G Erreger (Mikroorganismus), Krankheitserreger
S agente patógeno (microorganismo), patógeno

pathogénique
E pathogenic
G pathogen
S patógeno

pathologique
E pathological
G pathologisch
S patológico

patient
E patient
G Patient
S paciente

patron
E stencil, template
G Schablone
S modelo, patrón, plantilla

patte
E tab, tongue
G Einstecklasche
S cubrejunta de pestaña

paupière
E eye lid
G Augenlid
S párpado

pays rapporteur (UE)
E Reference Member State (EU) (RMS)
G Erstzulassender (EU) Mitgliedsstaat
S País Miembro (UE) de Referencia (para registro de medicamentos)

pelle
E blade
G Schaufel
S pala

pellet
E pellet
G Pellet
S pellet

pellicule
E coat, coating, film, layer
G Beschichtung, Überzug, Lage, Schicht
S estrato, cubierta, revestimiento

pénétration
E penetration, permeation
G Penetration, Durchdringung
S penetración

pénétrer
E penetrate, to
G eindringen
S penetrar

pente
E gradient, slope
G Gefälle, Neigung
S declive, gradiente, inclinación, pendiente

avec une pente
E sloped
G mit Gefälle, geneigt
S con inclinación, inclinado

peptone
E peptone
G Pepton
S peptona

percement
E bore
G Bohrung
S perforación

percolation
E percolation
G Perkolation
S percolación

perdre sa couleur
E fade, to
G verblassen
S empalidecer

perforation
E perforation
G Perforierung
S perforación

perforations d'aiguille
E pin holes
G Nadellöcher
S perforaciones de aguja

perforé
E perforated
G gelocht
S perforado

perforer
E perforate, to
G perforieren
S perforar

performance
E capacity, performance
G Leistung
S rendimiento

performance de séparation
E separation performance
G Trennungsleistung
S rendimiento separador

performance d'un moteur
E motor performance
G Motorleistung
S rendimiento de un motor

performance d'une colonne
E column performance
G Trennleistung der Säule
S rendimiento separador de la columna

périmé
E obsolete, out-dated
G überholt
S obsoleto, envejecido

périmètre
E circumference
G Umfang
S circunferencia, perímetro, extensión

période d'immersion
E immersion period
G Eintauchzeit
S tiempo de inmersión

période d'immobilisation en production
E production downtime
G Produktionsausfall, Produktionsausfallzeit
S pérdida de producción, tiempo de pérdida de producción

période d'incubation
E period of incubation
G Inkubationsdauer
S período de incubación

période d'utilisation
E standing time
G Standzeit
S período de funcionamiento

période d'utilisation (de filtres)
E period of use (of filters)
G Standzeit (von Filtern)
S período de uso (de filtros)

perméabilité
E transmittance, permeability
G Durchlässigkeit, Permeabilität
S permeabilidad

perméabilité à la vapeur d'eau
E water vapour permeability
G Wasserdampfdurchlässigkeit
S permeabilidad al vapor de agua

perméabilité à l'air
E air permeability
G Luftdurchlässigkeit
S permeabilidad al aire

perméable
E permeable
G durchlässig, permeabel
S permeable

perméable à l'air
E permeable to air
G luftdurchlässig
S permeable al aire

permis
E permissible
G zulässig
S permitido

peroxide d'hydrogène
E hydrogen peroxide
G Wasserstoffperoxid
S peróxido de hidrógeno

personne autorisée
E authorised individual (person)
G autorisierte Person, befugte Person
S persona autorizada

personne compétente
E qualified person
G Sachkundiger
S experto, perito

personne qualifiée
E qualified person
G sachkundige Person
S persona cualificada

personne responsable
E responsible person
G Verantwortlicher
S responsable

personne responsable de la pharmaco-vigilance
E pharmaco-vigilance manager, drug safety manager
G Stufenplanbeauftragter
S responsable de farmacovigilancia

personnel de service
E operating personnel
G Bedienungspersonal
S personal de servicio

personnel occupant un poste à responsabilités
E key personnel
G Personal in Schlüsselstellung
S personal en posición clave

perte
E loss
G Verlust
S pérdida

perte de poids (lors de la dessication)
E weight loss (on drying)
G Gewichtsverlust (bei der Trocknung)
S pérdida de peso (al desecar)

perte de qualité
E loss of quality
G Güteminderung
S pérdida de calidad

perte due à l'évaporisation
E evaporative loss
G Verdunstungsverlust
S pérdida de evaporación

pertes dues au séchage
E loss on drying
G Trocknungsverlust
S pérdidas por desecación

pertinent
E relevant, pertinent
G relevant
S relevante

perturbation
E malfunction, interference
G Störung
S avería, fallo

perturbation de fonctionnement
E breakdown
G Betriebsstörung
S interrupción del funcionamiento

peser
E weigh in, to
G einwiegen
S pesar

pesticide
E pesticide
G Pestizid, Schädlingsvertilgungsmittel
S pesticida

pétrir
E knead, to
G kneten
S amasar

English
German
French
Spanish

pH (potentiel hydrogène)
E pH
G pH-Wert
S pH

pharmacien
E pharmacist
G Apotheker
S farmacéutico

pharmacocinétique
E pharmacokinetics
G Pharmakokinetik
S farmacocinética

pharmacologie
E pharmacology
G Pharmakologie
S farmacología

pharmacopée
E pharmacopoeia
G Arzneibuch, Pharmakopöe
S farmacopea

pharmacopée américaine
E United States Pharmacopoeia (USP)
G Arzneibuch der USA
S farmacopea estadounidense

pharmacopée européenne (PhEur)
E European Pharmacopoeia (PhEur)
G Europäisches Arzneibuch (PhEur)
S Farmacopea Europea

phase
E coat, coating, film, layer
G Beschichtung, Überzug, Lage, Schicht
S estrato, cubierta, revestimiento

phase aqueuse
E aqueous phase
G wäßrige Phase
S fase acuosa

phase de développement
E development stage
G Entwicklungsstufe
S etapa de desarrollo, nivel de desarrollo

phase de recrutement
E recruitment phase
G Rekrutierungsphase
S fase de reclutamiento

phase de refroidissement
E cooling phase
G Abkühlphase
S fase de enfriamento

phase gazeuse
E gaseous phase
G Gasphase
S fase gaseosa

phase liquide
E liquid phase
G flüssige Phase
S fase líquida

phase mobile
E mobile phase (in chromotography)
G Fließmittel (in der Chromatographie)
S fase móvil (en cromatografía)

phase organique
E organic phase
G organische Phase
S fase orgánica

phase solide
E solid phase
G feste Phase
S fase sólida

phase stationnaire
E stationary phase
G stationäre Phase
S fase estacionaria

phase vapeur
E vapour phase
G Dampfphase
S fase vapor

pH-mètre
E pH meter
G pH-Meter
S pH metro

phosphorescence
E phosphorescence
G Phosphoreszenz
S fosforescencia

photochimique
E photochemical
G photochemisch
S fotoquímico

photolyse
E photolysis
G Photolyse
S fotólisis

photomètre
E photometer
G Photometer
S fotómetro

photomètre de flamme
E flame photometer
G Flammenphotometer
S fotómetro de llama

photométrie
E photometry
G Photometrie
S fotometría

photométrie de flamme
E flame photometry
G Flammenphotometrie
S fotometría de llama

photo-sensible
E light-sensitive
G lichtempfindlich
S fotosensible

phytochimie
E phytochemistry
G Phytochemie
S fitoquímica

phytopharmaceutiques
E phytopharmaceuticals, herbal medicines
G Phytopharmaka, pflanzliche Arzneimittel
S fitofármacos

pic
E peak
G Peak
S pico

pic double
E double peak
G Doppelpeak
S pico doble

pic étranger
E extraneous peak
G nicht zugehöriger Peak
S pico extraño

pic fantôme
E ghost peak
G Geisterpeak
S pico fantasma

pièce brute
E blank
G Rohling
S pieza bruta

pièce de rechange
E spare part, replacement part
G Ersatzteil, Austauschteil
S pieza de recambio

pièce sujette à l'usure
E part subject to wear
G Verschleißteil
S pieza desgastable

pièces mobiles
E movable parts
G bewegliche Teile
S piezas móviles

piège à insectes
E insect trap
G Insektenfalle
S trampa de insectos

pierre facilitant l'ébullition
E boiling chip
G Siedestein
S piedra de ebullición

English German French Spanish

pigment
E colouring agent, dye, stain, pigment
G Färbemittel, Farbstoff, Pigment
S colorante, tintura, pigmento

pigment végétal
E vegetable dye
G Pflanzenfarbstoff
S colorante vegetal, pigmento vegetal

pignon
E pinion
G Ritzel
S piñón

pile
E stack, pile
G Stapel
S montón, pila

piler
E crush, to; grind, to; mill, to
G zerstoßen
S machacar, pulverizar, triturar

pilon
E pestle
G Pistill
S pistilo

pilule
E pill
G Pille
S píldora

pince
E terminal, tongs
G Klemme, Zange
S borne, terminal, pinza

pince à creuset
E tongs
G Tiegelzange
S pinza de crisol

pinces
E clamp, crimping tongs
G Klammer, Falzzange
S pinzas, tenazas para cerrar tubos

pincettes
E crimping tongs
G Falzzange
S tenazas para cerrar tubos

pipette
E pipette
G Pipette
S pipeta

pipette calibrée
E calibrated pipette
G Vollpipette
S pipeta calibrada

pipette de prélèvement
E powder sampler, sampling device, sampling pipette
G Stechheber
S pipeta (de toma de muestras)

pipetter
E pipette off, to
G abpipettieren
S pipetear

piquant
E sharp
G scharf
S afilado, agudo, cortante

pissette
E wash bottle
G Spritzflasche
S matraz de lavado

pistolet chalumeau
E flame gun
G Flammpistole
S pistola de llama

piston
E piston
G Kolben (technisch)
S émbolo, pistón

piston doseur
E dosing piston
G Dosierkolben
S matraz de dosificación

pivotable
E hinged, pivotable
G schwenkbar
S giratorio

pivoté
E swivelled, pivotted
G ausgeschwenkt
S girado hacia fuera

pixel
E pixel
G Pixel
S píxel

placard de vestiaire
E locker
G Spind
S armario estrecho

placebo
E placebo
G Placebo
S placebo

placement
E placement
G Plazierung
S colocación

plafond
E ceiling
G Decke
S techo

faux plafond
E suspended ceiling, false ceiling
G abgehängte Decke, eingezogene Decke
S techo suspendido, techo falso

plafond en béton
E concrete ceiling
G Betondecke
S techo de hormigón

plage de confiance
E confidence area
G Vertrauensbereich
S área de confianza, intervalo de confianza

plage de fusion
E melting range
G Schmelzbereich
S márgenes de fusión

plage d'évaluation
E evaluation range
G Auswertebereich
S área de evaluación

plan
E schedule
G Zeitplan
S horario, calendario

plan (horizontal)
E plan
G Grundriß
S plano

plan de l'édifice
E building (facility) floor plan
G Gebäudeplan
S plan del edificio

plan de solutionnement d'un problème
E problem decision plan
G Problementscheidungsplan
S plan para decidir problemas

plan de stockage (entrepôt)
E stacking plan (in warehouse)
G Stapelplan (im Lager)
S plan de almacenamiento

plan d'étage
E floor plan
G Stockwerksplan
S plano de los pisos

plan échelonné
E graduated plan
G Stufenplan
S plan escalonado, plan graduado

plan incliné
E inclined plane
G schiefe Ebene
S plano inclinado

English German French Spanish

plancher
E floor, soil
G Boden
S suelo

planification des besoins
E requirements planning
G Bedarfsplanung
S planificación de necesidades

planification du travail
E work scheduling
G Arbeitsvorbereitung
S preparación del trabajo

plans du site
E site plan, layout
G Lageplan
S plano del lugar

plaque de CCM (chromatographie en couche mince)
E TLC plate (thin layer chromatography)
G DC-Platte (Dünnschichtchromatographie)
S placa para cromatografía en capa fina (CCF)

plaque de contact
E contact plate
G Abklatschplatte
S placa de contacto

plaque de sédimentation
E settling plate
G Sedimentationsplatte
S placa de sedimentación

plaque déflectrice
E baffle
G Ablenkplatte
S placa de desviación

plaquette (conditionnement)
E blister pack
G Durchdrückpackung
S blíster

plaquette en verre (pour diapositives)
E cover slip, cover glass (microscopy)
G Deckglas (Mikroskopie)
S cubreobjetos (microscopio)

plaquette thermoformée
E blister pack
G Blisterverpackung
S embalado en blísters

plasticité
E plasticity
G Plastizität
S plasticidad

plastifiant
E softening agent, plasticiser
G Weichmacher
S plastificante

plastique
E plastic, plastic material
G Kunststoff, plastisch
S plástico

plat
E plane, level
G eben
S liso, llano, plano

plateau
E rack, tray
G Tablett, Magazin (für Ampullen), Hordenblech
S bandeja (para ampollas)

plateau de balance
E weighing pan, weighing scale
G Waagschale
S platillo de balanza

plateau d'une matrice
E die plate
G Matrizenscheibe
S disco matriz

plateau tournant
E revolving plate feeder, turntable
G Drehteller, Aufgabedrehteller
S plato giratorio, placa giratoria

plate-forme de commande
E operating platform
G Bedienungsbühne
S plataforma de control

plate-forme de levage
E lifting platform
G Hebebühne
S plataforma elevadora

platine
E circuit board
G Platine
S platino

plein à ras-bord
E brimful
G randvoll
S lleno a rebosar

plexiglas
E Plexiglas, acrylic glass
G Plexiglas
S plexiglás

pli
E fold
G Falte
S arruga, pliegue

pliable
E flexible, pliable
G biegsam
S flexible, maleable, plegable

pliage
E bend, flexure
G Biegung
S flexión, curvatura

pliage spatial (par ex. des protéines)
E spatial folding (e. g. of protein)
G räumliche Faltung (z. B. eines Proteins)
S conformación espacial, plegamiento espacial (p. ej. de una proteína)

plier
E fold, to; crimp, to; seam, to
G falzen
S plegar

plieuse
E folding machine
G Falzmaschine
S plegadora

plieuse pour boîtes pliantes
E folding carton set-up machine
G Faltschachtelaufrichtmaschine
S máquina plegadora de cajas

plinthe à gorge arrondie
E fluted skirting
G Hohlkehlsockel
S rodapié en forma de garganta

plomb
E sinker
G Senkkörper
S lastre, plomo

plomberie
E plumbing
G Verrohrung
S instalación de conducciones

pneumatique
E pneumatic
G pneumatisch
S neumático

poche
E bag, tubular bag
G Beutel, Schlauchbeutel
S sobre, bolsa tubular

empaqueter, emballer
E package in bags, to
G in Beutel verpacken
S empaquetar en sobres

poche intérieure
E internal bag
G Innenbeutel
S bolsa interior

pochoir
E stencil, template
G Schablone
S modelo, patrón, plantilla

English German French Spanish

poids
E weight
G Gewicht
S peso

poids à vide
E dead weight, net weight, tare
G Leergewicht
S peso en vacío, tara

poids de remplissage
E filling weight, shot weight
G Füllgewicht
S peso al envasar

poids d'un comprimé
E tablet weight
G Tablettengewicht
S peso del comprimido

poids individuel
E individual weight
G Einzelgewicht
S peso individual

poids initial
E initial weight
G Einwaage
S peso inicial

poids maximum
E maximum weight
G Höchstgewicht
S peso máximo

poids moléculaire
E molecular weight
G Molekulargewicht
S peso molecular

poids sec
E dry weight
G Trockengewicht
S peso seco

poids spécifique
E specific gravity
G spezifisches Gewicht
S peso específico

poignée
E handle, grip
G Bügel, Griff
S asa, estribo, empuñadura, mango

poignée de porte
E latch, door handle
G Klinke, Türklinke
S picaporte, gatillo, trinquete

poinçon
E punch, hob
G Stempel (zum Tablettieren), Prägestempel, Stanze
S troquel, cuño, estampa, punzonadora, troqueladora

poinçon inférieur
E lower punch
G Unterstempel
S troquel inferior

poinçon supérieur
E upper punch
G Oberstempel
S troquel superior

poinçon de fabrication de comprimés
E tabletting punch
G Tablettierstempel
S troquel para comprimidos

poinçonner
E stamp, to; emboss, to; punch, to; die-cut, to, mark, to
G stempeln, prägen, stanzen, ausstanzen
S acuñar, estampar, troquelar, punzonar, perforar

poinçonneuse
E punching station
G Lochstanze
S perforadora, punzonadora, troquel

point de congélation
E freezing point
G Gefrierpunkt, Eispunkt
S punto de congelación

English German French Spanish

point de fusion
E melting point
G Schmelzpunkt
S punto de fusión

point de fusion instantané
E instant melting point
G Sofortschmelzpunkt
S punto de fusión inmediata

point de fusion (d'ampoules)
E fusion point (of ampoules)
G Abschmelzhöhe (von Ampullen)
S punto de fusión (de ampollas)

point de goutte
E dropping point
G Tropfpunkt
S punto de goteo

point de mesure
E measuring point
G Meßpunkt
S punto de medida

point de mesure de la pression
E pressure-measuring point
G Druckmeßdose
S punto de medida de presión

point de prélèvement
E sampling location, sampling point
G Probenahmestelle
S lugar de toma de muestras

point de ramollissement
E softening point
G Erweichungspunkt
S punto de reblandecimiento

point de référence
E reference point
G Bezugspunkt
S punto de referencia

point de retrait
E point of withdrawal
G Entnahmestelle
S lugar de extracción

point de rosée
E dewpoint
G Taupunkt
S punto de descongelación

point de rupture
E break point, breaking point
G Bruchstelle
S lugar de ruptura

point de rupture (d'une ampoule)
E cutting point (of an ampoule)
G Brechpunkt (einer Ampulle)
S punto de ruptura (de una ampolla)

point de solidification
E solidification point
G Erstarrungspunkt
S punto de solidificación

point d'ébullition
E boiling point
G Siedepunkt
S punto de ebullición

point d'eutexie
E eutectic point
G Eutektikum
S punto eutéctico

point d'inflammation
E flash point
G Flammpunkt
S punto de ignición

point le plus froid
E coldest spot (autoclave)
G kältester Punkt (beim Autoklav)
S punto más frío (en autoclave)

point zéro
E zero (in diagram)
G Nullpunkt (beim Diagramm)
S punto cero (en diagrama)

pointe
E spike
G Spike
S punta

pointe de pipette
E pipette tip
G Pipettenspitze
S punta de pipeta

pointe d'injection
E injection tip
G Injektionsspitze
S punta de jeringa

pointeau
E pin
G Stift (technisch)
S clavija, perno, pivote

poison
E poison, toxin
G Gift
S tóxico, veneno

polaire
E polar
G polar
S polar

polarimètre
E polarimeter
G Polarimeter
S polarímetro

polariseur
E polariser
G Polarisator
S polarizador

polarité
E polarity
G Polarität
S polaridad

poli
E smooth, ground
G glatt, geschliffen
S liso, pulido, resbaladizo, bruñido, tallado

poli-miroir
E highly polished
G hochglanzpoliert
S muy pulido

polir
E smooth, to; polish, to
G glätten, polieren
S alisar, pulir, bruñir

polissage de verre
E ground glass
G Glasschliff
S pulido del vidrio

politique d'élimination des déchets
E waste avoidance
G Abfallvermeidung
S evitación de desechos

polluant
E polluting, harmful
G umweltverschmutzend
S polucionante

pollution de l'environnement
E environmental waste
G Umweltverschmutzung
S desgaste ecológico, degradación ecológica

pollution des eaux résiduelles
E waste water pollution
G Abwasserverschmutzung
S polución de aguas residuales

pollution par le bruit
E noise
G Lärmbelastung
S ruido

pollution réductrice
E reducing impurity
G reduzierende Verunreinigung
S impureza reductora

polycyclique
E polycyclic
G polycyclisch
S policíclico

polymère
E polymer
G polymer
S polímero

polymère aqueux
E aqueous polymer
G wäßriges Polymer
S polímero acuoso

polystyrène expansé
E expanded polystyrene (EPS)
G expandiertes Polystyrol (EPS)
S poliesterol expandido

polyvalent
E multivalent
G mehrwertig
S polivalente

pommade
E ointment, fatty ointment
G Salbe, Fettsalbe
S pomada, pomada con elevado contenido en grasa, ungüento

pommade auriculaire
E ear ointment
G Ohrensalbe
S pomada auricular

pommade nasale
E nasal ointment
G Nasensalbe
S pomada nasal

pommade pour les yeux
E eye ointment
G Augensalbe
S pomada oftálmica

pommade rectale
E rectal ointment
G Rektalsalbe
S pomada rectal

pommade vaginale
E vaginal ointment
G Vaginalsalbe
S pomada vaginal

pompe
E pump
G Pumpe
S bomba

pompe à anneau d'eau
E water-ring pump
G Wasserringpumpe
S bomba de anillo de agua

pompe à gradient
E gradient pump
G Gradientenpumpe
S bomba de gradiente

pompe à valve rotatoire
E rotary valve pump
G Drehschieberpumpe
S bomba de válvula rotativa

pompe à vide
E vacuum pump
G Vakuumpumpe
S bomba de vacío

pompe de circulation
E circulatory pump
G Umwälzpumpe
S bomba de circulación

pompe doseuse
E peristaltic pump
G Dosierpumpe
S bomba de dosificación

pompe d'une trompe à eau
E water jet pump
G Wasserstrahlpumpe
S bomba de chorro de agua

pompe HPLC
E HPLC pump
G HPLC-Pumpe
S bomba de HPLC

pompe lubrifiante
E lubrication pump
G Schmierstoffpumpe
S bomba de lubri(fi)cante

pompe péristaltique
E peristaltic pump
G Schlauchpumpe
S bomba peristáltica

poncé et décapé
E pickled and blasted
G gebeizt und gestrahlt
S decapado y pulido

population de cellules
E cell population
G Zellpopulation
S población celular

poreux
E porous
G porös
S poroso

porosité
E porosity
G Porosität
S porosidad

porte coulissante
E sliding door
G Schiebetür
S puerta corrediza

porte coupée
E hatch
G Durchreiche
S postigo

porte de protection anti-incendie
E fire protection door
G Brandschutzklappe
S puerta de protección contra incendios

porte-objet (microscopie)
E slide (microscopy)
G Objektträger (Mikroskopie)
S portaobjetos (microscopio)

porte-parole
E chairman, spokesman
G Vorsitzender, Obmann
S portavoz, presidente

portion
E part, moiety
G Teil
S parte

portions insaponifiables
E unsaponifiable matter
G unverseifbare Anteile
S porciones insaponificables

portoir pour échantillons
E sample rack
G Probenständer
S estante de muestras

poser
E apply, to; attach, to
G anbringen
S instalar, montar

position de rejet
E reject position
G Ausschußposition
S posición de desecho

position d'une vanne
E valve setting
G Ventilstellung
S posición de la válvula

position inclinée
E in sloping position
G Schräglage
S inclinación

positionneur de clapet
E flap positioner
G Klappensteller
S posicionador de válvulas

posologie
E dosage
G Dosierung
S dosificación, posología

possibilité de lavage des mains
E hand wash facility
G Handwaschgelegenheit
S posibilidad de lavar las manos

poste de travail
E place of work
G Arbeitsplatz
S puesto de trabajo, empleo

pot fileté
E screw cap glass container
G Schraubglas
S recipiente de vidrio con cierre de rosca

potentialisation
E potentation
G Potenzierung
S potenciación

potentiel de danger
E hazard potential
G Gefahrenpotential
S potencial de riesgos

potentiel redox
E redox potential
G Redoxpotential
S potencial redox

potentiomètre
E potentiometer
G Potentiometer
S potenciómetro

poubelle
E waste disposal vessel
G Abfallbehälter
S recipiente de desechos

poudrage
E dusting powder
G Streupulver
S polvo vulnerario

poudre
E powder
G Pulver, Puder
S polvo

poudre à utilisation orale
E oral powder
G Pulver zum Einnehmen
S polvo oral

poudre en vrac
E loose powder
G loses Pulver
S polvo suelto

poudreux
E powdery
G pudrig
S pulverulento

poulie de guidage
E casters
G Laufrollen, Lenkrollen
S polea, roldana

pouvoir colorant
E dyeing power
G Färbkraft
S poder colorante

pouvoir d'adhésion
E adhesiveness
G Haftfähigkeit
S adherencia, adhesividad

préamplification
E pre-amplification
G Vorverstärkung
S preamplificación

pré-assemblé
E pre-assembly
G Vormontage
S montaje previo

précaution
E precaution
G Vorsichtsmaßnahme
S medida precautoria

précautions de sécurité
E safety precautions
G Sicherheitsmaßnahmen
S medidas de seguridad

précautions de stockage
E storage precautions
G Vorsichtsmaßnahmen bei der Lagerung
S medida precautoria al almacenar

précipitation
E precipitation, precipitate
G Ausfällung, Fällung
S precipitación, precipitado

précipité
E precipitate, precipitation
G Niederschlag, Fällung
S precipitado, precipitación

précipiter
E precipitate, to
G ausfällen
S precipitar

précis
E clear, exact, precise, unambiguous
G eindeutig, genau, präzise
S preciso

précision
E precision
G Präzision, Genauigkeit (einer Prüfmethode)
S precisión, exactitud (de un método de prueba)

précision de détection
E detection precision
G Detektionsgenauigkeit
S exactitud de detección

prédécesseur
E predecessor
G Vorgänger
S predecesor

pré-enrober
E precoat, to (tablets)
G andecken (beim Dragieren)
S prerrecubrir (grageas)

préformulation
E pre-formulation
G Präformulierung
S preformulación

pré-insertion
E pre-insertion
G Voreinschub
S preinserción

préjudice
E impairment, damage
G Beeinträchtigung
S merma, perjuicio

préjudice à la santé
E damage to health
G Gesundheitsschaden
S perjuicio para la salud

prélèvement d'un échantillon
E sampling
G Probenahme
S toma de muestra

pré-mélange
E pre-mix
G Vormischung
S mezcla previa

premiers secours
E first aid
G Erste Hilfe
S primeros auxilios

prendre le contrôle de
E take over, to
G übernehmen
S adquirir, comprar

préparation
E preparation, formulation
G Zubereitung
S formulación, preparación

préparation de référence
E reference medication (preparation)
G Referenzpräparat
S preparado de referencia

préparation de tourbe
E mud pack preparation
G Moorzubereitung
S preparación de turba

préparation des milieux de culture
E culture media preparation
G Nährmedienherstellung
S preparación de medio de cultivo

préparation d'un échantillon
E sample preparation
G Probenvorbereitung
S preparación de muestras

préparation d'une solution
E preparation of solution
G Lösungsherstellung
S preparación de una solución

préparation pharmaceutique
E medicinal product premix, drug premix
G Arzneimittelvormischung
S elaboración previa del medicamento

préparation pour essai en aveugle
E blinding
G Verblindung
S preparación para ensayo ciego

préparation pour test
E test preparation
G Prüfpräparat
S preparado de prueba

préparations injectables
E parenterals
G Parenteralia
S inyectables

préparations injectables de grand volume
E large volume parenterals (LVP)
G großvolumige Parenteralia
S inyectables voluminosos

préparations injectables de petit volume
E small volume parenterals (SVP)
G kleinvolumige Parenteralia
S inyectables de escaso volumen

pré-réglage
E pre-setting
G Voreinstellung
S prerreglaje

prescription
E medical prescription
G ärztliche Verordnung
S prescripción médica

pré-sélection
E pre-selection
G Vorauswahl
S preselección

présence
E presence
G Anwesenheit
S presencia

présence microbienne
E microbial load, bioburden
G mikrobielle Belastung
S carga microbiana

président directeur général (PDG)
E managing director, general manager
G Geschäftsführer
S gerente

presse à bascule
E lever press
G Hebelpresse
S prensa de palanca

presse à comprimés
E tablet press
G Tablettenpresse
S prensa de comprimidos

presse à comprimés avec instruments
E automated tablet press
G instrumentierte Tablettenpresse
S prensa automática de comprimidos

presse à comprimés haute vitesse
E high-speed tabletting press
G Hochgeschwindigkeitstablettenpresse
S prensa de alta velocidad

presse excentrique à comprimés
E eccentric tablet press
G Exzenterpresse
S prensa excéntrica

presse manuelle
E hand press
G Handpresse
S prensa manual

presse rapide
E high-speed press
G Hochleistungspresse
S prensa rápida

presse rotative
E rotary press
G Rundläuferpresse
S prensa rotatoria

presse rotative double
E double rotary press
G Doppelrundläuferpresse
S prensa rotatoria doble

presse-outil pour comprimés
E tablet tooling
G Tablettenwerkzeug
S utensilios para elaborar comprimidos

presser
E express, to
G auspressen
S exprimir, prensar

pression
E pressure
G Druck
S presión

souspression
E negative pressure
G Unterdruck
S presión baja

surpression
E positive pressure
G Überdruck
S sobrepresión

pression atmosphérique
E atmospheric pressure
G Atmosphärendruck
S presión atmosférica

pression d'air
E air pressure
G Luftdruck
S presión de aire

pression de fermeture
E sealing pressure
G Siegeldruck
S presión de sellado

pression de moulage
E moulding pressure
G Preßdruck
S presión de prensado

pression de pressage
E moulding pressure
G Preßdruck
S presión de prensado

pression de scellage
E sealing pressure
G Siegeldruck
S presión de sellado

pression de soutien
E support pressure
G Stützdruck
S presión de soporte

pression de travail
E working pressure
G Arbeitsdruck, Betriebsdruck
S presión de trabajo, presión empresarial

pression de vapeur
E steam pressure, vapour pressure
G Dampfdruck
S presión de vapor

pression d'éclatement
E bursting pressure
G Berstdruck
S presión de rotura

pression différentielle
E pressure differential
G Differenzdruck
S presión diferencial

pression interne
E internal pressure
G Innendruck
S presión interna

pression osmotique
E osmotic pressure
G osmotischer Druck
S presión osmótica

pression partielle
E partial pressure
G Partialdruck
S presión parcial

prêt à l'emploi
E ready-to-use, ready for operation
G gebrauchsfertig, betriebsbereit
S dispuesto para el servicio, listo para el uso, preparado para funcionar

prêt à l'utilisation
E ready for operation
G betriebsbereit
S preparado para funcionar

prêt au service
E ready for operation
G betriebsbereit
S preparado para funcionar

prêt-à-monter
E kit
G Bausatz
S kit

prétraitement d'échantillons
E sample pre-treatment
G Probenvorbehandlung
S pretratamiento de muestras

preuve
E detection, evidence, proof
G Nachweis, Beweis
S demostración, prueba

prévention
E prevention
G Vermeidung
S evitación

prévu pour
E designed for
G ausgelegt für
S construido para, diseñado para

principe actif (d'un médicament)
E medicinal substance, active substance, active pharmaceutical ingredient (API)
G Arzneistoff, Wirkstoff
S sustancia medicamentosa, principio activo (medicamento)

principes actifs naturels
E natural active substances
G Wirkstoffe, natürlich vorkommende
S sustancias activas naturales

prion bovin
E bovine prion
G Rinderprion
S prión bovino

prion cellulaire (prpc)
E cellular prion (prpc)
G Prion, zelluläres
S prión celular (prpc)

prions spécifiques à la scrapie (prpsc)
E scrapie-specific prions (prpsc)
G Scrapie-spezifische Proteine (prpsc)
S priones específicos de la encefalopatía espongiforme ovina

prise
E handle, grip
G Bügel, Griff
S estribo, asa, empuñadura, mango

prise de terre
E ground, grounding, earth, earthing
G Erdung, Ableitung
S toma de tierra, derivación

prise en masse
E caking, cake formation
G Kuchenbildung
S cuajamiento

English German French Spanish

prix d'achat
E purchase cost
G Kaufpreis
S precio de compra

procédé
E procedure
G Verfahren
S procedimiento

procédé aseptique
E aseptic process, aseptic technology
G aseptische Prozeßtechnik
S técnica de proceso aséptico

procédé de circulation des gaz
E gas flow-through process
G Gasdurchströmungsverfahren
S procedimiento de purga gaseosa

procédé de désinfection
E disinfecting procedure
G Desinfektionsverfahren
S procedimiento de desinfección

procédé de granulation
E granulating process
G Granulierverfahren
S procedimiento de granulación

procédé monocouche
E single coating process
G Einschichtverfahren
S procedimiento de cubierta simple

procédé par immersion
E by immersion
G im Tauchverfahren
S en procedimiento de inmersión

procédure de fabrication
E manufacturing procedure
G Herstellungsverfahren
S procedimiento de fabricación

procédure de nettoyage
E cleaning procedure
G Reinigungsvorschrift
S instrucción de limpieza

procédure de reconnaissance mutuelle
E Mutual Recognition Agreement (MRA), Mutual Recognition Procedure (MRP)
G Abkommen zur gegenseitigen Anerkennung, Gegenseitiges Anerkennungsverfahren bei der Zulassung von Arzneimitteln in der EU
S Acuerdo de Reconocimiento Mutuo de Procedimientos Administrativos en la UE, Procedimiento de Reconocimiento Mutuo en la UE

procédure de test
E analytical (testing) procedure
G Prüfverfahren
S procedimiento de prueba

procédure opératoire
E operating procedure, instruction
G Arbeitsvorschrift, Arbeitsanweisung
S instrucción de trabajo, norma de trabajo

procédures opératoires standards
E standard operating procedure (SOP)
G Standardarbeitsanweisung
S instrucción estándar de trabajo

processus
E operation, process
G Vorgang, Prozeß
S proceso

processus de distillation
E distillation process
G Destillationsprozeß
S proceso de destilación

processus de libération
E release procedure
G Freigabeverfahren
S proceso de autorización

processus non soumis à un contrôle
E unattended operation
G nicht unter Beobachtung stehender Vorgang
S proceso no observado

procès-verbal des défauts
E deficiency protocol
G Mängelprotokoll
S protocolo de deficiencias

procès-verbal d'un test
E test protocol
G Prüfprotokoll
S protocolo de prueba

producteur de spores
E spore former
G Sporenbildner
S productor de esporas

producteur sous-traintant
E contract manufacturer
G Auftragshersteller
S fabricante por comisión

production
E manufacture, production, extraction, generation (of)
G Herstellung, Produktion, Gewinnung, Erzeugung
S fabricación, producción, extracción, obtención, generación

production à l'échelle pilote
E pilot scale production
G Produktion im Versuchsmaßstab
S producción a escala piloto

production de mousse
E foam formation, foaming
G Schaumbildung
S formación de espuma

production de poussière
E dust production
G Staubentwicklung
S producción de polvo

production de vapeur
E steam generation
G Dampferzeugung
S producción de vapor

production par un sous-traitant
E contract manufacturing
G Auftragsherstellung, Auftragsproduktion
S producción por contrata, producción por encargo

produire
E compile, to
G erstellen
S elaborar, producir, redactar

produit à usage médical
E medical device
G Medizinprodukt
S producto médico

produit biopharmaceutique
E biopharmaceutical
G biotechnologisch hergestelltes Arzneimittel
S medicamento producido biotecnológicamente

produit brut
E raw product, crude product
G Rohprodukt
S materia prima, producto bruto

produit commercial
E commercial product
G Handelsware
S producto comercial

produit de contraste aux rayons X
E X-ray contrast medium
G Röntgenkontrastmittel
S medio de contraste radiológico

produit de décomposition
E decomposition product
G Zersetzungsprodukt
S producto de degradación

produit de dégradation
E degradation product
G Abbauprodukt, Zerfallsprodukt
S producto de degradación, producto de desintegración

produit de polissage
E polish
G Poliermittel
S producto para pulir

produit d'origine plasmatique
E blood plasma product, blood plasma derivative
G Blutplasmaderivat
S producto de plasma sanguíneo

produit en vente libre
E over-the-counter (OTC) product
G frei verkäufliches Produkt, OTC-Produkt
S producto de venta libre

produit fini
E finished product
G Fertigprodukt
S producto acabado

produit intermédiaire
E intermediate product, semi-manufactured product
G Zwischenprodukt, Halbfertigware
S producto intermediario, producto semiacabado

produit naturel
E natural product
G Naturprodukt
S producto natural

produit nutritif
E nutrient
G Nährstoff
S nutriente, sustancia nutricia

produit pharmaceutique
E medicinal product, drug
G Arzneimittel
S medicamento

produit pharmaceutique fini
E finished medicinal product
G Fertigarzneimittel
S medicamento manufacturado, especialidad farmacéutica manufacturada

produit recyclé
E reprocessed product
G wiederaufbereitetes Produkt
S producto reciclado

produit rejeté
E rejected product
G verworfenes Produkt
S producto desechado

produit sanguin
E blood product
G Blutprodukt
S producto sanguíneo

produit sans ordonnance
E over-the-counter (OTC) product, over-the-counter (OTC) medicament
G frei verkäufliches Produkt, OTC-Produkt, Selbstmedikationsprodukt
S producto de venta libre, producto para automedicación

produit secondaire
E by-product
G Nebenprodukt
S producto colateral, producto secundario

produit semi-fini
E semi-finished product
G Vorprodukt
S producto semiterminado

produit stérile
E sterile product
G Sterilprodukt
S producto estéril

produits chimiques
E chemicals
G Chemikalien
S productos químicos

produits d'hygiène grand public
E health care products
G Gesundheitsprodukte
S productos para la salud

produits en vrac
E bulk mixture
G Bulkmischung
S mezcla a granel

produits éthiques
E ethical products
G ethische Produkte
S productos éticos

produits homéopathiques
E homeopathic products
G homöopathische Erzeugnisse
S productos homeopáticos

produits injectables de grand volume
E large volume parenterals (LVP)
G großvolumige Parenteralia
S productos inyectables de gran volumen

produits injectables de petit volume
E small volume parenterals (SVP)
G kleinvolumige Parenteralia
S productos inyectables de poco volumen

produits inoffensifs
E harmless products
G unschädliche Mittel
S productos inocuos

produits manufacturés
E manufactured goods, finished goods
G Fertigwaren
S productos manufacturados

produits ophtalmiques
E ophthalmic products
G Ophthalmica
S productos oftálmicos

produits radiopharmaceutiques
E radio-pharmaceuticals
G Radiopharmazeutika
S productos radiofarmacéuticos

produits secondaires
E secondary products
G Sekundärprodukte
S productos secundarios

produits secondaires microbiens
E microbial by-products
G mikrobielle Nebenprodukte
S productos colaterales microbianos

profil chimique
E chemical profile
G chemisches Profil
S perfil químico

profil de contamination (d'un produit)
E contamination profile (of a product)
G Kontaminationsprofil (eines Produktes)
S perfil de contaminación (de un producto)

profil de libération
E release profile
G Freisetzungsprofil
S perfil de liberación

profil d'impuretés
E impurity profile
G Verunreinigungsprofil
S perfil de impurezas

profil du comprimé
E tablet profile
G Tablettenprofil
S perfil de comprimido

profondeur de pénétration
E penetration depth
G Eindringtiefe
S profundidad de penetración

profondeur d'immersion
E immersion depth
G Eintauchtiefe
S profundidad de inmersión

programmable
E programmable
G programmierbar
S programable

programmation
E programming
G Programmierung
S programación

programmation de la longueur d'onde
E wavelength programming
G Wellenlängenprogrammierung
S programación de la longitud de onda

programme
E schedule
G Zeitplan
S horario, calendario

programme de nettoyage
E cleaning schedule
G Reinigungsplan
S plan de limpieza

programme d'échantillonnage
E sampling plan
G Probenahmeplan
S plan de toma de muestras

programme sanitaire
E sanitation programme
G Hygieneplan
S plan higiénico, programa sanitario

programmeur
E programmer
G Programmierer
S programador

projet de loi
E draft bill
G Gesetzesentwurf
S proyecto de ley

prolifération de cellules
E cell proliferation
G Zellvermehrung
S proliferación celular

prolongation d'un délai
E deadline extension
G Fristverlängerung
S prolongación de un plazo

prolonger
E extend, to; prolong, to
G verlängern
S alargar, prolongar

promotion de la croissance
E growth promotion
G Wachstumsförderung
S estimulación del crecimiento

propagation
E spreading
G Spreizung
S extensión, propagación

prophylactique
E prophylactic
G prophylaktisch
S profiláctico

prophylaxe
E prophylaxis
G Prophylaxe
S profilaxia

proportions de mélange
E blending ratio
G Mischungsverhältnis
S proporción de mezcla

propreté
E cleanliness
G Sauberkeit
S limpieza

propriété
E property
G Eigenschaft
S característica, propiedad

propriété couvrante
E covering power, hiding power
G Deckkraft
S capacidad de cubrir

propriété d'écoulement
E flow property, flowing property, fluidity
G Fließeigenschaft, Rieselfähigkeit
S propiedad fluida, capacidad de fluir

propriété intellectuelle
E intellectual property
G intellektuelles Eigentum
S propiedad intelectual

propriété lubrifiante
E slip property
G Gleiteigenschaft
S propiedad deslizante

propriétés de surface
E surface properties
G Oberflächenbeschaffenheit
S características de superficie

prorogation d'un brevet
E patent prolongation
G Patentfristerneuerung
S prolongación del plazo de patente

prospective
E prospective
G prospektiv
S prospectivo

protéase
E protease
G Protease
S proteasa

protection (électrique)
E fuse (electrical)
G Schütz (elektrisch)
S protección (eléctrica)

protection anti-chocs
E impact protection
G Stoßschutz
S protección frente a la colisión

protection anti-gouttes
E drop protection
G Tropfschutz
S protección frente al goteo

protection cônique
E conical screener
G konischer Abschirmer
S protector cónico

protection contre la rouille
E rust protection
G Rostschutz
S protección antioxidante

protection contre les poussières
E dust guard
G Staubschutz
S protección contra el polvo

protection d'un brevet
E patent protection
G Patentschutz
S protección de patentes

protection faciale
E face protection
G Gesichtsschutz
S protección facial

protection pour les oreilles
E ear protector, ear defender
G Gehörschutz
S protección auricular

protection pour l'œil
E eye protection
G Augenschutz
S protección ocular

protégé contre les accidents
E accident-proof
G unfallsicher
S a prueba de accidentes

protégé contre une explosion
E explosion-protected
G explosionsgeschützt, Ex-geschützt
S protegido contra explosión,
protegido frente a explosión

protéines-prions (prp)
E prion proteins (prp)
G Prionproteine
S proteína priónica (prp)

protocole de fabrication
E batch processing record
G Herstellungsprotokoll
S protocolo de fabricación

English German French Spanish

protocole de validation
E validation protocol
G Validierungsplan
S plan de validación

protocole opératoire
E testing schedule
G Prüfplan
S plan de prueba, protocolo del ensayo

prototype
E prototype
G Erstausführung
S prototipo

protozoaires
E protozoa
G Protozoen
S protozoos

provoquer
E cause, to
G verursachen
S causar, provocar

publication
E publication
G Veröffentlichung
S publicación

puissance absorbée
E power input
G Leistungsaufnahme
S absorción de potencia

puits
E recess, cavity, well
G Vertiefung
S cavidad, depresión

puits d'évacuation d'air
E exhaust air shaft, exhaust air flue
G Abluftschacht
S pozo de evacuación de aire

pulvérisateur
E atomiser
G Zerstäuber, Nebelgenerator
S atomizador, pulverizador

pulvériser
E pulverise, to; powder, to; grind, to; atomise, to; vaporise, to
G pulverisieren, zerstäuben, aufsprühen
S pulverizar, atomizar

pupitre de commande
E operator console, panel, control panel
G Bedienpult, Schalttafel
S pupitre de mando, tablero de control, cuadro de distribución

pureté
E purity
G Reinheit
S pureza

pureté chimique
E chemical purity
G chemische Reinheit
S pureza química

pureté chirale
E chiral purity
G chirale Reinheit
S pureza quiral

pureté de pic
E peak purity
G Peakreinheit
S pureza del pico

pureté énantiomère
E enantiomeric purity
G enantiomere Reinheit
S pureza enantiómera

pureté optique
E optical purity
G optische Reinheit
S pureza óptica

purge au gaz rare
E inert gas purging
G Inertbegasung
S purga con gases inertes

purger
E flush, to (with); purge, to (with)
G durchströmen (mit), begasen
S inundar (con), purgar (con), gasear

purification
E purification
G Aufreinigung (chemisch)
S purificación (química)

purification d'un produit
E product purification
G Produktreinigung
S limpieza del producto

purifié
E purified
G gereinigt
S purificado

putréfaction
E putrefaction
G Fäulnis
S putrefacción

pycnomètre
E pycnometer, specific gravity meter
G Pyknometer
S picnómetro

pyrogènes
E pyrogens
G Pyrogene, fiebererzeugende Substanzen
S pirógenos

pyrogénicité
E pyrogenicity
G Pyrogenität
S pirogenicidad

pyrolyse
E pyrolysis
G Pyrolyse
S pirólisis

qualification
E qualification, suitability
G Qualifizierung, Eignung
S cualificación, aptitud, calificación, idoneidad

qualification de fournisseur
E supplier qualification
G Lieferantenqualifizierung
S cualificación del abastecedor

qualification de l'équipement
E equipment qualification
G Qualifizierung der Ausrüstung
S cualificación del equipamiento

qualification de l'installation
E installation qualification
G Installationsqualifizierung
S cualificación de una instalación

qualification des opérations, qualification opérationnelle
E operational qualification (OQ)
G Funktionsqualifizierung
S cualificación funcional

qualification des performances (d'un procédé)
E performance qualification
G Verfahrensqualifizierung, Leistungsqualifizierung
S cualificación de un procedimiento, cualificación del rendimiento

qualification d'un logiciel
E software qualification
G Softwarequalifizierung
S cualificación de la software

qualité
E quality
G Qualität, Güte
S calidad, cualidad

qualité alimentaire
E food grade
G lebensmittelecht
S calidad alimenticia

qualité pharmaceutique
E pharmaceutical grade
G entspricht Arzneibuchqualität
S calidad farmacéutica

qualité uniforme
E consistent quality
G gleichbleibende Qualität
S calidad invariable

quantifiable
E quantifiable
G quantitativ bestimmbar
S cuantificable

quantitatif
E quantitative
G quantitativ
S cuantitativo

quantité
E quantity, amount
G Menge
S cantidad

quantité (d'enduit) appliquée
E coating quantity
G Auftragsmenge (beim Coating)
S cantidad a aplicar (al recubrir)

quantité de remplissage
E filling quantity
G Füllmenge, Abfüllmenge
S cantidad de relleno, cantidad envasada

quantité en excès
E overfill(ing)
G Überfüllung
S repleción

quantité livrée
E quantity received
G Liefermenge
S cantidad suministrada

quantité produite
E quantity produced
G Produktionsmenge
S cantidad producida

quarantaine (entrepôt)
E quarantine (warehouse)
G Sperrlager, Quarantäne
S almacén para cuarentena, cuarentena, bloqueo, cierre

quartz
E quartz
G Quarz
S cuarzo

questionnaire
E questionnaire, trial form, case report form
G Fragebogen, Prüfbogen
S cuestionario

quittance
E receipt
G Empfangsbestätigung
S acuse de recibo

quotient
E quotient
G Quotient
S cociente

R & S (risque et sécurité)
E R & S (risk and safety)
G R & S (Risiko und Sicherheit)
S R & S (riesgo y seguridad)

phrases de R & S
E R & S phrases
G R & S-Sätze
S frases de R & S

R + D (recherche et développement)
E R + D (Research and Development)
G F + E (Forschung und Entwicklung)
S investigación y desarrollo

rabattable
E foldable, tiltable
G abklappbar
S plegable

raccord
E connector
G Verbindungsstück
S pieza de unión

raccordement de tuyau
E tube connector
G Schlauchkupplung
S acoplamiento de tubo

raccordement étanche
E leak-tight connection
G dichte Verbindung
S conexión hermética

raccourci
E abridgement
G Abkürzung, Verkürzung
S acortamiento, abreviatura, abreviación

racémate
E racemate
G Razemat
S racemado

racémique
E racemic
G racemisch
S racémico

racine carrée
E square root
G Quadratwurzel
S raíz cuadrada

racler
E scrape, to; scrape off, to
G schaben, abkratzen
S raer, rascar, raspar

racloir
E scraper
G Schaber, Abstreifer
S rascador, raspador

radiateur à reflux
E reflux condenser
G Rückflußkühler
S radiador, refrigerador de reflujo

radiation
E radiation
G Strahlung
S radiación

raide
E steep
G steil
S empinado, escarpado

rainure
E groove, slit
G Nut, Rille, Schlitz
S acanaladura, estría, muesca, ranura, fisura, hendidura, raja

rallonge
E extension
G Ansatzstück
S pieza de empalme, pieza insertable

rallonger
E extend, to; prolong, to
G verlängern
S alargar, prolongar

ramification
E branching
G Verzweigung
S ramificación

ramollir
E soften, to
G erweichen
S reblandecer

rampe de conditionnement
E packaging line
G Verpackungslinie
S cadena de empaquetado

rampe de remplissage
E filling line, bottling line
G Abfüllinie
S cadena de envasado

rance
E rancid
G ranzig
S rancio

randomisé
E randomised
G randomisiert
S randomizado

rappel
E recall, return
G Rückruf, Retoure
S retirada, retorno

rappel d'un produit
E product recall
G Produktrückruf
S retirada de un producto

English German French Spanish

rapport
E report, ratio
G Bericht, Verhältnis
S informe, proporción

rapport annuel de production
E annual product report
G jährlicher Produktbericht
S informe anual de producción

rapport de développement
E development report
G Entwicklungsbericht
S informe de desarrollo

rapport de réception technique
E technical acceptance report
G Abnahmebericht
S informe de recepción técnica

rapport de situation
E status report
G Statusbericht
S informe de la situación

rapport de validation
E validation report
G Validierungsbericht
S informe de validación

rapport expérimental
E test report
G Prüfbericht
S informe de prueba

rapport sur l'écologie
E environmental report
G Umweltschutzbericht
S informe ecológico

rapporter à quelqu'un
E report to someone, to
G berichten, jemandem
S informar a alguien

râteau d'agitateur
E stirrer rake
G Rührwerksrechen
S rastrillo del agitador

rayonnement infrarouge
E infrared radiation
G Infrarotstrahlung
S radiación infrarroja

rayonnement thermique
E convective heat
G Wärmestrahlung
S radiación térmica

rayons gamma
E gamma rays
G Gammastrahlen
S rayos gamma

réacteur
E reactor
G Reaktor
S reactor

réactif
E reagent
G Reagenz
S reactivo

réactif à composant unique
E single-component reagent
G Einkomponenten-Reagenz
S reactivo de componente único

réactif de Karl Fischer
E Karl Fischer reagent
G Karl-Fischer-Lösung
S reactivo de Karl Fischer

réactif prêt à l'emploi
E ready-to-use reagent
G gebrauchsfertiges Reagenz
S reactivo listo para el uso

réactifs à deux composants
E dual-component reagent
G Zweikomponenten-Reagenz
S reactivo de doble componente

réaction cinétique
E kinetic reaction
G kinetische Reaktion
S reacción cinética

réaction de premier ordre
E first-order reaction
G Reaktion 1. Ordnung
S reacción de primer orden

réaction de second ordre
E second-order reaction
G Reaktion 2. Ordnung
S reacción de segundo orden

réaction de substitution
E substitution reaction
G Substitutionsreaktion
S reacción de sustitución

réaction endothermique
E endothermic reaction
G endothermische Reaktion
S reacción endotérmica

réaction exothermique
E exothermic reaction
G exothermische Reaktion
S reacción exotérmica

réaction indésirable
E adverse reaction
G unerwünschte Reaktion
S reacción indeseable

réaction inflammatoire
E inflammatory reaction
G Entzündungsreaktion
S reacción inflamatoria

réaction ouvrant un anneau
E ring-opening reaction
G Ringöffnungsreaktion
S reacción de apertura de anillo

réaction secondaire
E side reaction
G Nebenreaktion
S reacción colateral

réaction spontanée
E spontaneous reaction
G Spontanreaktion
S reacción espontánea

réaction thermique
E thermal reaction
G thermische Reaktion
S reacción térmica

réalisation
E fulfilment, realisation
G Erfüllung
S cumplimiento, realización

réaliser
E carry out, to; execute, to
G durchführen
S ejecutar, llevar a cabo, realizar

réassemblage
E re-assembly
G Wiederzusammenbau
S reensamblaje

récepteur
E receptor
G Rezeptor
S receptor

réception
E acceptance
G Annahme
S aceptación

réception de marchandises
E central receiving
G Warenannahme, zentrale
S recepción central de mercancías

réception en usine
E factory acceptance test (FAT)
G Werksabnahme
S test de aceptación en fábrica

réception technique (d'une machine)
E final acceptance (of a machine)
G Abnahme (einer Maschine)
S recepción técnica (de una máquina)

réchauffement
E heating
G Erwärmung
S calentamiento

English German French Spanish

recherche clinique
E clinical research
G klinische Forschung
S investigación clínica

recherche et développement
E Research and Development
G Forschung und Entwicklung
S investigación y desarrollo

récipient
E container, reaction vessel, vial
G Behältnis, Ansatzbehälter, Gefäß, Fläschchen
S recipiente, contenedor, botellín, frasco, vial

récipient à dose unique
E single unit dose container
G Einzeldosisbehältnis
S recipiente de dosis única

récipient de collecte
E collection vessel
G Auffanggefäß
S recipiente colector

récipient de débordement
E overflow vessel
G Überlaufgefäß
S recipiente de desbordamiento

récipient de l'agitateur
E stirring vessel
G Rührkessel
S caldera de agitación

récipient de stockage
E holding tank, storage vessel, storage tank, reservoir
G Lagertank, Aufbewahrungstank, Vorratstank
S tanque depósito, tanque de conservación

récipient d'élimination des déchets
E waste disposal vessel
G Abfallbehälter
S recipiente de desechos

récipient final
E final container
G Endbehältnis
S recipiente final

récipient monodose
E single dose container
G Einzeldosisbehältnis
S recipiente de dosis única

récipient multi-doses
E multi-dose container
G Mehrdosenbehältnis
S recipiente de dosis múltiple

récipient pour échantillon
E sample vessel
G Probengefäß
S recipiente para muestras

récipient pressurisé
E pressurised container
G Druckbehälter
S recipiente presurizado

récipient servant à l'inactivation
E inactivation vessel
G Inaktivierungsgefäß
S recipiente de inactivación

récipient soumis à la pression
E pressurised container
G Druckbehälter
S recipiente presurizado

récipient sous pression
E pressure vessel
G Druckgefäß
S recipiente a presión

recirculation
E recirculation
G Umlauf
S circulación, rotación

réclamation
E complaint
G Reklamation, Beanstandung
S reclamación

récolte de cellules
E cell harvesting
G Zellernte
S recolección de células

récolter
E harvest, to
G ernten
S cosechar

recombinant
E recombinant
G rekombinant
S recombinante

reconstitution
E reconstitution
G Wiederherstellung
S reconstitución, restablecimiento

recouvert
E covered
G verkleidet
S recubierto, revestido

recouvrement
E overlap
G Überschneidung
S entrecruzamiento, interferencia

recristallisation
E recrystallisation
G Umkristallisation
S recristalización

rectangulaire
E rectangular
G rechtwinkelig
S rectangular

rectifié
E rectified
G rektifiziert
S rectificado

reçu
E receipt
G Empfangsbestätigung
S acuse de recibo

recueillir
E collect, to; entrap, to
G auffangen
S captar, colectar, recoger

recuire
E anneal, to
G glühen
S incandescer

récupération
E recovery
G Rückgewinnung, Wiedergewinnung
S recuperación

récupération de la chaleur
E heat recovery
G Wärmerückgewinnung
S recuperación de calor

récupération de solvant
E solvent recovery
G Lösungsmittelrückgewinnung
S recuperación de solvente

récupérer
E recover, to
G wiedergewinnen
S recuperar

recyclage
E re-cycling
G Wiederverwertung
S reciclaje

redresseur de courant
E rectifier
G Stromgleichrichter
S rectificador de corriente

réducteur
E reducer
G Reduzierstück
S reductor

réduction microbienne
E microbial reduction
G Keimreduktion
S reducción de gérmenes

réduire
E reduce, to
G reduzieren
S reducir

référence
E cross reference, record
G Querverweis, Protokoll
S referencia, protocolo

référence à
E reference to
G Verweis auf
S referencia a

reflux
E reflux, back flow
G Rückfluß
S reflujo

réfractomètre
E refractometer
G Refraktometer
S refractómetro

réfrigérant
E cooler, coolant, condenser
G Kühler, Kühlflüssigkeit
S refrigerador, líquido refrigerante

réfrigérant à boules
E bulb cooler
G Kugelkühler
S refrigerador a bolas

réfrigérateur
E refrigerator
G Kühlschrank
S nevera

réfrigération
E refrigeration, cooling
G Kälteerzeugung, Abkühlung
S refrigeración, enfriamiento

réfrigérer
E refrigerate, to
G kühl lagern
S conservar frío

réfringence
E refringence
G Brechungsvermögen
S refringencia

refroidir
E refrigerate, to
G kühl lagern
S conservar frío

refroidissement
E cooling
G Abkühlung
S enfriamiento

refus (par ex. d'un brevet)
E rejection (e. g. of a patent)
G Ablehnung (z. B. eines Patentes)
S rechazo (p. ej. de una patente)

régénération
E regeneration
G Regenerierung
S regeneración

registre
E index, contents, list
G Verzeichnis
S índice

registre d'évaluation d'erreurs
E defect (error, failure) evaluation list
G Fehlerbewertungsliste
S lista de evaluación de errores

réglage
E adjustment, setting
G Einstellung, Regulierung
S ajuste, regulación

réglage de la température
E temperature setting
G Temperatureinstellung
S ajuste de temperatura

réglage d'un régulateur
E controller set point
G Reglereinstellung
S ajuste de un regulador

réglage fin
E fine adjustment
G Feinregulierung, Feineinstellung
S regulación fina, ajuste fino

règlement de sécurité
E safety regulation
G Sicherheitsvorschriften
S reglamento de seguridad

régler
E adjust, to
G einstellen
S ajustar, regular

règles concernant les risques et la sécurité
E risk and safety phrases
G Risiko- und Gefahrensätze
S reglas concernientes a riesgos y peligros

règles d'étiquetage
E labelling rules
G Etikettierungsregeln
S reglas de etiquetado

règles GMP
E GMP guidelines
G GMP-Richtlinien
S directrices de GMP

mise en pratique des règles GMP
E implementation of GMP guidelines
G Umsetzung von GMP-Richtlinien
S puesta en práctica de directices de GMP

respect des règles GMP
E observance of GMP guidelines
G Befolgung von GMP-Richtlinien
S observancia de directrices de GMP

règles vestimentaires
E gowning procedure
G Bekleidungsvorschrift
S prescripción de vestuario

régleur pneumatique
E cross-bellows controller
G Kreuzbalgregler
S regulador de fuelle cruzado

régulateur
E controller, control valve, throttle
G Regler, Drossel
S regulador, estrangulador

régulateur de flux
E variable flowmeter
G variabler Volumenstromregler
S regulador variable de flujo

régulateur de pression
E pressure regulator, reducing valve
G Druckregler
S regulador de presión

régulateur de température
E temperature controller
G Temperaturregler
S regulador de temperatura

régulateur de tension
E voltage regulator
G Spannungsregler
S regulador de tensión

régulateur d'écoulement d'air
E air flow controller
G Luftstromwächter
S controlador de la corriente de aire

régulation du débit
E flow regulation
G Durchflußregulierung
S regulación del flujo

régulations concernant les rejets
E disposal regulations
G Entsorgungsvorschriften
S prescripciones de eliminación

régulations des activités de transport
E transport regulations
G Transportbestimmungen
S especificaciones de transporte

réintroduire
E reintroduce, to
G wiedereinschleusen
S reintroducir

rejet
E ejection, rejection, disposal
G Auswurf, Zurückweisung, Entsorgung, Ausstoß
S eyección, rechazo, desecho, eliminación

rejeter
E reject, to; eject, to
G zurückweisen, ausstoßen
S rechazar, emitir, expeler, expulsar

relais
E relay
G Relais
S relé, relevador

relais amplificateur
E relay amplifier
G Relaisverstärker
S amplificador de relé

relevé de la pression
E pressure reading
G Druckablesung
S lectura de la presión

relevé d'un lot
E batch record
G Chargenprotokoll
S protocolo de lotes

relève-plateau
E beam arrest (balance)
G Arretiervorrichtung (bei Waagen)
S dispositivo de fijación (en básculas)

relever
E read, to; read off, to
G ablesen
S leer

remanier
E review, to
G überarbeiten
S perfeccionar, revisar

remboursement
E reimbursement
G Erstattung
S devolución, restitución

remplaçant
E deputy
G Stellvertreter
S suplente, sustituto

remplacer
E replace, to
G ersetzen
S reemplazar, sustituir

remplir à l'aide d'un entonnoir
E funnel, to
G eintrichtern
S llenar con embudo

remplissage
E filling
G Abfüllung
S envasado, embotellamiento

remplissage aseptique
E aseptic filling
G aseptische Abfüllung
S envasado aséptico

remplissage des milieux de culture
E culture medium filling, media fill
G Nährmedienabfüllung
S relleno con medio de cultivo

remplissage d'une ampoule
E ampoule filling
G Ampullenabfüllung
S rellenado de una ampolla

remplissage uniforme
E uniform filling
G Füllung, gleichmäßige
S relleno uniforme

remplisseuse
E filling machine
G Abfüllmaschine
S máquina de envasado

rémunération
E remuneration
G Vergütung
S remuneración

rendement
E yield, recovery, throughput
G Ertrag, Ausbeute, Wiedergewinnung, Durchsatz
S rendimiento, recuperación

rendement brut
E raw yield
G Rohausbeute
S rendimiento bruto

rendement de transformation en granulé
E granulation performance
G Granulationsleistung
S rendimiento de granulación

rendement d'une production
E production output
G Produktionsleistung
S rendimiento de producción

rendement final
E final yield
G Endausbeute
S rendimiento final

rendement horaire
E output per hour
G Stundenleistung
S rendimiento horario

rendement réel
E actual yield
G Ausbeute, tatsächliche
S rendimiento real

rendement secondaire
E secondary yield
G Sekundärausbeute
S rendimiento secundario

rendement théorique
E theoretical yield
G theoretische Ausbeute
S rendimiento teórico

rendement total
E total yield
G Gesamtausbeute
S rendimiento total

renforcé
E reinforced
G verstärkt
S intensificado, reforzado

renouvellement d'air
E air exchange
G Luftwechsel
S renovación del aire

renverser
E spill, to
G verschütten
S derramar, verter

renvoi
E return
G Retoure
S retorno

renvoyer
E make redundant, to
G entlassen
S despedir

réorganisation
E re-equipping
G Umrüstung
S modernización, reorganización

réorganiser
E re-equip, to
G umrüsten
S modernizar, reorganizar

réorganiser les palettes
E re-pallet, to
G umpalettieren
S cambiar de paleta

répandre
E spill, to
G verschütten
S derramar, verter

réparation
E repair
G Reparatur, Instandsetzung
S reparación

répartition de la température
E heat distribution
G Temperaturverteilung
S distribución de temperatura

répertoire
E index, contents, list
G Verzeichnis
S índice

répétition
E repetition
G Wiederholung
S repetición

répétitivité
E repeatability
G Wiederholbarkeit
S repetitividad

répétitivité de la précision
E precision repeatability
G Wiederholbarkeit der Präzision
S repetitividad de la precisión

repiquage
E transfer inoculation
G Überimpfung
S sobreinoculación

report
E carryover
G Übertrag
S transporte

reproductibilité
E reproducibility
G Reproduzierbarkeit
S reproductibilidad

reproductible
E reproducible
G reproduzierbar
S reproducible

répulsant l'humidité
E moisture-repelling
G feuchtigkeitsabweisend
S repelente de la humedad

requalification
E requalification
G Requalifizierung
S recualificación

requête
E application
G Antrag
S solicitud, instancia

réseau
E network
G Netzwerk
S malla, obra de malla, retículo

réseau cristallin
E lattice
G Kristallgitter
S retículo cristalino

réseau de sprinkler
E sprinkler
G Sprinkleranlage
S aspersor

réservé
E retentive
G zurückhaltend
S reservado

réservoir
E reservoir, collector
G Vorratsgefäß, Sammelbehälter
S depósito (colector), recipiente de depósito

résidu
E residue
G Rückstand, Rest
S residuo, resto

résidu de distillation
E distillation residue
G Destillationsrückstand
S residuo de destilación

résidu de filtration
E filter residue
G Filterrückstand
S residuo de filtración

résidu de pressage
E residue
G Preßrückstand
S residuo de prensado

résidu de séchage
E residue on drying
G Trockenrückstand
S residuo seco

résidu de tamisage
E overs, residue
G Siebrückstand
S residuo de tamizado

résidu d'ignition
E residue on ignition
G Glührückstand
S residuo de ignición

résidu d'un produit
E product residue
G Produktrückstand
S residuo de un producto

résidu radioactif
E radioactive waste
G radioaktiver Abfall
S residuos radiactivos

résidu visible
E visible residue
G sichtbarer Rückstand
S residuo visible

résidus
E rubbish, waste
G Müll, Abfall, Ausschuß
S basura, desechos, residuos, desecho

résidus de vaporisation
E residue on evaporating
G Verdampfungsrückstand
S residuo de evaporación

résine
E resin
G Harz
S resina

résine acrylique
E acrylic resin
G Acrylharz
S resina acrílica

résine échangeuse d'ions
E ion exchange resin
G Austauscherharz
S resina de intercambio iónico

résine époxy
E epoxy resin
G Epoxidharz
S epoxirresina

résine synthétique
E synthetic resin
G Kunstharz
S resina sintética

résistance
E durability, resistance
G Beständigkeit
S estabilidad, inalterabilidad

résistance à la flexion
E flexional strength
G Beugungsfestigkeit
S resistencia a la flexión

résistance à la friction
E frictional resistance
G Reibungswiderstand, Abriebfestigkeit
S resistencia a la fricción, resistencia a la abrasión

résistance à la lumière
E light-fastness
G Lichtbeständigkeit
S resistencia a la luz

résistance à la plicature
E resistance to bending
G Knickechtheit
S resistencia al pandeo

English German French Spanish

résistance à la pression
E pressure resistance
G Druckfestigkeit
S resistencia a la presión

résistance à la rupture
E breaking strength, breaking resistance
G Bruchfestigkeit
S resistencia a la rotura

résistance à la traction et à la compression
E traction-compression resistance
G Zug- und Druckfestigekit
S resistencia a la tracción y a la presión

résistance à l'abrasion
E resistance to abrasion
G Reibeechtheit
S resistente a la fricción

résistance à l'éclatement
E bursting strength
G Berstdruckfestigkeit
S resistencia al estallido

résistance à l'usure
E resistance to wear
G Verschleißwiderstand
S resistencia al desgaste

résistance au choc
E impact resistance
G Schlagfestigkeit
S resistencia a los choques

résistance au déchirement
E resistance to tearing, tear strength, tensile strength
G Reißfestigkeit, Zerreißfestigkeit
S resistencia al desgarro

résistance au filtrage
E filtration resistance
G Filtrationswiderstand
S resistencia a la filtración

résistance au fléchissement
E flexural strength
G Biegefestigkeit
S resistencia a la flexión

résistance au frottement
E frictional resistance
G Reibungswiderstand
S resistencia a la fricción

résistance au pliage
E flexing resistance, flexural strength
G Biegefestigkeit, Falzechtheit
S resistencia a la flexión, resistencia al plegado

résistance du filtre
E filter resistance
G Filterwiderstand
S resistencia del filtro

résistance électrique
E electrical resistance
G elektrischer Widerstand
S resistencia eléctrica

résistance spécifique
E specific resistance
G spezifischer Widerstand
S resistencia específica

résistant
E resistant
G resistent, widerstandsfähig
S resistente, tenaz

résistant à la chaleur
E heat-resistant
G hitzebeständig
S resistente al calor

résistant à la corrosion
E resistant to corrosion
G korrosionsbeständig
S resistente a la corrosión

résistant à la décoloration
E resistant to fading
G lichtecht
S resistente a la decoloración

résistant à la lumière
E light-fast
G lichtbeständig
S resistente a la luz

résistant à la pression
E pressure-resistant
G druckfest
S resistente a la presión

résistant à l'abrasion
E non-abrasive, resistant to abrasion
G abriebfest
S resistente a la abrasión

résistant à l'humidité
E moisture-resistant
G feuchtigkeitsbeständig
S resistente a la humedad

résistant au suc gastrique
E gastro-resistant
G magensaftresistent
S resistente al jugo gástrico

résistant au vieillissement
E age-resistant
G alterungsbeständig
S resistente al envejecimiento

résistant aux acides
E acid-resistant
G säurebeständig
S resistente a los ácidos

résistant aux chocs
E shock-resistant, impact-resistant
G stoßfest, erschütterungsbeständig
S resistente a los golpes, resistente a la agitación

résistant aux solvants
E solvent-resistant
G lösungsmittelbeständig
S resistente a solventes

résorption
E resorption
G Resorption
S resorción

responsabilité
E responsibility
G Verantwortlichkeit
S responsabilidad

responsabilité (juridique)
E liability (legal)
G Haftung (rechtlich)
S responsabilidad (jurídica)

responsable
E person responsible, clerk
G Sachbearbeiter
S encargado, ponente

responsable du contrôle-qualité
E head of quality control
G Kontrolleiter
S director de control

ressort
E spring
G Feder (Sprung-)
S resorte

ressort d'ajustage (de poinçon)
E key (of punch)
G Paßfeder, Schlüssel (des Stempels)
S llave (de troquel)

ressort de rappel
E counter-spring, return spring
G Rückzugfeder
S muelle de retorno

ressort de torsion
E torsion spring
G Torsionsfeder
S muelle de torsión

résultat d'analyse
E analytical result
G Testergebnis
S resultado de la prueba

résultats
E result
G Ergebnis
S resultado

résultats escomptés
E expected results
G erwartete Ergebnisse
S resultados esperados

résumé des caractéristiques du produit
E summary of product characteristics (SPC)
G Zusammenfassung der Produktmerkmale
S resumen de características del producto

rétablissement
E reconstitution
G Wiederherstellung
S reconstitución, restablecimiento

retard
E delay, delay time, time lag
G Verzögerung, Verzögerungszeit, Zeitverzögerung
S retardo, retraso, tiempo de retraso

retardé
E delayed
G verzögert
S retardado, retrasado

retardement de l'ébullition
E boiling retardation
G Siedeverzug
S retraso de la ebullición

rétention
E retention
G Retention
S retención

réticent
E retentive
G zurückhaltend
S reservado

réticulaire
E reticular, net-like
G netzförmig, vernetzt
S reticular, integrado en una red

réticule
E crosswires
G Fadenkreuz
S retículo

retouche
E reprocessing
G Nacharbeitung
S reprocesado, retocado

retour
E reverse flow
G Rücklauf
S retorno

retrait
E withdrawal
G Entnahme
S extracción, toma

retraitement
E reprocessing, reworking
G Wiederaufbereitung, Umarbeitung
S reprocesado, adaptación, remodelación, transformación

rétrécir
E shrink, to
G schrumpfen
S contraerse, retraerse, reducirse

réutilisable
E returnable, re-usable
G wiederverwendbar, Mehrweg-
S reutilizable

réutilisation
E re-use
G Wiederverwendung
S reutilización

revalidation
E revalidation
G Revalidierung
S revalidación

revêtement
E cover, coating
G Verkleidung, Belag
S cubierta, revestimiento, recubrimiento

revêtement (de tuyauteries)
E cladding (of piping)
G Verkleidung (von Rohrleitungen)
S recubrimiento (de conducciones)

revêtement de couleur
E colour coating
G Farbüberzug
S revestimiento coloreado

revêtement de sol
E flooring, floor covering, floor finishing
G Bodenbelag, Fußbodenbelag
S pavimento, revestimiento del suelo

revêtement de surface
E surface coating
G Oberflächenbeschichtung
S revestimiento de superficies

revêtement plastique
E plastic coating
G Kunststoffbeschichtung
S revestimiento plástico

revêtu
E covered
G verkleidet
S recubierto, revestido

revêtu de plastique
E plastic-coated
G kunststoffbeschichtet
S revestido de plástico

révisé
E reviewed
G überarbeitet
S perfeccionado, revisado

réviser
E review, to
G überarbeiten, revidieren
S perfeccionar, revisar

rhéologie
E rheology
G Rheologie
S reología

rigide
E rigid
G starr, steif
S rígido

rigole d'alimentation
E feed chute
G Zufuhrrinne
S canal de alimentación

rigole d'écoulement
E drain duct
G Abflußrinne
S desaguadero

rigole d'écoulement pour comprimés
E tablet exit chute
G Tablettenablaufrinne
S canal de salida de los comprimidos

rincer
E rinse, to
G spülen
S enjuagar, irrigar, lavar

rincer (avec)
E flush, to (with); purge, to (with)
G durchströmen (mit)
S inundar (con), purgar (con)

risque biologique
E biohazard
G Biogefahr, Gefahr durch biologische Agenzien
S peligro biológico

risque de blessures
E risk of injury
G Verletzungsgefahr
S riesgo de lesión

risque d'incendie
E fire hazard
G Feuergefahr
S peligro de incendio

risque pour la santé
E health risk
G Gesundheitsrisiko
S riesgo para la salud

rivet
E rivet
G Niete
S remache

rivet conique
E countersunk rivet
G Senkniete
S remache avellanado

robinet
E stopcock
G Hahn
S grifo

robinet d'arrêt
E stopcock
G Absperrhahn
S grifo de cierre

robinet d'arrêt à trois voies
E three-way stopcock
G Dreiwegehahn
S grifo con tres vías

robinet de purge
E discharge cock, drain cock
G Ablaßhahn
S grifo de salida

robuste (par ex. instrument, méthode)
E rugged (e. g. instrument, method)
G robust (z. B. Gerät, Methode)
S robusto (p. ej. instrumento, método)

robustesse
E robustness
G Robustheit
S robustez

robustesse d'un procédé
E process robustness
G Robustheit des Prozesses
S robustez del proceso

rondelle
E washer
G Unterlegscheibe
S arandela

rongeur
E rodent
G Nagetier
S roedor

rotation optique
E optical rotation
G optische Drehung
S rotación óptica

rotation spécifique
E specific rotation
G spezifische Drehung
S rotación específica

rotations (par minute)
E revolutions (per minute)
G Umdrehungen (pro Minute)
S revoluciones (por minuto)

rotor
E rotor
G Rotor
S rotor

rotule
E ball + socket joint
G Kugelgelenk
S articulación de rótula, unión esférica

roue de dosage
E dosing wheel
G Dosierrad, Dosierstern
S rueda de dosificación

roue de ventilateur
E fan wheel
G Gebläserad
S rueda de ventilador

rouille
E rust
G Rost
S herrumbre, orín

rouiller
E rust, to
G rosten
S oxidarse

rouleau
E roller, drum
G Walze
S cilindro, rodillo

rouleau de gravure
E engraving roll
G Gravurrolle
S rollo de grabado

rouleau porteur
E casters
G Laufrollen, Lenkrollen
S polea, roldana

rouleau presseur
E pre-pressing roller
G Vordruckrolle (Tablettenpresse)
S rollo de prensado previo (comprimidos)

rouleau presseur principal
E main compression roll
G Hauptdruckrolle
S rollo principal de prensa

rouleaux de guidage
E guide rollers
G Führungsrollen
S poleas de guía

roulement à billes
E ball bearing
G Kugellager
S rodamiento a bolas

route de développement
E development route
G Entwicklungsweg
S vía de desarrollo, vía evolutiva

rugosité de la surface
E surface rawness
G Oberflächenrauhigkeit
S rugosidad de superficie

rupture de fil
E thread rupture
G Fadenbruch
S ruptura de hilo

rupture de trémie
E sieve rupture
G Siebbruch
S ruptura del tamiz

sabot distributeur
E feed shoe
G Füllschuh
S zueco distribuidor

sac
E bag
G Beutel
S sobre

sac à double paroi
E bag in bag
G Beutel in Außenbeutel
S sobre de pared doble

sac de filtration
E filter bag
G Filterbeutel
S bolsa filtro

sac filtrant
E sack filter
G Sackfilter
S saco filtrante

sac poubelle
E waste bag
G Abfallbeutel
S bolsa de desechos

sachet
E bag, sachet (as dosage form)
G Beutel (als Darreichungsform)
S sobre (como forma de administración)

sachet de séparation
E split bag
G Trennbeutel
S bolsa de separación

sachet hermétique
E sealed bag, sachet
G Siegelrandbeutel
S bolsa hermética

sachet plan
E flat bag
G Flachbeutel
S bolsa plana

sachet plat
E flat bag
G Flachbeutel
S bolsa plana

saillir
E project, to; protrude, to
G überhängen, überstehen
S pender sobre, sobresalir, resaltar

saisie de données
E data entry
G Dateneingabe
S entrada de datos

salinité
E salinity
G Salinität, Salzigkeit
S salinidad

salle de préparation des milieux de culture
E culture media preparation room
G Nährmedienküche
S sala de preparación de medios de cultivo

salle des machines
E machine room
G Maschinenraum
S sala de máquinas

sang conservé
E stored blood
G Blutkonserve
S conserva de sangre

sangsue
E leech
G Blutegel
S sanguijuela

saponification
E saponification
G Verseifung
S saponificación

saponifier
E saponify, to
G verseifen
S saponificar

sas
E lock
G Schleuse
S esclusa

sas réservé au personnel
E personnel lock
G Personenschleuse
S esclusa de personal

sas réservé aux fournitures, sas réservé au matériel
E material lock
G Materialschleuse
S esclusa de material

saturation
E saturation
G Sättigung
S saturación

saturé
E saturated
G gesättigt
S saturado

sauvegarde électronique de données
E electronic data storage
G Datenspeicherung
S almacenamiento de datos

scanner à luminescence
E luminescence scanner
G Lumineszenztaster
S sensor de luminiscencia

sceau en plomb
E seal
G Plombe
S empaste, marchamo, precinto

sceller (comprimés)
E seal, to (tablets)
G einsiegeln, siegeln, verschließen (Tabletten)
S estampar, precintar, sellar, cerrar (comprimidos)

schéma
E drawing, site plan, layout
G Zeichnung, Lageplan
S dibujo, plano del lugar

schéma de charge (pour autoclave)
E load pattern (for autoclaves)
G Beschickungsmuster (für Autoklaven)
S esquema de carga (para autoclave)

schéma de chargement
E loading configuration
G Beladungsschema
S esquema de carga

schéma de dosage
E dosing pattern
G Dosierungsschema
S muestra de dosificación

schéma de fabrication
E flow chart
G Ablaufschema, Fließschema
S esquema operacional, diagrama operacional

schéma de l'installation, des canalisations et diagrammes des instruments
E installation scheme, piping and instrument diagram
G R+I-Schema
S esquema de instalación, de canalización y diagramas de instrumentos

schéma de marche
E flow chart
G Ablaufschema, Fließschema
S esquema operacional, diagrama operacional

schéma de montage
E circuit diagram
G Schaltbild
S diagrama de circuito

schéma de principe
E flow chart
G Ablaufschema, Fließschema
S esquema operacional, diagrama operacional

schéma de production
E production schedule
G Produktionsplan
S plan de producción

schéma des connexions
E circuit diagram
G Schaltbild
S diagrama de circuito

schéma fonctionnel
E flow chart, process flow diagram (PFD)
G Flußdiagramm, Prozeßflußdiagramm
S diagrama de flujo, diagrama de flujo de procesos

schéma fonctionnel et instrumental
E piping and instrument diagram (P&ID)
G R+I-Schema
S esquema de procesos e instrumentos

schéma interne de suggestions pour employés
E employee suggestion scheme
G betriebliches Vorschlagswesen
S sistema empresarial de propuestas

schéma opérationnel
E flow chart
G Ablaufschema, Fließschema
S esquema operacional, diagrama operacional

schéma relationnel
E relationship diagram
G Relationsdiagramm
S diagrama de relaciones

science médicale
E medical science
G Medizinische Wissenschaft
S ciencia médica

scission endothermique
E endothermic split-off
G endothermische Abspaltung
S escisión endotérmica

English German French Spanish

screening
E screening
G Reihenuntersuchung, Abschirmung
S examen secuencial, serie de ensayos, apantallamiento, protección

screening à ultra-haut rendement
E ultra-high throughput screening (UHTS)
G Screenen mit ultrahohem Durchsatz (UHTS)
S detención con ultrarrendimiento

screening de principes actifs
E active substance screening
G Wirkstoffscreening
S detección de sustancias activas

screening d'une banque de données
E database screening
G Datenbankscreening
S búsqueda en banco de datos

séchage à micro-ondes
E microwave drying
G Mikrowellentrocknung
S desecación por microondas

séchage final
E final drying
G Nachtrocknen
S secado final

séchage par atomisation
E spray-dry, to
G sprühtrocknen
S secar atomizando

séché à l'air
E air-dried
G luftgetrocknet
S secado al aire

sécher
E dry, to; desiccate, to
G trocknen, eintrocknen
S desecar, secar

sécheur en lit fluidisé
E fluid bed dryer
G Wirbelschichttrockner
S secador de lecho fluidificado

séchoir
E drying oven
G Trockenschrank
S secador

séchoir à circulation d'air
E circulatory dryer
G Umlufttrockner
S secador de circulación de aire

séchoir à cylindres
E drum dryer
G Walzentrockner
S secador de cilindros

secouer
E shake, to; shake out, to; vibrate, to
G ausschütteln, rütteln
S sacudir, trepidar, vibrar

secoueur
E vibrator, shaker
G Rüttler, Schüttler
S vibrador, agitador

secoueuse
E vibrator, shaker
G Rüttler, Schüttlet, Schüttelmaschine
S vibrador, agitador

secours d'urgence
E first aid
G Erste Hilfe
S primeros auxilios

secret d'entreprise
E company secret
G Betriebsgeheimnis
S secreto empresarial

sécréter
E separate, to
G abscheiden
S precipitar, separar

section
E division
G Sparte
S especialidad, rama, sector

section transversale
E cross-section
G Querschnitt
S sección transversal

sécurité
E safety, security
G Sicherheit, Unbedenklichkeit
S seguridad

sécurité de dosage
E dosage security
G Dosierungssicherheit
S seguridad de dosificación

sécurité de prélèvement
E tamper-proof seal
G Entnahmesicherung
S precintado de un frasco

sécurité des données
E data security
G Datensicherheit
S seguridad de datos

sécurité du personnel
E personnel safety, personnel protection
G Personenschutz
S seguridad del personal

sécurité du travail
E safety at work
G Arbeitssicherheit
S seguridad en el trabajo

sécurité d'un produit
E product safety
G Produktsicherheit
S seguridad de un producto

sécurité informatique
E computer security
G Computersicherheit
S seguridad informática

sédatif
E sedative
G Beruhigungsmittel
S sedante, tranquilizante

sédiment
E sediment
G Ablagerung, Bodensatz
S depósito, sedimento

sédimenter
E sediment, to
G sedimentieren
S sedimentar

segment de tamisage
E sieve insert
G Siebeinsatz
S inserción del tamiz

ségrégation
E segregation, separation
G Abtrennung
S segregación, separación

ségrégation physique
E physical segregation
G räumliche Trennung
S separación espacial

sélection
E selection
G Auswahl, Auslese
S selección

sélectivité
E selectivity
G Selektivität
S selectividad

semi-conducteur
E semiconductor
G Halbleiter
S semiconductor

semi-solide
E semi-solid
G halbfest
S semisólido

English German French Spanish

sensibilité
E sensitivity
G Empfindlichkeit
S sensibilidad

sensibilité de détection
E detection sensitivity
G Detektionsempfindlichkeit
S sensibilidad de detección

sensible
E sensitive
G empfindlich
S sensible

sensible à la chaleur
E heat-sensitive, heat-labile
G hitzeempfindlich, hitzelabil
S sensible al calor, lábil al calor

sensible à la corrosion
E corrodible, sensitive to corrosion
G korrosionsempfindlich
S sensible a la corrosión

sensible à la lumière
E light-sensitive
G lichtempfindlich
S fotosensible

sensible à l'humidité
E moisture-sensitive
G feuchtigkeitsempfindlich
S sensible a la humedad

séparateur
E separator
G Abscheider
S precipitador, separador

séparateur à cyclone
E cyclone separation
G Zyklonabscheidung
S separación por centrifugación

séparateur de formes
E parting agent
G Formentrennmittel
S separador de formas

séparateur de vapeur
E steam separator
G Dampfabscheider
S separador de vapor

séparateur d'eau
E water separator
G Wasserabscheider
S separador de agua

séparateur d'huile
E oil separator, oil trap
G Ölabscheider
S separador de aceite

séparation
E segregation, separation
G Trennung, Abtrennung
S segregación, separación

séparation des solvants
E solvent separation
G Lösungsmittelabscheidung
S separación de solventes

séparé
E separated, segregated
G abgetrennt
S aislado, separado

séparer
E separate, to
G abscheiden
S precipitar, separar

septum
E septum
G Septum
S septo

séquençage
E sequencing
G Sequenzierung
S formación de secuencias, secuenciación

séquence
E sequence
G Reihenfolge
S secuencia

séquence de cycles
E cycle sequence
G Zyklussequenz
S secuencia de ciclos

série
E series
G Baureihe
S serie

série d'analyses
E screening
G Reihenuntersuchung
S examen secuencial, serie de ensayos

série de perforations
E row of perforations
G Lochreihe
S serie de perforaciones

série de poids
E set of weights
G Gewichtssatz
S juego de pesas

séries
E series
G Serien
S series

séries de dilution
E dilution series
G Verdünnungsreihe
S serie de dilución

seringue
E syringe
G Spritze
S jeringa

seringue à usage unique
E disposable syringe
G Einmalspritze
S jeringa de uso único

seringue à usage unique
E disposable syringe
G Einmalspritze
S jeringa de uso único

seringue d'injection
E injection syringe
G Injektionsspritze
S jeringuilla

seringue prête à l'emploi
E prefilled syringe
G Fertigspritze
S jeringa lista para el uso

seringue prête à l'usage
E prefilled syringe
G Fertigspritze
S jeringa dispuesta para el uso

serpentin chauffant
E heating coil
G Heizschlange, Aufheizspirale
S serpentín de calefacción, serpentín de calentamiento

serpentin chauffant immergé
E immersed heating coil
G Heizschlange, untergetauchte
S serpentín de calefacción sumergido

serpentin de refroidissement
E cooling coil
G Schlangenkühler
S serpentín refrigerador

serpillière
E cleaning cloth, cleaning tissue
G Reinigungstuch
S paño de limpieza

serre-fils
E cable clamp, cable terminal
G Kabelschelle, Kabelklemme
S abrazadera de cable, terminal de cable

sertir
E flange, to; bead, to; border, to
G umbördeln
S bordear, rebordear, redondear

sérum
E serum
G Serum
S suero

English German French Spanish

sérum de veau fœtal
E foetal calf serum (FCS)
G fötales Kälberserum
S suero bovino fetal

sérums d'origine animale
E animal sera
G tierische Seren
S sueros de origen animal

service
E department
G Abteilung
S departamento

serviette à usage unique
E disposable towels
G Einmalhandtücher
S toallas de uso único

shampooing
E shampoo
G Shampoo
S champú

signal acoustique
E acoustic signal
G akustisches Signal
S señal acústica

signal d'alarme
E alarm, alarm signal
G Alarm
S alarma

signal optique
E visual signal
G optisches Signal
S señal óptica

signature
E signature
G Unterschrift
S firma

signature d'autorisation
E approval signature
G Unterschrift zur Genehmigung
S firma autorizante

signature électronique
E electronic signature
G elektronische Unterschrift
S firma electrónica

signification
E significance
G Bedeutung
S importancia, significado

silencieux
E silencer, attenuator
G Schalldämpfer
S silenciador

silicate
E silicate
G Silikat
S silicato

silice
E silicic acid, silica
G Kieselsäure, Siliciumdioxid
S ácido silícico, dióxido de silicio

siliconisation
E siliconisation
G Silikonisierung
S siliconización

sillon
E groove
G Nut, Rille
S acanaladura, estría, muesca, ranura

simultanément
E simultaneous
G gleichzeitig
S simultáneo, simultáneamente

siphon
E stench trap, siphon
G Geruchsverschluß
S válvula de hedor

siphon de dépôt d'huile
E oil separator, oil trap
G Ölabscheider
S separador de aceite

sirop
E syrup
G Sirup
S jarabe

sirop contre la toux
E cough syrup
G Hustensaft
S jarabe antitusígeno

site d'application
E site of action
G Angriffspunkt
S lugar de aplicación

site de fabrication
E plant, factory, facility
G Betriebsstätte
S plantas empresariales

site de production
E manufacturing site
G Produktionsstätte
S lugar de producción

société
E company
G Gesellschaft
S sociedad

société anonyme
E public liability company
G Aktiengesellschaft
S sociedad anónima

société mère
E parent company
G Mutterfirma
S sociedad matriz

socle
E base, socket
G Sockel, Untergestell
S base, casquillo, zócalo, pie, soporte

sol
E floor, soil
G Boden
S suelo

solide
E solid
G Feststoff, fest
S sustancia sólida, duradero, estable, sólido

solidifier
E solidify, to
G erstarren
S solidificar

solidité
E firmness, solidity
G Festigkeit
S firmeza, solidez

sollicitation à la flexion
E flexional strain
G Biegebeanspruchung
S tensión de flexión

sollicitation du matériel
E material stress
G Materialbeanspruchung
S tensión sobre el material

solubilisant
E solubiliser
G Lösungsvermittler
S solubilizante

solubilité
E solubility
G Löslichkeit
S solubilidad

soluble
E soluble
G löslich
S soluble

difficilement soluble
E sparingly soluble
G schwer löslich
S difícilmente soluble

facilement soluble
E readily soluble
G leicht löslich
S fácilmente soluble

English
German
French
Spanish

English German French Spanish

insoluble
E insoluble
G unlöslich
S insoluble

peu soluble
E slightly soluble
G wenig löslich
S poco soluble

pratiquement insoluble
E practically insoluble
G praktisch unlöslich
S prácticamente insoluble

très difficilement soluble
E very slightly soluble
G sehr schwer löslich
S muy difícilmente soluble

très soluble
E very soluble
G sehr leicht löslich
S muy fácilmente soluble

solution
E solution
G Lösung
S solución

solucion non-saturée
E unsaturated solution
G ungesättigte Lösung
S solución insaturada

solution saturée
E saturated solution
G gesättigte Lösung
S solución saturada

solution sursaturée
E supersaturated solution
G übersättigte Lösung
S solución sobresaturada

solution colorimétrique
E colorimetric solution
G Farbvergleichslösung
S solución colorimétrica

solution de fixation
E fixing solution
G Fixierlösung
S solución fijadora

solution de lavage auriculaire
E ear wash
G Ohrenspüllösung
S solución de lavado auricular

solution de perfusion
E infusion solution
G Infusionslösung
S solución de infusión

solution de référence
E reference solution
G Vergleichslösung
S solución de referencia

solution de rinçage
E rinsing solution
G Spüllösung
S solución de lavado

solution de teinture
E staining liquid
G Färbelösung
S solución colorante

solution d'hémofiltration
E solution for haemofiltration
G Hämofiltrationslösung
S solución de hemofiltración

solution injectable
E injection solution
G Injektionslösung
S solución inyectable

solution mère
E stock solution
G Stammlösung
S solución madre

solution pour bain de bouche
E mouthwash
G Mundspüllösung
S solución de enjuague bucal

solution pour dialyse péritonéale
E solution for peritoneal dialysis
G Peritonealdialyselösung
S diálisis peritoneal

solution pour gargarisme
E gargle
G Gurgellösung
S solución para gargarismos

solution réactive
E reagent solution
G Reagenzlösung
S solución reactiva

solution saline
E saline solution
G Kochsalzlösung
S solución salina

solution saline physiologique
E physiological saline
G physiologische Kochsalzlösung
S solución salina fisiológica

solution tampon
E buffer solution
G Pufferlösung
S solución de tamponamiento

solution volumétrique
E volumetric solution
G Maßlösung
S solución volumétrica

solvant
E solvent
G Lösungsmittel
S solvente

solvant inorganique
E inorganic solvent
G anorganisches Lösungsmittel
S solvente inorgánico

solvant organique
E organic solvent
G organisches Lösungsmittel
S solvente orgánico

solvant visqueux
E viscous solvent
G viskoses Lösungsmittel
S solvente viscoso

solvants organiques halogènes
E halogen-containing organic solvents
G halogenhaltige organische Lösungsmittel
S diluyentes orgánicos halogenados

solvants organiques non halogènes
E halogen-free organic solvents
G halogenfreie organische Lösungsmittel
S diluyentes orgánicos no halogenados

somme intermédiaire
E carryover
G Übertrag
S transporte

sondage
E bearing
G Peilung
S sondeo

sonde
E probe, catheter
G Sonde, Katheter
S sonda, catéter

sonde de température
E temperature sensor
G Temperaturfühler
S sensor de temperatura

sonde d'échantillonnage
E removal probe, sampling probe
G Entnahmesonde
S sonda de toma (de muestras)

sonde thermique
E temperature sensor, thermocouple, heat sensor
G Temperatursensor, Thermofühler, Wärmefühler
S sensor de temperatura, sonda térmica, sensor térmico

sortie
E outlet, orifice, drain
G Auslaß, Austritt, Ablauf
S descarga, escape, salida

sortie d'air
E air outlet
G Luftaustrittsöffnung
S orificio de salida del aire

sortie de détecteur
E detector outlet
G Detektorauslaß
S salida del detector

sortie de purge
E outlet, discharge outlet
G Auslauf
S desagüe, salida

sortie de régulation de pression
E pressure release outlet
G Druckablaß
S salida de presión

sortie de vidange
E outlet, discharge outlet
G Auslauf
S desagüe, salida

sortie d'une colonne
E column outlet
G Auslaßöffnung einer Säule
S orificio de salida de una columna

sortiment
E product range
G Sortiment
S surtido

soude
E alkaline solution, lye, sodium hydroxide solution
G Lauge, Natronlauge
S lejía, sosa alcalina

soudé
E welded
G verschweißt
S soldado

soudé par soudure orbitale
E orbitally welded
G orbital geschweißt
S soldado orbitalmente

souder
E weld, to; seam weld, to
G schweißen, nahtschweißen
S soldar

souder par points
E spot-weld, to
G punktschweißen
S soldar por puntos

souder par rapprochement
E butt-weld, to
G stumpfschweißen
S soldar a tope

soudure
E welding seam, weld
G Schweißnaht
S soldadura

soudure orbitale
E orbital fusion welding
G Orbitalschweißen
S soldadura orbital

souffler
E blow out, to
G ausblasen
S apagar soplando

soufflet
E bellows
G Faltenbalg
S fuelle plegable

soulagement
E relief
G Entlastung
S alivio, descarga

soumettre (une demande d'autorisation de mise sur le marché)
E submit, to (application for marketing approval)
G einreichen (Zulassungsantrag)
S presentar (una solicitud de autorización)

soumission à un effort
E stress, strain
G Beanspruchung
S carga, tensión

soupape à billes
E ball valve
G Kugelventil
S válvula esférica

soupape de retenue
E throttle check valve, throttle non-return valve
G Drosselrückschlagventil
S válvula estranguladora de retención, válvula activada por reflujo

soupape de sûreté (pour la pression)
E pressure relief valve
G Druckentlastungsklappe
S válvula de descompresión

soupape de vapeur
E steam valve
G Dampfventil
S válvula de vapor

source
E source
G Quelle
S fuente

source de chaleur
E heating source
G Heizquelle
S fuente de calor

source de chauffage
E heating source
G Heizquelle
S fuente de calor

source de courant continu
E direct current source
G Gleichstromquelle
S fuente de corriente continua

source de lumière
E light source
G Lichtquelle
S fuente luminosa

source d'électricité
E power source
G Stromquelle
S fuente de electricidad

source d'erreur
E source of error (failure)
G Fehlerquelle
S fuente de errores

source d'inflammation
E ignition source
G Zündquelle
S fuente de ignición

source d'un courant électrique
E electrical power source
G elektrische Stromquelle
S fuente de corriente eléctrica

sous condition d'exploitation
E in process
G im Betriebszustand
S funcionando

à l'arrêt, immobilisé
E at rest
G im Ruhezustand
S parado

sous-cutanée
E subcutaneous
G subkutan
S subcutáneo

sous-lot
E partial batch, sub-batch
G Teilcharge
S lote parcial, sublote

English German French Spanish

sous-pression
E negative pressure
G Unterdruck
S depresión, hipotensión

sous-produit
E by-product
G Nebenprodukt
S producto colateral, producto secundario

sparadrap
E sticking plaster
G Pflaster, Heftpflaster
S esparadrapo

spatule
E spatula
G Spatel
S espátula

spécification
E instruction, specification
G Vorschrift
S prescripción

en conformité avec les spécifications
E complying with specification
G vorschriftsmäßig
S conforme a las prescripciones

hors spécification
E out of specification (OOS)
G außerhalb der Spezifikation
S fuera de la especificación

spécification de fonctionnement
E function specification
G Funktionsspezifizierung
S especificación funcional

spécification de l'instrument
E instrument specification
G Gerätespezifikation
S especificación de aparatos

spécification de qualité
E quality specification
G Gütebestimmung
S especificación de calidad

spécification du codage de couleurs
E colour code specification
G Farbcodierungsspezifikation
S especificación de la codificación de colores

spécification d'un système
E system specification
G Systemspezifikation
S especificación de un sistema

spécification standard
E standard specification
G Normvorschrift
S prescripción estándar

spécifications de l'usager
E user requirements, user specifications
G Lastenheft
S requerimientos del usuario

spécifications des matériaux
E material specifications
G Materialspezifikationen
S especificaciones del material

spécifications du fabricant
E manufacturer's specification
G Herstellerangaben
S especificaciones del fabricante

spécifications fonctionnelles
E required specification
G Pflichtenheft
S descripción de tareas

spécificité
E specificity
G Spezifität
S especificidad

spécifier
E specify, to
G spezifizieren
S especificar

spécifique au lot
E batch-related
G chargenspezifisch
S específico del lote

spécimen
E sample, specimen
G Probe, Muster
S muestra, espécimen

spectomètre de particules
E particle spectrometer
G Teilchenspektrometer
S espectrometría de partículas

spectre
E spectrum
G Spektrum
S espectro

spectre infrarouge
E IR spectrum
G IR-Spektrum
S espectro infrarrojo

spectrophotomètre
E spectrophotometry
G Spektralphotometrie
S espectrofotometría

spectroscopie à émission de flamme
E flame emission spectroscopy
G Flammenemissionsspektroskopie
S espectroscopia de emisión de llama

spectroscopie IR
E IR spectroscopy
G IR-Spektroskopie
S espectroscopia IR

spectroscopie IR par transformation de Fourier
E FTIR spectroscopy
G FTIR-Spektroskopie
S espectroscopia infrarroja en transformación de Fourier

spectroscopie nucléaire à résonance magnétique
E nuclear magnetic resonance (NMR) spectroscopy
G Kernresonanzspektroskopie
S espectroscopia de resonancia nuclear

spectroscopie par émission atomique
E atomic emission spectroscopy
G Atomemissionsspektroskopie
S espectroscopia de emisión atómica

sphérique
E spherical
G sphärisch
S esférico

spores
E spores
G Sporen
S esporas

sporicide
E sporicide
G sporozid
S esporicida

squameux
E scaly
G schuppig
S escamoso

stabilité
E stability
G Haltbarkeit
S conservabilidad, estabilidad

stabilité à court terme
E short-term stability
G Kurzzeitstabilität
S estabilidad a corto plazo

stabilité à long terme
E long-term stability, durability, resistance
G Langzeitstabilität, Beständigkeit
S estabilidad a largo plazo, inalterabilidad

stabilité au stockage (de stockage)
E storage stability, warehouse stability, shelf-life
G Lagerstabilität, Lagerfähigkeit
S estabilidad de almacén, capacidad de almacenamiento

stabilité d'un produit
E product stability
G Produktstabilität
S estabilidad de un producto

stabilité thermique
E thermal stability
G thermische Stabilität
S estabilidad térmica

stable
E durable, stable
G dauerhaft, haltbar
S duradero, consistente, estable

stable à la chaleur
E heat-stable
G hitzestabil
S estable al calor

stable au chargement
E load-resisting
G belastungsstabil
S estable a la carga

stagiaire
E apprentice, trainee, temporary help
G Auszubildender, Praktikant, Aushilfe
S aprendiz, pasante, practicante, ayuda temporal

standard
E scale, standard
G Maßstab, Norm
S escala, estándar, patrón, norma

standard de référence
E reference, standard
G Referenzstandard
S estándar de referencia

standard interne
E internal standard
G Hausstandard
S estándar interno

standardisation
E standardisation
G Normierung
S normalización, estandarización

standardisé
E standardised
G genormt
S estandarizado, normalizado

standardiser
E standardise, to
G standardisieren
S estandarizar

station de compression
E compression station
G Druckstation
S estación de compresión

station de mise en bouteilles
E filling station
G Abfüllstation
S estación de envasado

station de pliage
E folding station
G Falzstation
S estación de plegado

station de poinçonnage
E die-cutting station, punch station
G Stanzstation, Stempelstation
S estación de troquelado

station de remplissage
E filling station
G Abfüllort, Füllstation, Abfüllstation
S estación de llenado, estación de envasado

station de scellage
E sealing station
G Verschlußstation
S estación de cierre

station d'épuration
E waste water treatment plant
G Kläranlage
S estación depuradora

station d'estampage
E embossing station, coding station
G Prägestation
S estación de troquelado

station en bidons
E filling station
G Abfüllstation
S estación de envasado

statisticien
E statistician
G Statistiker
S estadístico

statistiques de prélèvement
E sampling statistics
G Probenahmestatistik
S estadística de toma de muestras

statut de libération
E release status
G Freigabestatus
S status de autorización

statut de sécurité
E safety status
G Sicherheitsstatus
S status de seguridad

stéréosélectif
E stereoselective
G stereoselektiv
S estereoselectivo

stérile
E sterile
G steril, keimfrei
S estéril

stérile-filtré
E sterile-filtered
G sterilfiltriert
S filtrado estérilmente

stérile-filtrer
E sterile-filter, to
G sterilfiltrieren
S filtrar estérilmente

stérilisateur à air chaud
E hot air steriliser
G Heißluftsterilisator
S esterilizador de aire caliente

stérilisateur à chaleur sèche
E dry heat steriliser
G Trockenhitzesterilisator
S esterilizador de calor seco

stérilisateur à flammes
E flame steriliser
G Flammensterilisator
S esterilizador a la llama

stérilisateur de milieu
E media steriliser
G Mediensterilisator
S esterilizador de medios

stérilisation
E sterilisation
G Sterilisation
S esterilización

stérilisation à la chaleur
E heat sterilisation
G Hitzesterilisation
S esterilización al calor

stérilisation à la vapeur
E steam sterilisation
G Dampfsterilisation
S esterilización al vapor

stérilisation à l'air chaud
E dry heat sterilisation
G Heißluftsterilisation
S esterilización por aire caliente

stérilisation au gaz
E gas sterilisation
G Gassterilisation
S esterilización por gas

stérilisation finale
E final sterilisation
G Endsterilisation
S esterilización final

stérilisation finale à la vapeur
E terminal steam sterilisation
G abschließende Dampfsterilisation
S esterilización final al vapor

stérilisation in situ
E in-situ sterilisation
G In-situ-Dämpfen
S esterilización in situ

stérilisation par irradiation
E radiation sterilisation
G Strahlensterilisation
S esterilización por irradiación

stéroïdes
E steroids
G Steroide
S esteroides

stock
E inventory, stock
G Lagerbestand
S existencias en almacén, stocks

stockable
E suitable for storage
G lagerfähig
S adecuado para almacenaje

stockage
E storage, retention
G Lagerung, Aufbewahrung
S almacenamiento, conservación, almacenaje

précautions de stockage
E storage precautions
G Vorsichtsmaßnahmen bei der Lagerung
S medidas de precaución al almacenar

stockage à froid
E cold store, cold storage
G Kühllager
S almacén frigorífico

stockage à très basse température
E frozen storage
G Tiefkühllager
S almacén congelador

stockage de solvants
E solvent storage
G Lösungsmittellager
S almacén de solventes

stockage d'échantillons
E sample storage
G Probenlagerung
S almacenamiento de muestras

stockage intermédiaire
E interim storage
G Zwischenlagerung
S almacenaje intermediario

stockage thermique
E heated storage
G Heißlagerung
S almacenamiento caliente

stocker
E store, to
G einlagern
S almacenar

stocker au sec
E store dry, to
G trocken lagern
S almacenar en seco

stoichiométrie
E stoichiometry
G Stöchiometrie
S estequiometría

stratégie zéro défaut
E zero defect strategy
G Null-Fehler-Strategie
S estrategia de ausencia total de errores

stress statique
E static stress
G statische Beanspruchung
S tensión estática

striage
E corrugation
G Riffelung
S acanaladura, estría, ranura

strie
E streaks, stria
G Schliere
S estría

strié
E corrugated
G geriffelt
S acanalado, estriado

strier
E corrugate, to
G riffeln
S acanalar, estriar

structure cristalline
E crystal structure
G Kristallaufbau
S estructura cristalina

structure spatiale
E spatial structure
G Raumstruktur, Tertiärstruktur
S estructura espacial, estructura terciaria (p. ej. de una proteína)

sublimation
E sublimation
G Sublimierung
S sublimación

substance à analyser
E analyte
G Analyt
S sustancia a analizar

substance amère
E bitter component
G Bitterstoff
S sustancia amarga

substance apparentée
E related substance
G verwandte Substanz
S sustancia emparentada

substance aromatique
E aromatic substance
G Aromastoff
S sustancia aromática

substance complexante
E complex former
G Komplexbildner
S agente secuestrante

substance de contraste
E contrast medium
G Kontrastmittel
S medio de contraste

substance de liaison
E bonding material
G Verbindungsmaterial
S material de unión

substance de référence standard
E standard reference material
G Standardreferenzsubstanz
S sustancia de referencia estándar

substance extractible
E extractable substance
G extrahierbare Substanz
S sustancia extraíble

substance irritante
E irritating substance
G reizende Substanz
S sustancia irritante

substance narcotique
E narcotic substance
G Betäubungsmittel
S sustancia narcótica

substance neutralisante
E neutralising substance, inactivating substance (for disinfectant)
G Enthemmer (zur Inaktivierung von Desinfektionsmitteln)
S sustancia neutralizante (para inactivar desinfectantes)

substance standard de titrimétrie
E volumetric standard
G Urtiter
S título estándar

substance toxique
E toxic compound
G toxische Verbindung
S compuesto tóxico

substances halogènes
E halogenated compounds
G halogenierte Verbindungen
S compuestos halogenados

English German French Spanish

substances pétrochimiques
E petrochemicals
G petrochemische Substanzen
S sustancias petroquímicas

substitution
E substitution
G Substitution
S sustitución

substitution nucléophilique
E nucleophilic substitution
G nukleophile Substitution
S sustitución nucleófila

substrat
E substrate
G Substrat
S sustrato

suc gastrique
E gastric juice, gastric fluid
G Magensaft
S jugo gástrico

sucre de canne
E cane sugar
G Rohrzucker
S azúcar de caña

superficie
E area
G Fläche
S superficie

superficie d'un filtre
E filter surface
G Filteroberfläche
S superficie del filtro

supervision
E supervision
G Aufsicht
S control, inspección, supervisión

suppléance
E deputisation
G Stellvertretung
S suplencia, sustitución

suppléant
E deputy
G Stellvertreter
S suplente, sustituto

supplément
E supplement, supplementation, overage
G Ergänzung, Aufschlag
S complemento, aumento, suplemento

support
E mount, support, support brace, stand, frame, bearing (mach.)
G Halterung, Stütze, Gestell, Stutzen, Lager (Maschinenteil)
S apoyo, soporte, armazón, bastidor, empalme, tubuladura, asiento, cojinete, soporte

support de cuvette
E cell mount, cell holder
G Küvettenhalter
S portacubetas

support de filtre
E filter insert, filter stand
G Filtereinsatz, Filtergestell
S inserción del filtro, soporte del filtro

support de poinçon
E punch holder
G Stempelhalter
S soporte del troquel

suppositoire vaginal
E vaginal suppository, pessary
G Vaginalzäpfchen
S supositorio vaginal

suppositoires
E suppositories
G Suppositorien
S supositorios

sûr à la marche
E non-crushing, hard-wearing
G trittsicher
S paso seguro, de

sur besoin
E as required
G bei Bedarf
S en caso necesario

sur demande
E as required
G bei Bedarf
S en caso necesario

sur site
E on-site
G vor Ort
S en el lugar

suranné
E obsolete, out-dated
G überholt
S obsoleto, envejecido

surcharge
E overload, overloading
G Überlastung
S sobrecarga

surcharge de la colonne
E column overloading
G Säulenüberladung
S sobrecarga de columna

surdosage
E overdose
G Überdosierung
S sobredosificación

surdose
E overdose
G Überdosierung
S sobredosificación

surdosé
E overdosed
G überdosiert
S sobredosificado

surface
E surface, area
G Oberfläche, Fläche
S superficie

surface au contact d'un produit
E product contact surface
G produktberührende Oberfläche
S superficie en contacto con el producto

surface de culture
E seed layer, culture surface
G Kulturrasen
S superficie de cultivo

surface de membrane
E membrane area
G Membranfläche
S superficie de la membrana

surface de pic
E peak area
G Peakfläche
S superficie del pico

surface de séparation
E interface
G Grenzfläche
S interfase, superficie limitante

surface de travail
E working surface
G Arbeitsoberfläche
S superficie de trabajo

surface d'un comprimé
E tablet surface
G Tablettenoberfläche
S superficie del comprimido

surface d'un filtre
E filter surface
G Filterfläche
S superficie del filtro

surface d'une installation
E plant area
G Betriebsfläche
S área de las instalaciones empresariales

surface plane
E flat surface
G ebene Fläche
S superficie plana

surface polie
E smooth surface
G glatte Oberfläche
S superficie lisa

surface rugueuse
E rough surface
G rauhe Oberfläche
S superficie rugosa

surface totale
E total area
G Gesamtfläche
S superficie total

surgélation
E deep freezing
G Tiefkühlung
S congelación

surnageant
E supernatant
G Überstand
S sobrenadante

surpression
E positive pressure, excess pressure
G Überdruck
S sobrepresión

surpression atmosphérique
E excess atmospheric pressure
G Atmosphärenüberdruck
S sobrepresión atmosférica

sursaturation
E supersaturation
G Übersättigung
S sobresaturación

surveillance
E monitoring, supervision
G Überwachung, Aufsicht
S supervisión, vigilancia, control, inspección

surveillance par les autorités
E monitoring by the authorities
G behördliche Überwachung
S control oficial

surveiller
E monitor, to; supervise, to; control, to; check, to
G überwachen, überprüfen
S supervisar, vigilar, comprobar

susceptible à la corrosion
E susceptible to corrosion
G korrosionsanfällig
S susceptible a la corrosión

suspenser
E suspend, to
G suspendieren
S suspender

suspensif
E suspendibility
G Suspendierbarkeit
S suspensibilidad

suspension
E suspension, suspension device
G Suspension, Suspendierung, Aufhängung
S suspensión

suspension à ressort
E spring suspension
G Federaufhängung
S suspensión mediante resorte

suspension dans l'air, en
E airborne
G aerogen
S aerógeno

suspension de laquage
E lacquering fluid
G Lackiersuspension
S suspensión de lacado

suture
E suture
G Nahtmaterial
S material de sutura

symbole CE
E CE symbol
G CE-Zeichen
S símbolo CE

symbole de danger
E hazard symbol
G Gefahrensymbol
S símbolo de peligro

synérèse
E synaresis
G Synärese
S sinéresis

synthèse
E synthesis
G Synthese
S síntesis

système d'aide au pipettage
E pipetting aid
G Pipettierhilfe
S sistema de ayuda para pipetear

système d'alarme
E alarm system
G Alarmsystem
S sistema de alarma

système d'alimentation
E feed system
G Eintragsvorrichtung
S sistema de alimentación

système d'amarrage
E docking system
G Andocksystem
S sistema de fijación, sistema de acoplamiento

système d'aspiration
E aspiration system, evacuation system
G Absaugvorrichtung
S sistema de aspiración, sistema de evacuación

système d'aspiration de la poussière
E dust exhausting device, dust extraction
G Staubabsauganlage
S sistema de aspiración de polvo

système de canalisation
E duct network, ducting, piping system, ducting system
G Kanalnetz, Rohrleitungssystem, Schachtsystem
S red de canales, sistema de canalización, sistema de conducciones

système de codage pour les numéros de lot
E batch number coding
G Chargenbezeichnungsschlüssel
S código de designación de lotes

système de collecte
E collection system
G Sammelsystem
S sistema colector

système de contrôle
E control system, monitoring system
G Leitsystem, Überwachungssystem
S sistema de control, sistema de vigilancia

système de contrôle d'une installation
E plant control
G Anlagensteuerung
S control de plantas e instalaciones

système de documentation électronique de lots
E electronic batch recording system
G elektronische Chargen-dokumentation
S documentación electrónica de lotes

système de fixation
E docking system
G Andocksystem
S sistema de fijación, sistema de acoplamiento

système de gestion des données de laboratoire (LIMS)
E laboratory information management system (LIMS)
G Laborinformations- und -management-System (LIMS)
S sistema de gestión de datos de laboratorio (LIMS)

système de gestion du stockage
E stock management system
G Lagerhaltung
S gestión de stocks

système de gestion d'un procédé
E process control system
G Prozeßleitsystem
S sistema de gestión de un proceso

système de pipettage
E pipetting system, pipettor
G Pipettiersystem
S sistema de pipeteo

système de pipettage à canaux multiples
E multi-channel pipetting system
G Vielfachkanalpipettiersystem
S sistema de pipeteo con canales múltiples

système de pressurisation
E pressurisation system
G Drucksystem
S sistema de presurización

système de pulvérisation
E spraying system
G Sprühsystem
S sistema de pulverización

système de ruissellement
E trickle installation, trickle plant
G Berieselungsanlage
S sistema de lavado

système de santé
E health care
G Gesundheitswesen
S sistema sanitario

système de suivi
E tracing system
G Rückverfolgungssystem
S sistema de retromarcado

système de surveillance
E monitoring system
G Überwachungssystem
S sistema de vigilancia

système de surveillance des comprimés
E tablet monitoring system
G Tablettenüberwachungssystem
S sistema de vigilancia de comprimidos

système de traitement de l'eau
E water treatment system
G Wasseraufbereitungsanlage
S sistema de tratamiento de agua

système de traitement électronique de données
E electronic data processing
G elektronische Datenverarbeitung
S proceso electrónico de datos

système de ventilation
E ventilation system
G Belüftungsanlage, Belüftungssystem, Lüftungsanlage, raumlufttechnische Anlage
S sistema de ventilación

système d'élimination
E disposal system
G Entsorgungssystem
S sistema de eliminación

système d'évacuation
E aspiration system, evacuation system
G Absaugvorrichtung
S sistema de aspiración, sistema de evacuación

système d'évacuation d'air
E air aspiration, air exhaust system
G Luftabsaugung
S aspiración de aire

système d'exploitation
E operating system
G Bedienungssystem
S sistema de servicio

système d'observation
E tracing system
G Rückverfolgungssystem
S sistema de retromarcado

système expert
E expert system
G Expertensystem
S sistema de expertos

système thérapeutique transdermique
E transdermal delivery system
G Transdermales Therapeutisches System
S sistema terapéutico transdérmico

systèmes logistiques
E logistic systems
G logistische Systeme
S sistemas logísticos

table
E table
G Tabelle
S tabla

table d'alimentation
E feed table
G Zuführtisch
S mesa de abastecimiento

table de chargement
E feed table
G Zuführtisch
S mesa de abastecimiento

table de travail
E bench, work bench
G Arbeitstisch
S mesa de trabajo

table d'une matrice
E die table
G Matrizentisch
S mesa para matriz

tableau
E table
G Tabelle
S tabla

tableau de bord
E panel
G Armaturentafel
S cuadro de mandos, tablero de instrumentos

tableau de commande
E operator console, panel, control panel
G Bedienpult, Schalttafel
S pupitre de mando, tablero de control, cuadro de distribución, cuadro de mando

tableau d'instruments
E instrument panel
G Instrumententafel
S tablero de instrumentos

tableau d'utilisation
E operating panel
G Bedienungsfeld
S panel de mandos

tablette à sucer
E lozenge, pastille
G Lutschtablette
S comprimido para chupar

tablier
E skirting, apron (of machine)
G Abhängung, Schürze
S delantal

tache
E stain
G Fleck
S mancha

tachymètre
E tachometer, velocimeter, tachymeter, revolution counter
G Geschwindigkeitsmesser, Drehzahlmesser
S taquímetro, contador de revoluciones

taille
E format, size
G Format, Format
S formato, tamaño, magnitud, tamaño

taille de l'emballage
E package size
G Packungsgröße
S tamaño del envase

taille des particules
E particle size
G Korngröße, Partikelgröße, Teilchengröße
S tamaño del grano, tamaño de las partículas

taille des particules uniforme
E uniform particle size
G Gleichkorn
S tamaño uniforme de las partículas

taille d'un lot
E batch size
G Chargengröße, Losgröße
S tamaño de un lote

taille d'un pore
E pore size
G Porengröße
S tamaño del poro

taille d'une capsule
E capsule size
G Kapselgröße
S tamaño de una cápsula

taillé en biais
E sloping
G abgeschrägt
S biselado

taille moléculaire
E molecular size
G Molekülgröße
S tamaño molecular

taille nominale
E nominal size
G Nenngröße
S tamaño nominal

tambour
E roller, drum
G Walze, Trommel
S cilindro, rodillo, tambor

tambour à fibres
E fibre drum
G Fibertrommel
S tambor de fibras

tamis
E sieve, sieve screen
G Sieb, Siebboden
S cedazo, criba, tamiz, suelo del tamiz

tamis bas
E bottom screen
G Bodensieb
S tamiz base

tamis en toile métallique
E wire sieve
G Drahtsieb
S tamiz de alambre

tamis fin
E fine sieve
G Feinsieb
S tamiz fino

tamis grossier
E coarse sieve
G Grobsieb
S tamiz de malla gruesa

tamis métallique
E mesh wire
G Drahtnetz
S red de alambre

tamis secoueur
E sieve shaker
G Siebschüttler
S tamiz agitador

tamis vibrant
E vibrating sieve, vibrating screen
G Rüttelsieb
S tamiz vibrante

tamisage d'air
E air sieving
G Luftstrahlsiebung
S tamizado del aire

tamisage humide
E wet sieving
G Naßsiebung
S tamizado húmedo

tamiser
E sieve, to; sift, to
G sieben
S cribar, tamizar

tampon
E plug, stopper, buffer, tampon
G Stopfen, Puffer, Tampon
S tapón, tampón

tampon (pour imprimer)
E stamp (for printing)
G Stempel (zum Drucken)
S estampadora (para imprimir)

tampon d'ouate
E cotton plug, swab, gauze, pad
G Wattebausch, Tupfer
S torunda, torunda de algodón

tampon vaginal
E medicated vaginal tampon
G Vaginaltampon
S tampón vaginal

tangente
E tangent
G Tangente
S tangente

tannin
E tanning agent
G Gerbstoff
S tanino

tapis roulant
E conveyor belt
G Fließband, Förderband, Transportband
S cinta transportadora

tare
E tare
G Tara
S tara

tarer
E tare, to
G tarieren, austarieren
S tarar

taux
E ratio
G Verhältnis
S proporción

taux de cisaillement
E shear gradient
G Schergefälle
S gradiente de cizallamiento

taux de concentration maximal de travail
E MAC value
G MAK-Wert
S valor de concentración máxima de trabajo

taux de mortalité
E mortality rate
G Absterberate
S tasa de extinción, tasa de mortalidad

taux de récupération
E recovery rate
G Wiederfindungsrate
S tasa de recuperación

taux de récupération d'un produit
E product yield
G Produktausbeute
S rendimiento en producto

taux de rendement
E recovery rate
G Wiederfindungsrate
S tasa de recuperación

taux de renouvellement d'air
E air exchange rate
G Luftwechselrate
S tasa de renovación de aire

taux de retenue des particules
E particle separation rate
G Partikelabscheiderate
S tasa de separación de partículas

taux d'erreur
E failure rate
G Fehlerrate
S tasa de errores

technicien
E service technician
G Servicetechniker
S técnico de servicio

technique
E technique, method
G Technik, Methode
S técnica, método

technique aseptique
E aseptic process, aseptic technology
G aseptische Prozeßtechnik
S técnica de proceso aséptico

technique d'encartonnage
E cartoning technology
G Kartoniertechnik
S técnica de encartonar

technique des procédés
E process technology
G Verfahrenstechnik
S técnica del procedimiento

techniques de mesure, de réglage et de contrôle
E measuring and control technology
G Meß-Steuer-Regel (MSR)-Technik
S técnica de medición, regulación y control

teindre
E stain, to
G färben
S colorear, teñir

teinte
E colour shade, hue
G Farbton
S matiz del color

teinter
E stain, to
G färben
S colorear, teñir

teinture
E dye, stain, pigment, tincture
G Farbe, Farbstoff, Färbung, Färbemittel, Tinktur
S pigmento, tintura, coloración, colorante

teinture standard
E tincture standard
G Urtinktur
S tintura madre

télécommande
E remote control, remote operation
G Fernbedienung, Fernsteuerung, Fernüberwachung
S telemando, control remoto

température
E temperature
G Temperatur
S temperatura

température adiabatique
E adiabatic temperature
G adiabatische Temperatur
S temperatura adiabática

température ambiante
E room temperature, ambient temperature
G Raumtemperatur, Umgebungstemperatur
S temperatura ambiente

température d'admission
E inlet temperature
G Eingangstemperatur, Einlaßtemperatur
S temperatura de entrada

température de liquéfaction
E dropping point
G Tropfpunkt
S punto de goteo

température de solidification
E solidification temperature
G Erstarrungstemperatur
S temperatura de solidificación

température de sortie
E outlet temperature
G Auslaßtemperatur
S temperatura de salida

température de stérilisation
E sterilisation temperature
G Sterilisationstemperatur
S temperatura de esterilización

température d'entrée
E inlet temperature
G Eingangstemperatur, Einlaßtemperatur
S temperatura de entrada

température d'un procédé
E process temperature
G Prozeßtemperatur
S temperatura de un proceso

temporaire
E temporary
G vorläufig
S provisional, temporal, transitorio

temps de contact
E contact time
G Kontaktzeit
S tiempo de contacto

temps de désintégration
E disintegration time
G Zerfallszeit
S tiempo de desintegración

temps de doublement
E doubling time
G Generationszeit
S tiempo de generación

temps de réchauffement
E heat-up time
G Aufheizzeit
S tiempo de calentamiento

temps de récupération
E recovery time (in clean room)
G Erholzeit (im Reinraum)
S tiempo de recuperación (en área estéril)

temps de refroidissement
E cool-down time
G Abkühlzeit
S tiempo de enfriamiento

temps de réorganisation
E re-equipping time
G Umrüstzeit
S tiempo de reequipamiento

temps de réponse
E response time
G Ansprechzeit
S tiempo de respuesta

temps de résidence
E residence time, dwell time
G Verweilzeit, Aufenthaltsdauer
S tiempo de permanencia, duración de la permanencia

temps de résidence moyen
E mean residence time (MRT)
G mittlere Verweilzeit
S tiempo promedio de permanencia

temps de rétention
E retention time
G Retentionszeit
S tiempo de retención

temps de séchage
E drying time
G Trocknungszeit
S tiempo de desecación

temps de solidification
E solidification time, setting time
G Erstarrungszeit, Abbindezeit
S tiempo de solidificación

temps de stérilisation
E sterilisation time
G Sterilisationszeit
S tiempo de esterilización

temps de traitement
E processing time
G Durchlaufzeit
S tiempo de paso

temps d'éjection
E ejection time
G Ausstoßzeit
S tiempo de eyección

temps d'immobilisation
E down time
G Stillstandzeit (wegen Reparatur)
S tiempo de detención (por avería)

temps d'incubation
E incubation time
G Bebrütungszeit
S tiempo de incubación

temps mort
E breakdown, downtime (machine), dead time, failure
G Ausfall, Totzeit
S avería, desperfecto, tiempo muerto, fallo

temps requis
E time required
G Zeitaufwand
S tiempo invertido

tenailles
E tongs, crimping tongs
G Zange, Falzzange
S pinza, tenazas para cerrar tubos

teneur en eau
E water content
G Wassergehalt
S contenido en agua

teneur en humidité
E moisture content
G Feuchtigkeitsgehalt
S contenido en humedad

teneur en matière solide
E solid matter content
G Feststoffgehalt
S contenido en materia sólida

teneur en micro-organismes
E bioburden, bacterial (microbial) content
G Keimbelastung, Keimgehalt
S carga de gérmenes, contenido en gérmenes

teneur en oxygène
E oxygen content
G Sauerstoffgehalt
S contenido en oxígeno

teneur totale en carbone
E total organic carbon (TOC)
G Gesamtkohlenstoffgehalt
S contenido total en carbono

teneur totale en carbone organique
E total organic carbon (TOC)
G gesamtorganischer Kohlenstoff
S contenido total en carbono orgánico

tenside
E tenside
G Tensid
S agente tensioactivo

tensioactif
E surfactant, tenside
G oberflächenaktive Verbindung, grenzflächenaktiver Stoff
S agente tensioactivo, sustancia tensioactiva

tension
E tension
G Spannung, Zug
S tensión, tracción

tension (électrique)
E voltage
G Spannung
S tensión

tension de fléchissement
E flexural stress
G Biegespannung
S tensión de flexión

tension de pliage
E flexural stress
G Biegespannung
S tensión de flexión

tension de régime
E operating voltage
G Betriebsspannung
S voltaje de funcionamiento

tension du secteur
E line voltage
G Netzspannung
S tensión de la red

tension superficielle
E surface tension
G Oberflächenspannung
S tensión superficial

tératogène
E teratogenic
G teratogen
S teratógeno

terme
E time limit, deadline
G Frist
S plazo

terminal de contrôle
E control panel
G Bedienterminal
S terminal de control

ternaire
E ternary
G ternär
S ternario

ternir, se (métal)
E tarnish, to (metal)
G anlaufen (Metall)
S deslustrarse, empañarse (metales)

test au bain bleu
E blue dye bath test
G Blaubadtest
S prueba de baño con colorante azul

test d'acceptance (par ex. pour logiciel)
E acceptance test (e. g. for software)
G Akzeptanztest (z. B. für Software)
S prueba de aceptación (p. ej. de software)

test d'appareils
E equipment test
G Gerätetest
S comprobación de aparatos

test de contact direct
E direct contact test
G Abklatschtest
S prueba de contacto directo

test de contrôle
E analysis, control test
G Prüfung
S examen, ensayo, prueba, test

test de limites
E limit test
G Grenzprüfung
S prueba de límites

test de maintien du vide
E vacuum test
G Vakuumhaltetest
S prueba de mantenimiento del vacío

test de pression de retenue
E pressure test
G Druckhaltetest
S prueba de retención de la presión

test de pureté
E purity test
G Reinheitsprüfung
S prueba de pureza

test de qualification
E suitability test
G Eignungsprüfung
S prueba de aptitud

test de solidité
E robustness testing
G Prüfung der Robustheit
S comprobación de la robustez

test de stabilité
E stability test
G Haltbarkeitsuntersuchung
S prueba de estabilidad

test de stabilité accéléré
E accelerated stability test
G Streßtest
S estudio acelerado de estabilidad

test de stérilité
E sterility test
G Steriltest
S prueba estéril

test de stimulation
E challenge test
G Belastungstest
S prueba de carga

test de stimulation microbien
E microbial challenge test
G Bakterienbelastungstest
S prueba de estimulación con bacterias

test d'efficacité anti-microbien
E anti-microbial effectiveness test
G Konservierungsmittelbelastungstest
S prueba de eficacia antimicrobiana

test d'étanchéité du blister
E blister tightness test
G Blisterdichtigkeitstest
S prueba de estanqueidad del blíster

test d'identité
E identity test
G Identitätsprüfung
S prueba de identidad

test d'intégrité
E integrity test, integrity testing
G Integritätstest, Integritätsprüfung
S prueba (test) de integridad

test d'intégrité de filtre
E filter integrity test
G Filterintegritätstest
S prueba de integridad del filtro

test organoleptique
E organoleptic testing
G Sinnesprüfung
S prueba organoléptica

tester
E test, to
G prüfen
S comprobar, ensayar, examinar, investigar, probar

tête d'analyse
E scanning head
G Tastkopf
S cabeza de exploración

tête de pompe
E pump head
G Pumpenkopf
S cabeza de bomba

tête du poinçon
E punch tip
G Stempelkopf
S cabeza de troquel

tête d'un poinçon
E punch head
G Stempelkopf
S cabeza del troquel

tête rotative de pulvérisation
E rotary spray
G Rotationssprühkopf
S cabeza rotatoria de pulverización

thérapeutique
E therapeutic
G therapeutisch
S terapéutico

thérapie à long terme
E long-term therapy
G Langzeittherapie
S terapia a largo plazo

thermocouple
E thermocouple
G Thermoelement
S elemento termoeléctrico, pila termoeléctrica

thermodilatation
E thermal expansion
G Wärmeausdehnung
S termodilatación

thermo-élastique
E thermo-elastic
G thermoelastisch
S termoelástico

thermoplastique
E thermo-plastic
G thermoplastisch
S termoplástico

thermosceller
E heat seal, to
G heißsiegeln
S sellar al calor

thermostat
E thermostat
G Thermostat
S termostato

tige
E shaft
G Schaft, Welle
S árbol, asta, eje

tige de piston
E piston rod
G Kolbenstange
S barra del émbolo

tige transversale
E cross bar
G Querstange
S barra transversal

tissu
E tissue
G Gewebe
S tejido

tissu d'une muqueuse
E mucosal tissue
G Schleimhautgewebe
S tejido mucoso

tissu en plastique
E synthetic tissue
G Kunststoffgewebe
S tejido sintético

tissu fragile
E fine tissue
G Feingewebe
S tejido fino

tissu synthétique
E synthetic tissue
G Kunststoffgewebe
S tejido sintético

titrage de précipitation
E precipitation titration
G Fällungstitration
S volumetría de precipitación

titration
E titration, blending ratio
G Titration, Mischungsverhältnis
S titulación, proporción de mezcla

dosage en retour
E back titration
G Rücktitration
S titulación inversa

titre
E titre
G Titer
S título

titulaire d'un doctorat
E graduate (with doctorate), PhD
G promoviert
S doctorado

English German French Spanish

toboggan
E chute
G Rutsche
S tobogán

toboggan d'alimentation
E charge chute
G Befüllrutsche
S tobogán de carga

toboggan de charge
E charge chute
G Befüllrutsche
S tobogán de carga

toile métallique
E wire mesh
G Drahtgewebe
S tela metálica

toison
E fleece
G Vlies
S vellocino

tôle
E sheet, plate, tray
G Blech
S chapa, lámina, plancha

tolérance
E tolerance
G Toleranz
S tolerancia

hors des limites de tolérance
E out of tolerance
G außer Toleranz
S fuera de la tolerancia

tolérances spécifiques
E specified tolerances
G festgelegte Toleranzen
S tolerancias prefijadas

tonicité
E tonicity
G Tonizität
S tonicidad

tonneau
E barrel
G Faß
S tonel

tonneau en acier inoxydable
E stainless steel drum
G Edelstahlfaß
S tonel de acero inoxidable

tonneau en plastique
E plastic barrel
G Kunststoffaß
S tonel de plástico

topique
E topical
G topisch
S tópico

torsion
E torsion
G Torsionskraft, Verdrillung
S torsión, fuerza de torsión

touche
E key
G Taste
S tecla

touche de fonctionnement
E function keys
G Funktionstasten
S botones de operación

touche marche-arrêt
E start/stop key
G An/Aus-Taste
S interruptor de encendido

tour d'arrosage
E washing tower, spray tower
G Rieselturm
S torre de lavado

tour de refroidissement
E cooling tower
G Kühlturm
S torre de refrigeración

tour de tamisage
E sieve tower
G Siebturm
S torre de tamizado

tournant
E rotating
G rotierend
S girando

tourner
E rotate, to
G rotieren
S girar

tournesol
E litmus
G Lackmus
S litmus, tornasol

toxicité
E toxicity
G Toxizität, Giftigkeit
S toxicidad

toxicologie
E toxicology
G Toxikologie
S toxicología

toxine
E toxin, poison
G Toxin, Giftstoff
S toxina, veneno, sustancia venenosa

toxique
E poisonous, toxic
G giftig, toxisch
S tóxico, venenoso

toxique au contact de la peau
E toxic in contact with skin
G giftig bei Hautkontakt
S tóxico si entra en contacto con la piel

toxique si ingéré
E toxic if swallowed
G giftig beim Verschlucken
S tóxico si se ingiere

toxique si inhalé
E toxic by inhalation
G giftig beim Einatmen
S tóxico si se inhala

traçabilité
E traceability
G Rückführbarkeit, Rückverfolgbarkeit
S trazabilidad, retromarcado

traçabilité d'un lot
E batch traceability
G Chargenrückverfolgbarkeit
S seguimiento de un lote

traçable
E traceable
G rückverfolgbar
S de traza determinable

trace
E trace
G Spur
S traza, vestigio

trace-témoin de l'audit
E audit trail
G Auditweg
S traza-testigo de la auditoría

traceur
E marker, tracer
G Leitsubstanz
S marcador

traction
E tension
G Zug, Spannung
S tracción, tensión

traitable
E processable
G verarbeitungsfähig
S procesable

traité au jet de sable
E sand-blasted
G sandgestrahlt
S tratado con chorro de arena

English German French Spanish

traitement
E processing, reprocessing, handling (of)
G Bearbeitung, Verarbeitung, Aufarbeitung, Handhabung, Umgang (mit)
S elaboración, transformación, proceso, manejo, tratamiento, trato (con)

traitement alcalin
E alkaline treatment
G alkalische Behandlung
S tratamiento alcalino

traitement automatique
E machine processing
G maschinelle Verarbeitung
S elaboración automática, proceso automático, transformación automática

traitement biologique
E biological treatment
G biologische Behandlung
S tratamiento biológico

traitement complémentaire
E reprocessing
G Nacharbeitung
S reprocesado, retocado

traitement de surface
E surface treatment
G Oberflächenbehandlung
S tratamiento de superficies

traitement des eaux usées
E water purification
G Wasseraufbereitung
S purificación de agua

traitement électronique des données
E electronic data processing, EDP
G elektronische Datenverarbeitung, EDV
S proceso electrónico de datos

traitement manuel
E manual processing
G manuelle Verarbeitung
S elaboración manual, proceso manual, transformación manual

traitement préalable
E pre-treatment
G Vorbehandlung
S pretratamiento

traitement secondaire
E secondary treatment
G Nachbehandlung
S tratamiento subsiguiente

traitement thermique
E heat treatment
G Wärmebehandlung
S tratamiento térmico

traiter
E process, to; reprocess, to
G aufarbeiten
S procesar

trame
E raster, screen
G Raster
S trama

transcription
E transcription
G Transkription
S transcripción

transcription de données
E data transcription
G Datentranskription
S transcripción de datos

transducteur
E transducer
G Meßwertaufnehmer
S registrador de valores medidos, transductor

transférer
E transfer, to; relocate, to
G übertragen, verlagern
S desplazar, transferir, trasladar

transfers de technologie
E technology transfer
G Technologietransfer
S transferencia tecnológica

transfert
E transfer
G Übertragung
S transferencia

transfert de chaleur
E heat transfer
G Wärmeübertragung
S transferencia térmica

transfert d'échantillons
E sample transfer
G Probenübertragung
S transferencia de muestras

transformer en pastilles
E pelletise, to
G pelletieren
S transformar en pellets

transition de phase
E phase transition
G Phasenübergang
S transición de fase

transition thermique uniforme
E uniform heat transfer
G gleichmäßiger Wärmeübergang
S transición térmica uniforme

translucide
E translucent
G lichtdurchlässig
S translúcido

transmetteur de pression
E pressure transmitter
G Druckaufnehmer
S transmisor de presión

transmission
E transmission, drive, gear ratio
G Getriebe, Übersetzung (im Getriebe), Antrieb
S engranaje, transmisión, impulso, propulsión, tracción

transmission UV
E UV transmittance
G UV-Transmission
S transmisión UV

transparence
E transparency, light transmittance
G Durchsichtigkeit, Lichtdurchlässigkeit
S transparencia, transparencia para la luz

transparent
E clear, transparent
G klar, durchsichtig
S claro, transparente

transpercer
E pierce, to
G durchstechen
S perforar

transporté par l'air
E airborne
G aerogen
S aerógeno

transporter
E convey, to
G fördern
S fomentar, promover

transvaser
E refill, to
G umfüllen
S transvasar, trasegar

travail en trois-huit
E shift
G Arbeitsschicht
S turno de trabajo

trémie
E funnel, hopper
G Trichter, Fülltrichter
S embudo, tolva, embudo de llenado

trémie d'alimentation
E hopper, funnel
G Schütttrichter
S tolva

trémie de charge
E feed silo, feed hopper, filling funnel, charging funnel
G Beschickungssilo, Beschickungstrichter, Einfülltrichter
S depósito de carga, embudo de relleno, embudo de carga

trémie de remplissage
E feed hopper
G Fülleinrichtung
S dispositivo de relleno

trempe
E curing
G Aushärtung
S curado

tremper
E cure, to
G aushärten
S curar

trépied
E stand
G Stativ
S soporte, trípode

très efficace
E highly potent, highly effective
G hochwirksam
S muy eficaz

très fluide
E non-viscous, thin-bodied
G dünnflüssig
S fluido

tri
E screening
G Erkennung
S detección

triple liaison
E trivalent bonding
G Dreifachbindung
S enlace triple

trituration
E trituration
G Trituration
S trituración

troncature d'un cône
E truncated cone
G Kegelstumpf
S tronco de cono

trou d'homme
E manhole
G Mannloch
S registro

trouble
E turbid, cloudy
G trüb
S turbio

tube
E tube
G Tube, Schlauch, Rohrbogen
S tubo

tube à essais
E test tube
G Reagenzglas
S probeta, tubo de ensayo

tube de congélation
E cryotube
G Gefrierröhrchen
S tubo de congelación

tube de fumée
E smoke tube
G Rauchröhrchen
S tubo de humo

tube de remplissage
E feed tube
G Füllrohr
S tubo de llenado

tube de silicone
E silicone tubing
G Silikonschlauch
S tubo de silicona

tube de verre
E glass tube
G Glasröhrchen
S tubo (de ensayo) de vidrio

tube en caoutchouc
E rubber tube
G Gummischlauch
S tubo de goma

tube en Y
E Y-duct
G Hosenrohr
S tubo en Y

tube plongeur
E dip tube
G Eintauchrohr
S tubo de inmersión

tubulure d'accès
E access port
G Eintrittsstutzen
S tubuladura de acceso

tubulure d'aspiration d'air
E air suction connection port
G Luftansaugstutzen
S empalme para aspiración de aire

tubulure de prélèvement d'échantillon
E sampling port
G Probeentnahmestutzen
S tubuladura de toma de muestra

tuer
E kill, to; destroy, to
G abtöten
S destruir, matar

tunnel de rétraction
E shrinking tunnel
G Schrumpftunnel
S túnel de retracción

tunnel de stérilisation
E tunnel steriliser
G Hitzetunnel
S túnel de esterilización

turbide
E turbid, cloudy
G trüb
S turbio

turbidité
E turbidity
G Trübung
S turbidez

turbulence
E turbulence
G Turbulenz
S turbulencia

turbulence d'air
E air turbulence
G Luftverwirbelung
S turbulencia del aire

tuyau
E tube
G Schlauch
S tubo

tuyau coudé
E pipe bend
G Knierohr
S tubo acodado

tuyau de rallonge
E extension pipe
G Ansatzrohr
S tubo de empalme

tuyau de remplissage
E filling tube
G Abfüllschlauch
S tubo de envasado

tuyau d'écoulement
E drain
G Abfluß
S desagüe

tuyauterie
E tubing
G Schlauchleitung
S tubería flexible

tuyauterie apte à la pression
E pressure tubing
G Druckschlauch
S tubo de presión

English
German
French
Spanish

English
German
French
Spanish

tuyauterie d'alimentation
E feed
G Zuleitung
S alimentación, tubería de alimentación

tuyauterie en inox
E stainless steel piping
G Edelstahlrohrleitung
S tubería de acero inoxidable

tuyère
E nozzle, nozzle head
G Düse, Sprühkopf
S aplicador, inyector, tobera, cabeza del inyector

tyndallisation
E fractional sterilisation
G Tyndallisation
S tindalización

type de liant
E binding agent type
G Bindemitteltyp
S tipo de aglutinante

type de membrane
E membrane type
G Membrantyp
S tipo de membrana

type de poinçon
E punch type
G Stempeltyp
S tipo de troquel

type de verre
E glass type
G Glasart
S tipo de vidrio

ultrafiltration
E ultrafiltration
G Ultrafiltration
S ultrafiltración

ultra-son
E ultrasound
G Ultraschall
S ultrasonido

ultraviolet
E ultraviolet
G ultraviolett
S ultravioleta

uniforme
E uniform
G einheitlich, gleichmäßig
S homogéneo, uniforme, constante

uniformité
E uniformity, consistency
G Einheitlichkeit, Gleichförmigkeit
S homogeneidad, uniformidad

uniformité de couleur
E colour uniformity
G Farbuniformität
S uniformidad cromática

uniformité du contenu
E content uniformity (CU)
G Einheitlichkeit des Gehaltes, Gehaltseinheitlichkeit
S uniformidad del contenido

uniformité du poids
E uniformity of weight
G Gewichtseinheitlichkeit
S uniformidad del peso

uniformité d'une dose
E dose uniformity
G Einheitlichkeit der Dosierung
S uniformidad de la dosificación

unité
E unit
G Einheit
S unidad

unité de distillation à plusieurs étages
E multi-stage distillation unit
G Mehrstufendestillationsanlage
S unidad de destilación a etapas múltiples

unité de dosage
E dosage unit
G Dosiereinheit
S unidad de dosificación

unité de mesure
E unit of measurement
G Maßeinheit, Meßgröße
S unidad de medida, unidad de medición, dimensión

unité de séquençage
E sequencing unit
G Sequenzierungseinheit
S unidad de secuenciación

unité de transmission
E drive unit
G Antriebseinheit
S unidad propulsora

unité d'expédition
E dispatch unit
G Versandeinheit
S unidad de envío

unité formant colonie
E colony-forming unit (CFU)
G koloniebildende Einheit (KBE)
S unidad formadora de colonias

unités défectueuses
E defective units
G fehlerhafte Einheiten
S unidades defectuosas

urgence
E emergency
G Notfall
S caso de urgencia

usage auriculaire
E auricular use
G Anwendung am Ohr
S uso otológico

usage bucco-mucosal
E oromucosal use
G Anwendung in der Mundhöhle
S uso bucal

usage cutané
E cutaneous use
G Anwendung auf der Haut
S uso cutáneo

usage dental
E dental use
G dentale Anwendung
S uso dental

usage endo-cervical
E endocervical use
G endozervikale Anwendung
S uso endocervical

usage épidural
E epidural use
G epidurale Anwendung
S uso epidural

usage gingival
E gingival use
G Anwendung am Zahnfleisch
S uso gingival

usage ophtalmique
E ocular use, ophthalmic use
G Anwendung am Auge
S uso oftálmico

usage sinusien
E endosinusial use
G Anwendung in den Nebenhöhlen
S uso endosinusal

usage unique, à
E disposable
G Einweg-
S uso único, de

usé
E worn out
G ausgeleiert
S desgastado

usine
E facility, plant (machines), factory
G Anlage (Maschine), Betriebsstätte
S equipo, instalación (máquina), plantas empresariales

usine automatique
E unmanned operation
G bedienerloser Betrieb
S funcionamiento automático

usine chimique
E chemical plant
G Chemiebetrieb
S planta química

usine clé en main
E turnkey plant
G schlüsselfertige Fabrik
S fábrica llave en mano

usine de production
E production facility, production plant
G Produktionsbetrieb
S empresa productora

usine pilote
E pilot plant
G Versuchsanlage
S instalación piloto

usure
E wear and tear
G Abnutzung, Verschleiß, Verschleißerscheinung
S desgaste, manifestación de desgaste

utilisateur
E user
G Benutzer
S usuario

utilisation gastro-intestinale
E gastro-enteral use
G gastrointestinale Anwendung
S aplicación gastrointestinal

utilisation nasale
E nasal use
G nasale Anwendung
S aplicación nasal

utilisation par inadvertance
E inadvertent use
G versehentlicher Gebrauch
S uso por inadvertencia

utilisation permamente (d'un instrument)
E sustained use
G Dauergebrauch
S uso duradero

utilisation sous-cutanée
E subcutaneous use
G subkutane Anwendung
S aplicación subcutánea

utilisation transcutanée
E transdermal use
G transdermale Anwendung
S aplicación transdérmica

utilisation vaginale
E vaginal use
G vaginale Anwendung
S aplicación vaginal

vaccin
E vaccine
G Impfstoff
S vacuna

vaccin viral
E viral vaccine
G Virusimpfstoff
S vacuna viral

vaccin vivant
E live vaccine
G Lebendimpfstoff
S vacuna viva

valence
E valency
G Wertigkeit
S valencia

valeur à blanc
E blank, blank value
G Leerwert, Blindprobe, Blindwert
S valor en blanco, muestra en blanco, valor testigo, testigo

valeur aberrante
E outlier
G Ausreißer
S elemento fuera de los márgenes habituales

valeur actuelle
E actual value
G Istwert
S valor real

valeur anormale
E outlier
G Ausreißer
S elemento fuera de los márgenes habituales

valeur nominale
E nominal value, required value
G Nennwert, Sollwert
S valor nominal

valeur témoin
E blank
G Blindprobe, Blindwert
S muestra en blanco, valor en blanco, valor testigo, testigo

validable
E validatable
G validierbar
S validable

validation
E validation
G Validierung
S validación

validation analytique
E analytical validation
G analytische Validierung
S validación analítica

validation concurrente
E concurrent validation
G begleitende Validierung
S validación acompañante

validation d'ordinateur
E computer validation
G Computervalidierung
S validación informática

validation du nettoyage
E cleaning validation
G Reinigungsvalidierung
S validación de la limpieza

validation d'un procédé
E process validation
G Prozeßvalidierung
S validación de un proceso

validation informatique
E computer validation
G Computervalidierung
S validación informática

validation prospective
E prospective validation
G prospektive Validierung
S validación prospectiva

validation retrospective
E retrospective validation
G retrospektive Validierung
S validación retrospectiva

valide à partir de
E valid from
G gültig ab
S válido a partir de

validité
E validity
G Gültigkeit
S validez

valve d'arrêt
E on/off valve
G Absperrventil
S válvula de cierre

valve de sortie
E outlet valve
G Auslaßventil
S válvula de salida

valve de ventilation
E ventilation valve
G Belüftungsventil
S válvula de ventilación

valve de vidange
E emptying valve
G Entleerventil
S válvula de vaciamiento

valve rotatoire
E rotary valve
G Drehschieber
S válvula rotativa

English German French Spanish

vanne
E valve
G Ventil
S válvula

vanne à billes
E ball valve
G Kugelventil
S válvula esférica

vanne à membrane
E diaphragm valve
G Membranventil
S válvula de membrana

vanne anti-retour
E non-return valve, check valve
G Rückschlagventil
S válvula de retención

vanne d'alimentation
E filling valve, charging valve
G Einfüllklappe
S válvula de relleno

vanne d'aspiration
E aspiration valve
G Ansaugventil
S válvula de aspiración

vanne de détente
E reducing valve
G Reduzierventil
S válvula reductora

vanne de pompe
E pump valve
G Pumpenventil
S válvula de bomba

vanne de purge
E drain valve, outlet valve
G Ablaßventil
S válvula de salida

vanne de régulation
E regulating valve
G Regelventil
S válvula reguladora

vanne de sécurité
E safety valve
G Sicherheitsventil
S válvula de seguridad

vanne de sortie
E drain valve, outlet valve
G Ablaßventil
S válvula de salida

vanne de verrouillage
E blocking valve
G Sperrventil
S válvula de bloqueo

vanne d'entrée
E inlet valve
G Einlaßventil
S válvula de entrada

vanne d'injection
E injection valve
G Einspritzventil
S válvula de inyección

vanne magnétique
E solenoid valve
G Magnetventil
S válvula magnética

vanne papillon
E butterfly valve
G Drosselventil
S válvula de mariposa

vanne solénoïde
E solenoid valve
G elektromagnetisches Ventil
S válvula electromagnética

vanne trois voies
E three-way valve
G Dreiwegeventil
S válvula con tres vías

vapeur d'eau
E steam, vapour
G Dampf
S vapor

vapeur d'eau saturée
E saturated steam
G gesättigter Wasserdampf
S vapor de agua saturado

vapeur d'une installation
E plant steam
G Betriebsdampf
S vapor de una planta

vapeur externe
E external steam
G externe Dampfzufuhr
S suministro de vapor externo

vapeur primaire
E primary steam
G Primärdampf
S vapor primario

vapeur pure
E clean steam, pure steam
G Reindampf, Reinstdampf
S vapor puro

vapeur purifiée
E purified steam
G gereinigter Dampf
S vapor purificado

vapeur saturée
E saturated steam
G Sattdampf
S vapor saturado

vapeur surchauffée
E super-heated steam
G gespannter Wasserdampf
S vapor sobrecalentado, vapor de agua sobrecalentado

vaporisation
E vaporisation
G Verdampfung
S evaporación, vaporización

variabilité
E variability
G Schwankung
S fluctuación

variabilité des résultats
E variability
G Variabilität
S variabilidad

variabilité du processus
E process variability
G Prozeßvariabilität
S variabilidad de un proceso

variation de température
E temperature fluctuation
G Temperaturschwankung
S fluctuación de la temperatura

variation de tension
E voltage variation, voltage fluctuation
G Spannungsänderung, Spannungsschwankung
S variación de la tensión, fluctuación de la tensión

variations de l'intensité du courant
E power supply fluctuation
G Stromversorgungsschwankungen, Netzschwankungen
S fluctuaciones de la intensidad de corriente eléctrica, fluctuaciones del suministro eléctrico

vaseline
E vaseline
G Vaselin
S vaselina

végétal
E plant, plant-based, phyto-
G pflanzlich
S vegetal

vendeur
E sales representative
G Außendienstmitarbeiter
S agente externo de ventas

vendu sans ordonnance
E non-prescription
G nicht verschreibungspflichtig
S de venta libre

vendu sur ordonnance
E prescription
G verschreibungspflichtig
S de receta obligatoria

vendu uniquement en pharmacie
E for sale in pharmacies only
G apothekenpflichtig
S de venta sólo en farmacias

ventes
E sales
G Absatz, Verkauf, Vertrieb
S ventas, volumen de ventas, distribución, venta

ventilateur
E ventilator, fan
G Ventilator, Gebläse
S ventilador

ventilateur aspirant
E suction ventilator
G Luftabsauger
S aspirador de aire

ventilateur centrifuge
E centrifugal fan
G Zentrifugalventilator
S ventilador centrífugo

ventilation
E ventilation
G Belüftung
S aireación, ventilación

ventiler
E deaerate, to; ventilate, to; vent, to
G entlüften, belüften
S airear, ventilar

vérification
E verification, check, reconciliation
G Überprüfung, Verifizierung, Bilanzierung
S comprobación, verificación, hacer balance

vérifié
E checked, inspected
G geprüft
S comprobado

vérifier
E monitor, to; supervise, to; control, to; check, to
G überwachen, überprüfen
S supervisar, vigilar, comprobar

vermine
E vermin
G Ungeziefer
S bichos

vernis
E varnish
G Lack
S barniz, laca

vernis de couverture
E coating lacquer
G Überzugslack
S barniz de cobertura

vernissage interne
E internal lacquer
G Innenlackierung
S barnizado interno

verre de borosilicate
E borosilicate glass
G Borosilikatglas
S vidrio de silicato bórico

verre de protection
E cover glass
G Abdeckplatte
S cubreobjetos

verre fritté
E fused glass
G Sinterglas
S vidrio sinterizado

verre stratifié
E laminated glass
G laminiertes Glas
S vidrio laminado

verrerie
E glassware
G Glasgeräte
S instrumental de vidrio

verser au goutte à goutte
E drip, to; trickle, to
G träufeln
S gotear

version
E edition, version, issue
G Ausgabe, Version, Ausführung
S edición, versión, realización, modelo

version spéciale
E special version
G Sonderausführung
S construcción especial, versión especial

vestiaire
E gowning room, locker room, changing room
G Ankleideraum, Spindraum, Umkleide
S vestuario

vêtement de protection
E protective clothing
G Schutzkleidung
S ropa protectora

vêtement de sécurité
E safety clothing
G Sicherheitskleidung
S ropa de seguridad

vêtement de travail
E working clothing
G Arbeitskleidung
S ropa de trabajo

corbeille pour vêtements de travail
E clothing receptacle
G Kleidungsaufnahmebehälter
S cesto para ropa de trabajo

vêtement pour zone stérile
E sterile gowns, sterile clothing
G Sterilraumkleidung
S vestuario estéril

vêtement protecteur pour zone d'atmosphère contrôlée
E clean room clothing
G Reinraumkleidung
S ropa para área estéril

vêtement qui ne peluche pas
E lint-free clothes
G fusselfreie Kleidung
S ropa sin pelusa

vêtements de ville
E street clothing
G Straßenkleidung
S ropa de calle

vétérinaire
E doctor of veterinary medicine, vet
G Tierarzt
S veterinario

viabilité
E viability
G Lebensfähigkeit
S viabilidad

viable
E viable
G lebensfähig
S viable

vibration
E vibration
G Erschütterung, Schwingung, Vibration
S vibración, trepidación, oscilación

vibreur
E vibrator, shaker
G Rüttler
S vibrador

vide
E vacuum
G Vakuum
S vacío

vide à diaphragme
E membrane vacuum
G Membranvakuum
S vacío de membrana

English
German
French
Spanish

vider
E empty, to; evacuate, to
G entleeren
S vaciar

vieillir
E age, to
G altern
S envejecer

vieillissement
E ageing, maturing
G Alterung
S envejecimiento

vieillissement (forcé) prématuré
E forced ageing
G beschleunigte Alterung (künstlich)
S envejecimiento acelerado (artificial)

vieillissement thermique
E thermal ageing
G thermische Alterung
S envejecimiento térmico

vieillot
E obsolete, out-dated
G überholt
S obsoleto, envejecido

virologie
E virology
G Virologie
S virología

virus
E viruses
G Viren
S virus

vis à oreilles
E wing screw
G Flügelschraube
S tornillo de aletas

vis à six pans creux femelle
E Allen screw
G Inbusschraube
S tornillo hexagonal

vis avec écrou
E screw with nut
G Schraube mit Mutter
S tornillo con tuerca

vis conique
E countersunk screw
G Senkschraube
S tornillo avellanado

vis d'Archimède
E worm gear, worm screw, worm drive
G Förderschnecke, Schneckenförderer
S tornillo sin fin, tornillo transportador, transportador de tornillo sin fin

vis de dosage
E dosing screw, feed screw
G Dosierschnecke
S tornillo dosificante

vis de mise au point
E adjusting screw
G Justierschraube
S tornillo de ajuste

vis doseuse pour poudre
E powder feeder
G Pulverdosierschnecke
S tornillo sin fin dosificador de polvo

vis micromètre
E fine adjusting screw, micrometer screw
G Mikrometerschraube
S tornillo micrométrico

vis moletée
E knurled screw
G Rändelschraube
S tornillo moleteado

vis sans fin
E worm gear, worm screw
G Schnecke, Förderschnecke
S tornillo sin fin, tornillo transportador

viscosimètre à sphère descendante
E falling sphere viscosimeter
G Kugelfallviskosimeter
S viscosímetro de esfera descendiente

viscosimétrie
E viscometry
G Viskositätsmessung
S medida de la viscosiad

viscosité
E viscosity, toughness
G Viskosität, Zähigkeit
S viscosidad

visite médicale périodique
E periodic health check
G regelmäßige Gesundheitsuntersuchung
S inspección médica periódica

visite sur site
E on-site visit
G Ortsbesichtigung
S visita del lugar

visqueux
E viscous, tough
G viskos, dickflüssig, zähflüssig, zäh
S viscoso, espeso, resistente, tenaz

visser
E screw on, to
G aufschrauben
S atornillar

visualiser
E visualise, to
G sichtbarmachen
S visualizar

vitesse d'absorption
E absorption rate
G Absorptionsgeschwindigkeit
S velocidad de absorción

vitesse d'agitation
E stirring speed, agitating speed
G Rührgeschwindigkeit
S velocidad de agitación

vitesse de compression
E compression speed
G Preßgeschwindigkeit
S velocidad de compresión

vitesse de diffusion
E diffusion speed
G Diffusionsgeschwindigkeit
S velocidad de difusión

vitesse de dissolution
E dissolution rate, dissolution speed
G Auflösegeschwindigkeit, Auflösungsrate
S velocidad de disolución, tasa de disolución

vitesse de hachoir
E chopper speed
G Zerhackergeschwindigkeit
S velocidad de troceo

vitesse de la table d'une matrice
E die plate speed
G Matrizentischgeschwindigkeit
S velocidad de la mesa para matriz

vitesse de l'air
E air velocity
G Luftgeschwindigkeit
S velocidad del aire

vitesse de libération
E release rate
G Freisetzungsrate
S tasa de liberación

vitesse de libération in-vitro
E in-vitro release rate
G In-vitro-Freisetzungsrate
S tasa de liberación in vitro

vitesse de machine
E machine speed
G Maschinengeschwindigkeit
S velocidad de una máquina

vitesse de pulvérisation
E spray rate
G Sprührate
S tasa de pulverización

vitesse de réaction
E reaction velocity, reaction speed
G Reaktionsgeschwindigkeit
S velocidad de reacción

vitesse de refroidissement
E cooling rate
G Abkühlungsgeschwindigkeit
S velocidad de enfriamiento

vitesse de rotation d'un moteur
E motor revolutions
G Motordrehzahl
S número de revoluciones del motor

vitesse de séparation
E separation rate
G Abscheiderate
S velocidad de separación

vitesse de solubilisation
E speed of solubility
G Lösungsgeschwindigkeit
S velocidad de disolución

vitesse de transmission
E impeller speed, drive speed
G Laufradgeschwindigkeit, Antriebsgeschwindigkeit
S velocidad de revolución, velocidad de propulsión, velocidad de rodamiento

vitesse du tapis
E belt speed
G Bandgeschwindigkeit
S velocidad de cinta

vitesse d'un poinçon
E punch speed, punch velocity
G Stempelgeschwindigkeit
S velocidad del troquel

vitesse initiale
E start speed, initial speed
G Anfangsgeschwindigkeit
S velocidad inicial

vitesse maximale
E maximum speed
G Höchstgeschwindigkeit
S velocidad máxima

vitesse moyenne
E average speed
G durchschnittliche Geschwindigkeit
S velocidad media

voie d'administration
E dosage form, administration form
G Darreichungsform
S forma de administración

voie d'application
E application route
G Applikationsweg
S vía de administración

voie de synthèse
E synthesis route
G Syntheseweg
S vía de síntesis

volatile
E volatile
G flüchtig
S volátil

composants volatiles
E volatile components
G flüchtige Bestandteile
S componentes volátiles

non-volatile
E non-volatile
G nicht flüchtig
S no volátil

volatilisation
E volatilisation
G Verflüchtigung
S volatilización

volatiliser
E volatilise, to
G sich verflüchtigen
S volatilizarse

volet
E flap
G Klappe
S tapa, válvula

volet de ventilation
E vent flap
G Entlüftungsklappe
S válvula de ventilación

volontaire
E volunteer
G Proband
S voluntario

volontaire sain
E healthy volunteer
G gesunder Freiwilliger
S voluntario sano

voltage
E operating voltage
G Betriebsspannung
S voltaje de funcionamiento

voltmètre
E voltmeter
G Spannungsmesser
S voltímetro

volume de charge
E filling volume
G Füllvolumen
S volumen de relleno

volume de course
E stroke volume
G Hubvolumen
S volumen de carrera del émbolo

volume de délivrance
E dispensing volume
G Verteilungsvolumen
S volumen de distribución

volume de la boucle
E loop volume
G Schleifenvolumen
S volumen de bucle

volume de remplissage
E filling quantity
G Abfüllmenge
S cantidad envasada

volume d'injection
E injection volume
G Einspritzvolumen
S volumen de inyección

volume d'un pore
E pore volume
G Porenvolumen
S volumen del poro

volume effectif
E effective volume
G Nutzungsvolumen
S volumen efectivo

volume mort
E dead volume
G Totvolumen
S volumen muerto

volume nominal
E nominal volume
G Nennvolumen
S volumen nominal

volume résiduel
E residual volume
G Restvolumen
S volumen residual

volumétrie
E volumetry
G Volumetrie
S volumetría

volumétrique
E volumetric
G volumetrisch
S volumétrico

volumineux
E voluminous
G voluminös
S voluminoso

vulnérabilité
E vulnerability
G Anfälligkeit
S vulnerabilidad

English German French Spanish

wagon-citerne
E tank wagon
G Tankwagen
S camión cisterna

zone
E range
G Bandbreite
S anchura de banda, gama, márgenes

zone séparée, zone isolée, zone de confinement
E segregated area
G abgetrennter Bereich
S área separada

zone aseptique
E clean area
G reiner Bereich
S área limpia

zone auxiliaire
E auxilary area
G Nebenbereich
S área auxiliar

zone d'accès contrôlé
E controlled access area
G kontrollierter Zugangsbereich
S zona de acceso controlado

zone d'accès limité
E limited access area
G Bereich mit eingeschränktem Zugang
S zona de acceso limitado

zone d'atmosphère contrôlée
E climate-controlled area, clean room, clean area
G Bereich mit kontrolliertem Klima, Reinraum
S zona de atmósfera controlada, área estéril

zone de détection
E detection range
G Detektionsbereich
S zona de detección

zone de fabrication
E manufacturing environment
G Herstellungsumgebung
S entorno de producción

zone de remplissage
E filling section
G Füllbereich
S zona de relleno

zone de rétention
E retention range
G Rückhaltebereich
S márgenes de retención

zone d'hygiène
E hygienic area
G Hygienezone
S área higiénica

Spanish A – Z

English

German

French

Spanish

Advertencias para el uso:
p. 14–15

abastecedor
E supplier, vendor
G Lieferant
F fournisseur

abastecer
E supply, to
G liefern, versorgen mit
F fournir, livrer

abastecimiento
E supply
G Versorgung
F alimentation

abastecimiento de agua potable
E tap water feed
G Trinkwasserzufuhr
F arrivée d'eau potable

abastecimiento de aire
E air supply
G Luftversorgung
F alimentation en air

abastecimiento de láminas
E film supply
G Folienbeschickung
F alimentation en feuilles

abastecimiento público de agua
E public water supply
G öffentliche Wasserversorgung
F approvisionnement public en eau

abertura
E opening
G Öffnung
F ouverture

abertura de matriz
E die opening, die bore
G Matrizenöffnung
F ouverture d'une matrice, cavité de matrice

abertura de relleno
E filling port
G Einfüllöffnung
F ouverture de chargement

abertura del embudo
E funnel opening
G Trichteröffnung
F ouverture d'un entonnoir, ouverture d'un trémie

ablandar (agua)
E soften, to (water)
G enthärten (Wasser)
F adoucir (eau)

abono
E fertiliser
G Düngemittel
F engrais

abrasión
E friability, abrasion
G Abrieb, Abtrag
F abrasion

abrazadera
E clip
G Schelle
F collier

abrazadera de cable
E cable clamp
G Kabelschelle
F serre-fils

abreviación
E abridgement
G Abkürzung, Verkürzung
F raccourci

abreviatura
E abridgement
G Abkürzung, Verkürzung
F raccourci

absolutamente
E absolute
G absolut
F absolu

absoluto
E absolute
G absolut
F absolu

absorbedor de fuerza
E power absorber
G Kraftaufnehmer
F absorbeur d'énergie

absorbente
E absorbent
G Absorbens
F absorbant

absorber
E absorb, to
G absorbieren
F absorber

absorción
E absorption
G Absorption
F absorption

absorción de humedad
E moisture uptake
G Feuchtigkeitsaufnahme
F absorption d'humidité

absorción de potencia
E power input
G Leistungsaufnahme
F puissance absorbée

absorción del principio activo
E absorption of medicinal substance
G Arzneistoffaufnahme
F adsorption d'un principe actif

absorción UV
E UV absorption
G UV-Absorption
F absorption UV

abuso
E abuse
G Mißbrauch
F abus

acanalado
E corrugated
G geriffelt
F cannelé, strié

acanaladura
E corrugation, groove
G Riffelung, Rille
F cannelure, striage, rainure, sillon

acanalar
E corrugate, to
G riffeln
F canneler, strier

accesibilidad
E accessibility
G Zugänglichkeit
F accessibilité

acceso
E access
G Zugang, Zutritt
F accès

acceso al sistema
E system access
G Zugang zum System
F accès au système

acceso autorizado
E authorised access
G autorisierter Zugang
F droit d'accès

acceso controlado
E controlled access
G kontrollierter Zugang
F accès contrôlé

acceso limitado
E limited access, restricted access
G eingeschränkter Zugang
F accès limité, accès restrictif

accesorio
E accessory
G Ausrüstungsteil
F accessoire

accesorios
E accessory, fitting
G Zubehör, Armatur
F accessoire, garniture

accesorios del aparato
E instrument accessories
G Gerätezubehör
F accessoires d'un équipement

accidente
E accident
G Unfall
F accident

acción correctora
E corrective action
G Korrekturmaßnahme
F action corrective

acción recíproca
E interaction
G Wechselwirkung
F interaction, action réciproque

aceite etérico
E essential oil
G ätherisches Öl
F huile essentielle

aceite transmisor de calor
E heat-transmitting oil
G wärmeübertragendes Öl
F huile conductrice de chaleur

acelerador
E accelerator
G Beschleuniger
F accélérateur

acelerador de haz de electrones
E electron beam accelerator
G Elektronenstrahlbeschleuniger
F accélérateur de faisceau d'électrons

acelerar
E accelerate, to
G beschleunigen
F accélérer

aceptación
E acceptance
G Annahme
F réception, acceptation, acceptance

acero
E steel
G Stahl
F acier

acero al carbono
E carbon steel
G Karbonstahl
F acier au carbone

acero cromado
E chrome steel
G Chromstahl
F acier chromé

acero cromado y niquelado
E nichrome steel
G Chromnickelstahl
F acier chromé et nickelé

acero inoxidable
E stainless steel
G Edelstahl
F acier inoxydable, inox

acidez
E acidity
G Azidität
F acidité

acidificar
E acidify, to
G ansäuern
F acidifier

ácido
E acid
G Säure, sauer
F acide

ácido carbónico
E carboxylic acid
G Carbonsäure
F acide carboxylique

ácido clorhídrico
E hydrochloric acid
G Salzsäure
F acide chlorhydrique

ácido concentrado
E concentrated acid
G starke Säure
F acide concentré

ácido débil
E weak acid
G schwache Säure
F acide faible

ácido fumante
E fuming acid
G rauchende Säure
F acide fumant

ácido graso
E fatty acid
G Fettsäure
F acide gras

ácido nítrico
E nitric acid
G Salpetersäure
F acide nitrique

ácido nucleico
E nucleic acid
G Nukleinsäure
F acide nucléique

ácido silícico
E silicic acid
G Kieselsäure
F silice, acide silicique

ácido sulfúrico
E sulphuric acid
G Schwefelsäure
F acide sulfurique

ácido sulfúrico crómico
E chromosulphuric acid
G Chromschwefelsäure
F acide sulfurique chromique

aclarar (una estructura)
E elucidate, to (a structure)
G aufklären (Struktur)
F élucider (une structure)

acodadura de un tubo
E tube kink
G Schlauchknick
F coude d'un tuyau

acondicionamiento de la columna
E column conditioning
G Säulenkonditionierung
F conditionnement d'une colonne

acoplamiento
E coupling
G Kupplung
F couplage

acoplamiento de tubo
E tube connector
G Schlauchkupplung
F raccordement de tuyau

acoplamiento magnético
E magnetic clutch
G Magnetkupplung
F embrayage magnétique

acoplar
E couple, to
G ankuppeln
F accoupler, accrocher

acople de columna
E column coupling
G Säulenverbindung
F couplage de colonnes

acortamiento
E abridgement
G Verkürzung
F raccourci

acreditar
E accredit, to
G akkreditieren
F accréditer

acta personal
E personnel file
G Personalakte
F acte du personnel

activación
E actuation, activation
G Aktivierung
F activation

actividad de superficie
E surface activity
G Oberflächenaktivität
F activité de surface

actividad farmacológica
E pharmacological activity
G pharmakologische Aktivität
F activité pharmacologique

activo
E effective, potent
G wirksam
F efficace

actualizar
E update, to
G aktualisieren
F actualiser

acuerdo
E agreement
G Vereinbarung
F accord, convention

acuerdo de licencia
E licensing agreement
G Lizenzabkommen
F contrat de licence

Acuerdo de Reconocimiento Mutuo de Procedimientos Administrativos en la UE
E Mutual Recognition Agreement (MRA)
G Abkommen zur gegenseitigen Anerkennung
F procédure de reconnaissance mutuelle

acumulación
E accumulation
G Anhäufung
F accumulation

acumulación de partículas
E accumulation of particles
G Partikelansammlung
F accumulation de particules

acuñado
E embossment, embossed
G Prägung, geprägt
F estampage, estampé

acuñar
E stamp, to; emboss, to
G prägen
F poinçonner, estamper

acuoso
E aqueous
G wäßrig
F aqueux

acuse de recibo
E receipt
G Empfangsbestätigung
F reçu, quittance

adaptación
E reworking
G Umarbeitung
F retraitement

adaptador de guiaondas
E stub
G Stichleitung
F bout

adecuado
E suitable, appropriate, adequate
G angemessen, geeignet, passend
F approprié, adéquat, convenable

adecuado para almacenaje
E suitable for storage
G lagerfähig
F stockable, apte à l'emmagasinage

adherencia
E adherence, adhesiveness
G Adhärenz, Haftfähigkeit
F adhérence, pouvoir d'adhésion

adherir (comprimidos)
E adhere, to; stick, to (tablets)
G kleben (bei Tabletten)
F adhérer

adhesión (física)
E adhesion
G Haftung (physikalisch)
F adhésion

adhesividad
E adhesiveness
G Haftfähigkeit
F pouvoir d'adhésion

adhesivo para láminas
E film laminating adhesive
G Folienverbundkleber
F adhésif pour feuilles

adhesivo termofusible
E heat-sealing adhesive
G Heißsiegelkleber
F adhésif thermofusible

adicción
E addiction
G Sucht
F accoutumance

adición
E addition
G Zugabe
F adjonction

adición al final de la cadena
E tailings
G Nachlauf
F addition en bout de chaîne

adiestramiento
E training
G Schulung
F éducation, entraînement

aditivo
E additive
G Zusatzstoff
F additif, adjuvant

aditivo alimentario
E food additive
G Nahrungsergänzungsmittel
F additif alimentaire

administración
E administration
G Verwaltung
F administration

administración (de un medicamento)
E administration (of a drug)
G Darreichung, Verabreichung (eines Medikaments)
F administration (d'un médicament)

administración del material
E materials handling, materials management
G Materialwirtschaft
F manipulation des matériaux

administración peroral
E oral administration
G perorale Darreichung
F administration orale

adobar
E marinate, to; pickle, to
G beizen
F mariner

adquirir
E acquire, to; take over, to
G aufkaufen, übernehmen
F acquérir, prendre le contrôle de

adquisición
E procurement
G Beschaffung
F achats

adsorción
E adsorption
G Adsorption
F adsorption

aerobio
E aerobic
G aerob
F aérobie

aerógeno
E airborne
G aerogen
F aéroporté, transporté par l'air, en suspension dans l'air

aerosol de espuma
E foam spray
G Schaumspray
F aérosol pour mousse

aerosol dosificante
E metered dose inhaler
G Dosieraerosol
F inhalateur doseur

afilado
E sharp
G scharf
F coupant, aiguisé, piquant

afinidad
E affinity
G Affinität
F affinité

agar
E agar
G Agar
F agar, agar-agar

agar chocolate
E chocolate agar
G Schokoladenagar
F gélose chocolat

agar oblicuo
E sloping agar
G Schrägagar
F agar oblique

agencia de autorización de licencias sanitarias
E regulatory authorities
G Zulassungsbehörde
F autorités compétentes responsables des autorisations de mise sur le marché

agente antiespumante
E anti-foaming agent, defoamer
G Entschäumer, Antischaummittel
F antimousse, agent antimousse

agente de precipitación
E precipitating agent
G Fällungsmittel
F agent de précipitation

agente de resorción
E resorption agent
G Resorptionsvermittler
F agent de résorption

agente descalcificante
E decalcifier
G Entkalker
F détartrant

agente desecante
E drying agent
G Trockenmittel
F agent de dessication

agente desinfectante
E disinfectant
G Desinfektionsmittel
F désinfectant

agente desnaturalizante
E denaturing agent
G Denaturierungsmittel, Vergällungsmittel
F agent dénaturant

agente dispersor
E dispersion agent
G Dispersionsmittel
F agent de dispersion

agente externo de ventas
E sales representative
G Außendienstmitarbeiter
F commercial, vendeur

agente formador de películas
E film-forming agent
G Filmbildner
F agent filmogène

agente inactivador
E inactivation agent
G Inaktivierungsmittel
F agent d'inactivation

agente levigante
E eluant
G Elutionsmittel
F éluant

agente nocivo
E harmful agent
G schädliches Mittel
F agent nocif

agente patógeno (microorganismo)
E pathogen
G Erreger (Mikroorganismus)
F pathogène

agente patógeno atenuado
E attenuated pathogen
G abgeschwächter Erreger
F agent pathogène atténué

agente precipitador
E precipitation agent
G Ausfällungsmittel
F agent de précipitation

agente quelante
E chelating agent
G Komplexiermittel
F agent chélatant

agente químico
E chemical agent
G chemisches Mittel
F agent chimique

agente saporífero
E flavouring agent, flavour
G Geschmackstoff
F agent aromatique

agente secuestrante
E complex former
G Komplexbildner
F substance complexante

agente tensioactivo
E surfactant, tenside
G oberflächenaktive Verbindung, Tensid
F tensioactif, tenside

agente terapéutico
E therapeutic agent
G Heilmittel
F agent thérapeutique

agente viral
E viral agent
G virales Agens
F agent viral

agentes citostáticos
E cytostatics
G Zytostatica
F cytostatiques

agentes diagnósticos
E diagnostics
G Diagnostica
F diagnostiques

agentes químicos
E chemical agents
G chemische Agenzien
F agents chimiques

agitación intensa
E vigorous stirring
G kräftiges Rühren
F agitation vigoureuse

agitador
E stirrer, agitator, shaker
G Rührwerk, Rührer, Schüttelmaschine, Schüttler
F agitateur, secoueuse, secoueur

agitador de aletas
E blade stirrer
G Flügelrührer
F agitateur à pales

agitador de ancla
E anchor stirrer
G Ankerrührer
F agitateur à ancre

agitador magnético
E magnetic stirrer, magnetic stirring bar
G Magnetrührer, Rührfisch
F agitateur magnétique, barreau aimanté

agitar
E stir, to
G rühren
F agiter

aglomerado
E agglomerate
G Agglomerat
F aggloméra

aglomerante
E binding agent
G Bindemittel
F liant

aglomerar
E agglomerate, to; sinter, to
G agglomerieren, sintern
F agglomérer, fritter

aglutinación
E agglutination
G Agglutination
F agglutination

aglutinante
E binding agent
G Bindemittel
F liant

agrandamiento
E enlargement
G Vergrößerung
F agrandissement

agregado
E aggregate
G Aggregat
F agrégat

agua
E water
G Wasser
F eau

agua bidestilada
E redistilled water, double-distilled water
G Aqua bidest.
F eau pour préparation injectable (PPI)

agua clorada
E chlorinated water
G Chlorwasser
F eau chlorée

agua completamente desmineralizada
E demineralised water
G VE-Wasser
F eau déminéralisée

agua condensada
E condense water
G Kondenswasser
F eau condensée

agua corriente
E tap water
G Leitungswasser
F eau du robinet

agua corriente potable
E potable water
G Trinkwasser
F eau potable

agua de alimentación
E feed water
G Speisewasser
F eau d'alimentation

agua de cristalización
E water of crystallisation
G Kristallwasser
F eau de cristallisation

agua de inyección
E splash water
G Spritzwasser
F eau de ruissellement

agua de lavado
E rinsing water
G Spülwasser
F eau de rinçage

agua de procesado
E process water
G Prozeßwasser
F eau pour opérations

agua de refrigeración
E cooling water
G Kühlwasser
F eau de refroidissement

agua de rociado
E splash water
G Spritzwasser
F eau de ruissellement

agua del lavado final
E final rinse
G letztes Spülwasser
F rinçage final

agua desalinizada mediante ósmosis inversa
E reverse osmosis water
G Wasser, durch Umkehrosmose entsalztes
F eau désalinisée par osmose inverse

agua desionizada
E deionised water
G entionisiertes Wasser
F eau déionisée

agua desmineralizada
E demineralised water
G demineralisiertes Wasser, entmineralisiertes Wasser
F eau déminéralisée

agua destilada
E distilled water
G destilliertes Wasser, Aqua dest.
F eau distillée

agua farmacéutica
E pharmaceutical water
G Pharma-Wasser
F eau pharmaceutique

agua helada
E ice water
G Eiswasser
F eau glacée

agua medicinal
E medicinal water
G Heilwasser
F eau médicinale

agua para inyección
E water for injection (WFI)
G Wasser für Injektionszwecke
F eau PPI

agua potable
E drinking water
G Trinkwasser
F eau potable

agua purificada
E purified water
G gereinigtes Wasser, Reinstwasser, Aqua purificata
F eau purifiée, eau PPI

agua sin nucleasas
E nuclease-free water
G nukleasefreies Wasser
F eau dénuée de nucléase

agua ultrapurificada
E high purity water, ultrapure water
G Reinstwasser, hochreines Wasser
F eau de haute pureté, eau ultra pure

aguas residuales
E waste water
G Abwasser
F eaux résiduelles, eaux usées, eaux d'égouts

agudo
E sharp
G scharf
F coupant, aiguisé, piquant

aguja de envasado
E filling needle
G Abfüllnadel
F aiguille de remplissage

aguja de inyección
E injection needle, filling nozzle
G Injektionsnadel, Düsennadel
F aiguille pour injection, aiguille d'injection, injecteur à aiguillle

ahorro de tiempo
E time-saving
G Zeitersparnis
F économie de temps

aire acondicionado
E air conditioner
G Klimaanlage
F appareil de climatisation

aire circulante
E recirculating air
G Umluft
F air de recirculation

aire comprimido
E compressed air
G Druckluft, Preßluft
F air comprimé

aire de atomizador
E atomising air
G Zerstäuberluft
F air d'atomiseur

aire de escape
E exhaust air, outlet air
G Abluft, Raumabluft
F air d'évacuation, air d'échappement

aire de escape de un proceso
E exhaust air
G Prozeßabluft
F air d'évacuation

aire fresco
E outside air, external air
G Außenluft
F air frais, air libre

aire libre
E outside air, external air
G Außenluft
F air frais, air libre

aire limpio
E clean air
G Reinluft
F air filtré

aireación
E ventilation
G Belüftung
F ventilation

airear
E deaerate, to; ventilate, to; vent, to
G entlüften, belüften
F désaérer, aérer, ventiler

aislado
E separated, segregated
G abgetrennt
F séparé, détaché, isolé

aislamiento
E insulation
G Isolierung
F isolation

aislamiento sonoro
E noise insulation
G Geräuschisolierung
F insonorisation du bruit

aislamiento térmico
E heat insulation
G Wärmeisolierung
F isolation thermique

aislante
E glove box, isolator
G Isolator
F isolateur

ajustable
E adjustable
G einstellbar
F ajustable

ajustar
E adjust, to; align, to
G einstellen, ausrichten, justieren
F ajuster, régler, aligner, centrer, étalonner

ajuste
E adjustment, alignment, setting
G Einstellung, Regulierung, Justierung
F ajustement, réglage, étalonnement

ajuste de la velocidad
E speed adjustment
G Geschwindigkeitseinstellung
F ajustement de la vitesse

ajuste de temperatura
E temperature setting
G Temperatureinstellung
F réglage de la température

ajuste de un proceso
E operational adjustment, process adjustment
G betriebliche Anpassung, Prozeßanpassung
F ajustement de fonctionnement, ajustement d'un procédé

ajuste de un regulador
E controller set point
G Reglereinstellung
F réglage d'un régulateur

ajuste del funcionamiento
E operational adjustment, process adjustment
G betriebliche Anpassung, Prozeßanpassung
F ajustement de fonctionnement, ajustement d'un procédé

ajuste del pH
E pH adjustment
G pH-Wert-Einstellung
F ajustement du pH

ajuste fino
E fine adjustment
G Feineinstellung
F réglage fin, mise au point précise

alambique
E flask, still
G Kolben (Glasgefäß), Destille
F ballon, flacon, appareil de distillation

alambre
E wire
G Draht
F fil métallique

alargadera
E extension cable
G Verlängerungskabel
F câble de rallonge

alargar
E extend, to; prolong, to
G verlängern
F prolonger, rallonger

alarma
E alarm, alarm signal
G Alarm
F signal d'alarme

alarma de incendio
E fire alarm
G Feuermelder
F alarme d'incendie

alcalinidad
E alkalinity, basicity
G Alkalinität, Basizität
F alcalinité, basicité

alcalinizar
E deacidify, to
G entsäuern
F alcaliniser

alcalino
E alkaline, basic
G alkalisch, basisch
F alcalin, basique

aldehído
E aldehyde
G Aldehyd
F aldéhyde

aleación
E alloy
G Legierung
F alliage

alergeno
E allergen
G Allergen
F allergène

alergizante
E sensitising
G allergisierend
F allergisant

aleta de agitación
E stirring blade
G Rührflügel
F pale d'agitation

algodón
E cotton, cotton wool
G Baumwolle, Watte
F coton, ouate

algodón de vendaje
E cotton wool
G Verbandwatte
F ouate à pansement

alicuotar
E aliquot, to
G aliquotieren
F aliquoter

alimentación
E load, feed
G Beschickung, Zufuhr, Zuleitung
F charge, alimentation, tuyauterie d'alimentation

alimentación de gas
E gas supply
G Gaszufuhr
F alimentation en gaz

alimentación de vacío
E vacuum feed
G Vakuumbeschickung
F alimentation du vide

alimentación por gravedad
E gravity feed
G Zufuhr durch Gefälle
F alimentation par gravité

alimentador a la red
E power supply
G Netzgerät
F alimentation en courant électrique

alimento
E food, nutrient
G Lebensmittel, Nährstoff
F aliment, nourriture, produit nutritif, nutriment

alinear
E align, to
G ausrichten
F aligner, ajuster, centrer

alisar
E smooth, to
G glätten
F polir

alivio
E relief
G Entlastung
F soulagement, décharge

allanar
E roll, to
G walzen
F passer au rouleau

almacén
E warehouse, storage room, storage area
G Lagerraum, Lager(bereich)
F entrepôt, aire d'entreposage, aire de stockage

almacén congelador
E frozen storage
G Tiefkühllager
F stockage à très basse température

almacén de estanterías altas
E high-bay storage
G Hochregallager
F étagère de stockage

almacén de medios de envasado
E packaging warehouse
G Packmittell-Lager
F magasin d'articles de conditionnement

almacén de mercancías
E warehouse
G Warenlager
F entrepôt

almacén de solventes
E solvent storage
G Lösungsmittellager
F stockage de solvants

almacén frigorífico
E cold store, cold storage
G Kühllager
F stockage à froid

almacén para cuarentena
E quarantine (warehouse)
G Sperrlager
F quarantaine (entrepôt)

almacén para paletas
E pallet store
G Palettenstellplatz
F dépôt de palettes

almacenaje
E retention, storage, archiving
G Aufbewahrung
F conservation, stockage, archivage

almacenaje intermediario
E interim storage
G Zwischenlagerung
F stockage intermédiaire

almacenamiento
E storage
G Lagerung
F stockage

almacenamiento caliente
E heated storage
G Heißlagerung
F stockage thermique

almacenamiento de datos
E electronic data storage
G Datenspeicherung
F sauvegarde électronique de données

almacenamiento de muestras
E sample storage
G Probenlagerung
F stockage d'échantillons

almacenar
E store, to; stack, to
G einlagern, stapeln
F stocker, empiler

almacenar en seco
E store dry, to
G trocken lagern
F stocker au sec

almidón
E starch
G Stärke
F amidon

almidón de maíz
E corn starch
G Maisstärke
F amidon du maïs

alquilación
E alkylation
G Alkylierung
F alkylation

alta resolución, de
E high-resolution
G hochauflösend
F haute-résolution

altamente dosificado
E highly dosed
G hoch dosiert
F à haute dose

altura
E height
G Höhe
F hauteur

altura de banda de un comprimido
E tablet web height, band height
G Tablettensteghöhe
F hauteur de bande d'un comprimé

altura de caída
E drop height
G Fallhöhe
F hauteur de chute

altura de carga (p. ej. de autoclave)
E loading height (e. g. of autoclave)
G Beladungshöhe (z. B. eines Autoklaven)
F hauteur de chargement (p. ex. d'un autoclave)

altura de la mesa para matriz
E die plate height
G Matrizentischhöhe
F hauteur du plateau d'une matrice

altura de presión
E pressurisation level
G Druckhöhe
F niveau de pressurisation

altura del pico
E peak height
G Peakhöhe
F hauteur de pic

altura del relleno
E filling depth
G Fülltiefe
F hauteur de remplissage

altura regulable, de
E height-adjustable
G höhenverstellbar
F à hauteur ajustable

altura total
E overall height
G Gesamthöhe
F hauteur totale

alumbrado de techo
E ceiling lighting
G Deckenbeleuchtung
F éclairage plafonnier

amargo
E bitter
G bitter
F amer

amasar
E knead, to
G kneten
F pétrir, malaxer

aminas
E amines
G Amine
F amines

aminas aromáticas
E aromatic amines
G aromatische Amine
F amines aromatiques

aminas primarias
E primary amines
G primäre Amine
F amines primaires

aminas secundarias
E secondary amines
G sekundäre Amine
F amines secondaires

aminas terciarias
E tertiary amines
G tertiäre Amine
F amines tertiaires

aminoácido
E amino acid
G Aminosäure
F acide aminé

aminoácido esencial
E essential amino acid
G essentielle Aminosäure
F acide aminé essentiel

amontonar
E stack, to
G stapeln
F empiler

amorfo
E amorphous
G amorph
F amorphe

amperaje
E amperage
G Stromstärke
F ampérage

amperímetro
E ammeter
G Amperemeter, Strommesser
F ampèremètre

ampliación
E expansion
G Ausdehnung
F expansion

ampliación de la empresa
E plant expansion
G Betriebserweiterung
F agrandissement d'une installation

amplificación
E amplification
G Verstärkung
F amplification

amplificador
E amplifier
G Verstärker
F amplificateur

amplificador de relé
E relay amplifier
G Relaisverstärker
F relais amplificateur

amplificador de señal
E signal amplifier
G Signalverstärker
F amplificateur de signal

amplitud
E amplitude, width
G Amplitude, Weite
F amplitude, largeur, étendue

ampolla
E ampoule, bubble, blister
G Ampulle, Blase
F ampoule, bulle

ampolla bebible
E oral ampoule
G Trinkampulle
F ampoule buvable

ampolla de apertura manual
E one-point cut (OPC) ampoule
G Brechampulle
F ampoule autocassable

ampolla de plástico
E plastic ampoule
G Kunststoffampulle
F ampoule en plastique

ampolla de vidrio
E glass ampoule
G Spießampulle
F ampoule de verre

añadir
E add, to
G zugeben
F ajouter

anaerobio
E anaerobic
G anaerob
F anaérobe

análisis
E analysis, determination
G Analyse, Bestimmung
F analyse, détermination, évaluation

análisis coulométrico
E coulometric analysis
G coulometrische Analyse
F analyse coulométrique

análisis de activación de neutrones
E neutron activation analysis
G Neutronenaktivierungsanalyse
F analyse par activation neutronique

análisis de autorización
E release analysis
G Freigabeuntersuchung
F analyse de libération

análisis de datos en mátrix
E matrix data analysis
G Matrixdatenanalyse
F analyse de données matricielles

análisis de hidrocarburos totales (de petróleo)
E total petroleum hydrocarbon (tph) analysis
G Analyse auf Gesamt-(Petroleum)-Kohlenwasserstoffe
F analyse de la teneur totale du pétrole en hydrocarbures

análisis de influencia y posibilidad de defectos
E failure mode and effect analysis (FMEA)
G Fehlermöglichkeits- und Einflußanalyse (FMEA)
F analyse de modes et effets des pannes (FMEA)

análisis de muestras
E sample assay, sample analysis
G Probenanalyse
F analyse d'échantillon

análisis de peso seco
E dry weight analysis
G Trockengewichtanalyse
F analyse à poids sec

análisis de repetición
E replicate analysis
G Wiederholungsanalyse
F analyse répétée

análisis de tendencias
E trend analysis
G Trendermittlung
F analyse des tendances

análisis de vestigios
E trace analysis
G Spurenanalyse
F analyse de traces

análisis del medio ambiente
E environmental analysis
G Umweltanalyse
F analyse de l'environnement

análisis del peso
E gravimetric analysis
G Gewichtsanalyse
F analyse du poids

análisis del producto
E product assay, product analysis
G Produktanalyse
F analyse d'un produit

análisis del riesgo
E risk analysis
G Risikoanalyse
F analyse des risques

análisis elemental
E elementary analysis
G Elementaranalyse
F analyse élémentaire

análisis estructural
E structural analysis
G Strukturaufklärung
F analyse structurelle

análisis volumétrico
E volumetric analysis
G volumetrische Analyse
F analyse volumétrique

analítica de desarrollo
E analytical development
G Entwicklungsanalytik
F développement analytique

analítico
E analytical
G analytisch
F analytique

anchura
E width
G Breite, Weite
F largeur, étendue

anchura de banda
E range
G Bandbreite
F échelle, intervalle, gamme, zone

anchura de la fisura
E slit width
G Spaltbreite
F largeur d'une fissure, largeur d'une fente

anchura del pico
E peak width
G Peakbreite
F largeur de pic

anchura nominal
E nominal width
G Nennweite
F largeur nominale

anchura total
E overall width
G Gesamtbreite
F largeur totale

andamio
E supporting structure
G Gerüst
F échafaudage

anemómetro de resistencia eléctrica
E hot-wire anemometer
G Hitzedrahtanemometer
F anémomètre à résistance électrique

anemómetro de rueda de aletas
E fan wheel anemometer
G Flügelradanemometer
F anémomètre à moulinet, anémomètre à ailettes

anexo
E insert
G Beilage
F annexe

anexo (de un documento)
E enclosure, appendix
G Anlage (zur Dokumentation), Anhang
F annexe, appendice

angulado
E angled, angular
G abgewinkelt
F à angles, angulaire

ángulo
E angle
G Winkel
F angle

ángulo de incidencia
E angle of incidence
G Einfallswinkel
F angle d'incidence

ángulo de inclinación
E angle of slope, angle of gradient
G Neigungswinkel
F angle de pente

ángulo de la pendiente
E angle of slide
G Böschungswinkel
F angle de pente

ángulo de reflexión
E angle of reflection
G Reflektionswinkel
F angle de réflexion

ángulo de refracción
E angle of refraction
G Brechungswinkel
F angle de réfraction

anhídrido carbónico
E carbon dioxide
G Kohlendioxyd
F dioxyde de carbone

anhidro
E anhydrous
G wasserfrei
F anhydre

añicos de vidrio
E glass splinters
G Glassplitter
F éclats de verre

anillo de soporte
E retaining ring
G Haltering
F anneau de support

anillo hermético
E sealing ring
G Dichtring
F joint d'étanchéité

anillo tórico
E O-ring
G O-Ring
F joint torique

anomalía celular
E cellular anomaly
G zelluläre Anomalie
F anomalie cellulaire

anorgánico
E inorganic
G anorganisch
F anorganique

antibiótico
E antibiotic
G Antibioticum
F antibiotique

anticuerpo
E antibody
G Antikörper
F anticorps

anticuerpo monoclonal
E monoclonal antibody
G monoklonaler Antikörper
F anticorps monoclonal

antideslizante
E slip-proof, non-slip
G rutschsicher
F anti-dérapant

antídoto
E antidote
G Gegengift
F antidote

antiestático
E anti-static agent
G Antistatikum
F agent antistatique

antifúngico
E anti-fungal
G pilzabtötend
F antifongique

antioxidante
E anti-oxidant
G Antioxidans
F antioxydant

antípodas ópticos
E optical antipodes
G optische Antipoden
F antipodes optiques

anuncio
E tender
G Ausschreibung
F appel d'offres

anuncio de enmienda
E amendment
G Änderungsanzeige
F amendement

apagar soplando
E blow out, to
G ausblasen
F souffler, éteindre

apantallamiento
E screening
G Abschirmung
F screening, tri, dépistage

aparato de análisis
E analytical apparatus
G Analysengerät
F appareil d'analyses

aparato de calefacción
E heating aggregate
G Heizaggregat
F appareil de chauffage

aparato de cesto
E basket apparatus
G Korbgerät
F appareil à corbeille

aparato de destilación a columna de presión
E pressure column distillation plant
G Druckkolonnendestillationsanlage
F appareil de distillation à colonnes multiples

aparato de iluminación
E light, light fittings
G Beleuchtungskörper
F appareil d'éclairage

aparato de limpieza
E cleaning equipment
G Reinigungsgerät
F équipement de nettoyage

English German French Spanish

aparato de medición
E measuring instrument
G Meßgerät
F instrument de mesure

aparato de medición de partículas
E particle measuring instrument
G Partikelmeßgerät
F appareil de mesure des particules

aparato de toma de muestras
E sampling equipment, sampler
G Probenahmegerät, Probengeber
F équipement pour le prélèvement d'un échantillon, échantillonneuse

aparatos
E apparatus, equipment
G Geräte
F appareillage expérimental

aparatos periféricos
E peripheral instrumentation
G periphere Geräte
F appareils périphériques

apatógeno
E apathogenic
G apathogen
F apathogène

apéndice (de un documento)
E enclosure, appendix
G Anlage (zur Dokumentation), Anhang
F annexe, appendice

apilador
E stacker
G Stapler
F chariot élévateur

apilamiento
E stacking
G Stapelung
F empilage

apilamiento de envases
E package stacking
G Packungsstapelung
F empilage de conditionnement

apilar
E stack, to
G stapeln
F empiler

aplanado
E flattened
G abgeflacht
F aplati

aplanamiento
E flattening
G Abflachung
F aplatissement

aplanar
E roll, to
G walzen
F passer au rouleau

aplastar
E pinch, to; squeeze, to
G quetschen
F écraser

aplicabilidad
E applicability
G Anwendbarkeit
F applicabilité

aplicación
E application
G Anwendung
F application

aplicación dental
E dental use
G dentale Anwendung
F usage dental

aplicación externa, para
E for external application
G zur äußerlichen Anwendung
F pour application externe

aplicación gastrointestinal
E gastro-enteral use
G gastrointestinale Anwendung
F utilisation gastro-intestinale

aplicación nasal
E nasal use
G nasale Anwendung
F utilisation nasale

aplicación subcutánea
E subcutaneous use
G subkutane Anwendung
F utilisation sous-cutanée

aplicación transdérmica
E transdermal use
G transdermale Anwendung
F utilisation transcutanée

aplicación vaginal
E vaginal use
G vaginale Anwendung
F utilisation vaginale

aplicaciones potenciales
E potential applications
G potentielle Anwendungen
F applications potentielles

aplicador
E applicator, nozzle
G Applikator, Düse
F applicateur, buse, gicleur, tuyère

aplicador binario
E binary nozzle
G Zweistoffdüse
F buse binaire

aplicador de bola
E ball nozzle
G Kugeldüse
F buse à billes

aplicador de lavado
E cleaning nozzle
G Waschdüse
F buse de nettoyage

aplicador nasal
E nasal applicator
G Nasenolive
F applicateur nasal

aplicar
E apply, to
G aufbringen, auftragen
F appliquer, étendre

aplicar (una muestra)
E apply, to (sample)
G aufgeben (Probe)
F appliquer (un échantillon)

apoderado general
E executive with power of procuration
G Prokurist
F fondé de pouvoirs

apoyo
E support brace
G Stütze
F support

aprendiz
E apprentice
G Lehrling, Auszubildender
F apprenti, stagiaire

aprendizaje
E apprenticeship
G Lehre
F apprentissage

aprobación
E approval
G Billigung
F approbation

aprobación del producto
E product release
G Produktfreigabe
F libération de produit

aprobar
E approve, to
G billigen
F approuver

apropiado
E suitable, appropriate, adequate
G angemessen, geeignet
F approprié, adéquat

English German French Spanish

aptitud
E suitability
G Eignung
F qualification

arandela
E washer, lamella
G Unterlegscheibe, Lamelle
F rondelle, lamelle

arandela hermética
E sealing ring
G Dichtring
F joint d'étanchéité

arandela para junta hermética
E gasket ring
G Dichtungsring
F joint torique en forme de rondelle

árbol
E shaft
G Schaft, Welle
F arbre, essieu, tige

árbol de levas
E camshaft
G Nockenwelle
F arbre à cames

árbol motor
E drive shaft
G Antriebswelle
F arbre de transmission

archivado
E archiving
G Archivierung
F archivage

archivo
E archive
G Archiv
F archives

área auxiliar
E auxilary area
G Nebenbereich
F zone auxiliaire

área central de pesado
E central weighing area
G zentrale Einwaage
F aire centrale de pesage

área de confianza
E confidence area
G Vertrauensbereich
F plage de confiance

área de encartonamiento
E cartoning section
G Kartonierteil
F aire d'encartonnage

área de evaluación
E evaluation range
G Auswertebereich
F plage d'évaluation

área de fermentación
E fermentation room
G Fermentationsraum
F aire de fermentation

área de las instalaciones empresariales
E plant area
G Betriebsfläche
F surface d'une installation

área de pulverización
E spray area
G Sprühbereich
F aire de pulvérisation

área estéril
E clean room, clean area
G Reinraum
F zone d'atmosphère contrôlée

área higiénica
E hygienic area
G Hygienezone
F zone d'hygiène

área limpia
E clean area
G reiner Bereich
F zone aseptique

área lineal
E linear range
G Linearbereich
F intervalle linéaire

área separada
E segregated area
G abgetrennter Bereich
F zone séparée, zone isolée, zone de confinement

argumentación
E rationale, reasoning
G Begründung
F exposé des motifs, explication

arista
E edge
G Rand
F arête, bord

armadura
E fitting
G Armatur
F garniture

armario de secado en bandeja
E tray dryer
G Hordentrockenschrank
F dessicateur à plateaux, dessicateur à claies

armario estrecho
E locker
G Spind
F placard de vestiaire

armazón
E stand, frame, supporting structure
G Gestell, Gerüst
F échafaudage, support, cadre

armazón del filtro
E filter housing
G Filtergehäuse
F boîtier de filtre

aroma
E fragrance, odour
G Duft
F odeur

arriesgar (la calidad)
E endanger, to (quality)
G gefährden (Qualität)
F mettre en danger, compromettre (la qualité)

arruga
E fold
G Falte
F pli

artesano
E workman, tradesman
G Handwerker
F ouvrier, artisan

articulación de rótula
E ball + socket joint
G Kugelgelenk
F rotule, joint à rotule

artículo de laboratorio
E lab ware
G Laborartikel
F matériel de laboratoire

asa
E handle, grip
G Griff
F prise, poignée

asbesto
E asbestos
G Asbest
F amiante

ascensor
E lift, elevator
G Aufzug
F ascenseur

aseguramiento de conformidad
E conformity assurance
G Konformitätssicherung
F assurance de conformité

aseguramiento de la calidad
E quality assurance (QA)
G Qualitätssicherung (QS)
F assurance-qualité

English German French Spanish

asegurar
E guarantee, to; secure, to; ensure, to
G sicherstellen
F assurer, garantir

aséptico
E aseptic
G aseptisch
F aseptique

asesor
E expert, assessor
G Begutachter
F expert

asiento
E bearing (mach.)
G Lager (Maschinenteil)
F assise, support

asistente de laboratorio
E laboratory assistant
G Laborant
F assistant de laboratoire, laborantin

asistido por ordenador
E computerised, computer-assisted
G computergestützt
F assisté par ordinateur

asociación profesional
E trade association
G Berufsgenossenschaft
F association professionelle

aspecto externo
E appearance
G äußere Beschaffenheit
F aspect, apparence

aspecto general
E appearance, general
G allgemeines Aussehen
F apparence (générale)

aspereza
E roughness
G Rauhigkeit
F grossièreté

áspero
E rough
G rauh
F grossier

aspersor
E sprinkler
G Sprinkleranlage
F réseau de sprinkler

aspiración de aire
E air aspiration, air exhaust system
G Luftabsaugung
F système d'évacuation d'air

aspirador de aire
E suction ventilator
G Luftabsauger
F ventilateur aspirant

aspirar
E aspirate, to
G ansaugen, absaugen
F aspirer

asta
E shaft
G Schaft, Welle
F arbre, essieu, tige

ástil
E weighing beam
G Wiegebalken
F fléau de balance

atenuación (de una señal)
E attenuation (of a signal)
G Abschwächung (eines Signals)
F atténuation (d'un signal)

atomizador
E atomiser
G Zerstäuber, Nebelgenerator
F atomiseur, pulvérisateur

atomizar
E atomise, to; vaporise, to
G zerstäuben
F atomiser, pulvériser

atornillado hermético
E bulkhead connection
G Schottverschraubung
F connexion étanche

atornilladura
E screw fitting
G Verschraubung
F connexion à filetage

atornillar
E screw on, to
G aufschrauben
F visser, dévisser

auditoría
E audit
G Audit
F audit, inspection

auditoría de empresa
E plant audit
G Betriebsprüfung
F audit d'une installation

auditoría interna
E internal audit
G internes Audit
F audit interne

aumento
E magnification, supplement, overage
G Vergrößerung, Aufschlag
F agrandissement, supplément, majoration

aumento a escala (de un proceso)
E scale-up (of a procedure)
G Maßstabsvergößerung (eines Verfahrens)
F extrapolation (d'un procédé)

aumento de presión
E pressure increase
G Druckanstieg
F augmentation de pression

aumento de temperatura
E temperature increase
G Temperaturerhöhung
F augmentation de température

aumento del rendimiento
E yield enhancement
G Ausbeutesteigerung
F augmentation du rendement

ausencia
E absence
G Abwesenheit
F absence

autoadhesivo
E self-adhesive
G selbstklebend
F auto-adhésif

autoclave
E autoclave
G Autoklav
F autoclave

autoclave vertical
E vertical autoclave
G Vertikalautoklav
F autoclave vertical

autocomprobación
E self-check
G Selbstüberprüfung
F auto-inspection

autoinspección
E self-inspection
G Selbstinspektion
F auto-inspection

automa(tiza)ción
E automation
G Automation
F automatisation

automa(tiza)ción de un proceso
E process automation
G Prozeßautomatisierung
F automatisation d'un procédé

automatizar
E automate, to
G automatisieren
F automatiser

English German French Spanish

automedicación
E self-medication
G Selbstmedikation
F automédication

autoridades
E authorities
G Behörde
F autorité réglementaire

autoridades de protección del medio ambiente
E environmental protection agency (EPA)
G Umweltschutzbehörde
F agence pour la protection de l'environnement

autorización
E authorisation, approval, authority
G Genehmigung, Befugnis
F autorisation

autorización como genérico
E generic marketing authorisation
G Zulassung als Generikum
F autorisation de mise sur le marché comme médicament générique

autorización electrónica
E electronic approval
G elektronische Genehmigung
F autorisation électronique

autorización oficial
E licence, approval, authorisation
G behördliche Genehmigung
F autorisation d'une autorité réglementaire

autorización para imprimir
E print release
G Druckfreigabe
F autorisation d'imprimer

autorización para venta en el mercado
E marketing authorisation, approval
G Marktzulassung
F autorisation de mise sur le marché (A.M.M.)

autorizar
E authorise, to; approve, to
G genehmigen
F autoriser

avería
E breakdown, downtime (machine), fault, failure, accident, malfunction, interference
G Ausfall, Störfall, Störung, Panne
F panne, temps mort, défaillance, incident, perturbation, dérangement

avería de una máquina
E machine breakdown
G Maschinenausfall
F défaillance de machine

avería eléctrica
E electrical interference
G elektrische Störung
F interférence électrique

averiguar
E determine, to
G ermitteln, bestimmen
F déterminer, évaluer

aviso de alarma
E warning
G Warnhinweis
F avertissement

aviso de avería
E malfunction indication, malfunction alarm, failure alarm
G Störungsmeldung
F alarme de mauvais fonctionnement

aviso de errores
E failure message
G Fehlermeldung
F message d'erreur

aviso de peligro
E hazard indication
G Gefahrenhinweis
F mise en garde

causa (graves) quemaduras
E causes (severe) burns
G verursacht (schwere) Verbrennungen
F peut provoquer de (sévères) brûlures

irrita las vías respiratorias
E irritating to respiratory system
G reizt die Atemwege
F peut irriter le système respiratoire

irrita los ojos
E irritating to eyes
G reizt die Augen
F peut provoquer des irritations aux yeux

peligroso para el feto
E may cause harm to unborn child
G gefährdet ungeborene Kinder
F dangereux pour les enfants pendant une grossesse

puede causar cáncer
E may cause cancer
G kann Krebs erzeugen
F peut provoquer un cancer

puede dañar la fertilidad
E may impair fertility
G kann die Fruchtbarkeit beeinträchtigen
F peut altérer la fertilité

puede originar daños genéticos hereditarios
E may cause heritable genetic damage
G kann vererbliche Genschäden verursachen
F peut être la cause de dommages génétiques héréditaires

tóxico si se ingiere
E toxic if swallowed
G giftig beim Verschlucken
F toxique si ingéré

tóxico si se inhala
E toxic by inhalation
G giftig beim Einatmen
F toxique si inhalé

tóxico, venenoso
E toxic
G toxisch, giftig
F toxique

aviso de seguridad
E safety instructions
G Sicherheitshinweis
F instructions de sécurité

ayuda temporal
E temporary help
G Aushilfe
F stagiaire, aide temporaire

ayudas de funcionamiento
E operative aids
G Bedienhilfen
F aides au fonctionnement

azúcar de caña
E cane sugar
G Rohrzucker
F sucre de canne

bacterias
E bacteria
G Bakterien
F bactérie

bactericida
E bactericidal
G bakterizid
F bactéricide

bajar
E lower, to; reduce, to
G senken
F abaisser, baisser

balance de etiquetas
E label reconciliation
G Etikettenbilanzierung
F bilan d'étiquettes

balanza
E balance
G Waage
F balance

balanza de carga superior
E top-loading balance
G oberschalige Waage
F balance à plat en haut

balanza de precisión
E precision balance
G Feinwaage, Präzisionswaage
F balance de précision

balanza de resorte
E spring balance
G Federwaage
F balance à ressort

balanza de torsión
E torsion balance
G Torsionswaage
F balance de torsion

baldosa
E tile
G Fliese
F carreau

balón de vidrio
E glass balloon
G Glasballon
F ballon de verre

bálsamo
E embrocation, liniment
G Einreibemittel
F beaume, onguent, liniment

banco de células germinales
E stem cell bank
G Stammzellbank
F banque de cellules souches

banco de sangre
E blood bank
G Blutbank
F banque du sang

banco de trabajo
E work bench
G Werkbank
F établi

banco de trabajo estéril
E clean bench
G reine Werkbank
F paillasse sous flux laminaire

banda de esporas
E spore strip
G Sporenstreifen
F bande de spores

banda de láminas
E sheet of film
G Folienbahn
F bande d'étoffe

bandas de interferencia
E interfering bands
G Störbanden, interferierende Banden
F bandes d'interférence

bandeja
E tray
G Tablett, Hordenblech
F plateau

bandeja (para ampollas)
E rack, tray
G Magazin (für Ampullen)
F plateau

baño de aceite
E oil bath
G Ölbad
F bain d'huile

baño de agua
E water bath
G Wasserbad
F bain-marie

baño de sumersión
E immersion bath
G Tauchbad
F bain d'immersion

baño ultrasónico
E ultrasonic bath
G Ultraschallbad
F bain à ultra-sons

baricentro
E centre of gravity
G Schwerpunkt
F centre de gravité

barniz
E varnish, lacquer
G Lack
F vernis, laque

barniz de cobertura
E coating lacquer
G Überzugslack
F vernis de couverture

barniz de inmersión
E immersion lacquer
G Tauchlack
F laque par immersion

barniz externo
E outer lacquer
G Außenlack
F laque extérieure

barniz interno
E internal lacquer
G Innenlack
F laque interne

barniz protector interno
E internal protective lacquer
G Innenschutzlack
F laque interne de protection

barnizado de superficies
E surface lacquer
G Oberflächenlackierung
F laquage superficiel

barnizado interno
E internal lacquer
G Innenlackierung
F vernissage interne

barnizar
E lacquer, to
G lackieren
F laquer

barra de vidrio
E glass rod
G Glasstab
F baguette de verre

barra del émbolo
E piston rod
G Kolbenstange
F tige de piston

barra transversal
E cross bar
G Querstange
F tige transversale

barras de código
E code bars
G Codestriche
F code à barres

barrera líquida
E barrier fluid
G Sperrflüssigkeit
F barrière fluidique

barrera luminosa
E optical barrier, light barrier
G Lichtschranke
F barrière optique

barrera óptica
E optical barrier, light barrier
G Lichtschranke
F barrière optique

báscula de análisis
E analytical balance
G Analysenwaage
F balance d'analyse

báscula de cinta
E band balance, conveyor balance
G Bandwaage
F balance de convoyeur

báscula de control
E control balance
G Kontrollwaage
F balance de contrôle

base
E base, basis, socket
G Base, Basis, Sockel
F base, socle

base de absorción (para pomadas)
E absorption base (for ointments)
G Absorptionsgrundlage (für Salben)
F base d'absorption (pour pommades)

base orgánica
E organic base
G organische Base
F base organique

basicidad
E basicity, alkalinity
G Basizität, Alkalinität
F basicité, alcalinité

básico
E basic, alkaline
G basisch, alkalisch
F basique, alcalin

bastidor
E stand, frame, trolley
G Gestell, Fahrgestell
F support, cadre, chassis mobile

bastón de vidrio
E glass rod
G Glasstab
F baguette de verre

bastoncillos de prueba
E test strip
G Teststäbchen
F bâtonnet de test

basura
E rubbish, waste
G Müll
F déchets, résidus

bata
E lab coat, gown
G Kittel
F blouse

bata de laboratorio
E lab coat, gown
G Laborkittel
F blouse de laboratoire

biberón
E aspirator bottle
G Saugflasche
F biberon

bichos
E vermin
G Ungeziefer
F vermine

bimetal
E bimetal
G Bimetall
F bimétal

biocompatible
E biocompatible
G biokompatibel
F biocompatible

biodisponibilidad
E bioavailability
G Bioverfügbarkeit
F biodisponibilité

bioequivalencia
E bioequivalence
G Bioäquivalenz
F bioéquivalence

biogenerador
E biogenerator
G Biogenerator
F biogénérateur

biogénesis
E biogenesis
G Biogenese
F biogenèse

biógeno
E biogenic
G biogen
F biogène

bioindicador
E bioindicator
G Bioindikator
F indicateur biologique

biología molecular
E molecular biology
G Molekularbiologie
F biologie moléculaire

bioluminiscencia
E bioluminescence
G Biolumineszenz
F bioluminescence

biomasa
E biomass
G Biomasse
F biomasse

biosíntesis
E biosynthesis
G Biosynthese
F biosynthèse

biotecnología
E biotechnology
G Biotechnologie
F biotechnologie

bisel
E bevel
G Abschrägung, Facette
F biseau

bisel (del troquel de comprimidos)
E punch chamfer (of tablet punch)
G Fase (am Tablettenstempel)
F biseau (d'un poinçon à comprimés)

biselado
E sloping
G abgeschrägt
F taillé en biais, en biseau, biseauté

blíster
E blister, blister pack
G Blister, Durchdrückpackung
F blister, plaquette (conditionnement)

bloque de inyección
E injection block
G Einspritzblock
F bloc d'injection

bloque de moldeo
E die block
G Formblock
F bloc de moulage

bloquear
E block, to; jam, to
G blockieren
F bloquer

bloqueo
E blockage, quarantine
G Blockierung, Sperrung
F blocage, quarantaine

blusa
E smock
G Kurzkittel
F blouse

bobina de resistencia
E resistance coil
G Widerstandsspule
F bobine de résistance

bolsa de desechos
E waste bag
G Abfallbeutel
F sac poubelle

bolsa de separación
E split bag
G Trennbeutel
F sachet de séparation

bolsa filtro
E filter bag
G Filterbeutel, Filtersack
F sac de filtration, filtre à poches

bolsa hermética
E sealed bag, sachet
G Siegelrandbeutel
F sachet hermétique

bolsa interior
E internal bag
G Innenbeutel
F poche intérieure

bolsa plana
E flat bag
G Flachbeutel
F sachet plat, sachet plan

bolsa tubular
E tubular bag
G Schlauchbeutel
F poche

bomba
E pump
G Pumpe
F pompe

bomba de anillo de agua
E water-ring pump
G Wasserringpumpe
F pompe à anneau d'eau

bomba de chorro de agua
E water jet pump
G Wasserstrahlpumpe
F pompe d'une trompe à eau

bomba de circulación
E circulatory pump
G Umwälzpumpe
F pompe de circulation

bomba de dosificación
E peristaltic pump
G Dosierpumpe
F pompe doseuse

bomba de gradiente
E gradient pump
G Gradientenpumpe
F pompe à gradient

bomba de HPLC
E HPLC pump
G HPLC-Pumpe
F pompe HPLC

bomba de lubri(fi)cante
E lubrication pump
G Schmierstoffpumpe
F pompe lubrifiante

bomba de vacío
E vacuum pump
G Vakuumpumpe
F pompe à vide

bomba de válvula rotativa
E rotary valve pump
G Drehschieberpumpe
F pompe à valve rotatoire

bomba peristáltica
E peristaltic pump
G Schlauchpumpe
F pompe péristaltique

boquilla
E mouthpiece
G Mundstück
F embout

boquilla lubri(fi)cante
E lubricating nipple
G Schmiernippel
F bouchon graisseur

borde
E edge
G Rand
F arête, bord

borde (de un comprimido)
E rim, bur (of a tablet)
G Grat (einer Tablette)
F arête (d'un comprimé)

bordear
E flange, to; bead, to; border, to
G umbördeln
F sertir

borne
E terminal
G Klemme
F pince, borne

bosquejo
E draft
G Entwurf
F ébauche

bote
E can, tin
G Dose
F canne

botella
E bottle
G Flasche
F bouteille

botella con cierre de rosca
E screw-cap bottle
G Schraubflasche, Flasche mit Schraubverschluß
F bouteille munie d'un bouchon à vis

botella de aluminio
E aluminium bottle
G Aluminiumflasche
F bouteille d'aluminium

botella de cuello ancho
E wide-necked bottle
G Weithalsflasche
F bouteille à col large

botella de gas
E gas cylinder
G Gasflasche
F bouteille de gaz

botella de gas a presión
E gas cylinder
G Druckgasflasche
F bouteille de gaz

botella de plástico
E plastic bottle
G Kunststoff-Flasche
F bouteille en plastique

botella perforable
E perforable bottle
G Durchstechflasche
F bouteille perforable

botellín
E vial
G Fläschchen
F flacon, récipient

botón de ajuste
E adjusting knob
G Einstellknopf
F bouton d'ajustement

botones de operación
E function keys
G Funktionstasten
F touche de fonctionnement

brazo de horquilla
E yoke
G Joch, Gabelarm
F bras de levier

brazo de robot
E robotic arm
G Roboterarm
F bras d'un robot

brazo giratorio
E swivel arm
G Schwenkarm
F bras pivotant

brida
E flange
G Flansch
F bride, collerette

bridar
E flange, to
G flanschen
F brider

brillante
E glossy
G glänzend
F brillant, lustré

brillante como seda
E silk glossy
G seidenglänzend
F brillant (comme de la soie)

brillo
E gloss
G Glanz
F lustre, brillance

bromado
E bromination
G Bromierung
F bromage

brotar
E swell, to
G quellen
F gonfler

bruñido
E ground
G geschliffen
F moulu, poli

bruñir
E polish, to
G polieren
F polir

bucle de dosificación
E dosing loop
G Dosierschleife
F boucle de dosage

bucle de pruebas
E test loop
G Testschleife
F boucle de test

bucle para toma de muestras
E sample loop
G Probenschleife
F boucle d'échantillon

bultos sueltos
E itemised goods
G Stückgut
F colis

burbuja
E bubble, blister
G Blase
F bulle

burbuja de aire capturada
E air bubble, entrapped
G eingeschlossene Luftblase
F bulle d'air piégée

burbuja de gas
E gas bubble
G Gasblase
F bulle de gaz

bureta
E burette
G Bürette
F burette

burlete rebordeado
E bead
G Bördelrand
F bourrelet

búsqueda en banco de datos
E database screening
G Datenbankscreening
F screening d'une banque de données

cabeza de bomba
E pump head
G Pumpenkopf
F tête de pompe

cabeza de exploración
E scanning head
G Tastkopf
F tête d'analyse

cabeza del inyector
E nozzle head
G Sprühkopf
F gicleur, buse

cabeza del troquel
E punch head, punch tip
G Stempelkopf
F tête d'un poinçon

cabeza rotatoria de pulverización
E rotary spray
G Rotationssprühkopf
F tête rotative de pulvérisation

cabina de pesado
E weighing cubicle
G Wägekabine
F cabine de pesée

cable
E cable
G Kabel
F câble

cable de prolongación
E extension cable
G Verlängerungskabel
F câble de rallonge

cables
E wiring
G Verkabelung
F câblage

cables de conducción eléctrica
E electrical cables
G elektrische Zuleitungen
F câbles électriques

cadena carbonada
E carbon chain
G Kohlenstoffkette
F chaîne carbonée

cadena de empaquetado
E packaging line
G Verpackungslinie
F chaîne de conditionnement, rampe de conditionnement

cadena de envasado
E filling line, bottling line
G Abfüllstraße, Abfüllinie
F chaîne de remplissage, ligne de remplissage, rampe de remplissage

cadena de producción
E production line
G Produktionslinie
F chaîne de production

cadena de refrigeración
E refrigerating chain
G Kühlkette
F chaîne de réfrigération

cadena larga, de
E long-chained
G langkettig
F à chaîne longue

caducar
E expire, to
G verfallen
F expirer

caja
E can, tin, box, carton, outer carton, housing
G Dose, Schachtel, Umkarton, Gehäuse
F canne, carton, boîte, boîtier

caja de ampollas
E ampoule box
G Ampullenschachtel
F boîte d'ampoules

caja de apilamiento
E stacking box
G Stapelkasten
F boîte de stockage

caja de cartón
E carton
G Pappschachtel
F carton

caja de distribución
E switch box, control box, wiring box, junction box
G Schaltkasten, Verteilerkasten
F armoire électrique, boîte de distribution

caja de fusibles
E fuse box
G Sicherungskasten
F boîte de fusibles

caja de madera
E wooden case
G Holzkiste
F caisse en bois

caja de terminales
E terminal box
G Klemmkasten
F boîte de bornes

English German French Spanish

caja del sensor
E sensor housing
G Sensorgehäuse
F étui du capteur

caja plegable
E folding carton
G Faltschachtel
F boîte pliante

calcinar
E ignite, to
G ausglühen
F faire rougir, se calciner

calcular
E calculate, to
G berechnen
F calculer

cálculo
E calculation
G Rechnung, Berechnung
F calculation, calcul

cálculo del rendimiento
E yield calculation
G Ausbeuteberechnung
F calcul du rendement

caldear
E heat, to
G beheizen
F chauffer

caldera
E vessel, boiler
G Kessel
F chaudière, bouilloire

caldera de agitación
E stirring vessel
G Rührkessel
F récipient de l'agitateur

caldera de fermentación
E fermentation vessel
G Fermentationskessel
F cuve de fermentation

caldera para gragear
E coating pan
G Dragierkessel
F dragéification (à la turbine)

caldera presurizada de reacción
E pressurised reaction vessel
G Druckreaktionskessel
F cuve à réaction sous pression

caldo de cultivo
E culture broth
G Kulturbouillon, Nährbouillon
F bouillon de culture

calefacción con suministro de vapor externo
E external steam heating
G Beheizung mit externer Dampfzufuhr
F chauffage avec apport de vapeur externe

calendario
E schedule
G Zeitplan
F plan, programme

calentado al vapor
E steam-heated
G dampfbeheizt
F chauffé à la vapeur

calentador de inmersión
E immersion heater
G Tauchsieder
F chauffe-liquide

calentamiento
E heating
G Erwärmung
F réchauffement

calibración
E calibration
G Kalibrierung, Eichung
F calibration

calibración por punto único
E single point calibration
G Ein-Punkt-Kalibrierung
F calibration par un point de mesure

calibración por varios puntos
E multiple point calibration
G Kalibrierung anhand mehrerer Meßpunkte
F calibration par points de mesure multiples

calibración de aparatos
E instrument calibration
G Gerätekalibrierung
F calibration de l'équipement

calibrar
E calibrate, to; meter, to; dose, to
G eichen, kalibrieren, dosieren
F calibrer, doser

calibre
E gauge
G Meßlehre
F jauge

calibre de grosores
E thickness gauge
G Dickenmeßgerät
F jauge d'épaisseur, palmer

calidad
E quality
G Qualität
F qualité

calidad alimenticia
E food grade
G lebensmittelecht
F qualité alimentaire

calidad farmacéutica
E pharmaceutical grade
G entspricht Arzneibuchqualität
F qualité pharmaceutique

calidad invariable
E consistent quality
G gleichbleibende Qualität
F qualité uniforme

calificación
E suitability
G Eignung
F qualification

calor
E heat
G Wärme
F chaleur

calor de escape
E waste heat
G Abwärme
F chaleur perdue

calor de evaporación
E heat of evaporation
G Verdampfungswärme
F chaleur d'évaporation

calor de reacción
E heat of reaction
G Reaktionswärme
F chaleur due à la réaction

calor específico
E specific heat
G spezifische Wärme
F chaleur spécifique

calorímetro
E calorimeter
G Kalorimeter
F calorimètre

calorímetro de flujo de calor
E heat flow calorimeter
G Wärmeflußkalorimeter
F calorimètre à flux de chaleur

calota de rebordeo
E crimping cap
G Bördelkappe
F bouchon, couvercle, calotte

calzado de laboratorio
E laboratory shoes
G Laborschuhe
F chaussures de laboratoire

cámara
E chamber
G Kammer
F chambre

cámara cromatográfica
E developing chamber (chromatography)
G Chromatographiekammer
F chambre de développement (chromatographie)

cámara de aclimat(iz)ación
E climatic chamber
G Klimaprüfkammer
F chambre de climatisation

cámara de compresión
E compression chamber
G Preßkammer
F chambre de compression

cámara de cromatografía en capa fina
E thin layer chromatography developing chamber
G Dünnschichtchromatographiekammer
F chambre de développement pour chromatographie sur couche mince

cámara de dosificación
E metering chamber, dosing chamber
G Dosierkammer
F chambre de dosage

cámara de esterilización
E autoclave (sterilisation) chamber
G Sterilisierkammer
F chambre d'autoclave

cámara de incubación
E incubation room
G Inkubationsraum
F chambre d'incubation

cámara frigorífica
E cold room
G Kühlraum
F chambre froide

cámara tropical
E tropical chamber
G Tropenkammer
F chambre tropicale

cambiar de paleta
E re-pallet, to
G umpalettieren
F réorganiser les palettes

cambio
E change, variation
G Wechsel, Änderung
F changement

cambio de bobina
E reel changes
G Rollenwechsel
F changement de bobine

cambio de color
E colour change
G Farbumschlag
F changement de couleur

cambio de emplazamiento
E change of site, change of location
G Standortwechsel
F déménagement

cambio de formato
E size changeover
G Formatumstellung
F modification d'un format

camión cisterna
E tank wagon
G Tankwagen
F wagon-citerne

camisa de agua
E water jacket
G Wassermantel
F chemise d'eau

camisa de refrigeración
E cooling jacket
G Mantelkühlung
F chemise de refroidissement

camisa refrigerante
E cooling jacket
G Kühlmantel
F manteau de refroidissement

campaña
E campaign
G Kampagne
F campagne

campana de extracción de gases
E ventilated hood, fume cupboard
G Abzug
F hotte à flux laminaire, hotte chimique

campo de aplicación
E area of application, scope, validity
G Anwendungsgebiet, Geltungsbereich
F champ d'application, domaine d'application

canal
E duct, channel, recess, gutter
G Kanal, Rinne, Hohlkehle
F canal, canalisation, voie, moulure creuse, gouttière

canal de alimentación
E feed chute
G Zufuhrrinne
F rigole d'alimentation, conduit d'alimentation

canal de cables
E cable duct
G Kabelkanal
F canal de câbles

canal de descompresión
E pressure relief duct
G Druckentlastungskanal
F canalisation de décompression

canal de distribución
E sales channel
G Vertriebsweg
F canal de distribution

canal de salida
E waste duct
G Ablaufrinne
F canalisation d'élimination des déchets

canal de salida de los comprimidos
E tablet exit chute
G Tablettenablaufrinne
F rigole d'écoulement pour comprimés

canal del aire de escape
E exhaust air duct
G Abluftkanal
F canal d'évacuation de l'air

canalización
E pipe(work), pipeline
G Rohrleitung
F canalisation

canalización de aire
E air duct, air shaft
G Luftschacht
F canalisation d'air

cancerógeno
E carcinogenic
G krebserregend, cancerogen
F carcinogène, cancérogène

cancerógeno si se inhala
E may cause cancer by inhalation
G kann beim Einatmen Krebs erzeugen
F cancéreux si inhalé

candela filtrante
E filter cartridge
G Filterkerze
F chandelle filtrante

cañería en anillo
E main ring
G Ringleitung
F boucle de recirculation

cantidad
E quantity, amount
G Menge
F quantité

cantidad a aplicar (al recubrir)
E coating quantity
G Auftragsmenge (beim Coating)
F quantité (d'enduit) appliquée

English German French Spanish

cantidad de relleno
E filling quantity
G Füllmenge
F quantité de remplissage

cantidad envasada
E filling quantity
G Abfüllmenge
F quantité de remplissage, volume de remplissage

cantidad producida
E quantity produced
G Produktionsmenge
F quantité produite

cantidad suministrada
E quantity received
G Liefermenge
F quantité livrée

cantina
E canteen
G Kantine
F cantine

canto rebordeado
E bead
G Bördelrand
F bourrelet

cánula
E cannula, injection needle
G Kanüle
F canule

capa aislante
E insulating layer
G Isolierschicht
F couche d'isolation

capacidad
E capacity, volume
G Kapazität, Fassungsvermögen
F capacité, contenance

capacidad colorante
E colour capacity
G Färbevermögen
F capacité de coloration

capacidad de absorción
E absorptivity, absorption capacity, absorbing capacity, absorptive capacity, absorbing power
G Absorptionsfähigkeit, Absorptionsvermögen, Saugfähigkeit
F capacité d'absorption

capacidad de absorción de agua
E water absorption capacity
G Wasseraufnahmevermögen
F capacité d'absorption d'eau

capacidad de adsorción
E adsorptivity, adsorption capacity
G Adsorptionsfähigkeit
F capacité d'adsorption

capacidad de almacenamiento
E storage stability, shelf-life
G Lagerfähigkeit
F stabilité au stockage

capacidad de carga
E loading capacity, load capacity
G Tragfähigkeit, Belastbarkeit
F limite de charge, force portante, capacité de chargement

capacidad de cubrir
E covering power, hiding power
G Deckkraft
F propriété couvrante

capacidad de enlace
E binding capacity
G Bindungsvermögen
F capacité de fixation

capacidad de fijación
E binding capacity
G Bindungsvermögen
F capacité de fixation

capacidad de fluir
E flowing property, fluidity
G Rieselfähigkeit
F propriété d'écoulement

capacidad de hinchamiento
E swelling capacity
G Quellfähigkeit
F capacité de gonflement

capacidad de recuperación
E recovery capability
G Erholungsfähigkeit
F capacité de récupération

capacidad de retención (de un filtro)
E retention efficiency (in filters)
G Rückhaltevermögen (bei Filtern)
F efficacité de rétention (pour un filtre)

capacidad de separación
E separation capacity
G Trennungskapazität
F capacité de séparation

capacidad de tamponamiento
E buffering capacity
G Pufferkapazität
F capacité d'un tampon

capacidad funcional
E operability, functionality
G Funktionsfähigkeit
F fonctionnalité

capataz
E foreman
G Vorarbeiter
F contremaître

capaz de fluir
E capable of flowing, flowable
G rieselfähig
F capable d'écoulement

capilar
E capillary
G Kapillare
F capillaire

capilar de ebullición
E boiling capillary
G Siedekapillare
F capillaire d'ébullition

cápsula
E capsule, sleeve
G Kapsel, Hülse
F capsule, douille, coussinet, manchon

cápsula amilácea
E cachet
G Oblatenkapsel
F cachet

cápsula de evaporación
E evaporating dish
G Abdampfschale
F capsule d'évaporation

cápsula de gelatina
E gelatine capsule
G Gelatinekapsel
F capsule de gélatine

cápsula de gelatina blanda
E soft gelatine capsule
G Weichgelatinekapsel
F gélule molle

cápsula de gelatina dura
E hard gelatine capsule
G Hartgelatinekapsel
F gélule

cápsula gelatinosa dura
E hard capsule
G Steckkapsel
F gélule

cápsula mordible
E biting capsule
G Zerbeißkapsel
F capsule à croquer

capsular
E encapsulate, to
G verkapseln
F encapsuler

captador de fibras
E fibre catcher
G Faserfänger
F capteur de fibres

captar
E collect, to; entrap, to
G auffangen
F capter, recueillir

capucha
E head covering, cap
G Kopfhaube
F bonnet

característica
E property, feature, curve
G Eigenschaft, Merkmal, Kennlinie
F propriété, caractéristique, particularité

característica de aceptación
E acceptance graph
G Annahmekennlinie
F courbe d'acceptance

característica de calidad
E quality attribute
G Qualitätsmerkmal
F caracteristique de qualité

característica de defecto
E defect characteristic
G Fehlermerkmal
F caractéristique du défaut

característica de seguridad
E safety feature
G Sicherheitsmerkmal
F caractéristique de sécurité

característica individual
E individual characteristic
G Einzelmerkmal
F caractéristique individuelle

características de compresión
E compression characteristics
G Preßeigenschaften
F caractéristiques de compression

características de superficie
E surface properties
G Oberflächenbeschaffenheit
F propriétés de surface

caracterización (de un compuesto)
E characterisation (of a compound)
G Charakterisierung (einer Verbindung)
F caractérisation (d'un composé organique)

caracterización de aparatos
E apparatus designation
G Gerätekennzeichnung
F marquage de l'appareil

caracterización de cañerías
E piping designation
G Rohrleitungskennzeichnung
F marquage des tuyaux

carbón
E carbon
G Kohle
F carbone

carbón activado
E activated charcoal
G Aktivkohle
F charbon actif

carcinógeno
E carcinogenic
G karzinogen
F carcinogène, cancérogène

carencia
E deficiency
G Mangel
F déficience, carence, insuffisance

carga
E loading, load, feed, loading, stress, strain
G Belastung, Beschickung, Beladung, Ladung, Beanspruchung
F chargement, charge, soumission à un effort

carga dinámica
E dynamic load
G dynamische Belastung
F charge dynamique

carga microbiana
E microbial load, bioburden
G mikrobielle Belastung
F présence microbienne

carga (electricidad)
E charge (electricity)
G Ladung (Elektrizität)
F charge (électricité)

carga a granel
E bulk material
G Schüttgut
F matériau en vrac

carga de gérmenes
E bioburden
G Keimbelastung
F teneur en micro-organismes

carga de presión
E pressure loading
G Druckbelastung
F charge de pression

carga eléctrica
E electrical charge
G elektrische Ladung
F charge électrique

carga electrostática
E electrostatic charge
G elektrostatische Aufladung
F charge électrostatique

carga estática
E static charge, static load
G statische Aufladung, statische Belastung
F charge statique

carga máxima
E maximum load
G Höchstlast
F charge maximale

carga previa
E preliminary batch
G Vorcharge
F lot préliminaire

carga térmica
E thermal load
G thermische Belastung
F charge thermique

cargar con paleta
E palletise, to
G palettieren
F palettiser

carrera del émbolo
E stroke
G Hub, Kolbenweg
F course de piston

carretilla elevadora de horquilla
E fork-lift truck
G Gabelstapler
F chariot élévateur

carril de ascenso (del troquel superior)
E lifting cam (of upper punch)
G Aufzugsschiene (des Oberstempels)
F came (de poinçon) ascendante

carril de tracción inferior
E pull-down cam
G Niederzugsschiene
F came de poinçon descendante

carro de montaje
E mounting trolley
G Montagewagen
F chariot de montage

carro de transporte
E transport cart
G Transportwagen
F chariot de transport

carro elevador
E lifting truck
G Hubwagen
F chariot élévateur

carta de aviso (de la FDA)
E warning letter (from FDA)
G Verwarnung (der FDA)
F lettre d'avertissement (de la FDA)

English German French Spanish

cartel con avisos de seguridad
E safety poster
G Plakat mit Sicherheitshinweisen
F affiche avec consignes de sécurité

cárter
E sump
G Ölwanne
F carter à huile

cárter del motor
E motor housing
G Motorgehäuse
F carter d'un moteur

cartón
E carton, outer carton, pasteboard, cardboard
G Karton, Umkarton, Pappe
F carton, boîte

cartón barnizado
E varnished cardboard
G lackierte Pappe
F papier vernis

cartón de envío
E shipping carton
G Versandkarton
F conteneur

cartón de fibra
E fibre cardboard
G Fiberkarton
F carton à fibres

cartón externo
E outer carton
G Umkarton
F carton d'expédition

cartón ondulado
E corrugated cardboard (carton)
G Wellpappe
F carton ondulé

cartucho
E cartridge
G Kartusche, Patrone
F cartouche

cartucho de filtro
E filter cartridge
G Filterpatrone
F cartouche de filtre

cáscara
E sleeve
G Hülse
F douille, coussinet, manchon

casco protector
E safety helmet, hard hat
G Schutzhelm
F casque de protection

caso de urgencia
E emergency
G Notfall
F urgence

caso necesario, en
E as required
G bei Bedarf
F sur besoin, sur demande

casquete
E cover, hood
G Haube, Abdeckung
F couvercle, capuchon

casquillo
E base, socket
G Sockel, Buchse
F socle, borne

catalizador
E catalyst
G Katalysator
F catalyseur

cataplasma
E poultice
G Umschlagpaste
F cataplasme

categoría de comprimido
E tablet category
G Tablettenkategorie
F catégorie du comprimé

catéter
E catheter
G Katheter
F cathéter, sonde

catión
E cation
G Kation
F cation

cátodo
E cathode
G Kathode
F cathode

causa de error
E cause of failure
G Fehlerursache
F cause du défaut

causar
E cause, to
G verursachen
F provoquer

cáustico
E caustic
G ätzend
F caustique

cauterizar
E marinate, to; pickle, to
G beizen
F mariner

cavidad
E recess, cavity, well, hollow space
G Vertiefung, Hohlraum
F cavité, puits, espace creux

cazo
E ladle, scoop
G Schöpfkelle
F louche

cedazo
E sieve
G Sieb
F tamis

célula
E cell
G Zelle
F cellule

célula de detección
E detector cell
G Detektorzelle
F cellule de détection

célula de fluxometría
E flow-through cell, flow cell
G Durchflußzelle
F cellule de mesure du débit

célula de medida de la conductividad
E conductivity cell
G Leitfähigkeitsmeßzelle
F cellule de mesure de conductivité

célula fotoeléctrica
E photo cell, photoelectric cell
G Photozelle
F cellule photoélectrique

celulosa
E cellulose
G Zellstoff
F cellulose

ceniza
E ash
G Asche
F cendre

ceniza sulfatada
E sulphate ash
G Sulfatasche
F cendre sulfatée

cenizas residuales
E residue on ignition, residue on annealment
G Verbrennungsrückstand, Glührückstand
F cendres résiduelles

censado
E censored
G zensiert
F censuré

English German French Spanish

central energética
E power station
G Kraftwerk
F centrale énergétique

centrar
E centre, to
G zentrieren
F centrer

centrífuga
E centrifuge
G Zentrifuge
F centrifugeuse

centrifugación
E centrifugation
G Zentrifugation
F centrifugation

centrifugar
E centrifuge, to
G zentrifugieren
F centrifuger

centro de gravedad
E centre of gravity
G Schwerpunkt
F centre de gravité

centro de investigación clínica
E clinical trial location
G klinische Prüfeinrichtung
F emplacement des essais cliniques

cepa (microbiología)
E strain
G Stamm
F lignée

cepillo
E brush
G Bürste
F brosse

cepillo rotativo
E revolving brush
G Bürstenwalze
F brosse de laminage

cepillo rotatorio
E revolving brush
G Walzenbürste
F brosse rotative

cera
E wax
G Wachs
F cire

cerrado
E locked location
G unter Verschluß
F enfermé

cerrar
E seal, to; close off, to
G verschließen, absperren
F sceller, clore, fermer

cerrar ampollas a la llama
E flame-seal, to (ampoules)
G zuschmelzen (Ampullen)
F obturer par vitrification (ampoules)

cerrar herméticamente
E tighten, to; seal, to
G abdichten
F colmater, boucher, étanchéifier

cerrar una ampolla
E seal an ampoule, to
G Ampulle verschließen
F fermer une ampoule,
obturer une ampoule

certificación
E certification
G Zertifizierung
F certification

certificado
E certificate
G Zertifikat
F certificat

certificado de análisis
E certificate of analysis
G Analysenzertifikat
F certificat d'analyse

certificado de calibración
E calibration certificate
G Eichschein, Kalibrierschein
F certificat de calibration

certificado de conformidad
E certificate of conformity
G Konformitätszertifikat
F certificat de conformité

certificado de prueba
E test certificate
G Prüfzertifikat
F certificat d'analyse

certificar
E certificate, to
G zertifizieren
F certifier

cesto colector
E retaining basket
G Fangkorb
F corbeille

cesto para autoclave
E autoclave basket
G Korbeinsatz für Autoklaven
F corbeille d'autoclave

cesto rotatorio
E rotary basket
G Drehkörbchen
F corbeille rotative

champú
E shampoo
G Shampoo
F shampooing

chanclos
E overshoe
G Überschuhe
F couvre-chaussure

chapa
E sheet, plate, tray
G Blech
F tôle

chapa de revestimiento
E cover, casing
G Verkleidungsblech
F couvercle, capuchon

chapa desviadora
E baffle
G Umlenkblech
F chicane de déviation

chasis
E trolley
G Fahrgestell
F chassis mobile

chispas
E sparks
G Funken
F étincelles

choque
E impact
G Schlag, Stoß
F impact, coup

choque térmico
E thermal shock
G Wärmeschock
F choc thermique

chorro de aire
E air jet
G Luftstrahl
F jet d'air

ciclo
E cycle, run
G Zyklus, Lauf
F cycle, opération, expérience

ciclo de desecación
E drying cycle
G Trocknungszyklus
F cycle de séchage

ciclo de funcionamiento
E operational cycle
G Arbeitsablauf
F cycle de fonctionnement

ciclo de mezcla
E blending cycle
G Mischzyklus
F cycle de mélange

ciclo de pulverización
E spray cycle
G Sprühzyklus
F cycle de pulvérisation

ciclo de validación
E validation run
G Validierungslauf
F cycle de validation

ciclo vital
E life cycle
G Lebenszyklus
F cycle de vie

ciencia médica
E medical science
G Medizinische Wissenschaft
F science médicale

cierre
E closure, seal, cap, quarantine
G Verschluß, Sperrung
F bouchon, capuchon, couvercle, quarantaine

cierre a prueba de niños
E child-resistant closure
G kindersicherer Verschluß
F fermeture de sécurité pour enfants

cierre con cuentagotas
E dropper applicator
G Verschluß mit Tropfer
F applicateur compte-gouttes

cierre de botella
E bottle cap
G Flaschenverschluß
F capsule à bouteilles

cierre de rosca
E screw cap, screw connection
G Schraubkappe, Schraubverschluß
F bouchon à vis, fermeture à vis

cierre de tornillo
E wrench
G Schraubenschlüssel
F clef de serrage

cierre de un tubo
E tube closure
G Tubenverschluß
F bouchon de tube

cierre hermético
E hermetic seal
G hermetischer Verschluß
F fermeture hermétique

cierre hermético de un filtro
E filter seal
G Filterabdichtung
F étanchement d'un filtre

cierre inflable de silicona
E inflatable silicone seal
G aufblasbare Silikondichtung
F joint de silicone gonflable

cierre mecánico
E mechanical seal
G mechanischer Verschluß
F fermeture mécanique

cierre por gel
E gel seal
G Gelverschluß
F fermeture pour gel

cierre rápido
E quick-flange connection
G Schnellverschluß
F connexion à collerette instantanée

cilindrar
E roll, to
G walzen
F passer au rouleau

cilíndrico
E cylindrical
G zylindrisch
F cylindrique

cilindro
E roller, drum
G Walze
F rouleau, cylindre, tambour

cilindro cepillador
E revolving brush
G Bürstenwalze
F brosse de laminage

cilindro compresor (en la prensa de comprimidos)
E compression roll, compaction roll (tablet press)
G Druckrolle (an der Tablettenpresse)
F cylindre de compression

cilindro de aire comprimido
E compressed air cylinder
G Druckluftzylinder
F cylindre de compression

cilindro de jeringa
E syringe cylinder
G Spritzenzylinder
F cylindre de seringue

cinética
E kinetics
G Kinetik
F cinétique

cinta adhesiva
E adhesive tape
G Klebeband
F bande adhésive

cinta clasificadora
E sorting belt
G Sortierband
F bande de triage

cinta excéntrica
E eccentric band
G Exzenterband
F courroie excentrique

cinta magnética
E magnetic tape
G Magnetband
F bande magnétique

cinta sin fin
E continuous band
G Endlosbahn
F bande continue

cinta transportadora
E conveyor belt
G Fließband, Förderband, Transportband
F convoyeur à bande, tapis roulant

circuito eléctrico
E circuit, loop
G Stromkreis
F circuit

circuito eléctrico principal
E main circuit
G Hauptstromkreis
F circuit principal

circuito regulador
E control loop
G Regelkreis
F boucle d'asservissement

circulación
E recirculation
G Umlauf
F recirculation

circulación cerrada
E closed loop
G geschlossener Kreislauf
F circulation fermée

circunferencia
E circumference
G Umfang
F circonférence, périmètre, étendue

cistometría
E bubble point test
G Blasendrucktest
F essai de point de bulle

citometría de flujo
E flow cytometry
G Durchflußzytometrie
F cytométrie à débit liquide

citostáticos
E cytostatics
G Zytostatica
F cytostatiques

claridad
E clarity
G Klarheit
F clareté

claro
E distinct, clear, transparent, unambiguous
G deutlich, klar, eindeutig
F distinct, clair, transparent, précis

clase de peligro
E hazard class
G Gefahrenklasse
F classe de dangers

clase inflamable
E inflammability class
G Brandklasse
F classe d'inflammables

clasificación
E grade
G Einstufung
F classification

clasificar
E classify, to; grade, to
G klassieren, sichten, einstufen
F classifier

clavija
E bolt, pin
G Bolzen, Stift (technisch)
F boulon, cheville, broche, pointeau, goupille

cliché
E printing block
G Klischee
F cliché

cliente
E customer, client, contract provider, principal
G Abnehmer, Kunde, Auftraggeber
F client, donneur d'ordre, commettant

clientes de referencia
E reference customers
G Referenzkunden
F clientèle de référence

climatizado
E air-conditioned
G klimatisiert
F air conditionné

climatizador
E air-conditioning
G Klimatisierung
F climatisation

clonación
E cloning
G Klonierung
F clonage

clorar
E chlorinate, to
G chlorieren
F chlorurer

cloro
E chlorine
G Chlor
F chlor

cloruro de polivinilo
E polyvinyl chloride (PVC)
G Polyvinylchlorid (PVC)
F chlorure de polyvinyl (PVC)

coagulación
E coagulation
G Koagulation, Gerinnung
F coagulation

coagular
E coagulate, to
G gerinnen
F coaguler

cobre
E copper
G Kupfer
F cuivre

cocción (p. ej. de cristales)
E baking (e. g. of crystals)
G Zusammenbacken (z. B. von Kristallen)
F agglomération (par ex. de cristaux)

cociente
E quotient
G Quotient
F quotient

codificación de colores
E colour code
G Farbcodierung
F codage de couleurs

codificación de la fecha de caducidad
E expiration coding
G Codierung des Verfalldatums
F codage de la date d'expiration

código de designación de lotes
E batch number coding
G Chargenbezeichnungsschlüssel
F système de codage pour les numéros de lot

código de entrada de mercancías
E receiving code
G Wareneingangscode
F code d'entrée de marchandises

código de un lote
E batch code
G Chargencode
F codage d'un lot

código regional
E local code
G regionales Regelwerk
F code régional

coeficiente de absorción
E absorption coefficient
G Absorptionskoeffizient
F coefficient d'absorption

coeficiente de dilatación
E coefficient of expansion
G Dehnungskoeffizient
F coefficient d'expansion

coeficiente de extinción
E coefficient of absorbance
G Extinktionskoeffizient
F coefficient d'absorption

coeficiente de extinción UV
E UV coefficient of absorbance
G UV-Extinktionskoeffizient
F coefficient d'extinction UV

coeficiente de fricción
E coefficient of friction
G Reibungskoeffizient
F coefficient de friction, coefficient de frottement

coeficiente de validación
E coefficient of variation
G Variationskoeffizient
F coefficient de variation

coenzima
E coenzyme
G Koenzym
F coenzyme

cofia
E head covering, cap
G Kopfhaube
F bonnet

coherente
E coherent
G kohärent
F cohérent

cohesión
E cohesion
G Kohäsion
F cohésion

coincidencia
E conformity
G Übereinstimmung
F conformité

coincidir con
E conform with, to
G übereinstimmen mit
F être en conformité avec

English German French Spanish

cojinete
E bearing (mach.)
G Lager (Maschinenteil)
F assise, support

cola
E glue
G Leim
F colle

colectar
E collect, to; entrap, to
G auffangen
F capter, recueillir

colector de fracciones
E fraction collector
G Fraktionssammler
F collecteur de fractions

colector de gérmenes del aire
E microbial collector
G Luftkeimsammler
F échantillonneur d'air

colector de solvente
E solvent collector
G Lösungsmittelauffangbehälter
F collecteur de solvant

collar
E clip, flange
G Schelle, Flansch
F collier, bride, collerette

colocación
E placement
G Plazierung
F placement

colodión
E film-forming liquid, collodion
G filmbildende Flüssigkeit
F collodion

color
E dye, stain, pigment
G Farbe
F colorant, teinture, pigment

color de fabricación de comprimidos
E tablet dye
G Tablettierfarbe
F couleur de fabrication de comprimés

coloración
E colouration
G Färbung
F coloration, teinture

colorante
E colouring agent, stain, dye
G Färbemittel, Farbstoff
F colorant, pigment, teinture

colorante vegetal
E vegetable dye
G Pflanzenfarbstoff
F pigment végétal

colorear
E stain, to
G färben
F colorer, teinter, teindre

columna
E column
G Kolonne
F colonne

columna a presión
E pressure column
G Druckkolonne
F colonne sous pression

columna analítica
E analytical column
G analytische Säule
F colonne analytique

columna de agua
E water column
G Wassersäule
F colonne d'eau

columna previa
E pre-column
G Vorsäule
F colonne préalable

combustibilidad
E flammability
G Brennbarkeit
F combustibilité

combustible
E combustible, flammable
G brennbar
F combustible

combustión
E combustion, incineration
G Verbrennung
F combustion, incinération

comenzar (un proceso)
E start, to (a process)
G starten (Ablauf)
F démarrer (un procédé)

comienzo del estudio
E start of study, start of trial
G Studienstart
F démarrage d'un essai clinique

comisión ética
E ethics committee
G Ethikkomission
F commission d'éthique

comisión fiscal de validación
E validation review committee
G Steuerungsausschuß zur Validierung
F comité directeur de validation

comisionista
E contract acceptor, client
G Auftragnehmer
F client

comitente
E contract provider, principal, client
G Auftraggeber
F donneur d'ordre, commettant, client

compactador
E compactor
G Kompaktierer
F compacteur

compacto
E thick
G dick
F épais

compatibilidad
E compatibility
G Verträglichkeit, Kompatibilität
F compatibilité

compatibilidad de materiales
E material compatibility
G Materialverträglichkeit
F compatibilité des matériaux

compatible
E compatible
G kompatibel
F compatible

compensación de temperatura
E temperature equalisation
G Temperaturausgleich
F compensation de température

competencia
E authority
G Befugnis
F autorisation

competidor
E competitor
G Mitbewerber
F compétiteur

complejo de quelatos
E chelate, chelate complex
G Chelatkomplex
F chélate, complexe de chélation

complemento
E supplementation
G Ergänzung
F complément, supplément

completamente automático
E fully automatic
G vollautomatisch
F entièrement automatique

completetamente desmineralizado
E demineralised
G vollentsalzt
F complètement désalinisé

componente
E component, constituent, ingredient
G Bestandteil
F composant, constituant, ingrédient

componente activo
E active substance, active ingredient
G wirksamer Bestandteil
F composant actif

componente clave
E key component
G Schlüsselkomponente
F composant clé

componente formador (de una prensa de comprimidos)
E component (of a tablet press)
G Formatteil (bei einer Tablettenpresse)
F composant (d'une presse à comprimés)

componente moldeado por inyección
E injection-moulded component
G Spritzgußteil
F composant moulé par injection

componentes
E components
G Einzelteile
F composants

componentes del envase
E packaging components
G Bestandteile der Packung
F constituants d'un emballage

comportamiento
E behaviour
G Verhalten
F comportement

comportamiento de liberación
E release behaviour
G Freisetzungsverhalten
F comportement de libération

comportamiento en disolución
E dissolution behaviour
G Auflösungsverhalten
F comportement de dissolution

comportamiento térmico
E thermal behaviour
G thermisches Verhalten
F comportement thermique

composición
E composition
G Zusammensetzung
F composition

comprar
E purchase, to; take over, to
G kaufen, übernehmen
F acheter, acquérir, prendre le contrôle de

comprensible
E comprehensible
G verständlich
F compréhensible

compresa
E compress, wound dressing
G Kompresse, Wundauflage
F compresse, pansement

compresión
E compression, concentration
G Verdichtung
F compression, concentration

compresión de doble capa
E double-layer compression
G Zweischichtverpressung
F compression à double couche

compresión directa
E direct tablet compression
G Direkttablettierung
F compression directe

comprimido
E tablet, moulded
G Tablette, geformt, gepreßt
F comprimé, moulu

English German French Spanish

aspecto de un comprimido
E tablet appearance
G Aussehen der Tablette
F apparence d'un comprimé

heterogeneidad de los comprimidos
E tablet inconsistency
G Uneinheitlichkeit von Tabletten
F hétérogénéité des comprimés

resistencia a la ruptura de un comprimido
E tablet crushing strength
G Bruchfestigkeit einer Tablette
F résistance à la rupture d'un comprimé

uniformidad del color de los comprimidos
E tablet colour uniformity
G Einheitlichkeit der Tablettenfarbe
F uniformité de la couleur d'un comprimé

comprimido de cubierta estratificada
E laminated tablet
G Manteltablette
F comprimé multicouche

comprimido efervescente
E effervescent tablet
G Brausetablette
F comprimé effervescent

comprimido elongado
E oblong tablet
G längliche Tablette
F comprimé allongé

comprimido oblongo
E oblong tablet
G Oblongtablette
F comprimé oblong

comprimido para chupar
E lozenge, pastille
G Lutschtablette
F pastille, tablette à sucer

comprimido redondo
E round tablet
G Rundtablette
F comprimé rond

comprimido retard
E retard tablet, delayed action tablet
G Retardtablette
F comprimé à libération retardée

comprimido vaginal
E vaginal tablet
G Vaginaltablette
F comprimé vaginal

comprimidos
E compressed tablets
G Preßtabletten
F comprimés

comprimidos defectuosos
E faulty tablets
G fehlerhafte Tabletten
F comprimés défectueux

comprimidos masticables
E chewing tablet
G Kautablette
F comprimé à mâcher

comprimir
E compress, to; concentrate, to
G verdichten
F comprimer, concentrer

comprobación
E verification, check
G Überprüfung
F vérification

comprobación de aparatos
E equipment test
G Gerätetest
F test d'appareils

comprobación de datos
E collation of data
G Datenüberprüfung
F collation de données

comprobación de la robustez
E robustness testing
G Prüfung der Robustheit
F test de solidité

comprobado
E checked, inspected
G geprüft
F contrôlé, inspecté, vérifié

comprobar
E control, to; check, to; test, to
G überprüfen, prüfen
F contrôler, vérifier, tester

compuerta
E cursor
G Schieber
F curseur

compuesto
E compound
G Verbindung
F combinaison

compuesto organometálico
E organo-metallic compound
G metallorganische Verbindung
F composé organo-métallique

compuesto quelado
E chelated compound
G Chelatverbindung
F composé organique chélaté

compuesto químico
E chemical compound
G chemische Verbindung
F combinaison chimique

compuesto tóxico
E toxic compound
G toxische Verbindung
F substance toxique

compuestos halogenados
E halogenated compounds
G halogenierte Verbindungen
F substances halogènes

cóncavo
E concave
G konkav, nach innen gewölbt
F concave

concentración
E concentration, compression, enrichment
G Konzentration, Verdichtung, Anreicherung
F concentration, compression

concentración crítica de micelas
E critical micelle concentration
G kritische Micellkonzentration
F concentration critique de micelles

concentración de colorante
E dye concentration
G Farbstoffkonzentration
F concentration d'un colorant

concentración máxima de puestos de trabajo
E maximum allowable concentration (MAC)
G maximale Arbeitsplatz-konzentration (MAK)
F concentration maximale de postes de travail

concentración micelar crítica
E critical micelle concentration
G kritische Mizellkonzentration
F concentration critique de micelles

concentrado seco
E dried concentrate
G Trockenextrakt
F concentré sec

concentrar
E concentrate, to; compress, to; thicken, to; enrich, to
G verdichten, eindicken, anreichern, einengen
F concentrer, comprimer, épaissir

concepción por zonas
E zonal concept
G Zonenkonzept
F concept de zones

conciencia del medio ambiente
E environmental awareness
G Umweltbewußtsein
F conscience de l'environnement

conclusión
E completion
G Beendigung
F achèvement

concordancia
E conformity
G Übereinstimmung
F conformité

concurso
E tender
G Ausschreibung
F appel d'offres

condensación
E condensation
G Kondensation
F condensation

condensado
E condensate
G Kondensat
F condensat

condensador
E condenser
G Kondensator
F condenseur

condensar
E concentrate, to; thicken, to
G eindicken
F épaissir

condiciones
E conditions
G Bedingungen
F conditions

condiciones adiabáticas de reacción
E adiabatic reaction conditions
G adiabatische Reaktionsbedingungen
F conditions de réaction adiabatiques

condiciones ambientales
E environmental conditions
G Umgebungsbedingungen
F conditions de l'environnement

condiciones de almacenamiento
E storage conditions
G Lagerungsbedingungen
F conditions de stockage

condiciones de funcionamiento
E operating conditions
G Betriebsbedingungen
F conditions de service

condiciones de producción
E manufacturing conditions
G Herstellungsbedingungen
F conditions de production

condiciones de reacción
E reaction conditions
G Reaktionsbedingungen
F conditions de réaction

condiciones experimentales
E experimental conditions
G Versuchsbedingungen
F conditions expérimentales

condiciones simuladas de ensayo
E simulated test condition
G Testbedingung, simulierte
F condition de test simulée

conducción (gas, agua)
E piping (gas, water)
G Leitung (Gas, Wasser)
F conduite (de gaz, d'eau)

conducción de agua
E water piping
G Wasserleitung
F conduite d'eau

conducción de aguas residuales
E waste water line
G Abwasserleitung
F conduite destinée aux eaux résiduelles

conducción de vapor
E steam line
G Dampfleitung
F conduite de vapeur

conducción de ventilación
E venting line
G Entlüftungsleitung
F canalisation de ventilation, canalisation d'aération

conducción térmica
E conductive heat
G Wärmeleitung
F conduction thermique

conducir
E guide, to
G leiten
F diriger

conductibilidad
E conductivity
G Leitfähigkeit
F conductivité

conductímetro
E conductivity meter
G Leitfähigkeitsmesser
F conductimètre

conductividad eléctrica
E conductivity
G elektrische Leitfähigkeit
F conductivité électrique

conductividad térmica
E thermal conductivity
G Wärmeleitfähigkeit
F conductivité thermique

conducto
E duct, channel
G Kanal, Schacht
F canal, canalisation, voie, conduite, bouche

conducto de alimentación
E charge tube
G Befüllrohr
F conduite de charge, conduite d'alimentation

conducto de carga
E charge tube
G Befüllrohr
F conduite de charge, conduite d'alimentation

conducto de envasado
E filling hose, filling pipe
G Abfüllrohr
F conduite de remplissage

conducto de evacuación de aire
E exhaust line
G Abluftleitung
F conduite d'évacuation

conductor
E conductive
G leitfähig
F conducteur

conectado
E connected
G angeschlossen
F connecté

mal conectado
E wrongly connected
G falsch angeschlossen
F faussement connecté

conectar
E connect, to; wire, to; switch on, to
G anschließen, schalten, verdrahten, einschalten
F connecter, enclencher, brancher

conectar a tierra
E ground, to; earth, to
G erden
F mettre à la terre

conexión
E connection
G Anschluß, Verbindung
F connexion

conexión (eléctrica)
E circuit (electrical)
G Schaltung (elektrisch)
F circuit, connexion (électrique)

conexión de abastecimiento
E supply connection, supply input
G Versorgungsanschluß
F connection de charge

conexión de bayoneta
E bayonet connection
G Bajonettverschluß
F fermeture à baïonnette

conexión de conducción de vapor
E steam connection
G Dampfleitungsverbindung
F connexion de conduite à vapeur

conexión de enchufe
E plug connection
G Steckkupplung
F connexion à fiche(s)

conexión de pared
E wall connection
G Wandanschluß
F connexion murale

conexión hermética
E leak-tight connection
G dichte Verbindung
F raccordement étanche

conexión lateral
E cross-linking
G Quervernetzung
F connexion latérale

conexión paralela
E parallel connection
G Parallelschaltung
F connection parallèle

conexión rápida
E quick coupling, instant coupling
G Schnellkupplung
F connexion instantanée

conexión sanitaria
E sanitary joint
G Sanitärverbindung
F joint sanitaire

conexiones sanitarias
E sanitary fittings
G Sanitäranschlüsse
F connections sanitaires

confiabilidad
E reliability
G Zuverlässigkeit
F fiabilité

confiable
E reliable
G zuverlässig
F fiable

confidencialidad
E confidentiality
G Vertraulichkeit
F confidentialité

configuración de aparatos
E instrument configuration
G Gerätekonfiguration
F configuration de l'instrument

configuración estérica
E sterical arrangement
G sterische Anordnung
F configuration stérique

conformación espacial (p. ej. de una proteína)
E spatial folding (e. g. of protein)
G räumliche Faltung (z. B. eines Proteins)
F pliage spatial (par ex. des protéines)

conforme a GMP
E GMP-conform
G GMP-gerecht
F conforme aux bonnes pratiques de fabrication

conformidad
E conformity
G Konformität
F conformité

conformidad con GMP
E GMP compliance
G GMP-Entsprechung
F conformité aux bonnes pratiques de fabrication

confortable para el usuario
E user-friendly
G bedienerfreundlich
F convivial pour l'utilisateur, adapté à l'utilisateur

confusión
E confusion, misidentification
G Verwechslung
F méprise, erreur

congelación
E deep freezing
G Tiefkühlung
F surgélation

congelado
E deep-frozen
G tiefgefroren
F congelé

congelador
E freezer
G Gefrierschrank
F congélateur

congelar
E deep-freeze, to
G tieffrieren
F congeler

conicidad
E conicalness, conicity
G Verjüngung, Konizität
F amincissement

cónico
E tapered, conical
G verjüngt, konisch, kegelförmig
F conique

conmutación de la longitud de onda
E wavelength switching
G Wellenlängenumschaltung
F changement de longueur d'onde

conmutador
E switch
G Schalter
F interrupteur

conmutar
E wire, to
G schalten, verdrahten
F enclencher, brancher, connecter

cono
E cone
G Kegel, Konus
F cône

conserva de sangre
E stored blood
G Blutkonserve
F sang conservé

conservabilidad
E stability
G Haltbarkeit
F stabilité

conservación
E preservation, retention, storage, archiving
G Konservierung, Aufbewahrung
F conservation, stockage, archivage

conservado
E preserved
G konserviert
F conservé

conservar
E preserve, to; retain, to; store, to
G konservieren, aufbewahren
F conserver, garder

conservar frío
E refrigerate, to
G kühl lagern
F réfrigérer, refroidir

consigna
E password
G Paßwort
F mot de passe

consistencia
E consistency
G Konsistenz
F consistance

consistencia de un lote
E batch consistency
G Chargenkonsistenz
F consistance d'un lot

consistente
E stable
G haltbar
F stable

consorcio
E company, concern
G Konzern
F compagnie, consortium

constancia del peso
E constant weight
G Gewichtskonstanz
F constance d'un poids

constante
E uniform
G gleichmäßig
F uniforme

constante de tiempo
E time constant
G Zeitkonstante
F constante de temps

constricción
E constriction
G Verengung
F constriction

construcción de sostén
E supporting construction
G Stützkonstruktion
F construction de soutien

construcción especial
E special version
G Sonderausführung
F version spéciale

construido para
E designed for
G ausgelegt für
F prévu pour, construit pour

consumidor
E consumer
G Verbraucher
F consommateur

consumo
E consumption
G Verbrauch
F consommation

consumo de electricidad
E power consumption
G Stromaufnahme
F consommation d'électricité

consumo de energía
E power consumption
G Leistungsverbrauch
F consommation d'énergie

consumo de vapor
E steam consumption
G Dampfverbrauch
F consommation de vapeur

consumo energético
E energy consumption
G Energieverbrauch
F consommation d'énergie

contador
E counter
G Zähler
F compteur

contador de células
E cell counter
G Zellzähler
F compteur de cellules

contador de comprimidos
E tablet counter
G Zählbrett (für Tabletten)
F compteur de comprimés

contador de etiquetas
E label counter
G Etikettenzähler
F compteur d'étiquettes

contador de horas de funcionamiento
E running time meter
G Betriebsstundenzähler
F compteur d'heures de mise en service

contador de partículas
E particle counter
G Partikelzähler
F compteur de particules

contador de revoluciones
E revolution counter, tachymeter
G Drehzahlmesser
F compte-tours, tachymètre

contaminación
E impurity, contamination
G Verunreinigung
F impureté, contamination

contaminación cruzada
E cross-mix, cross-contamination
G Untermischung, Kreuzkontamination
F contamination croisée

contaminación de un producto
E product contamination
G Produktverunreinigung
F contamination d'un produit

contaminación primaria
E primary contamination
G Primärkontamination
F contamination primaire

contaminación procedente del aire
E contamination, airborne
G aus der Luft stammende Kontamination
F contamination transportée par l'air, contamination aéroportée

contaminación secundaria
E secondary contamination
G Sekundärkontamination
F contamination secondaire

contaminado
E contaminated
G kontaminiert
F contaminé

contaminantes microbianos
E microbial contaminants
G mikrobielle Kontaminanten
F contaminants microbiens

contaminar
E contaminate, to
G kontaminieren, verschmutzen
F contaminer

contenedor
E container, reaction vessel
G Ansatzbehälter, Gebinde
F container, récipient, conditionnement

contenedor portátil
E mobile vessel, mobile container
G fahrbarer Ansatzbehälter
F cuve sur roues, cuve mobile

contenido
E content
G Inhalt, Gehalt
F contenu

contenido en agua
E water content
G Wassergehalt
F teneur en eau

contenido en gérmenes
E bacterial (microbial) content
G Keimgehalt
F teneur en micro-organismes

contenido en humedad
E moisture content
G Feuchtigkeitsgehalt
F teneur en humidité

contenido en materia sólida
E solid matter content
G Feststoffgehalt
F teneur en matière solide

contenido en oxígeno
E oxygen content
G Sauerstoffgehalt
F teneur en oxygène

contenido mínimo
E minimum contents
G Mindestinhalt
F contenu minimal

contenido total en carbono
E total organic carbon (TOC)
G Gesamtkohlenstoffgehalt
F teneur totale en carbone

contenido total en carbono orgánico
E total organic carbon (TOC)
G gesamtorganischer Kohlenstoff
F teneur totale en carbone organique

continuo
E continuous
G stufenlos
F continu

contrabrida
E counter-flange
G Gegenflansch
F contre-bride

contraerse
E shrink, to
G schrumpfen
F rétrécir

contraindicación
E contraindication
G Kontraindikation, Gegenanzeige
F contre-indication

contraindicado
E contraindicated
G kontraindiziert
F contre-indiqué

contraión
E counter-ion
G Gegenion
F contre-ion, ion complémentaire

contrapeso
E counter-weight
G Gegengewicht
F contrepoids

contrapresión
E support pressure
G Stützdruck
F contre-pression

contrapresión (en cromatografía)
E back pressure
G Gegendruck (in der Chromatographie)
F contre-pression

contrato
E contract
G Vertrag
F contrat

contrato de confidencialidad
E secrecy agreement
G Geheimhaltungsvertrag
F accord de confidentialité

control
E control, check, supervision
G Kontrolle, Aufsicht, Steuerung
F contrôle, supervision, surveillance

control antes de entrega
E pre-delivery check, factory acceptance test
G Vorabnahme (beim Hersteller)
F contrôle avant livraison

control de calidad
E quality control (QC)
G Qualitätskontrolle (QK)
F contrôle-qualité, contrôle de la qualité

control de comprimidos
E tablet checking
G Tablettenkontrolle
F contrôle d'un comprimé

English German French Spanish

control de desgarro de láminas
E film tear sensor
G Folienrißkontrolle
F contrôle des déchirures de feuilles

control de entrada de mercancías
E inspection of incoming goods
G Wareneingangsprüfung
F contrôle des livraisons de marchandises

control de fragmentos
E fragment control
G Bruchstückkontrolle
F contrôle des fragments

control de impresos
E print control (printed matter)
G Druckkontrolle (von Aufdruckdaten)
F contrôle de l'impression

control de la cantidad de relleno
E quantity control
G Füllmengenkontrolle
F contrôle de la quantité de remplissage

control de la expulsión
E ejection control
G Auswurfgegenkontrolle
F contrôle de l'éjection

control de las válvulas
E flap control
G Klappensteuerung
F guidage de clapet

control de lotes
E batch control
G Chargenkontrolle
F contrôle des lots

control de modificaciones
E change control, change management
G Änderungskontrolle
F contrôle des changements, contrôle des modifications

control de partículas
E particle monitoring
G Partikelmonitoring
F contrôle des particules

control de plagas
E pest control
G Schädlingsbekämpfung
F lutte antiparasitaire

control de plantas e instalaciones
E plant control
G Anlagensteuerung
F système de contrôle d'une installation

control de polvo
E dust control
G Staubkontrolle
F contrôle de la poussière

control de presión (en caso de sobrepresión)
E pressure control (excess pressure)
G Druckkontrolle (bei Überdruck)
F contrôle de la pression

control de un proceso
E process control
G Prozeßsteuerung
F contrôle d'un procédé

control del contenido
E content control
G Füllgutkontrolle
F contrôle du contenu

control del entorno
E environmental monitoring
G Umgebungskontrolle
F contrôle de l'environnement

control del peso
E weight control
G Gewichtskontrolle
F contrôle du poids

control del programa
E programme control
G Programmsteuerung
F contrôle d'un programme

control durante el proceso
E in-process control (IPC)
G In-Prozeß-Kontrolle
F contrôle lors de la fabrication

control ecológico
E environmental control
G Umweltkontrolle
F contrôle de l'environnement

control intermediario
E intermediate control
G Zwischenkontrolle
F contrôle intermédiaire

control microbiano
E microbial control
G mikrobielle Kontrolle
F contrôle microbien

control oficial
E monitoring by the authorities
G behördliche Überwachung
F surveillance par les autorités

control óptico
E visual control
G optische Kontrolle
F contrôle visuel

control programable mediante memoria
E programmable logic control (PLC)
G speicherprogrammierbare Steuerung (SPS)
F automate programmable industriel

control remoto
E remote control
G Fernsteuerung, Fernüberwachung
F télécommande, télécontrôle

control visual
E visual control, visual observation
G optische Kontrolle, Sichtkontrolle, visuelle Überwachung
F contrôle visuel

controlado por ordenador
E computer-controlled
G computergesteuert
F contrôlé par ordinateur

controlado por placebo
E placebo-controlled
G placebokontrolliert
F contrôlé par placebo

controlador de la corriente de aire
E air flow controller
G Luftstromwächter
F régulateur d'écoulement d'air

controles de interruptor unipolar
E lever switch controls
G Kippschalter-Kontrollen
F interrupteurs à bascule

convección de aire
E air convection
G Luftkonvektion
F convection de l'air

conveniente
E suitable
G passend
F convenable

convenio
E agreement
G Vereinbarung
F accord, convention

conversión
E conversion
G Umrechnung
F conversion

conversión térmica
E thermal conversion
G thermische Umwandlung
F conversion thermique

convertibilidad (de una sustancia en una reacción)
E convertibility (of a substance in a reaction)
G Umwandlungsfähigkeit (einer Substanz in einer Reaktion)
F convertibilité (d'une substance en une réaction)

convertidor de mediciones
E measurement converter
G Meßumformer
F convertisseur

convexo
E convex
G nach außen gewölbt, konvex
F convexe

English
German
French
Spanish

convocatoria
E tender
G Ausschreibung
F appel d'offres

copia de seguridad
E back-up file
G Sicherheitskopie
F copie de sauvegarde

copia de seguridad de un banco de datos
E data base backup
G Datenbanksicherheitskopie
F backup d'une base de données

copo
E floc
G Flocke
F bourre

correa trapezoidal
E fan belt
G Keilriemen
F courroie trapézoïdale

corrección
E correction
G Korrektur, Berichtigung
F correction

corrección (de un método de prueba)
E accuracy
G Richtigkeit
F exactitude

corrección de errores
E trouble-shooting, failure rectification
G Fehlerbehebung
F dépannage, action de corriger

corredera
E cursor
G Schieber
F curseur

corredera de tracción inferior
E pull-down cam
G Niederzugsschiene
F came de poinçon descendante

corredor
E corridor
G Flur
F corridor

corredor de servicio
E service corridor
G Technikgang
F corridor de service

corresponder
E correspond, to
G entsprechen
F correspondre (à)

no corresponder
E not corresponding to
G nicht entsprechen
F différent de

corriente
E current
G laufend
F courant

corriente alterna
E alternating current (AC)
G Wechselstrom
F courant alternatif

corriente continua
E direct current
G Gleichstrom
F courant continu

corriente de aire
E air current
G Luftstrom
F écoulement d'air

corriente de alimentación
E power supply
G Versorgungsstrom
F courant d'alimentation

corriente de desconexión
E breaking current
G Ausschaltstrom
F courant de coupure

corriente de fuga
E leakage current
G Kriechstrom
F courant de cheminement

corriente eléctrica
E current, electricity
G Strom
F courant, électricité

corriente gaseosa
E gas flow
G Gasstrom
F débit de gaz

corriente laminar
E laminar air flow
G Laminarströmung
F flux d'air laminaire

corriente trifásica
E three-phase current
G Drehstrom
F courant triphasé

corroer
E corrode, to
G korrodieren
F corroder

corrosión
E corrosion
G Korrosion
F corrosion

corroyente
E corrosive
G korrodierend
F corrosif

cortacircuito
E fuse
G Sicherung (elektrisch)
F fusible

cortante
E sharp
G scharf
F coupant, aiguisé, piquant

cortar
E close off, to
G absperren
F fermer

corte de corriente
E power failure
G Stromausfall
F coupure de courant

corte intermitente de corriente
E intermittent power interruption
G zeitweiser Stromausfall
F coupure de courant intermittente

corte transitorio de corriente
E intermittent power interruption
G zeitweiser Stromausfall
F coupure de courant intermittente

cortocircuito
E short circuit
G Kurzschluß
F court-circuit

cosechar
E harvest, to
G ernten
F récolter

cosméticos
E cosmetics
G Kosmetika
F cosmétiques

costes de adquisición
E purchase price
G Anschaffungskosten
F frais d'achat

costes de explotación
E current cost
G laufende Kosten
F coûts d'exploitation

costes de funcionamiento
E operational costs
G Betriebskosten
F coûts de fonctionnement

costes de instalación
E installation costs
G Installationskosten
F coûts d'une installation

costes de inversión
E investment costs
G Investitionskosten
F coûts d'investissements

costes del personal
E personnel cost
G Personalkosten
F coûts du personnel

costes preliminares
E up-front costs
G Vorauskosten
F coûts préalables

costura
E seam
G Naht
F couture, ourlet

covalente
E covalent
G kovalent
F covalent

crecimiento celular
E cell growth
G Zellwachstum
F croissance de cellules

crecimiento de moho
E mould growth
G Schimmelbefall
F formation de moisissure

crecimiento microbiano
E microbial growth
G mikrobielles Wachstum
F croissance microbienne

crema
E cream
G Creme
F crème

crema auricular
E ear cream
G Ohrencreme
F crème auriculaire

crema nasal
E nasal cream
G Nasencreme
F crème nasale

crema oftálmica
E eye cream
G Augencreme
F crème ophtalmique

crema rectal
E rectal cream
G Rektalcreme
F crème rectale

crema vaginal
E vaginal cream
G Vaginalcreme
F crème vaginale

cremado (de emulsiones)
E creaming (of emulsions)
G Aufrahmung (bei Emulsionen)
F crémage (d'une émulsion)

crematorio
E incinerator
G Verbrennungsanlage
F incinérateur

criba
E sieve
G Sieb
F tamis

cribar
E sieve, to; sift, to
G sieben
F tamiser

crisol
E crucible
G Tiegel
F creuset

cristal de sembrado
E seed crystal
G Impfkristall
F germe cristallin

cristales secundarios
E secondary crystals
G Sekundärkristalle
F cristaux secondaires

cristalino
E crystalline
G kristallin
F cristallin

cristalización
E crystallisation
G Kristallisierung, Auskristallisierung
F cristallisation

cristalización de inclusión
E inclusion crystallisation
G Einschlußkristallisation
F cristallisation occlusive

cristalizar
E crystallise, to
G kristallisieren
F cristalliser

cristalizar completamente
E crystallise out, to
G auskristallisieren
F se cristalliser complètement

criterio
E criterion
G Kriterium
F critère

siguiendo criterios estrictos (p. ej. test)
E according to stringent criteria (e. g. testing)
G gemäß strengen Kriterien (z. B. Test)
F selon des critères sévères (par ex. un test)

criterio de aceptación
E acceptance criterion
G Akzeptanzkriterium
F critère d'acceptation

criterio de dosificación
E dose criterion
G Dosiskriterium
F critère de dosage

cromado
E chromium plated
G verchromt
F chromé

cromatografía
E chromatography
G Chromatographie
F chromatographie

cromatografía ascendente
E ascending chromatography
G aufsteigende Chromatographie
F chromatographie ascendante

cromatografía descendente
E descending chromatography
G absteigende Chromatographie
F chromatographie descendante

cromatografía de adsorción
E adsorption chromatography
G Adsorptionschromatographie
F chromatographie d'adsorption

cromatografía de afinidad
E affinity chromatography
G Affinitätschromatographie
F chromatographie d'affinité

cromatografía de cationes
E cation chromatography
G Kationenchromatographie
F chromatographie sur résine échangeuse de cations

cromatografía de exclusión
E size exclusion chromatography
G Ausschlußchromatographie
F chromatographie par limite d'exclusion

cromatografía de exclusión iónica
E ion exclusion chromatography
G Ionenausschlußchromatographie
F chromatographie d'exclusion ionique

English German French Spanish

cromatografía de gases
E gas chromatography
G Gaschromatographie
F chromatographie en phase gazeuse

cromatografía de intercambio de ligandos ópticamente activos
E chiral ligand exchange chromatography
G chirale Ligandenaustausch-chromatographie
F chromatographie d'échange de ligands optiquement actifs

cromatografía de intercambio iónico
E ion exchange chromatography
G Ionenaustauschchromatographie
F chromatographie par échange d'ions

cromatografía de pares de iones
E ion pair chromatography
G Ionenpaarchromatographie
F chromatographie par paires d'ions

cromatografía en capa fina
E thin layer chromatography (TLC)
G Dünnschichtchromatographie (DC)
F chromatographie sur couche mince

cromatografía en fase inversa
E reverse-phase chromatography
G Umkehrphasenchromatographie
F chromatographie en phase inverse

cromatografía líquida a alta presión
E high pressure liquid chromatography (HPLC)
G Hochdruckflüssigkeitschromato-graphie
F chromatographie liquide sous haute pression

cromatografía sobre gel
E gel chromatography
G Gelchromatographie
F chromatographie sur gel

cromatograma
E chromatogram
G Chromatogramm
F chromatogramme

croquis transversal
E sectional drawing
G Querschnittszeichnung
F croquis de section

cruz de la balanza
E weighing beam
G Wiegebalken
F fléau de balance

cuaderno de bitácora
E log book
G Logbuch
F cahier de route

cuadro de distribución
E control panel
G Schalttafel
F pupitre de commande, tableau de commande

cuadro de mandos
E panel, control panel
G Armaturentafel, Schalttafel
F tableau de bord, pupitre de commande, tableau de commande

cuajamiento
E caking, cake formation
G Kuchenbildung
F prise en masse

cualidad
E quality
G Qualität
F qualité

cualificación
E qualification
G Qualifizierung
F qualification

cualificación de la software
E software qualification
G Softwarequalifizierung
F qualification d'un logiciel

cualificación de un procedimiento
E performance qualification
G Verfahrensqualifizierung
F qualification des performances (d'un procédé)

cualificación de una instalación
E installation qualification
G Installationsqualifizierung
F qualification de l'installation

cualificación del abastecedor
E supplier qualification
G Lieferantenqualifizierung
F qualification de fournisseur

cualificación del equipamiento
E equipment qualification
G Qualifizierung der Ausrüstung
F qualification de l'équipement

cualificación del rendimiento
E performance qualification
G Leistungsqualifizierung
F qualification des performances (d'un procédé)

cualificación funcional
E operational qualification (OP)
G Funktionsqualifizierung
F qualification des opérations, qualification opérationnelle

cuantía
E dimensions
G Abmessungen, Ausmaß
F dimensions

cuantificable
E quantifiable
G quantitativ bestimmbar
F quantifiable

cuantitativo
E quantitative
G quantitativ
F quantitatif

cuarentena
E quarantine
G Quarantäne, Sperrung
F quarantaine

cuarzo
E quartz
G Quarz
F quartz

cubeta
E cuvette, cell
G Küvette
F cuvette

cubeta de vidrio
E glass cuvette
G Glasküvette
F cuvette en verre

cubierta
E cover, hood, coat, film
G Haube, Abdeckung, Überzug, Verkleidung
F couvercle, capuchon, couche, pellicule, revêtement

cubierta de la máquina
E machine cover
G Maschinenabdeckung
F couvercle de machine

cubierta de polietileno
E polyethylene coating
G Polyethylenbeschichtung
F couverture en polyéthylène

cubierta de una cápsula
E capsule shell
G Kapselhülse
F gousse d'une capsule

cubierta de uso único
E disposable cover
G Einmalabdeckung
F couvercle à usage unique, capuchon à usage unique

cubierta del orificio de seguridad
E explosion relief duct cover
G Ex-Kanalabdeckung
F couvercle de canalisation anti-déflagrant

cubierta doble
E double jacket
G Doppelmantel
F double manchon, double manteau

English German French Spanish

cubierta resistente al jugo gástrico, con
E enteric-coated
G magensaftresistent überzogen
F à enrobage entérique

cubo del agitador
E stirrer hub
G Rührwerksnabe
F moyeu d'agitateur

cubrejunta de pestaña
E tab, tongue
G Einstecklasche
F languette, attache, patte

cubreobjetos (microscopio)
E cover glass, cover slip (microscopy)
G Deckglas, Abdeckplatte (Mikroskopie)
F lame de protection, plaquette en verre, verre de protection (microscopie)

cubrir (comprimidos)
E cap, to (tablets)
G deckeln (Tabletten)
F capsuler (comprimés)

cuchara de medida
E measuring spoon
G Meßlöffel
F cuillère-mesure

cuello de ampolla
E ampoule neck
G Ampullenhals
F col d'une ampoule

cuello de botella
E bottle neck
G Flaschenhals
F goulot, col de bouteille

cuello de troquel
E punch neck
G Stempelhals
F collet du poinçon

cuentagotas
E drop counter
G Tropfenzähler
F compte-gouttes

cuerpo extraño
E foreign body
G Fremdkörper
F corps étranger

cuerpo hueco
E hollow article, hollow body
G Hohlkörper
F corps creux

cuestionario
E questionnaire, trial form, case report form
G Fragebogen, Prüfbogen
F questionnaire

cultivo celular
E cell culture
G Zellkultur
F culture de cellules

cultivo celular heteroploide
E heteroploid cell culture
G heteroploide Zellkultur
F culture de cellules hétéroploïde

cultivo continuo
E continuous culture
G kontinuierliche Kultur
F culture en continu

cultivo de células de mamífero
E mammalian cell culture
G Säugetierzellkultur
F culture de cellules de mammifère

cultivo de células diploides
E diploid cell culture
G diploide Zellkultur
F culture de cellules diploides

cultivo de células tisulares
E tissue cell culture
G Gewebezellkultur
F culture de cellules tissulaires

cultivo madre (de organismos)
E stock culture
G Stammkultur
F culture mère

cumplimiento
E compliance, fulfilment, realisation
G Einhaltung, Erfüllung
F conformité, réalisation

cuño
E hob, punch
G Prägestempel
F poinçon

curado
E curing
G Aushärtung
F trempe

curar
E cure, to
G aushärten
F tremper

cursor
E cursor
G Schieber
F curseur

curva ascendente
E ascending curve
G Aufwärtskurve
F courbe ascendante

curva de calibración
E calibration curve
G Kalibrierkurve
F courbe de calibration

curva de expulsión (de prensa de comprimidos)
E ejector cam
G Auswerfkurve, Auswurfkurve
F came d'éjection

curva de relleno (prensa de comprimidos)
E filling cam (tablet press)
G Füllkurve (bei der Tablettenpresse)
F came de remplissage

curva de titulación
E titration curve
G Titrationskurve
F courbe de titrage, courbe de dosage

curvatura
E bend, flexure
G Biegung
F courbure, pliage

dañado
E defective, damaged
G beschädigt
F défectueux, endommagé

dañino
E harmful, hazardous
G schädlich
F nocif

daño
E damage
G Beschädigung
F dommage, dégâts

daño ecológico
E environmental damage
G Umweltschaden
F atteinte à l'environnement

daños de transporte
E transport damage
G Transportschaden
F dégâts dûs au transport

dar la primera capa
E prime, to
G grundieren
F amorcer

dar salida
E drain, to; discharge, to (liquids)
G ablassen (Flüssigkeiten)
F faire couler, laisser s'écouler

datos
E data, specifications
G Daten, Angaben
F données, spécifications

datos brutos
E raw data
G Rohdaten
F données brutes

datos de producción
E production data
G Produktionsdaten
F données de production

datos de validación
E validation data
G Validierungsdaten
F données de validation

datos genómicos
E genomic data
G Genomdaten
F données génomiques

decantación
E drain
G Abguß
F conduit d'écoulement, drain

decantar
E decant, to
G abgießen, dekantieren
F décanter, transvaser

decapado
E pickled
G gebeizt
F décapé

decapado y pulido
E pickled and blasted
G gebeizt und gestrahlt
F poncé et décapé

declive
E gradient, slope
G Gefälle
F pente, inclinaison

decocción
E decoction
G Abkochung, Decoct
F décoction

decoloración
E discoloration
G Verfärbung
F décoloration

decreto
E regulation
G Verordnung
F décret

decreto sobre narcóticos
E narcotics regulation
G Betäubungsmittelgesetz
F décret concernant les narcotiques

decreto sobre sustancias peligrosas
E regulations for hazardous goods, toxic chemical ordinance
G Gefahrstoffverordnung
F décret concernant les matières dangereuses

defecto
E deficiency
G Mangel
F déficience, carence, insuffisance

defecto de calidad
E defect, shortcoming
G Qualitätsmangel
F défaut de qualité

defecto de crecimiento
E growth defect
G Wachstumsdefekt
F défaut de croissance

defecto de embalaje
E packaging defect
G Verpackungsfehler
F défaut de conditionnement

defecto de registro
E register defect
G Passerfehler
F défaut de registre

defectuoso
E defective, faulty
G fehlerhaft
F défectueux

deficiencia
E deficiency
G Mangel
F déficience, carence, insuffisance

deflector
E baffle, deflector
G Leitblech
F déflecteur

deformación
E deformation
G Verformung
F déformation

deformación de láminas
E film forming
G Folienverformung
F façonnage de feuilles

deformación térmica
E thermoforming
G Thermoverformung
F emboutissage

degradable
E degradable
G abbaubar
F dégradable

degradable biológicamente
E biodegradable
G biologisch abbaubar
F biodégradable

degradación
E degradation, decomposition
G Abbau, Zersetzung
F dégradation, décomposition

degradación biológica
E biodegradation
G biologischer Abbau
F biodégradation

degradación ecológica
E environmental waste
G Umweltverschmutzung
F pollution de l'environnement

dejar escapar
E drain, to; discharge, to (liquids)
G ablassen (Flüssigkeiten)
F faire couler, laisser s'écouler

dejar precipitar
E allow to stand, to
G absetzen lassen
F laisser sédimenter,
laisser se déposer

dejar sedimentar
E allow to stand, to
G absetzen lassen
F laisser sédimenter,
laisser se déposer

delantal
E skirting, apron (of machine)
G Abhängung, Schürze
F tablier

demostración
E detection, evidence, proof
G Nachweis
F détection, preuve

denominación
E designation
G Bezeichnung
F désignation, appellation

denominar
E label, to; designate, to
G bezeichnen
F étiqueter

densidad
E density
G Dichte
F densité

densidad absoluta
E absolute density
G absolute Dichte
F densité absolue

English
German
French
Spanish

densidad aparente
E apparent density
G scheinbare Dichte
F densité apparente

densidad de apisonamiento
E packed density, tapped density
G Stampfdichte
F densité de tassement

densidad de células
E cell density
G Zelldichte
F densité de cellules

densidad de compresión
E tapped density, packed density
G Stampfdichte
F densité de package, densité de damage

densidad de la masa comprimida
E bulk density
G Schüttdichte
F densité apparente

densidad del polvo
E powder density
G Pulverdichte
F densité d'une poudre

densidad real
E true density
G wahre Dichte
F densité réelle

densidad relativa
E relative density
G relative Dichte
F densité relative

departamento
E department
G Abteilung
F département, service

departamento citado
E Notified Body
G Benannte Stelle
F organisme cité

departamento de farmacia galénica
E galenical development department
G Galenikabteilung
F département de développement galénique

departamento de personal
E personnel department
G Personalabteilung
F service de personnel

departamento de registros y licencias sanitarias
E regulatory affairs department
G Zulassungsabteilung
F département des affaires réglementaires

departamento técnico
E engineering
G Technik (als Abteilung)
F ingénierie

depósito
E warehouse, storage room, sediment, deposit
G Lagerraum, Ablagerung, Wandbelag
F entrepôt, dépôt, sédiment

depósito (colector)
E reservoir, collector
G Sammelbehälter
F réservoir, collecteur

depósito de carga
E feed silo
G Beschickungssilo
F trémie de charge

depósito de muestras (como mancha sobre la placa de cromatografía en capa fina)
E sample spotting (on TLC plate)
G Probenauftrag (als Fleck auf DC-Platte)
F application d'échantillons (sur plaque de CCM)

depresión
E recess, cavity, well, negative pressure
G Vertiefung, Unterdruck
F cavité, puits, sous-pression, depression

derecho de acceso
E authorised access
G Zugangsberechtigung
F autorisation d'accès

derivación
E ground, earth
G Ableitung, Erdung
F mise à la terre, prise de terre

derivado
E derivative
G Abkömmling, Derivat
F dérivé

derivado de aminoácido
E amino acid derivative
G Aminosäurederivat
F dérivé d'acide aminé

derramar
E spill, to
G verschütten
F renverser, répandre

derroche de material
E material wastage
G Materialverschwendung
F gaspillage

desacidificar
E deacidify, to
G entsäuern
F alcaliniser

desaguadero
E drain duct
G Abflußrinne
F rigole d'écoulement

desagüe
E outlet, discharge outlet, drain
G Auslauf, Abfluß
F sortie de vidange, sortie de purge, tuyau d'écoulement, drain

desalinizar
E desalt, to
G entsalzen
F dessaler

desarrollo
E development
G Entwicklung
F développement

desarrollo de resistencia
E development of resistance
G Resistenzentwicklung
F développement d'une résistance

desarrollo de un procedimiento
E process development
G Verfahrensentwicklung
F développement d'un procédé

desarrollo de un producto nuevo
E new product development
G Entwicklung eines neuen Produktes
F développement d'un nouveau produit

desbarbado
E deburring
G Entgratung
F ébarbage

desbarbador
E deburrer
G Entgrater
F ébarbeur

desbarbar
E deburr, to
G entgraten
F ébarber

desbastador
E deburrer
G Entgrater
F ébarbeur

desbloquear
E unlock, to
G entriegeln
F déverrouiller

desbordamiento
E overflow
G Überlauf
F débordement

descalcificar
E decalcify, to
G entkalken
F détartrer

descarga
E outlet, orifice, sink, relief
G Auslaß, Ausguß, Entlastung
F sortie, orifice, évier, soulagement, décharge

descarga de explosión
E explosion relief
G Explosionsentlastung
F décharge d'explosion

descargar
E discharge, to
G entladen
F décharger

descargar (pomada del contenedor)
E discharge, to (ointment from container)
G austragen (Salbe aus Container)
F décharger (la pommade du conteneur)

descenso de presión
E pressure drop
G Druckabfall
F chute de pression, dépressurisation

descenso de temperatura
E temperature decrease
G Temperaturabfall
F baisse de température

descodificador
E decoder
G Entschlüssler
F décodeur

descomposición
E decomposition
G Zersetzung
F décomposition

desconectar
E switch off, to
G abschalten
F couper, arrêter

desconexión (de una máquina)
E shut down (of a machine)
G Abschaltung (einer Maschine)
F arrêt (d'une machine)

descongelar
E defrost, to; thaw, to
G auftauen
F dégeler

descontaminar
E decontamination
G Dekontamination
F décontamination

descripción
E description
G Beschreibung
F description

descripción de tareas
E required specification
G Pflichtenheft
F spécifications fonctionnelles

descripción de un producto
E product description
G Produktbeschreibung
F caractérisation d'un produit

descripción de un puesto de trabajo
E job description
G Stellenbeschreibung
F description d'un emploi

desecación por microondas
E microwave drying
G Mikrowellentrocknung
F séchage à micro-ondes

desecante
E desiccator, desiccant
G Exsiccator, Trocknungsmittel
F dessicateur, déshydratant, desséchant

desecar
E dry, to; dry out, to; desiccate, to
G trocknen, austrocknen, eintrocknen
F sécher, dessiquer

desecho
E waste, disposal
G Abfall, Ausschuß, Entsorgung
F ordures, déchets

desecho de filtración
E filtrate waste
G Filtrationsabfall
F effluent de filtration

desecho fluido
E aqueous waste
G Flüssigabfall
F effluent aqueux

desechos
E rubbish, waste
G Müll
F déchets, résidus

desembocadura
E orifice
G Mündung
F orifice

desempolvamiento
E dedusting
G Entstaubung
F action de dépoussiérer, dépoussiérage

desempolvante
E deduster
G Entstauber
F dépoussiéreur

desengrasar
E degrease, to
G entfetten
F dégraisser

desgarro
E crack, tear
G Riß
F déchirure, fissure

desgasificación (de líquidos)
E degassing, deaeration (of liquids)
G Entgasung (von Flüssigkeiten)
F dégazage

desgasificador de vacío
E vacuum degasification
G Vakuumentgaser
F dégasification à vide

desgasificar
E degas, to; deaerate, to
G entgasen
F dégazer, désaérer

desgastado
E worn out
G ausgeleiert
F usé

desgaste
E wear and tear, stress, strain
G Abnutzung, Beanspruchung, Verschleiß
F usure, soumission à un effort

desgaste ecológico
E environmental waste
G Umweltverschmutzung
F pollution de l'environnement

deshidratación
E dehydration
G Dehydratisierung
F déhydratation

deshidratante
E desiccant
G Trocknungsmittel
F déshydratant, desséchant

designado (para algo)
E designated (for)
G bestimmt (für)
F désigné pour

desinfección
E disinfection
G Desinfektion
F désinfection

desinfección de instrumentos
E instrument disinfection
G Gerätedesinfektion
F désinfection des instruments

desinfección de la sala
E room disinfection
G Raumdesinfektion
F désinfection de locaux

desinfección de manos
E hand disinfection
G Händedesinfektion
F désinfection des mains

desinfectable
E disinfectable
G desinfizierbar
F désinfectable

desinfectantes autorizados
E approved disinfectants
G Desinfektionsmittel, zugelassene
F désinfectants autorisés

desinfectar
E disinfect, to; marinate, to; pickle, to
G desinfizieren, entkeimen, beizen
F désinfecter, mariner

desintegración
E disintegration
G Zerfall
F désintégration

desintegración radiactiva
E radioactive decay
G radioaktiver Zerfall
F désintégration radioactive

desintegrante
E disintegrant, tablet disintegrant
G Sprengmittel
F agent délitant, désintégrant

desintegrar(se)
E disintegrate, to
G zerfallen
F se désintégrer, se désagréger

deslizamiento de una lámina
E film slippage
G Folienschlupf
F glissement d'une feuille

deslizar
E slip, to
G gleiten
F couler, glisser

deslustrarse (metales)
E tarnish, to (metal)
G anlaufen (Metall)
F ternir, se ternir (métal)

desmineralizar
E deionise, to
G entmineralisieren
F déminéraliser

desmontable
E detachable, removable
G entfernbar, abnehmbar
F amovible, démontable, détachable

desmontaje
E disassembly, dismantling, removal
G Demontage, Zerlegung, Ausbau
F démontage

desmontaje de un filtro
E filter removal
G Filterausbau
F démontage de filtre

desnaturalización
E denaturing
G Denaturierung
F dénaturation

desnaturalizado
E denatured
G denaturiert, vergällt
F dénaturé

desocupado
E unmanned
G mannlos
F inoccupé

despedir
E make redundant, to
G entlassen
F renvoyer, licencier, congédier

desperfecto
E breakdown, downtime (machine), failure
G Ausfall
F panne, temps mort, défaillance

despido
E redundancy
G Entlassung
F licenciement

despirogenación
E depyrogenation
G Entpyrogenisierung
F dépyrogénation

despirogenar
E depyrogenate, to
G entpyrogenisieren
F dépyrogéner

desplazar
E transfer, to; relocate, to
G verlagern
F transférer, déplacer

despojos
E debris
G Bruch
F débris

desprotonización
E deprotonation
G Deprotonierung
F déprotonation

destilación en vacío
E vacuum distillation
G Vakuumdestillation
F distillation sous vide

destilado
E distillate
G Destillat
F distillat

destilar
E distil, to; distil off, to
G destillieren, abdestillieren
F distiller

destrucción
E destruction, killing
G Vernichtung, Abtötung
F destruction, action de tuer

destruir
E destroy, to; kill, to
G vernichten, abtöten
F détruire, tuer

desviación
E deviation
G Abweichung
F déviation, écart

desviación (de una aguja indicadora)
E deflection (of pointer)
G Ausschlag (eines Zeigers)
F déviation (d'une aiguille)

desviación de la línea de base
E baseline drift
G Basisliniendrift
F dérive de la ligne de base

desviación de temperatura
E temperature deviation
G Temperaturabweichung
F déviation de température

desviación del punto cero
E zero drift
G Nullpunktabweichung
F dérive du point zero

desviación estándar
E standard deviation
G Standardabweichung
F déviation standard

English German French Spanish

English German French Spanish

desviación estándar máxima permitida
E maximum permitted standard deviation
G maximal zulässige Standardabweichung
F déviation standard maximum permise

desviación estándar relativa
E relative standard deviation
G relative Standardabweichung
F écart-type relatif

desviar
E deflect, to
G ablenken
F dévier

detección amperométrica
E amperometric detection
G amperometrische Detektion
F détecteur ampérométrique

detección de sustancias activas
E active substance screening
G Wirkstoffscreening
F screening de principes actifs

detectable
E detectable
G nachweisbar, detektierbar
F détectable

detector de captura electrónica
E electron capture detector (ECD)
G Elektroneneinfangdetektor
F détecteur à capture électronique

detector de conductividad térmica
E conductivity detector
G Wärmeleitfähigkeitsdetektor
F conductimètre

detector de humedad
E humidity detector
G Feuchtesensor
F détecteur d'humidité

detector de humo
E smoke detector
G Rauchmelder
F détecteur de fumée

detector de ionización de llama
E flame ionisation detector (FID)
G Flammenionisationsdetektor (FID)
F détecteur à ionisation de flamme

detector de luz dispersa
E light-scattering detector
G Streulicht-Detektor
F détecteur de lumière diffuse

detector de metales
E metal detector
G Metallsuchgerät
F détecteur de métaux

detector de nitrógeno fosforado
E nitrogen-phosphorous detector (NPD)
G Stickstoff-Phosphor-Detektor
F détecteur d'azote phosphorisé

detector de nivel de relleno
E level detector
G Füllstandsmelder
F détecteur de niveau

detector UV/VIS
E UV/VIS detector
G UV/VIS-Detektor
F détecteur UV/VIS

detención con ultrarrendimiento
E ultra-high throughput screening (UHTS)
G Screenen mit ultrahohem Durchsatz (UHTS)
F screening à ultra-haut rendement

detención de la máquina
E machine stoppage
G Maschinenstillstand
F arrêt de machine

detergente
E cleansing agent, detergent
G Reinigungsmittel
F agent de nettoyage

deteriorar(se)
E deteriorate, to
G verderben
F se détériorer, s'abîmer

deterioro
E deterioration
G Verderb
F détérioration, altération

determinación
E determination
G Bestimmung
F détermination, évaluation

determinación del contenido
E determination of content
G Gehaltsbestimmung
F détermination du contenu

determinación del contenido en agua
E water determination
G Wasserbestimmung
F détermination de la teneur en eau

determinante de la calidad
E quality-determining
G qualitätsbestimmend
F qui détermine la qualité

determinar
E determine, to
G ermitteln, bestimmen
F déterminer, évaluer

devolución
E reimbursement
G Erstattung
F remboursement

dextrógiro
E dextro-rotatory
G rechtsdrehend
F dextrogyre

diafragma
E aperture, diaphragm
G Lochblende
F diaphragme

diagnóstico
E diagnosis, report, finding
G Befund
F diagnose

diagnóstico in vitro
E in-vitro diagnosis
G In-vitro-Diagnose
F diagnostic in-vitro

diagrama
E diagram
G Diagramm
F diagramme

diagrama circular
E pie chart
G Kreisdiagramm
F diagramme à secteurs

diagrama de afinidad
E affinity diagram
G Affinitätsdiagramm
F diagramme d'affinité

diagrama de circuito
E circuit diagram, wiring diagram
G Schaltbild, Schaltdiagramm
F schéma de montage, schéma des connexions, diagramme des connexions

diagrama de fases
E phase diagram
G Phasendiagramm
F diagramme de phases

diagrama de flujo
E flow chart
G Flußdiagramm
F schéma fonctionnel

diagrama de flujo de procesos
E process flow diagram (PFD)
G Prozeßflußdiagramm
F schéma fonctionnel

diagrama de relaciones
E relationship diagram
G Relationsdiagramm
F schéma relationnel

diagrama en árbol
E tree diagram
G Baumdiagramm
F diagramme arborescent

diagrama en mátrix
E matrix diagram
G Matrixdiagramm
F diagramme matriciel

diagrama operacional
E flow chart
G Fließdiagramm
F schéma opérationel, schéma de marche, schéma de principe

diálisis peritoneal
E solution for peritoneal dialysis
G Peritonealdialyselösung
F solution pour dialyse péritonéale

diámetro
E diameter
G Durchmesser
F diamètre

diámetro de bobina
E reel diameter
G Rollendurchmesser
F diamètre de bobine

diámetro de la columna
E column diameter
G Säulendurchmesser
F diamètre de colonne

diámetro de poro
E pore diameter
G Porendurchmesser
F diamètre d'un pore

diámetro de una superficie
E surface diameter
G Oberflächendurchmesser
F diamètre d'une surface

diámetro del comprimido
E tablet diameter
G Tablettendurchmesser
F diamètre d'un comprimé

diámetro del disco matriz
E die plate diameter
G Matrizenscheibendurchmesser
F diamètre du plateau d'une matrice

diámetro interno
E internal diameter
G lichter Durchmesser
F diamètre interne

diario
E daily
G täglich
F journalier

diario de laboratorio
E laboratory notebook, log book
G Laborjournal
F cahier de laboratoire

dibujo
E drawing
G Zeichnung
F dessin, figure, schéma

dibujo técnico
E engineering drawing
G technische Zeichnung
F dessin technique

dictamen
E expertise, expert opinion
G Gutachten, Begutachtung
F expertise, avis d'expert, opinion d'expert

diferencia de presión
E pressure differential
G Druckdifferenz
F différence de pression

diferencia de registro
E register difference
G Passerdifferenz
F différence de registre

diferenciación de gérmenes
E microbial differentiation
G Keimdifferenzierung
F différentiation microbienne

dificultad de deslizamiento del troquel
E punch sticking
G Stempelschwergängigkeit
F difficulté de glissement d'un poinçon

difracción luminosa
E diffraction
G Lichtbeugung
F diffraction de la lumière

difusión
E diffusion
G Diffusion
F diffusion

digno de confianza
E reliable
G verläßlich
F fiable

dilatación
E expansion
G Ausdehnung
F expansion

dilución
E dilution, dissolution
G Verdünnung, Auflösung
F dilution, dissolution

dilución máxima permitida
E maximum valid dilution (MVD)
G maximal zulässige Verdünnung (MZV)
F dilution maximale autorisée

diluido
E dilute
G verdünnt
F dilué

diluir
E dilute, to; dissolve, to
G verdünnen, auflösen, lösen
F diluer, dissoudre

diluyente
E diluent, dissolution medium
G Verdünnungsmittel, Auflösemedium
F diluant, milieu de dissolution

diluyente orgánico
E organic solvent
G organisches Lösungsmittel
F solvant organique

diluyentes orgánicos halogenados
E halogen-containing organic solvents
G halogenhaltige organische Lösungsmittel
F solvants organiques halogènes

diluyentes orgánicos no halogenados
E halogen-free organic solvents
G halogenfreie organische Lösungsmittel
F solvants organiques non halogènes

dimensión
E dimensions, unit of measurement
G Abmessungen, Ausmaß, Meßgröße
F dimensions, unité de mesure

dimensión interna
E internal dimension
G Innenmaß
F dimension interne

dimensiones
E dimensions
G Ausmaß
F dimensions

dimensiones del comprimido
E tablet dimensions
G Tablettenabmessungen
F dimensions d'un comprimé

dimensiones externas
E external dimensions
G Außenmaße
F dimensions externes

dimensiones totales
E overall dimensions
G Gesamtabmessungen
F dimensions totales

dióxido de silicio
E silica
G Siliciumdioxid
F silice

English German French Spanish

dirección del flujo aéreo
E air flow direction
G Luftströmungsrichtung
F direction de l'écoulement d'air

directiva
E policy, guideline
G Leitlinie
F directive

directivo
E executive
G Führungskraft
F directeur, cadre dirigeant

director
E director, head (person)
G Direktor, Leiter (als Person)
F directeur

director de control
E head of quality control
G Kontrolleiter
F responsable du contrôle-qualité

director de departamento
E head of department
G Abteilungsleiter
F chef de département, chef de service

director de grupo
E group manager
G Gruppenleiter
F chef de département

director de producción
E head of production
G Herstellungsleiter
F directeur de production

director de taller
E plant manager
G Werksleiter
F directeur d'usine

director de ventas
E sales manager
G Vertriebsleiter
F directeur des ventes

director del departamento técnico
E head of engineering department
G Technischer Leiter
F directeur du département d'ingénierie

director técnico de la empresa
E Plant Manager
G Betriebsleiter
F directeur technique

directrices de GMP
E GMP guidelines
G GMP-Richtlinien
F règles GMP

observancia de directrices de GMP
E observance of GMP guidelines
G Befolgung von GMP-Richtlinien
F respect des règles GMP

puesta en práctica de directices de GMP
E implementation of GMP guidelines
G Umsetzung von GMP-Richtlinien
F mise en pratique des règles GMP

directriz
E directive, guideline
G Richtlinie
F directive

directriz general
E cross-functional guideline
G abteilungsübergreifende Richtlinie
F lignes directrices générales

dirigido por minuta
E menu-controlled
G menügesteuert
F commandé par menu

dirigir
E guide, to
G leiten
F diriger

disco
E lamella
G Lamelle
F lamelle

disco de ruptura
E bursting disk, rupture disk
G Berstscheibe
F disque de rupture

disco matriz
E die plate
G Matrizenscheibe
F plateau d'une matrice

disco para cierre hermético
E washer, gasket
G Dichtungsscheibe
F joint (rondelle)

discrepancia
E discrepancy
G Diskrepanz
F disparité, écart

diseminación de (polvo)
E dissemination of (dust)
G Verbreitung von (Staub)
F dissémination de (poussière)

diseñado para
E designed for
G ausgelegt für
F prévu pour, construit pour

diseño
E draft
G Entwurf
F ébauche

diseño de un envase
E package design
G Verpackungsdesign
F design du conditionnement

diseño de un estudio (clínico)
E study design, trial design
G Studiendesign
F design d'un essai clinique

diseño modular
E modular design
G Modularbauweise
F design modulaire

disfunción
E malfunction
G Funktionsstörung
F dysfonctionnement

disminución
E conicalness, conicity
G Verjüngung, Konizität
F amincissement

disminuido
E tapered, conical
G verjüngt, konisch
F conique

disminuir
E diminish, to
G vermindern
F diminuer

disociación
E dissociation
G Dissoziation
F dissociation

disolución
E dissolution
G Auflösung
F dissolution

disolvente
E dissolution medium
G Lösemedium
F milieu de dissolution

disolver
E dissolve, to
G auflösen, lösen
F dissoudre

dispersar
E disperse, to
G dispergieren
F disperser

dispersión
E dispersion, stray range
G Dispersion, Streubreite
F dispersion

dispersión (de valores)
E spread, distribution (of values)
G Streuung (von Werten)
F diffusion, dispersion (de valeurs)

dispersión coloidal
E colloidal dispersion
G Kolloiddispersion
F dispersion colloïdale

dispersión cromática
E colour dispersion
G Farbdispersion
F dispersion de la couleur

dispersión luminosa
E light scattering, stray light
G Lichtstreuung
F dispersion de la lumière

dispersión refringente
E refractive dispersion
G Brechungsdispersion
F dispersion refractive

disponible
E available
G verfügbar
F disponible

disposición de matrices
E die alignment
G Matrizenausrichtung
F ajustage de la matrice

disposición del ensayo
E trial design
G Versuchsanordnung
F design d'un essai clinique

dispositivo
E device
G Vorrichtung
F appareillage, dispositif

dispositivo basculante
E tilting device
G Kippvorrichtung
F dispositif de basculement

dispositivo de apilamiento
E stacking device
G Stapelvorrichtung
F dispositif de stockage

dispositivo de control por transiluminación
E see-through scanner
G Durchlichtkontrolleinrichtung
F analyseur à balayage

dispositivo de enfriamiento
E cooling device
G Abkühlvorrichtung
F dispositif de refroidissement

dispositivo de fijación (en básculas)
E beam arrest (balance)
G Arretiervorrichtung (bei Waagen)
F relève-plateau

dispositivo de guía
E guide, guiding device, guiding mechanism
G Führungsvorrichtung
F guide, dispositif de guidage, mécanisme de guidage

dispositivo de limpieza de filtros
E filter cleaning device
G Filterabreinigungsvorrichtung
F dispositif de nettoyage de filtre

dispositivo de medición
E measuring device
G Meßmittel
F instrument de mesure

dispositivo de relleno
E filling device, charging device, feed hopper
G Einfüllvorrichtung, Fülleinrichtung
F trémie de remplissage, dispositif d'alimentation, appareillage d'alimentation

dispositivo de seguridad
E safety device
G Sicherheitsvorrichtung
F dispositif de sécurité

dispositivo de suspensión de filtros
E filter suspension rack
G Filteraufhängevorrichtung
F crémaillère pour filtre

dispositivo de vigilancia
E monitoring device
G Überwachungseinrichtung
F appareil de contrôle, appareil de surveillance

dispositivo dosificante
E metering device, dosing device
G Dosiereinrichtung
F appareil doseur

dispositivo elevador
E lifting device
G Hebevorrichtung, Hubvorrichtung
F dispositif de levage, appareillage élévateur

dispositivo giratorio
E swing-out device, swivelling device
G Ausschwenkvorrichtung
F dispositif d'orientation

dispositivo para dosificar
E metering aid, dosing aid
G Dosierhilfe
F dispositif d'aide au dosage

dispositivo tensor rápido
E fast-clamping device
G Schnellspannvorrichtung
F dispositif de serrage rapide

dispuesto para el servicio
E ready-to-use
G gebrauchsfertig
F prêt à l'emploi

disruptor
E baffle, deflector
G Leitblech
F déflecteur

distancia entre placas
E plate spacing
G Plattenabstand
F distance entre plateaux

distinto
E distinct, clear
G deutlich
F distinct, clair

distribución
E distribution, delivery, sales
G Verteilung, Ausgabe, Auslieferung, Vertrieb
F distribution, livraison, ventes

distribución (de un líquido)
E dispensing (of a liquid)
G Verteilung (einer Flüssigkeit)
F délivrance (d'un liquide)

distribución aleatoria
E random distribution
G Zufallsverteilung
F distribution randomisée

distribución de calor
E heat distribution
G Wärmeverteilung
F distribution de chaleur

distribución de fases
E phase distribution
G Phasenverteilung
F distribution de phases

distribución de frecuencias
E frequency distribution
G Häufigkeitsverteilung
F distribution de fréquences

distribución de material de embalaje
E packaging material dispensary
G Packmittelausgabe
F distribution du matériel d'emballage

distribución de partículas
E particle distribution
G Partikelverteilung
F distribution des particules

distribución de sumas
E sum distribution
G Summenverteilung
F distribution des sommes

distribución de temperatura
E heat distribution
G Temperaturverteilung
F répartition de la température

distribución del calor
E heat distribution
G Hitzeverteilung
F distribution de chaleur

distribución del tamaño de los granos
E particle size distribution
G Korngrößenverteilung
F distribution de la taille des particules

distribuidor
E dispenser
G Verteiler, Spender
F distributeur

distribuir
E dispense, to
G ausgeben
F dépenser, distribuer

doblado
E angled, angular
G abgewinkelt
F à angles, angulaire

doblar
E bend, to; buckle, to
G knicken
F casser, couder

doble ciego
E double-blind
G doppelblind
F en double aveugle

doctorado
E graduate (with doctorate), PhD
G promoviert
F titulaire d'un doctorat

documentación
E documentation
G Dokumentation
F documentation

documentación de un proceso
E process documentation
G Prozeßdokumentation
F documentation d'un procédé

documentación electrónica de lotes
E electronic batch recording
G elektronische Chargendokumentation
F documentation électronique de lots

documentar
E document, to
G dokumentieren
F documenter

documento
E certificate
G Urkunde
F certificat

donante
E donor (person)
G Spender (als Person)
F donneur (personne)

dosier de solicitud de autorización
E submission file for marketing authorisation
G Zulassungsdossier
F dossier de demande d'autorisation de mise sur le marché

dosificación
E dosage
G Dosierung
F posologie

dosificar
E meter, to; dose, to
G abmessen, dosieren
F doser

dosis
E dose
G Dosis
F dose

dosis baja
E low dosage
G niedrige Dosis
F dose faible

dosis de mantenimiento
E maintenance dosage
G Erhaltungsdosis
F dose de maintien

dosis diaria
E daily dosage
G Tagesdosis
F dose journalière

dosis liminar
E threshold dosage
G Schwellendosis
F dose liminaire

dosis máxima
E maximum dosage
G Höchstdosis
F dose maximale

dosis mortal
E fatal dose
G tödliche Dosis
F dose mortelle

dosis reducida
E low-dosed
G niedrig dosiert
F à dose faible

dosis umbral
E threshold dosage
G Schwellendosis
F dose liminaire

dosis única
E single dose
G Einzeldosis
F dose unique

duplicado
E duplicate
G Duplikat
F duplicata

duración
E duration
G Dauer
F durée

duración de conservación
E shelf-life
G Haltbarkeitsdauer
F durée de conservation, durée de stockage

duración de la irradiación
E duration of exposure to radiation
G Bestrahlungsdauer
F durée d'exposition à l'irradiation

duración de la permanencia
E dwell time, residence time
G Aufenthaltsdauer
F temps de résidence

duración de la validez de una patente
E patent duration, patent life
G Patentgültigkeitsdauer
F durée de validité d'un brevet

duración de prueba
E duration of trial
G Studiendauer
F durée d'un essai

duradero
E durable, stable, solid
G dauerhaft, haltbar, fest
F durable, stable, solide

dureza
E hardness
G Härte
F dureté

dureza de la bola
E ball hardness
G Kugeldruckhärte
F dureté à la bille

dureza del agua
E water hardness
G Wasserhärte
F dureté de l'eau

dureza del comprimido
E tablet hardness
G Tablettenhärte
F dureté d'un comprimé

English German French Spanish

dureza permanente (del agua)
E permanent hardness (of water)
G permanente Härte (von Wasser)
F dureté permamente (de l'eau)

dureza residual (p. ej. del agua)
E residual hardness (e. g. of water)
G Resthärte (z. B. von Wasser)
F dureté résiduelle (par ex. de l'eau)

dureza Rockwell (de herramientas)
E Rockwell hardness (of tools)
G Rockwell-Härte (von Werkzeug)
F dureté Rockwell (outils)

dureza temporal (del agua)
E temporary hardness (of water)
G temporäre Härte (von Wasser)
F dureté temporaire (de l'eau)

ebonita
E hard rubber, vulcanite
G Hartgummi
F caoutchouc durci, ébonite

ecológico
E environmentally friendly, non-polluting
G umweltfreundlich
F écologique

ecologista
E environmentalist, ecologist
G Umweltschützer
F écologiste

económico
E cost-efficient
G kosteneffizient
F économique

ecuación (matemática)
E equation
G Gleichung (mathematisch)
F équation

edición
E edition, version, issue
G Version
F édition, version

edición digital
E digital read out
G digitale Ausgabe
F édition numérique

edificio
E building
G Gebäude
F bâtiment, édifice

educación
E education, training
G Ausbildung
F éducation

edulcorante
E sweetener
G Süßstoff
F édulcorant

efecto
E effect
G Einwirkung
F effet

efecto colateral
E side effect
G Nebenwirkung
F effet secondaires

efecto secundario
E side effect
G Nebenwirkung
F effet secondaires

eficacia
E efficacy
G Wirksamkeit
F efficacité

eficacia desinfectante
E disinfecting effectiveness
G desinfizierende Wirksamkeit
F efficacité de la désinfection

eficaz
E effective, potent
G wirksam
F efficace

eficiencia
E efficiency
G Effizienz
F efficacité

eje
E shaft
G Schaft, Welle
F arbre, essieu, tige

eje de rotación
E axis of rotation
G Drehachse
F axe de rotation

eje longitudinal
E longitudinal axis
G Längsachse
F axe longitudinal

eje X
E X-axis
G X-Achse
F axe des abscisses

eje Y
E Y-axis
G Y-Achse
F axe des ordonnées

ejecutante
E operator
G Durchführender
F exécutant, opérateur

ejecutar
E carry out, to; execute, to
G durchführen
F réaliser, exécuter

ejecutivo
E executive
G Führungskraft
F directeur, cadre dirigeant

elaboración
E processing
G Verarbeitung, Bearbeitung
F fabrication, mise en forme, traitement

elaboración automático
E machine processing
G maschinelle Verarbeitung
F traitement automatique

elaboración manual
E manual processing
G manuelle Verarbeitung
F traitement manuel

elaboración previa del medicamento
E medicinal product premix, drug premix
G Arzneimittelvormischung
F préparation pharmaceutique

elaborar
E compile, to
G erstellen
F compiler, produire

elasticidad
E elasticity
G Elastizität
F élasticité

elástico
E elastic
G elastisch
F élastique

electrodo
E electrode
G Elektrode
F électrode

electrodo de vidrio
E glass electrode
G Glaselektrode
F électrode de verre

electroforesis capilar
E capillary electrophoresis
G Kapillarelektrophorese
F électrophorèse capillaire

electroforesis horizontal
E horizontal electrophoresis
G Horizontalelektrophorese
F électrophorèse horizontale

electroforesis vertical
E vertical electrophoresis
G Vertikalelektrophorese
F électrophorèse verticale

electrólisis
E electrolysis
G Elektrolyse
F électrolyse

electrólito
E electrolyte
G Elektrolyt
F électrolyte

electrotécnica y técnicas de medida y regulación
E measuring and control technology
G Elektro-, Meß- und Regeltechnik (EMR)
F électrotechnique et techniques de mesure et de réglage

elemento calefactor
E heating element
G Heizelement
F élément chauffant

elemento de manejo
E control knob
G Bedienungselement
F bouton de contrôle

elemento fuera de los márgenes habituales
E outlier
G Ausreißer
F valeur aberrante, anormale

elemento interruptor
E switch module
G Schaltelement
F élément commutateur

elemento termoeléctrico
E thermocouple
G Thermoelement
F thermocouple

eliminación
E disposal, removal, deconcentration
G Beseitigung, Entsorgung, Entfernung, Abreicherung
F élimination, rejet

eliminación de desechos
E waste disposal
G Abfallbeseitigung, Abfallentsorgung
F élimination des déchets, élimination des résidus

eliminación de pirógenos
E depyrogenation
G Entpyrogenisierung
F dépyrogénation

eliminación de virus
E removal of viruses, virus removal
G Virusabreicherung, Virusentfernung
F élimination des virus

eliminación del principio activo
E excretion of medicinal substance
G Arzneistoffausscheidung
F élimination d'un principe actif

eliminar (p. ej. virus)
E deplete, to; reduce, to (e. g. viruses)
G abreichern (z. B. Viren)
F éliminer (par exemple des virus)

eliminar errores
E eliminate a failure (fault), to
G Fehler beseitigen
F éliminer une erreur

eliminar pirógenos
E depyrogenate, to
G entpyrogenisieren
F dépyrogéner

eluado
E eluate
G Eluat
F éluat

eludir
E avoid, to
G vermeiden
F éviter

embalado en blísters
E blister pack
G Blisterverpackung
F conditionnement à bulles, conditionnement blister, plaquette thermoformée

embalaje
E package, pack, packaging
G Packung, Verpackung (als Vorgang)
F emballage, conditionnement

embalaje a prueba de niños
E child-proof packaging
G kindersichere Verpackung
F emballage de sécurité pour enfants

embalaje con gas inerte
E inert gas packaging
G Schutzgasverpackung
F emballage avec gaz inerte

embalaje de exportación
E export package
G Exportverpackung
F emballage à l'export

embalaje de plástico
E plastic packaging
G Kunststoffverpackung
F emballage plastique

embalaje de uso único
E disposable packaging
G Einwegverpackung, Wegwerfpackung
F conditionnement à usage unique

embalaje externo
E outer packaging
G Umverpackung
F emballage externe

embalaje impermeable al aire
E air-tight pack
G Verpackung, luftdichte
F emballage étanche à l'air

embalaje para clínica
E hospital pack
G Klinikpackung
F conditionnement pour hôpitaux

embalaje por comisión
E contract packaging
G Lohnverpackung
F empaquetage par sous-traitance

embalaje sellado
E sealed packaging
G Versiegelungsverpackung
F emballage hermétique

embalar
E pack, to; package, to
G einpacken, verpacken, konfektionieren
F emballer

embeber
E soak, to; impregnate, to
G tränken, imprägnieren
F imprégner

embocadura
E mouthpiece
G Mundstück
F embout

émbolo
E piston
G Kolben (technisch)
F piston

embotelladora
E bottling machine
G Flaschenabfüllmaschine
F machine de remplissage des bouteilles

embotellamiento
E filling
G Abfüllung
F remplissage

embrague
E coupling
G Kupplung
F couplage

embudo
E funnel, hopper
G Trichter
F entonnoir, trémie

embudo de Buechner
E Buchner funnel
G Nutsche
F entonnoir de Büchner

embudo de carga
E feed hopper
G Beschickungstrichter
F trémie de charge

embudo de llenado
E hopper
G Fülltrichter
F trémie

embudo de relleno
E filling funnel, charging funnel
G Einfülltrichter
F trémie de charge

embudo de separación
E separating funnel
G Scheidetrichter
F entonnoir séparateur

embutir a profundidad
E deep draw, to
G tiefziehen
F emboutir

emisión
E emission
G Emission
F émission

emitir
E eject, to
G ausstoßen
F éjecter, expulser, rejeter

empalidecer
E fade, to
G verblassen
F perdre sa couleur, se défraîchir

empalme
E support
G Stutzen
F support, embout

empalme de aspiración
E aspiration nipple
G Ansaugstutzen
F manchon d'aspiration

empalme de conexión
E connection port, connection nipple
G Anschlußstutzen
F douille de connexion, manchon de connexion

empalme de eliminación
E waste output
G Entsorgungsanschluß
F conduite destinée aux déchets

empalme de salida
E discharge nipple, drain nipple, outlet nipple, discharge port, outlet port
G Ablaßstutzen, Ablaufstutzen, Auslaufstutzen
F manchon d'écoulement, manchon de drainage, manchon de purge

empalme para aspiración de aire
E air suction connection port
G Luftansaugstutzen
F tubulure d'aspiration d'air

empañarse (metales)
E tarnish, to (metal)
G anlaufen (Metall)
F ternir, se ternir (métal)

empapar
E soak, to; impregnate, to
G tränken, imprägnieren
F imprégner

empaquetado
E packaging
G Verpackung (als Vorgang)
F conditionnement, emballage

empaquetado manual
E manual packaging
G Handverpackung
F emballage manuel

empaquetador comisionado
E contract packager
G Lohnabpacker
F empaqueteur

empaquetadora
E packaging machine
G Verpackungsmaschine
F conditionneuse

empaquetar
E pack, to; package, to
G einpacken, verpacken, konfektionieren
F emballer

empaste
E seal
G Plombe
F sceau en plomb

empinado
E steep
G steil
F raide, escarpé

empírico
E empirical
G empirisch
F empirique

emplasto transdérmico
E transdermal patch
G transdermales Pflaster
F pansement transcutané

emplazamiento
E site, location
G Standort
F emplacement

empleado
E employee
G Angestellter
F employé

empleado a tiempo parcial
E part-time employee
G Teilzeitkraft
F employé à mi-temps

empleo
E place of work
G Arbeitsplatz
F poste de travail

empresa de eliminación de desechos
E waste disposal company
G Abfallentsorgungsfirma
F entreprise de traitement des résidus

empresa de limpieza
E contract cleaner
G Reinigungsfirma
F entreprise de nettoyage

empresa filial
E subsidiary company
G Tochterfirma
F filiale (société)

empresa productora
E production facility, production plant
G Produktionsbetrieb
F usine de production

empresa subsidiaria
E subsidiary company
G Tochterfirma
F filiale (société)

empuñadura
E handle, grip
G Bügel, Griff
F prise, poignée

emulsión
E emulsion
G Emulsion
F émulsion

emulsión de aceite en agua
E oil/water emulsion
G Öl-in-Wasser-Emulsion
F émulsion d'huile dans l'eau

English German French Spanish

emulsión de agua en aceite
E water/oil emulsion
G Wasser-in-Öl-Emulsion
F émulsion d'eau dans l'huile

emulsión de silicona
E silicone emulsion
G Silikonemulsion
F émulsion de silicone

emulsionar
E emulsify, to
G emulgieren
F émulsionner

emulsivo
E emulsifier, emulsifying agent
G Emulgator
F émulsifiant

emulsor
E emulsifier
G Emulgiergerät
F émulseur

enantiómero
E enantiomer
G Enantiomere
F énantiomère

encaje (de un tubo)
E crimp, seam (of a tube)
G Falz (einer Tube)
F joint (d'un tube)

encargado
E person responsible, clerk
G Sachbearbeiter
F responsable

encargo de embalaje
E packaging order
G Verpackungsauftrag
F commande de conditionnement

encargo de fabricación por comisión
E contract manufacturer order
G Lohnherstellungsauftrag
F commande de fabrication par sous-traitance

encargo de producción
E manufacturing order
G Herstellungsauftrag
F commande de fabrication

encartonar
E carton, to
G kartonieren
F cartonner

encender
E switch on, to
G einschalten
F allumer

encendido
E ignition
G Zündung
F inflammation

encendido piezoeléctrico
E piezo ignition
G piezoelektrische Zündung
F allumage piezoélectrique

encolar
E glue, to
G leimen, kleben
F coller

encontrar errores
E locate a failure (fault), to
G Fehler finden
F identifier une erreur

enderezar
E prime, to
G grundieren
F amorcer

endotoxina
E endotoxin
G Endotoxin
F endotoxine

endotoxina bacteriana
E bacterial endotoxin
G Bakterienendotoxin
F endotoxine bactérienne

endurecimiento
E hardening
G Härten
F durcissage

enema
E enema
G Darmspülung, Klistier
F lavement, lavement intestinal

energía de activación
E activation energy
G Aktivierungsenergie
F énergie d'activation

enfardador
E bundling machine
G Bündelpacker
F lieuse

enfardar
E bundle, to
G bündeln
F lier ensemble

enfermedad contagiosa
E infectious disease
G ansteckende Krankheit
F maladie infectieuse

enfriamiento
E cooling
G Abkühlung
F refroidissement, réfrigération

engomar
E gum, to
G gummieren
F gommer

engranaje
E transmission, drive
G Getriebe
F transmission, engrenage

engranaje de tornillo si fin
E worm gear box
G Schneckengetriebe
F engrenage à vis sans fin

engrasar
E grease, to; lubricate, to
G einfetten, schmieren
F graisser, lubrifier

enjuagar
E rinse, to
G spülen
F rincer

enjuague bucal
E mouthwash
G Mundwasser
F bain de bouche

enlace
E bond
G Bindung
F liaison

enlace iónico
E ion bonding
G ionische Bindung
F liaison ionique

enlace triple
E trivalent bonding
G Dreifachbindung
F triple liaison

enlucido
E plastered
G verputzt
F crépi

enmascaramiento
E masking
G Maskierung
F masque

enmascaramiento del sabor
E taste masking
G Geschmacksüberdeckung
F masquage d'une saveur

enmascarar
E mask, to
G maskieren
F masquer

enmienda
E correction
G Berichtigung
F correction

enmohecido
E mouldy, mildewed
G schimmelig
F moisi

enrasado
E flush
G bündig
F lié

enriquecer
E concentrate, to; enrich, to
G anreichern
F concentrer

enriquecimiento
E concentration, enrichment
G Anreicherung
F concentration

ensamblaje
E assembly, set-up
G Zusammenbau
F assemblage, montage

ensamblar
E assemble, to
G zusammensetzen
F assembler

ensanchamiento de una botella
E shoulder section (of a bottle)
G Schulter (einer Flasche)
F collet d'une bouteille

ensanchamiento del pico
E peak spreading
G Peakverbreiterung
F étalement de pic

ensayar
E test, to
G prüfen
F tester

ensayo
E trial, experiment, analysis, control test
G Versuch, Prüfung
F essai, expérience, analyse, test de contrôle

ensayo clínico
E clinical trial
G klinische Prüfung
F essai clinique

reservado para ensayos clínicos
E for clinical trial use
G zur klinischen Prüfung bestimmt
F réservé aux essais cliniques

ensayo de adecuación de un sistema
E system suitability test
G Systemeignungstest
F essai d'aptitude d'un système

ensayo de compresión
E moulding trial
G Preßversuch
F essai de compression

ensayo de desintegración
E disintegration test
G Zerfallsprüfung
F essai de désintégration

ensayo de doble ciego
E double-blind study
G Doppelblindversuch
F essai en double aveugle

ensayo de estabilidad
E stability study
G Stabilitätsuntersuchung
F étude de stabilité

estabilidad a corto plazo
E short-term stability
G Kurzzeitstabilität
F étude de stabilité à court terme

estabilidad a largo plazo
E long-term stability
G Langzeitstabilität
F étude de stabilité à long terme

ensayo de repetición
E re-test
G Wiederholungsprüfung
F essai répété

enseñanza
E apprenticeship
G Lehre
F apprentissage

ensuciar
E contaminate, to
G verschmutzen
F contaminer

entorno
E environment
G Umgebung, Umwelt
F environnement

entorno no acuoso
E non-aqueous environment
G nicht-wäßrige Umgebung
F milieu non aquatique

entorno no controlado
E uncontrolled environment
G nicht kontrollierte Umgebung
F environnement non controlé

entorno de producción
E manufacturing environment
G Herstellungsumgebung
F zone de fabrication

entorno de un proceso
E process environment
G Prozeßumgebung
F environnement d'un procédé

entrada al detector
E detector inlet
G Detektoreinlaß
F entrée de détecteur

entrada de aire
E inlet air
G Zuluft
F entrée d'air

entrada de aire fresco
E fresh air inlet
G Frischluftzufuhr
F arrivée d'air frais

entrada de datos
E data entry
G Dateneingabe
F saisie de données

entrada de mercancías
E receipt (of goods)
G Wareneingang
F entrée des marchandises

entrada de un comando
E command, entry
G Befehlseingabe
F entrée d'une commande

entrada de una bomba
E pump inlet
G Pumpeneinlaß
F entrée d'une pompe

entrada para el personal
E personnel lock
G Personalschleuse
F sas réservé au personnel

entrecruzamiento
E overlap
G Überschneidung
F chevauchement, recouvrement

entrega
E delivery
G Ausgabe, Auslieferung, Lieferung
F livraison

entremezcla
E mix in, mix
G Untermischung, Vermischung
F mélange

entretenimiento
E maintenance
G Wartung
F entretien, maintenance

English German French Spanish

envasado
E packaging, filling
G Konfektionierung, Abfüllung
F conditionnement, remplissage

envasado aséptico
E aseptic filling
G aseptische Abfüllung
F remplissage aseptique

envasar
E pack, to; package, to; fill, to; charge, to
G einpacken, verpacken, konfektionieren, einfüllen
F emballer, charger, alimenter

envasar de nuevo
E re-pack, to
G umpacken
F changer l'emballage

envase
E package, pack
G Packung
F emballage, conditionnement

envase a prueba de niños
E child-resistant pack
G kindergesicherte Verpackung
F conditionnement de sécurité pour enfants

envase abierto
E open case, open package
G Anbruch
F emballage ouvert, emballage entamé

envase blíster
E blister pack
G Tiefziehverpackung
F conditionnement sous blister

envase clínico
E hospital pack
G Anstaltspackung
F emballage pour hôpitaux

envase original
E original package
G Orginalpackung
F conditionnement d'origine

envase porcionado
E portioned packaging
G portionierte Abpackung
F conditionnement en plusieurs phases

envase terminado
E finished pack
G Fertigpackung
F emballage fini

envase termoformado
E blister pack
G Tiefziehverpackung
F conditionnement thermoformé

envejecer
E age, to
G altern
F vieillir

envejecido
E obsolete, out-dated
G überholt, veraltet
F obsolète, périmé, suranné, vieillot

envejecimiento
E ageing, maturing
G Alterung
F vieillissement

envejecimiento acelerado (artificial)
E forced ageing
G beschleunigte Alterung (künstlich)
F vieillissement (forcé) prématuré

envejecimiento térmico
E thermal ageing
G thermische Alterung
F vieillissement thermique

enviar
E dispatch, to; ship, to
G versenden
F expédier

envío
E dispatch, shipment, shipping
G Versand
F expédition, envoi

envoltura
E package, pack, sheath, bush
G Packung, Hülle
F emballage, conditionnement, douille, coussinet, manchon

enzima
E enzyme
G Enzym
F enzyme

enzima modificador del ADN
E DNA-modifying enzyme
G DNA-modifizierendes Enzym
F enzyme de modification de l'ADN

enzima restrictivo
E restriction enzyme
G Restriktionsenzym
F enzyme de restriction

epimerización
E eperimisation
G Epimerisierung
F épimérisation

epitaxia de un estrato atómico
E atomic layer epitaxy (ALE)
G Atomschichtepitaxie
F épitaxie d'une couche d'atomes

epoxirresina
E epoxy resin
G Epoxidharz
F résine époxy

equilibrio
E equilibrium
G Gleichgewicht
F équilibre

reequilibrio
E re-equilibrium
G erneutes Gleichgewicht
F rééquilibre

equilibrio de presión
E pressure equilibrium
G Druckausgleich
F compensation de pression

equipamiento
E equipment
G Ausrüstung
F équipement

para diferentes productos
E multipurpose (equipment)
G für verschiedene Produkte
F (équipement) multi-usage

sólo para un producto
E dedicated (equipment)
G nur für ein Produkt
F (équipement) dédié

equipar
E provide with, to; equip, to
G ausrüsten
F équiper, outiller

equipo (máquina)
E facility, plant (machines)
G Anlage (Maschine)
F usine, établissement industriel, installation

equipo de instrumentos para el proceso de producción
E process equipment
G Produktionsanlagen
F équipement d'un procédé de fabrication

equipo de lavado oftálmico
E eye wash equipment
G Augendusche
F douche de rinçage pour les yeux

equivalencia
E equivalency
G Äquivalenz
F équivalence

equivalente
E equivalent
G äquivalent
F équivalent

eritrocito
E blood corpuscle
G Blutkörperchen
F globule sanguin

English German French Spanish

error
E defect, error, failure, fault, mistake
G Fehler
F défaut, erreur

error casual
E random error
G zufälliger Fehler
F erreur aléatoire

error de cálculo
E calculation error
G Rechenfehler
F erreur de calcul

error de medición
E measuring error
G Meßfehler
F erreur de mesure

error de transferencia
E transfer error
G Übertragungsfehler
F erreur de transfer

error humano
E human error
G menschlicher Fehler
F erreur humaine

esbozo
E draft
G Entwurf
F ébauche

escala
E scale, standard
G Skala, Maßstab
F échelle, standard

escala cromática
E colour scale
G Farbskala
F gamme de couleurs

escala de laboratorio
E laboratory scale
G Labormaßstab
F échelle de laboratoire

escala de medida
E measuring scale
G Meßskala
F échelle de mesure

dentro de la escala de medida
E on-scale
G innerhalb des Anzeigebereichs
F dans l'échelle de mesure

fuera de la escala de medida
E off-scale
G außerhalb des Anzeigebereichs
F en dehors de l'échelle de mesure

escala de producción
E production scale
G Produktionsmaßstab
F échelle de production

escala piloto
E pilot scale
G Versuchsmaßstab
F échelle pilote

escala, a
E true to scale
G maßstabgerecht
F à l'échelle

escalera de la casa
E stairs
G Treppenhaus
F escaliers

escamoso
E scaly
G schuppig
F squameux, couvert d'écailles

escaparse
E run off, to
G auslaufen
F couler, s'écouler

escape
E outlet, drain, orifice, leak, leakage, ventilated hood, fume cupboard
G Ablauf, Austritt, Leck, Abzug
F sortie, orifice, fuite, hotte à flux laminaire, hotte chimique

escarpado
E steep
G steil
F raide, escarpé

escisión endotérmica
E endothermic split-off
G endothermische Abspaltung
F scission endothermique

esclarecer (una estructura)
E elucidate, to (a structure)
G aufklären (Struktur)
F élucider (une structure)

esclusa
E lock
G Schleuse
F sas

esclusa de material
E material lock
G Materialschleuse
F sas réservé au matériel

esclusa de personal
E personnel lock
G Personenschleuse
F sas réservé au personnel

escombros
E debris
G Trümmer
F débris

escuadrado
E angled, angular
G abgewinkelt
F à angles, angulaire

esférico
E spherical
G sphärisch
F sphérique

esmaltado
E enamelled
G emailliert
F émaillé

esmalte
E enamel
G Email
F émail

espacio (intermedio)
E space
G Zwischenraum
F espace

espacio hueco
E cavity, hollow space
G Hohlraum
F cavité, espace creux

espacio libre
E clearance
G Freiraum
F espace libre

espacio muerto
E dead space
G Totraum
F espace mort

espacio para la cabeza
E head space
G Kopfraum, Gasraum
F espace de tête

espacios muertos, sin
E dead volume-free
G totraumfrei
F dépourvu de volume mort

esparadrapo
E sticking plaster
G Pflaster, Heftpflaster
F sparadrap

espátula
E spatula
G Spatel
F spatule

especialidad
E division
G Sparte
F département, section

English German French Spanish

especialidad farmacéutica manufacturada
E finished medicinal product
G Fertigarzneimittel
F médicament fini, produit pharmaceutique fini

especie
E species
G Art, Spezies, Gattung
F espèce

especie de origen
E origin of species
G Ursprungsart
F espèce d'origine

especificación
E specification, bill of materials, list of items
G Spezifikation, Stückliste
F spécification, liste-inventaire, liste détaillée

fuera de la especificación
E out of specification (OOS)
G außerhalb der Spezifikation
F hors spécification

especificación de aparatos
E instrument specification
G Gerätespezifikation
F spécification de l'instrument

especificación de calidad
E quality specification
G Gütebestimmung
F spécification de qualité

especificación de la codificación de colores
E colour code specification
G Farbcodierungsspezifikation
F spécification du codage de couleurs

especificación de un sistema
E system specification
G Systemspezifikation
F spécification d'un système

especificación funcional
E function specification
G Funktionsspezifizierung
F spécification de fonctionnement

especificaciones
E data, specifications
G Angaben
F données, spécifications

especificaciones de transporte
E transport regulations
G Transportbestimmungen
F régulations des activités de transport

especificaciones del fabricante
E manufacturer's specification
G Herstellerangaben
F spécifications du fabricant

especificaciones del material
E material specifications
G Materialspezifikationen
F spécifications des matériaux

especificar
E specify, to
G spezifizieren
F spécifier

especificidad
E specificity
G Spezifität
F spécificité

específico del lote
E batch-related
G chargenspezifisch
F spécifique au lot

espécimen
E sample, specimen
G Muster
F échantillon, spécimen

espectro
E spectrum
G Spektrum
F spectre

espectro infrarrojo
E IR spectrum
G IR-Spektrum
F spectre infrarouge

espectrofotometría
E spectrophotometry
G Spektralphotometrie
F spectrophotomètre

espectrometría de partículas
E particle spectrometer
G Teilchenspektrometer
F spectomètre de particules

espectroscopia de emisión atómica
E atomic emission spectroscopy
G Atomemissionsspektroskopie
F spectroscopie par émission atomique

espectroscopia de emisión de llama
E flame emission spectroscopy
G Flammenemissionsspektroskopie
F spectroscopie à émission de flamme

espectroscopia de resonancia nuclear
E nuclear magnetic resonance (NMR) spectroscopy
G Kernresonanzspektroskopie
F spectroscopie nucléaire à résonance magnétique

espectroscopia infrarroja en transformación de Fourier
E FTIR spectroscopy
G FTIR-Spektroskopie
F spectroscopie IR par transformation de Fourier

espectroscopia IR
E IR spectroscopy
G IR-Spektroskopie
F spectroscopie IR

espesante
E thickener, thickening agent
G Verdickungsmittel
F épaississant

espesar
E concentrate, to; thicken, to
G eindicken, einengen (Konzentration), verdicken
F épaissir, concentrer

espeso
E thick, viscous
G dick, zähflüssig
F épais, visqueux

espesor
E thickness
G Dicke
F épaisseur

espesor de la capa
E coating thickness
G Auftragsdicke
F épaisseur de l'enduit, épaisseur de la couche

espesor de lámina
E film thickness
G Foliendicke
F épaisseur de feuille

espesor de tabique
E wall thickness
G Wanddicke
F épaisseur d'un mur

espesor del comprimido
E tablet thickness
G Tablettendicke
F épaisseur d'un comprimé

espiraliforme
E spiral
G spiralförmig
F en forme d'hélice

esponja
E sponge
G Schwamm
F éponge

English
German
French
Spanish

esporas
E spores
G Sporen
F spores

esporicida
E sporicide
G sporozid
F sporicide

espuma
E foam, foam plastic
G Schaum, Schaumstoff
F mousse, mousse en plastique

espuma cutánea
E cutaneous foam
G Schaum zur Anwendung auf der Haut
F mousse pour utilisation cutanée

espuma rectal
E rectal foam
G Rektalschaum
F mousse rectale

espumante
E effervescent
G schäumend
F effervescent

espumar
E foam, to
G schäumen
F mousser

esputo
E sputum
G Sputum
F crachat

esqueleto
E supporting structure
G Gerüst
F échafaudage

esquema de carga
E loading configuration
G Beladungsschema
F schéma de chargement

esquema de carga (para autoclave)
E load pattern (for autoclaves)
G Beschickungsmuster (für Autoklaven)
F schéma de charge (pour autoclave)

esquema de instalación, de canalización y diagramas de instrumentos
E installation scheme, piping and instrument diagram
G R+I-Schema
F schéma de l'installation, des canalisations et diagrammes des instruments

esquema de procesos e instrumentos
E piping and instrument diagram (P&ID)
G R+I-Schema
F schéma fonctionnel et instrumental

esquema operacional
E flow chart
G Ablaufschema
F schéma opérationnel, schéma de marche, schéma de principe, schéma de fabrication

esquina
E corner
G Ecke
F coin

estabilidad
E stability, durability, resistance
G Haltbarkeit, Beständigkeit
F stabilité, stabilité à long terme, résistance

estabilidad a corto plazo
E short-term stability
G Kurzzeitstabilität
F stabilité à court terme

estabilidad a largo plazo
E long-term stability
G Langzeitstabilität
F stabilité à long terme

estabilidad de almacén
E warehouse stability
G Lagerstabilität
F stabilité de stockage

estabilidad de un producto
E product stability
G Produktstabilität
F stabilité d'un produit

estabilidad térmica
E thermal stability
G thermische Stabilität
F stabilité thermique

estabilizador
E stabilising agent
G Stabilisator
F agent stabilisant

estable
E stable, solid
G haltbar, fest
F stable, solide

estable a la carga
E load-resisting
G belastungsstabil
F stable au chargement

estable al calor
E heat-stable
G hitzestabil
F stable à la chaleur

establecer
E implement, to
G implementieren
F implémenter, établir

estación de cierre
E sealing station
G Verschlußstation
F station de scellage

estación de compresión
E compression station
G Druckstation
F station de compression

estación de envasado
E filling station
G Abfüllstation
F station de remplissage, station de mise en bouteilles, station en bidons

estación de llenado
E filling station
G Füllstation, Abfüllort
F station de remplissage

estación de plegado
E folding station
G Falzstation
F station de pliage

estación de troquelado
E punch station, die-cutting station, embossing station, coding station
G Stempelstation, Stanzstation, Prägestation
F station de poinçonnage, station d'estampage

estación depuradora
E waste water treatment plant
G Kläranlage
F station d'épuration

estadística de toma de muestras
E sampling statistics
G Probenahmestatistik
F statistiques de prélèvement

estadístico
E statistician
G Statistiker
F statisticien

estado (actual) de la técnica
E state-of-the-art
G Stand der Technik
F dernier cri de la technique

English German French Spanish

estado miembro
E member state
G Mitgliedstaat
F état membre

estallar
E burst, to
G bersten
F éclater

estampa
E punch
G Stanze
F poinçon

estampado
E embossment, embossed
G Prägung, geprägt
F estampage, estampé

estampadora (para imprimir)
E stamp (for printing)
G Stempel (zum Drucken)
F tampon (pour imprimer)

estampar
E die-cut, to; punch, to; stamp, to; emboss, to; imprint, to; stamp, to; print, to
G ausstanzen, prägen, aufprägen, einprägen, stanzen, einstanzen, bedrucken
F découper à l'emporte-pièce, poinçonner, imprimer, empreindre, estamper

estampar (comprimidos)
E seal, to (tablets)
G einsiegeln (Tabletten)
F sceller, clore (comprimés)

estándar
E scale, standard
G Maßstab
F échelle, standard

estándar de referencia
E reference, standard
G Referenzstandard
F standard de référence

estándar interno
E internal standard
G interner Standard, Hausstandard
F étalon interne, standard interne

estándares de seguridad
E safety standards
G Sicherheitsstandards
F normes de sécurité

estandarización
E standardisation
G Normierung
F standardisation

estandarizado
E standardised
G genormt
F standardisé

estandarizar
E standardise, to
G standardisieren
F standardiser

estanqueidad
E tightness
G Dichtigkeit
F étanchéité

estanqueidad del troquel
E punch tightness
G Stempeldichtigkeit
F étanchéité d'un poinçon

estante
E shelf
G Regal
F étagère

estante de almacén
E shelf
G Lagerregal
F étagère de stockage, étagère d'entreposage

estante de muestras
E sample rack
G Probenständer
F portoir pour échantillons

estar encargado de
E be in charge of, to
G beauftragt sein mit
F être chargé (d'une affaire)

estequiometría
E stoichiometry
G Stöchiometrie
F stoichiométrie

estereoselectivo
E stereoselective
G stereoselektiv
F stéréosélectif

esterificación
E esterification
G Veresterung
F estérification

estéril
E sterile
G steril, keimfrei
F stérile

esterilizabilidad
E sterilisability
G Sterilisierbarkeit
F aptitude à être stérilisé

esterilizable en autoclave
E autoclavable
G autoklavierbar
F autoclavable

esterilización
E sterilisation
G Sterilisation
F stérilisation

esterilización al calor
E heat sterilisation
G Hitzesterilisation
F stérilisation à la chaleur

esterilización al vapor
E steam sterilisation
G Dampfsterilisation
F stérilisation à la vapeur

esterilización final
E final sterilisation
G Endsterilisation
F stérilisation finale

esterilización final al vapor
E terminal steam sterilisation
G abschließende Dampfsterilisation
F stérilisation finale à la vapeur

esterilización in situ
E in-situ sterilisation
G In-situ-Dämpfen
F stérilisation in situ

esterilización por aire caliente
E dry heat sterilisation
G Heißluftsterilisation
F stérilisation à l'air chaud

esterilización por gas
E gas sterilisation
G Gassterilisation
F stérilisation au gaz

esterilización por irradiación
E radiation sterilisation
G Strahlensterilisation
F stérilisation par irradiation

esterilizador
E autoclave, steriliser
G Sterilisator
F autoclave

esterilizador a la llama
E flame steriliser
G Flammensterilisator
F stérilisateur à flammes

esterilizador de aire caliente
E hot air steriliser
G Heißluftsterilisator
F stérilisateur à air chaud

esterilizador de calor seco
E dry heat steriliser
G Trockenhitzesterilisator
F stérilisateur à chaleur sèche

esterilizador de medios
E media steriliser
G Mediensterilisator
F stérilisateur de milieu

esterilizar en autoclave
E autoclave, to
G autoklavieren
F autoclaver

esteroides
E steroids
G Steroide
F stéroïdes

estimulación del crecimiento
E growth promotion
G Wachstumsförderung
F promotion de la croissance

estrangulador
E throttle
G Drossel
F régulateur

estrategia de ausencia total de errores
E zero defect strategy
G Null-Fehler-Strategie
F stratégie zéro défaut

estrato
E layer
G Schicht, Lage
F couche, phase

estrato barrera
E barrier layer
G Sperrschicht
F couche de barrage

estrechado
E tapered, conical
G verjüngt, konisch
F conique

estrechamiento
E constriction
G Verengung
F constriction

estría
E streaks, stria, corrugation, groove
G Schliere, Riffelung, Rille
F strie, cannelure, striage, rainure, sillon

estriado
E corrugated
G geriffelt
F cannelé, strié

estriar
E corrugate, to
G riffeln
F canneler, strier

estribo
E handle, grip
G Bügel, Griff
F prise, poignée

estropeado
E defective, damaged
G beschädigt
F défectueux, endommagé

estructura cristalina
E crystal structure
G Kristallaufbau
F structure cristalline

estructura espacial (p. ej. de una proteína)
E spatial structure
G Raumstruktur, Tertiärstruktur
F structure spatiale

estructura terciaria (p. ej. de una proteína)
E spatial structure
G Raumstruktur, Tertiärstruktur
F structure spatiale

estuche
E housing
G Gehäuse
F boîtier

estudio acelerado de estabilidad
E accelerated stability test
G Streßtest
F test de stabilité accéléré

estudio clínico
E clinical study, clinical trial
G Studie, klinische
F essai clinique

estudio de dilución
E dissolution study
G Auflösungsstudie
F essai de dissolution

estufa de secado
E dry heat oven
G Trockenofen
F étuve

etapa crítica de un proceso
E critical processing step
G kritischer Prozeßschritt
F étape critique d'un procédé

etapa de conmutación
E switching stage
G Schaltstufe
F étape de permutation

etapa de desarrollo
E development stage
G Entwicklungsstufe
F phase de développement

etapa de producción
E manufacturing step
G Herstellungsstufe
F étape de fabrication

ético
E ethical
G ethisch
F éthique

etiqueta separable
E transferable label
G Abziehetikett
F étiquette prédécoupée

etiquetado
E labelling, lettering
G Beschriftung, Kennzeichnung, Etikettierung
F étiquetage, marquage

etiquetar
E mark, to; label, to
G kennzeichnen
F étiqueter, marquer

etiquetas
E labels
G Etiketten
F étiquettes

etiquetas autoadhesivas
E self-adhesive labels
G selbstklebende Etiketten
F étiquettes autoadhésives

etiquetas en rollo
E roll-fed labels
G Etiketten auf Rollen
F étiquettes en rouleaux

etiquetas sueltas
E loose labels, cut labels
G lose Etiketten
F étiquettes prédécoupées

eutéctico
E eutectic
G eutektisch
F eutectique

evaluación (de datos)
E evaluation, interpretation, assessment (of data)
G Bewertung, Auswertung (von Daten)
F interprétation, évaluation (de données)

evaluar
E evaluate, to; assess, to
G bewerten
F évaluer

evaporación
E evaporisation, effluvium
G Verdampfung, Verdunstung, Ausdünstung
F évaporation, évaporisation, effluent, efflux

evaporación del solvente
E solvent evaporation
G Verdampfen des Lösungsmittels
F évaporation du solvant

evaporador
E evaporator
G Verdampfer
F évaporateur

evaporador de vacío
E vacuum evaporation
G Vakuumverdampfer
F évaporateur sous vide

evaporador Kestner
E rising film evaporator
G Klettererverdampfer
F évaporateur Kestner

evaporador rotatorio
E rotatory evaporator
G Rotationsverdampfer
F évaporateur rotatif

evaporar(se)
E evaporate, to; strip, to
G verdampfen, verdunsten, ausdampfen, abdampfen, eindampfen
F évaporer, passer à la vapeur, faire évaporer, faire s'évaporer

evitación
E prevention
G Vermeidung
F prévention

evitación de desechos
E waste avoidance
G Abfallvermeidung
F politique d'élimination des déchets

evitar
E prevent, to; avoid, to
G verhindern, vermeiden
F empêcher, éviter

evolución
E development
G Entwicklung
F développement

exactitud (de un método de prueba)
E precision, accuracy
G Genauigkeit, Richtigkeit (einer Prüfmethode)
F précision, exactitude

exactitud de detección
E detection precision
G Detektionsgenauigkeit
F précision de détection

exactitud de la dosificación
E metering accuracy
G Dosiergenauigkeit
F exactitude de dosage

exactitud de la longitud de onda
E wavelength accuracy
G Wellenlängengenauigkeit
F exactitude de longueur d'onde

exactitud de la regulación
E control accuracy
G Regelgenauigkeit
F exactitude de réglage, exactitude de contrôle

exactitud del peso
E weight accuracy
G Gewichtsgenauigkeit
F exactitude d'un poids

exacto
E exact
G genau
F exact

examen
E investigation, analysis, control test
G Untersuchung, Prüfung
F inspection, analyse, test de contrôle

examen adicional
E subsequent test
G Nachuntersuchung
F examen supplétif

examen de heces
E faeces test
G Stuhluntersuchung
F analyse des selles

examen inicial
E examination on receipt
G Eingangsprüfung
F examen d'entrée

examen secuencial
E screening
G Reihenuntersuchung
F screening, série d'analyses

examinar
E investigate, to; test, to
G untersuchen, prüfen
F inspecter, tester

excedente
E excess
G Überschuß
F excès

excedente de peso
E excess weight
G Mehrgewicht
F excédent de poids

exceder
E exceed, to (a limit)
G überschreiten
F excéder

excipiente
E excipient, adjuvant
G Hilfsstoff
F excipient, adjuvant

excipiente de un supositorio
E suppository base
G Suppositoriengrundlage
F composant de base d'un suppositoire

excipiente de una pomada
E ointment base
G Salbengrundlage
F ingrédient de base d'une pommade

excreción
E excretion
G Exkretion
F excrétion

exicante
E desiccator
G Exsiccator
F dessicateur

exigencia
E requirement
G Anforderung, Erfordernis
F exigence

exigido
E required
G gefordert
F exigé

exigir
E require, to; demand, to
G erfordern, fordern
F exiger, nécessiter

existencias en almacén
E inventory, stock
G Lagerbestand
F inventaire, stock

expansión
E expansion
G Ausdehnung
F expansion

expansión longitudinal
E linear extension
G Längenausdehnung
F extension longitudinale

expedición
E dispatch, shipment, shipping
G Versand
F expédition, envoi

expedir
E dispatch, to; ship, to
G versenden
F expédier

expeler
E eject, to
G ausstoßen
F éjecter, expulser, rejeter

experimento
E trial, experiment
G Versuch
F essai, expérience

experimento con animales
E animal experiment
G Tierversuch
F expériences réalisées sur animaux

experto
E qualified person, expert, assessor
G Sachkundiger, Sachverständiger, Begutachter
F personne compétente, expert

expiración de una patente
E patent expiry
G Auslaufen des Patentes
F expiration d'un brevet

expirar
E expire, to
G verfallen
F expirer

exploración
E investigation
G Untersuchung
F inspection

exploración física
E physical inspection, physical examination
G körperliche Untersuchung
F inspection physique

exploración médica
E medical examination
G ärztliche Untersuchung
F examen médical

exploración médica al ser empleado
E medical examination on starting a new job
G Einstellungsuntersuchung
F examen médical suite à une embauche

explorar
E investigate, to
G untersuchen
F inspecter

explosividad
E explosiveness
G Explosivität
F explosivité

exprimir
E express, to
G auspressen
F presser

expulsar
E eject, to
G ausstoßen
F éjecter, expulser, rejeter

expulsión automática
E automatic ejection
G automatischer Auswurf
F éjection automatique

expulsión de comprimidos
E tablet ejection
G Tablettenauswurf
F éjection d'un comprimé

extender
E apply, to
G auftragen, auftragen
F appliquer, étendre

extensímetro de resistencia
E wire strain gauge
G Dehnungsmeßstreifen
F jauge de contrainte

extensión
E expansion, width, circumference, spreading, smear
G Ausdehnung, Weite, Umfang, Spreizung, Ausstrich
F expansion, largeur, étendue, circonférence, périmètre, propagation, ensemencement

extensión de una patente
E patent scope
G Patentumfang
F étendue d'un brevet

externo
E external
G äußerlich
F externe

extinción
E absorbance
G Extinktion
F absorption

extintor (de incendios)
E fire extinguisher
G Feuerlöscher
F extincteur

extracción
E extraction, production, withdrawal
G Extraktion, Gewinnung, Entnahme
F extraction, production, retrait

extracción en fase sólida
E solid phase extraction
G Festphasenextraktion
F extraction en phase solide

extracción líquido-líquido
E liquid-liquid extraction
G flüssig-flüssig-Extraktion
F extraction liquide-liquide

extracto
E extract
G Extrakt, Auszug
F extrait

extracto alcohólico
E alcoholate
G Alkoholauszug
F alcoolate

extracto concentrado
E concentrate
G Dickextrakt
F concentré

extracto fluido
E liquid extract
G Flüssigextrakt
F extrait liquide

extracto líquido
E liquid extract
G Flüssigextrakt
F extrait liquide

extracto seco
E dry extract
G Trockenextrakt
F extrait sec

extracto sólido
E solid extract
G Dickextrakt
F extrait solide

extraer
E extract, to
G extrahieren
F extraire

extremos de desecho
E dead spots
G tote Enden
F extrémités

extrudir
E extrude, to
G extrudieren
F extruder

extrusión
E extrusion
G Extrusion
F extrusion

extrusor
E extruder
G Extruder
F extrudeuse

eyección
E ejection
G Auswurf, Ausstoß
F éjection, rejet

eyección automática
E automatic ejection
G automatischer Auswurf
F éjection automatique

fábrica llave en mano
E turnkey plant
G schlüsselfertige Fabrik
F usine clé en main

fabricación
E manufacture, production
G Herstellung
F fabrication, production

fabricación a escala industrial
E industrial scale manufacture
G Herstellung im industriellen Maßstab
F fabrication à l'échelle industrielle

fabricación aséptica
E aseptic processing
G aseptische Herstellung
F fabrication aseptique

fabricación de comprimidos
E tabletting, compression, compaction
G Tablettierung
F fabrication de comprimés

fabricación informatizada
E computer-integrated manufacturing (CIM)
G computerintegrierte Herstellung
F fabrication informatisée

fabricación informatizada de comprimidos
E computer-integrated tabletting (CIT)
G computerintegrierte Tablettierung
F fabrication de comprimés informatisée

fabricación por comisión
E contract manufacture
G Herstellung im Lohnauftrag, Lohnherstellung
F fabrication en sous-traitance, fabrication par sous-traitance

fabricado biotecnológicamente
E manufactured biotechnologically
G biotechnologisch hergestellt
F manufacturé par biotechnologie

fabricante
E manufacturer
G Hersteller
F fabricant

fabricante de aparatos
E equipment manufacturer
G Gerätehersteller
F fabricant d'équipement

fabricante de material de embalaje
E packaging material manufacturer
G Packmittelhersteller
F fabricant de matériel d'emballage

fabricante de recipientes
E vessel manufacturer
G Behälterbauer
F fabricant de cuves

fabricante farmacéutico
E pharmaceutical manufacturer
G pharmazeutischer Unternehmer
F industriel de la pharmacie

fabricante por comisión
E contract manufacturer
G Auftragshersteller
F producteur sous-traintant

faceta
E bevel
G Abschrägung, Facette
F biseau

facilidad de deslizamiento del troquel
E easy punch sliding
G Stempelleichtgängigkeit
F facilité de glissement d'un poinçon

factor de retención
E retention factor
G Retentionsfaktor
F facteur de rétention

factor estándar
E standardisation factor
G Standardfaktor
F facteur de standardisation

factores de crecimiento
E growth factors
G Wachstumsfaktoren
F facteurs de croissance

fallo
E breakdown, downtime (machine), failure, malfunction, interference, fault, accident
G Ausfall, Störung, Störfall
F panne, temps mort, défaillance, perturbation, dérangement, incident

falsificación
E falsification
G Fälschung, Verfälschung
F falsification

falsificar
E falsify, to
G verfälschen
F falsifier

falta de peso
E short weight, underweight
G Untergewicht
F insuffisance de poids

farmacéutico
E pharmacist
G Apotheker
F pharmacien

farmacocinética
E pharmacokinetics
G Pharmakokinetik
F pharmacocinétique

farmacología
E pharmacology
G Pharmakologie
F pharmacologie

farmacopea
E pharmacopoeia
G Arzneibuch, Pharmakopöe
F pharmacopée

farmacopea estadounidense
E United States Pharmacopoeia (USP)
G Arzneibuch der USA
F pharmacopée américaine

Farmacopea Europea
E European Pharmacopoeia (PhEur)
G Europäisches Arzneibuch (PhEur)
F pharmacopée européenne (PhEur)

fase acuosa
E aqueous phase
G wäßrige Phase
F phase aqueuse

fase de enfriamento
E cooling phase
G Abkühlphase
F phase de refroidissement

fase de reclutamiento
E recruitment phase
G Rekrutierungsphase
F phase de recrutement

fase estacionaria
E stationary phase
G stationäre Phase
F phase stationnaire

fase gaseosa
E gaseous phase
G Gasphase
F phase gazeuse

fase líquida
E liquid phase
G flüssige Phase
F phase liquide

fase móvil (en cromatografía)
E mobile phase
G Fließmittel
F phase mobile

fase orgánica
E organic phase
G organische Phase
F phase organique

English
German
French
Spanish

English German French Spanish

fase sólida
E solid phase
G feste Phase
F phase solide

fase vapor
E vapour phase
G Dampfphase
F phase vapeur

fatiga del material
E material fatigue
G Materialermüdung
F fatigue du matériel

fecha de caducidad
E expiration date, expiry date
G Verfallsdatum
F date d'expiration

fecha de entrega
E due date, delivery date
G Lieferdatum
F date de livraison

fecha de expiración
E expiration date, expiry date
G Verfallsdatum
F date d'expiration

fecha de liberación
E release date
G Freigabedatum
F date de libération

fecundidad
E non-sterility
G Unsterilität
F fécondité

fermentación
E fermentation
G Fermentation, Gärung
F fermentation

fermentador
E fermenter
G Fermenter
F fermenteur

fermentar
E ferment, to
G fermentieren
F faire fermenter

fertilidad
E non-sterility
G Unsterilität
F fécondité

fertilizante
E fertiliser
G Düngemittel
F engrais

fiabilidad
E reliability
G Verläßlichkeit, Zuverlässigkeit
F fiabilité

fiabilidad de la dosificación
E dose reliability
G Zuverlässigkeit der Dosierung
F fiabilité d'une dose

fiable
E reliable
G zuverlässig
F fiable

fibra
E fibre
G Faser
F fibre

fibra artificial
E artificial fibre
G Kunstfaser
F fibre artificielle

fibra de vidrio
E fibreglass
G Glasfaser
F fibre de verre

ficha de control de calidad
E quality control card
G Qualitätsregelkarte
F carte de contrôle de qualité

ficha técnica (de un medicamento)
E technical information
G Fachinformation
F information technique

fijación
E fixing, attachment
G Befestigung
F fixation

fijar
E lock, to
G arretieren
F fermer à clef

filete
E thread
G Gewinde
F filetage

de paso derecho
E right-handed
G rechtsgängig
F à droite

de paso izquierdo
E left-handed
G linksgängig
F à gauche

filete de tornillo
E screw thread
G Schraubgewinde
F filetage

filtrable
E filterable
G filtrierbar
F pouvant être filtré

filtración
E filtration
G Filtration
F filtration

filtración estéril
E sterile filtration
G Sterilfiltration
F filtration stérile

filtración por gel
E gel filtration
G Gelfiltration
F filtration sur gel

filtración por membrana
E membrane filtration
G Membranfiltration
F filtration par membrane

filtrado
E filtrate
G Filtrat
F filtrat

filtrado estérilmente
E sterile-filtered
G sterilfiltriert
F stérile-filtré

filtrar
E filter, to
G filtrieren, abnutschen, kolieren
F filtrer

filtrar estérilmente
E sterile-filter, to
G sterilfiltrieren
F stérile-filtrer

filtro
E filter
G Filter
F filtre

filtro acanalado
E fluted filter
G Faltenfilter
F filtre nervuré, filtre cannelé

filtro antipolvo de gran rendimiento
E high efficiency particulate air (HEPA) filter
G Hochleistungsschwebstoffilter
F filtre antipoussières à haute performance

filtro biológico
E biological filter
G Biofilter
F filtre biologique

filtro de aire
E air filter
G Luftfilter
F filtre à air

filtro de asbesto
E asbestos filter
G Asbestfilter
F filtre en amiante

filtro de carbón
E carbon filter
G Kohlefilter
F filtre au carbone

filtro de coalescencia
E coalescing filter
G Koaleszenzfilter
F filtre coalescent

filtro de descarga
E outlet filter
G Auslaßfilter
F filtre de sortie

filtro de entrada
E inlet filter
G Eingangsfilter, Einlaßfilter
F filtre d'entrée, filtre d'admission

filtro de grava
E gravel filter
G Kiesbettfilter
F filtre de graviers

filtro de membrana
E membrane filter
G Membranfilter
F filtre à membrane, filtre microporeux

filtro de partículas
E particle filter
G Partikelfilter
F filtre à particules

filtro de polvo fino
E fine dust filter
G Feinstaubfilter
F filtre à poussières fines

filtro de profundidad
E depth filter
G Tiefenfilter
F filtre profondeur

filtro de salida
E outlet filter
G Auslaßfilter
F filtre de sortie

filtro de separación de aceite
E oil-separating filter
G Ölabscheidefilter
F filtre de retenue d'huile

filtro de ventilación
E vent filter
G Belüftungsfilter
F filtre de ventilation

filtro del aire de escape
E exhaust air filter
G Abluftfilter
F filtre à air d'évacuation

filtro estéril terminal
E terminal sterile filter
G endständiger Sterilfilter
F filtre stérile terminal

filtro HEPA (high efficiency particulated air)
E hepa filters
G HEPA-Filter
F filtres HEPA

filtro previo
E pre-filter
G Vorfilter
F filtre préalable

filtro reforzado con fibra de vidrio
E fibreglass-reinforced filter
G glasfaserverstärkter Filter
F filtre renforcé à la fibre de verre

filtro terminal
E terminal filter
G endständiger Filter
F filtre terminal

fin del estudio
E end of study, end of trial
G Studienende
F fin d'un essai clinique

firma
E signature
G Unterschrift
F signature

firma autógrafa
E signature
G eigenhändige Unterschrift
F autographe

firma autorizante
E approval signature
G Unterschrift zur Genehmigung
F signature d'autorisation

firma electrónica
E electronic signature
G elektronische Unterschrift
F signature électronique

firmeza
E firmness, solidity
G Festigkeit
F solidité

fisura
E crack, tear, slit, cleft
G Riß, Spalte, Schlitz, Spalt
F déchirure, fissure, fente, crevasse, rainure

fisura capilar
E hairline crack
G Haarriß
F fissure capillaire

fitofármacos
E phytopharmaceuticals, herbal medicines
G Phytopharmaka, pflanzliche Arzneimittel
F phytopharmaceutiques

fitoquímica
E phytochemistry
G Phytochemie
F phytochimie

flexible
E flexible, pliable
G biegsam
F flexible, pliable

flexión
E bend, flexure
G Biegung
F courbure, pliage

floculación
E flocculation
G Flockung
F floculation

flocular
E flocculate, to; flake, to; flaky
G ausflocken, flockig
F floculer, floconneux

flóculo
E floc
G Flocke
F bourre

flor
E blossom
G Blüte
F fleur

fluctuación
E variability
G Schwankung
F variabilité

fluctuación de la temperatura
E temperature fluctuation
G Temperaturschwankung
F variation de température

fluctuación de la tensión
E voltage fluctuation
G Spannungsschwankung
F variation de tension

fluctuación de presión
E pressure fluctuation
G Druckschwankung
F fluctuation de pression

English German French Spanish

fluctuación del peso de los comprimidos
E tablet weight variation
G Schwankung des Tablettengewichts
F écart entre les poids d'un comprimé, écart entre les poids d'un cachet

fluctuaciones de la intensidad de corriente eléctrica
E power supply fluctuation
G Stromversorgungsschwankungen, Netzschwankungen
F variations de l'intensité du courant

fluctuaciones del suministro eléctrico
E power supply fluctuation
G Netzschwankungen
F variations de l'intensité du courant

fluctuar
E vary, to; fluctuate, to
G schwanken
F fluctuer

fluidez
E flowability
G Fließfähigkeit
F fluidité

fluidificante (fabricación de comprimidos)
E flow promoter
G Fließmittel
F fluidifiant

fluido, muy fluido
E non-viscous, thin, thin-bodied
G dünnflüssig
F fluide, très fluide

flujo
E flow
G Durchfluß
F débit

flujo de aire
E air flow
G Luftströmung
F circulation d'air

flujo de difusión
E diffusion flow
G Diffusionsfluß
F débit de diffusion

flujo de material
E material flow
G Materialfluß
F flux des matériaux

flujo de personal
E personnel flow
G Personalfluß
F flux du personnel

flujo laminar
E laminar flow
G Laminarfluß, laminare Strömung
F flux laminaire

flujo turbulento
E turbulent flow
G turbulente Strömung
F flux turbulent

fluoración
E fluorination
G Fluorierung
F fluoruration

fluorescencia
E fluorescence
G Fluoreszenz
F fluorescence

fluorescente
E fluorescent
G fluoreszierend
F fluorescent

fluorometría
E fluorometry
G Fluorometrie
F fluorométrie

fluoruro de polivinilideno
E polyvinylidene fluoride (PVDF)
G Polyvinylidenfluorid
F fluorure de polyvinylidène (PVDF)

fluxómetro
E flowmeter
G Durchflußmesser, Strömungswächter
F débimètre

fluyendo libremente
E free flowing
G freifließend
F fluide, s'écoulant librement

folleto de información del paciente
E patient information leaflet
G Patientenbroschüre
F brochure d'information pour patient

fomentar
E convey, to
G fördern
F transporter

fondo de destilación
E distillation bottom
G Destillationsboden
F bas de la colonne de distillation

forma (p. ej. de partículas)
E shape (of particles)
G Form (z. B. von Partikeln)
F forme (de particules)

forma de administración
E dosage form, administration form
G Darreichungsform
F forme du dosage, voie d'administration

forma de la partícula
E particle form, particle shape
G Teilchenform, Partikelform
F forme d'une particule

forma del troquel
E punch shape, punch form
G Stempelform
F forme d'un poinçon

forma estéril
E sterile form
G sterile Zubereitung
F forme stérile

forma farmacéutica
E dosage form
G Arzneiform
F forme pharmaceutique

forma farmacéutica de dosis única
E single dose unit
G einzeldosierte Arzneiform
F une dose d'utilisation, forme d'une unité de prise

forma líquida de administración
E liquid form
G flüssige Form
F forme liquide (spécialités pharmaceutiques)

formación
E education, training
G Ausbildung
F éducation

formación de arrugas
E wrinkling
G Faltenbildung
F formation de plis, formation de rides

formación de espuma
E foam formation, foaming
G Schaumbildung
F formation de mousse, moussage, production de mousse

formación de frente (HPLC)
E fronting (in HPLC)
G Frontbildung (HPLC)
F formation d'un front (HPLC)

formación de pliegues
E wrinkling
G Faltenbildung
F formation de plis, formation de rides

formación de quelatos
E chelate formation
G Chelatbildung
F formation de chélate

formación de secuencias
E sequencing
G Sequenzierung
F séquençage

formación de un granuloma
E granuloma formation
G Bildung eines Granuloms
F formation d'un granulome

formación del personal
E personnel training
G Personalschulung
F formation du personnel

formación profesional
E vocational training
G Berufsausbildung
F formation professionnelle

formas sólidas de dosificación
E solid dosage forms
G feste Formen
F forme de dosage solide

formato
E format, size
G Format
F taille, format

formato de compresión
E compression format
G Preßformat
F format de compression

fórmula
E formula
G Formel
F formule

fórmula empírica
E empirical formula
G empirische Formel
F formule empirique

fórmula estructural
E structural formula
G Strukturformel
F formule développée

fórmula galénica
E formulation
G Galenik
F formulation

fórmula molecular
E molecular formula
G Molekularformel
F formule brute

formulación (galénica)
E formulation, preparation
G Formulierung, Zubereitung, Rezeptur, Formgebung, Galenik
F formulation, préparation

formulación con liberación controlada
E controlled release formulation
G Formulierung mit kontrollierter Freisetzung
F formulation avec libération contrôlée

formulación básica
E basic formulation
G Basisformulierung
F formulation de base

formulación de base
E basic formulation
G Basisformulierung
F formulation de base

formulación monolítica
E single dose form
G monolithische Arznei-form
F forme pharmaceutique monolithique

formulación primaria
E primary formulation
G Primärformulierung
F formulation primaire

formulario
E form, pre-printed form
G Formular, Vordruck
F formulaire

fosforescencia
E phosphorescence
G Phosphoreszenz
F phosphorescence

fotólisis
E photolysis
G Photolyse
F photolyse

fotometría
E photometry
G Photometrie
F photométrie

fotometría de llama
E flame photometry
G Flammenphotometrie
F photométrie de flamme

fotómetro
E photometer
G Photometer
F photomètre

fotómetro de llama
E flame photometer
G Flammenphotometer
F photomètre de flamme

fotoquímico
E photochemical
G photochemisch
F photochimique

fotosensible
E light-sensitive
G lichtempfindlich
F photo-sensible, sensible à la lumière

fracasar
E fail, to
G versagen
F faillir à sa tâche

fracción
E fraction
G Fraktion
F fraction

fracción de polvo
E powder fraction
G Pulverfraktion
F fraction de poudre

fracción de tamizado
E sieve fraction
G Siebfraktion
F fraction de tamisage

fraccionar
E fractionate, to
G fraktionieren
F fractionner

fractura de un metal
E metal fracture
G Metallbruch
F fracture du métal

frágil
E fragile, brittle
G zerbrechlich, spröde
F fragile, cassant

fragilidad
E brittleness
G Brüchigkeit
F fragilité

fragmento
E fragment, piece, fraction
G Bruchstück
F morceau, fragment

frasco
E vial
G Fläschchen
F flacon, récipient

frasco cuentagotas
E dropping bottle
G Tropfflasche
F flacon compte-gouttes, flacon doseur

frasco de lavado
E wash bottle
G Waschflasche
F flacon laveur

frasco de pipeteo
E pipette bottle
G Pipettenflasche
F flacon de pipette

frasco espolvoreador
E sprinkler can
G Streudose
F flacon saupoudreur

frecuencia
E frequency
G Häufigkeit
F fréquence

freno de discos múltiples
E multiple disk brake
G Lamellenbremse
F frein à disques multiples

frente de migración del solvente
E solvent front
G Fließmittelfront
F front de migration du solvant

friabilidad
E brittleness
G Brüchigkeit
F fragilité

fricción
E friction
G Reibung
F friction

frotamiento
E embrocation, friction
G Einreibung
F embrocation

frotis
E smear
G Ausstrich
F ensemencement

fuelle plegable
E bellows
G Faltenbalg
F soufflet

fuente
E source
G Quelle
F source

fuente (descendente) de recogida
E catch basin, drain
G Sinkkasten
F bassin de descente

fuente de calor
E heating source
G Heizquelle
F source de chauffage, source de chaleur

fuente de corriente continua
E direct current source
G Gleichstromquelle
F source de courant continu

fuente de corriente eléctrica
E electrical power source
G elektrische Stromquelle
F source d'un courant électrique

fuente de electricidad
E power source
G Stromquelle
F source d'électricité

fuente de errores
E source of error (failure)
G Fehlerquelle
F source d'erreur

fuente de ignición
E ignition source
G Zündquelle
F source d'inflammation

fuente luminosa
E light source
G Lichtquelle
F source de lumière

fuerza
E force
G Kraft
F force

fuerza (p. ej. de un comprimido)
E strength (e. g. of a tablet)
G Stärke (z. B. einer Tablette)
F dureté (par ex. d'un comprimé)

fuerza adhesiva
E adhesive force, adhesive power, adhesive strength
G Bindekraft, Haftkraft, Klebekraft
F force d'adhésion, force d'adhérence

fuerza centrífuga
E centrifugal force
G Zentrifugalkraft, Fliehkraft
F force de centrifugation

fuerza de atracción
E force of attraction
G Anziehungskraft
F force d'attraction

fuerza de cizallamiento
E shear strength
G Scherkraft
F force de cisaillement

fuerza de cohesión
E cohesive power
G Kohäsionskraft
F force de cohésion

fuerza de compresión
E compaction force
G Preßkraft
F force de compression

fuerza de compresión previa
E pre-compression force
G Vorpreßkraft
F force de compression préalable

fuerza de eyección
E ejection force
G Ausstoßkraft
F force d'éjection

fuerza de fricción
E frictional force
G Reibungskraft
F force de friction, force de frottement

fuerza de gravedad
E gravity
G Schwerkraft
F force de gravité

fuerza de percusión
E impact force
G Schlagkraft
F force de frappe, force d'impact

fuerza de rotación
E torsion force
G Drehkraft
F force de torsion

fuerza de torsión
E torsion
G Torsionskraft
F torsion

fuerza de tracción
E tensile force
G Zugkraft
F force de traction

fuerza impactante
E impact force
G Schlagkraft
F force de frappe, force d'impact

fumigación
E fumigation, flushing, purging
G Begasung, Raumbegasung
F fumigation

fumigante
E fumigant
G Begasungsmittel
F fumigant

función de la auditoría
E audit function
G Auditfunktion
F fonction d'audit

función sobreescribir
E overwrite function
G Überschreibfunktion
F fonction d'écrasement

funcionamiento automático
E automatic operation, unmanned operation
G automatischer Betrieb, bedienerloser Betrieb
F fonctionnement automatique, usine automatique

funcionamiento continuo
E continuous operation
G Dauerbetrieb, kontinuierlicher Betrieb
F fabrication en continu, opération continue

funcionamiento electroneumático
E electro-pneumatic operation
G elektro-pneumatischer Betrieb
F opération électro-pneumatique

funcionando
E in process
G im Betriebszustand
F à condition d'exploitation, sous condition d'exploitation

parado
E at rest
G im Ruhezustand
F à l'arrêt, immobilisé

fundición
E melt
G Schmelze
F fusion

fundir
E melt, to; fuse, to
G schmelzen, einschmelzen
F fondre, faire fondre

fungicida
E anti-fungal, fungicidal, fungicide
G pilzabtötend, fungizid, Fungizid
F antifongique, fongicide

fusible
E fuse
G Sicherung (elektrisch)
F fusible

fusible lento
E slow fuse
G träge Sicherung
F fusible à action retardée

fusible rápido
E fast fuse
G flinke Sicherung
F fusible à action instantanée

fusión
E melt
G Schmelze
F fusion

fusión de empresas
E merger, fusion
G Zusammenschluß von Firmen
F fusion (d'entreprises)

gabinete de seguridad biológica
E biohazard cabinet
G Biosicherheitskabinett
F enceinte de risques biologiques

gafas de seguridad
E safety spectacles
G Sicherheitsbrille
F lunettes de sécurité

gafas protectoras
E safety spectacles
G Schutzbrille
F lunettes de protection

galga
E gauge
G Meßlehre
F jauge

gálibo
E gauge
G Meßlehre
F jauge

galvanizado con zinc
E galvanised
G verzinkt
F galvanisé au zinc

gama
E range
G Bandbreite
F échelle, intervalle, gamme, zone

garantía
E guarantee, warranty
G Garantie
F garantie

garantía de esterilización
E sterility assurance
G Sterilisationssicherheit
F garantie de stérilité

garantizar
E guarantee, to; secure, to; ensure, to
G sicherstellen
F assurer, garantir

garganta
E recess
G Hohlkehle
F moulure creuse

gas
E gas
G Gas
F gaz

gas de escape
E exhaust gas, waste gas
G Abgas
F gaz d'échappement, gaz d'évacuation

gas diluido a presión
E pressure-dissolved gases
G unter Druck gelöste Gase
F gaz dissous sous pression

gas inerte
E inert gas
G Schutzgas
F gaz inerte

gas líquido
E liquid gas
G Flüssiggas
F gaz liquide

gas noble
E inert gas, rare gas
G Edelgas
F gaz inerte, gaz rare

gas portador
E carrier gas
G Trägergas
F gaz porteur

gas purgante
E purge gas
G Spülgas
F gas de purge

gasa
E gauze
G Mull
F gaze

gasear
E purge, to
G begasen
F purger

gaseoso
E gaseous
G gasförmig
F gazeux

gases comprimidos
E compressed gases
G komprimierte Gase
F gaz comprimés

gases licuados
E liquified gases
G verflüssigte Gase
F gaz liquéfiés

gastar
E dispense, to
G ausgeben
F dépenser, distribuer

gatillo
E latch, door handle
G Klinke
F loquet, poignée de porte

gel
E gel
G Gel
F gel

gel auricular
E ear gel
G Ohrengel
F gel auriculaire

gel azul de sílice
E blue silica gel
G Blaugel
F gel bleu

gel de sílice
E silica gel
G Kieselgel, Silicagel
F gel de silice

gel de uso endocervical
E endocervical gel
G Gel zur endozervikalen Anwendung
F gel pour utilisation endo-cervicale

gel nasal
E nasal gel
G Nasengel
F gel nasal

gel oftálmico
E eye gel
G Augengel
F gel pour œil

gel oral
E oral gel
G Gel zum Einnehmen
F gel pour administration orale

gel rectal
E rectal gel
G Rektalgel
F gel rectal

gel vaginal
E vaginal gel
G Vaginalgel
F gel vaginal

gelación
E gel formation
G Gelbildung
F formation de gel

gelar
E gel, to
G gelieren
F geler

gelificante
E gel-forming agent, gelling agent, gellant
G Gelbildner, Geliermittel
F gélifiant

generación
E generation (of)
G Erzeugung
F engendrement, production

generador
E generator
G Generator
F générateur

generador aleatorio
E random number generator
G Zufallsgenerator
F générateur de hasard

generador de humo
E smoke generator
G Raucherzeuger
F générateur de fumée

generador de impulsos
E pulse generator
G Impulsgeber
F générateur d'impulsions

English German French Spanish

generador de vapor puro
E pure steam generator
G Reindampferzeuger
F générateur de vapeur pure

generador eléctrico de emergencia
E emergency power supply
G Notstromaggregat
F générateur de courant d'urgence

genérico
E generic
G Genericum
F générique

género
E species
G Gattung
F espèce

gerencia
E company management
G Geschäftsleitung
F direction d'une société

gerente
E managing director, general manager
G Geschäftsführer
F président directeur général (PDG)

germen
E organism
G Keim
F germe, organisme microbien

germen de prueba
E test organism
G Prüfkeim
F organisme de contrôle

germen indicador
E indicator organism
G Indikatorkeim
F organisme indicateur

germinación (de esporas)
E germination
G Auskeimung (von Sporen)
F germination

gestión de la calidad
E quality management (QM)
G Qualitätsmanagement (QM)
F gestion de la qualité

gestión de la calidad absoluta
E total quality management (TQM)
G umfassendes Qualitätsmanagement
F gestion absolue de la qualité

gestión de stocks
E stock management system
G Lagerhaltung
F système de gestion du stockage

gestión de stocks caótica
E random location storage system
G Lagerhaltung, chaotische
F entreposage non ordonné

gestión ecológica
E environmental management
G Umweltschutzmanagement
F gestion de l'environnement

gestión empresarial
E plant management
G Betriebsführung
F management d'une installation

girado hacia fuera
E swivelled, pivotted
G ausgeschwenkt
F pivoté

girando
E rotating
G rotierend
F tournant

girar
E rotate, to
G rotieren
F tourner

giratorio
E hinged, pivotable
G schwenkbar
F pivotable

gobierno civil
E regional government
G Regierungspräsidium
F gouvernement régional

gollete
E bottle neck
G Flaschenhals
F goulot, col de bouteille

golpe
E impact
G Schlag, Stoß
F impact, coup

goma
E rubber
G Gummi
F caoutchouc

goma de mascar medicamentosa
E medicated chewing gum
G medizinisches Kaugummi
F chewing-gum médicamenté

goma limpia cristales (p. ej. en mezclador)
E wiper paddle (e. g. of a mixing vessel)
G Wischblatt (z. B. im Mischbehälter)
F lame d'essuyage (dans la cuve de mélange)

gotas antitusivas
E cough drops
G Hustentropfen
F gouttes antitussives

gotas auriculares
E ear drops
G Ohrentropfen
F gouttes auriculaires

gotas nasales
E nose drops
G Nasentropfen
F gouttes nasales

gotas oftálmicas
E eye drops
G Augentropfen
F gouttes ophtalmiques

gotas orales
E oral drops
G Tropfen zum Einnehmen
F gouttes pour voie orale

gotear
E drip, to; trickle, to; drop, to
G träufeln, tropfen
F verser au goutte à goutte, fuire

gotita
E droplet
G Tröpfchen
F gouttelettes

grabar
E engrave, to
G eingravieren
F graver

grabar (al aguafuerte)
E etch, to
G einätzen
F corroder, décaper

gradación de colores
E colour scale
G Farbabstufung
F gradation de couleurs

gradiente
E gradient, slope
G Gefälle, Gradient
F pente, inclinaison, gradient

gradiente de cizallamiento
E shear gradient
G Schergefälle
F taux de cisaillement

gradiente de flujo
E flow gradient
G Fließgradient
F gradient d'écoulement

gradiente de temperatura
E temperature gradient
G Temperaturgefälle
F gradient de température

grado de brillantez
E grade of gloss, grade of lustre
G Glanzgrad
F degré de lustre

grado de calidad
E quality grade
G Güteklasse
F degré de qualité

grado de contaminación
E contamination level
G Kontaminationsgrad
F niveau de contamination

grado de libertad
E degree of freedom
G Freiheitsgrad
F degré de liberté

grado de limpieza
E cleanliness grade
G Reinigungsgrad
F niveau de propreté

grado de novedad (p. ej. de un producto)
E novelty (e. g. of a product)
G Neuheitsgrad (z. B. eines Produktes)
F degré d'innovation (par ex. d'un produit)

grado de pureza
E cleanliness grade (e. g. room), purity (product)
G Reinheitsgrad
F niveau de propreté, niveau de pureté

grado de seguridad biológica
E biosafety level
G biologische Sicherheitsstufe
F niveau de bio-sécurité

grado hidrolítico
E hydrolytic grade
G hydrolytischer Grad
F degré hydrolytique

graduación
E scale
G Gradeinteilung
F graduation

graduación de una escala
E graduation
G Skaleneinteilung
F graduation

graduado
E graduated
G graduiert
F gradué

gradualmente
E stepwise
G stufenweise
F par étapes, échelonné

gragea
E coated tablet, sugar-coated tablet, capsule, cachet
G Filmtablette, Dragee, Zuckerdragee, Oblate
F comprimé pelliculé, comprimé dragéifié, dragée, capsule, cachet

gragea azucarada
E sugar-coated tablet
G Zuckerdragee
F comprimé dragéifié, dragée

gragear
E pan-coat, to
G dragieren
F dragéifier

Gram negativo
E Gram-negative
G Gram-negativ
F Gram-négatif

Gram positivo
E Gram-positive
G Gram-positiv
F Gram-positif

gran rendimiento
E high performance
G Hochleistungs-
F haute performance

grano fino, de
E fine-grained
G feinkörnig
F à grain fin

grano grueso
E coarse particle
G Grobkorn
F particule grossière

granulación
E grain
G Körnung
F granulation

granulación de degradación
E degradation granulation
G Abbaugranulierung
F granulation de dégradation

granulación en seco
E dry granulation
G Trockengranulierung
F granulation par séchage

granulación fina
E fine particles, fine grain
G feine Körnung
F granulation fine

granulación húmeda
E wet granulation
G Feuchtgranulierung
F granulation (par voie) humide

granulación sintética
E synthetic granulation
G Aufbaugranulierung
F granulation hors taille

granulado
E granulate
G Granulat
F granulé

granulado con liberación modificada de la sustancia activa
E modified release granules
G Granulat mit veränderter Wirkstoff-Freisetzung
F libération modifiée de granules

granulado de compresión
E moulding granulate
G Preßgranulat
F granule moulée

granulado grueso
E coarse granules
G Grobgranulat
F granulés grossiers

granulado resistente al jugo gástrico
E gastro-resistant granules
G magensaftresistentes Granulat
F granules gastro-résistantes

granulado retard
E prolonged release granules
G Retardgranulat
F granules à libération retardée

granulador de lecho fluidificado
E fluid bed spray granulator
G Wirbelschichtgranulator
F granulateur en lit fluidisé

granulador vertical
E vertical granulator
G Vertikalgranulator
F granulateur vertical

granular
E granulate, to; granular
G granulieren, körnig
F granuler, granulaire

gránulo
E granule
G Granulatkorn
F granule

granulometría
E sieve analysis
G Siebanalyse
F granulométrie

grasa lubri(fi)cante
E grease
G Schmierfett
F graisse

grifo
E stopcock
G Hahn (technisch)
F robinet

grifo con tres vías
E three-way stopcock
G Dreiwegehahn
F robinet d'arrêt à trois voies

grifo de cierre
E stopcock
G Absperrhahn
F robinet d'arrêt

grifo de salida
E discharge cock, drain cock
G Ablaßhahn
F robinet de purge

groseramente cristalino
E course-grained
G grobkristallin
F grossièrement cristallin

grosero
E coarse
G grob
F brut, grossier

grosor
E thickness
G Dicke
F épaisseur

grueso
E thick, coarse
G dick, grob
F épais, brut, grossier

grupo de trabajo
E working group, task force
G Arbeitsgruppe
F groupe de travail

guante
E gloves
G Handschuhe
F gants

guantes de uso único
E disposable gloves
G Einmalhandschuhe
F gants à usage unique

guantes protectores
E protective gloves
G Schutzhandschuhe
F gants protecteurs

guardar
E retain, to; store, to
G aufbewahren
F conserver, garder

guía
E guide, guiding device, guiding mechanism
G Führungsvorrichtung
F guide, dispositif de guidage, mécanisme de guidage

guía del troquel
E punch guide
G Stempelführung
F guidage d'un poinçon

guía para la junta
E gasket channel
G Dichtungsführung
F cannelure pour joint

gusto
E taste, flavour
G Geschmack
F goût

hacer balance
E reconciliation
G Bilanzierung
F vérification, bilancer

halogenación
E halogenation
G Halogenierung
F halogénation

haz
E pack
G Gebinde
F emballage

haz comprimido
E shrink-pack
G eingeschrumpftes Gebinde
F emballage sous film rétractable

haz contraído
E shrink-pack
G eingeschrumpftes Gebinde
F emballage sous film rétractable

haz doble
E double beam
G Doppelstrahl
F double faisceau

hélice alfa (p. ej. de proteína)
E alpha helix (e. g. of protein)
G Alpha-Helix (z. B. eines Proteins)
F hélice alpha (structure des protéines)

hembrilla
E socket
G Buchse
F borne

hendidura
E slit
G Schlitz, Spalt
F fente, fissure, rainure

herbicida
E herbicide
G Unkrautvernichtungsmittel
F herbicide

herméticamente cerrado
E tightly closed
G dicht verschlossen
F hermétiquement fermé

hermeticidad
E tightness
G Dichtigkeit
F étanchéité

hermeticidad para el aire
E air tightness
G Luftdichtheit
F imperméabilité à l'air

hermético
E leak-tight, air-tight
G dicht, luftdicht
F étanche, étanche à l'air

hermético para el polvo
E dust-tight
G staubdicht
F étanche à la poussière

herrumbre
E rust
G Rost
F rouille

hervir
E boil, to
G aufkochen, sieden
F bouillir

heterocíclico
E heterocyclic
G heterozyklisch
F hétérocyclique

heterogeneidad de comprimidos
E tablet inconsistency
G Uneinheitlichkeit von Tabletten
F hétérogénéité des comprimés

hidrato
E hydrate
G Hydrat
F hydrate

hidratos de carbono
E carbohydrates
G Kohlenhydrate
F hydrates de carbone, glucides

hidrocarburo
E hydrocarbon
G Kohlenwasserstoff
F composé hydrocarboné

hidrocarburos poliaromáticos
E polyaromatic hydrocarbons (PAH)
G polyaromatische Kohlenwasserstoffe (PAK)
F hydrocarbures polyaromatiques

hidrófilo
E hydrophilic, hygroscopic
G hydrophil, wasseranziehend
F hydrophile, hygroscopique

hidrófobo
E hydrophobic, water-repellent
G hydrophob, wasserabweisend
F hydrophobe

hidrófugo
E hydrophobic, water-repellent
G wasserabweisend
F hydrophobe

hidrogenación
E hydrogenation
G Hydrogenierung
F hydrogénation

hidrógeno
E hydrogen
G Wasserstoff
F hydrogène

hidrólisis
E hydrolysis
G Hydrolyse
F hydrolyse

hidrólisis parcial
E partial hydrolysis
G Hydrolyse, partielle
F hydrolyse partielle

higiene de la empresa
E plant hygiene, plant sanitation
G Betriebshygiene
F hygiène des installations

higiene personal
E personnel hygiene
G Personalhygiene
F hygiène du personnel

higrómetro
E hygrometer
G Hygrometer, Feuchtigkeitsmesser, Feuchtemesser
F hygromètre

higrómetro capilar
E hair hygrometer
G Haarhygrometer
F hygromètre à cheveux

higroscopicidad
E hygroscopicity
G Hygroskopizität
F hygroscopie

higroscópico
E hygroscopic
G hygroskopisch
F hygroscopique

hilo
E thread
G Faden
F fil

hinchable
E inflatable
G aufblasbar
F gonflable

hincharse
E swell, to
G quellen
F gonfler

hipertónico
E hypertonic
G hypertonisch
F hypertonique

hipotensión
E negative pressure
G Unterdruck
F sous-pression, depression

hipotónico
E hypotonic
G hypotonisch
F hypotonique

hoja
E foil, film
G Folie
F feuille

hoja de aluminio
E aluminium foil
G Aluminiumfolie
F feuille d'aluminium

hoja de datos de seguridad
E safety data sheet, material safety data sheet (MSDS)
G Sicherheitsdatenblatt
F feuillet de données sur la sécurité, feuille de données de sécurité

hoja de recubrimiento
E cover foil
G Deckfolie
F feuille de protection

hoja laminada
E laminated foil, composite foil
G Verbundfolie
F feuille stratifiée

hombro del pico
E peak shoulder
G Peakschulter
F épaulement de pic

homogeneidad
E homogeneity, uniformity, consistency
G Homogenität, Einheitlichkeit, Gleichförmigkeit
F homogénéité, uniformité, consistance

homogéneo
E homogeneous, uniform
G homogen, gleichmäßig, einheitlich
F homogène, uniforme

homogenizador
E homogeniser
G Homogenisator
F homogénéiseur

homogenizar
E homogenise, to
G homogenisieren
F homogénéiser

homólogo
E homologous
G homolog
F homologue

hongos
E fungi, moulds
G Pilze
F champignons

horario
E schedule
G Zeitplan
F plan, programme

horizontal
E horizontal
G waagerecht
F horizontal

horno de aire caliente
E hot air oven
G Heißluftofen
F four à air chaud

horno de columna
E column oven
G Säulenofen
F four pour colonne

horno de manguito
E muffle furnace
G Muffelofen
F four à moufle

horno de secado
E dry heat oven
G Trockenofen
F étuve

horno fundidor
E furnace
G Schmelzofen
F four

hueco
E recess, hollow
G Aussparung, hohl
F évidure, échancrure, creux

huella dactilar IR
E IR fingerprint
G IR-Fingerabdruck
F empreinte digitale IR

humectación
E humidification
G Befeuchtung
F humidification

humectante
E wetting agent
G Benetzungsmittel, Netzmittel, Feuchthaltemittel
F mouillant

humectar
E moisten, to; wet, to; humidify, to; humidise, to
G befeuchten, anfeuchten
F humidifier

humedad
E humidity, moisture
G Feuchtigkeit
F humidité

humedad adherente
E bound moisture
G gebundene Feuchtigkeit
F humidité adhérente

humedad no adherente
E unbound moisture
G nicht gebundene Feuchtigkeit
F humidité non liée

humedad atmosférica relativa
E relative humidity
G relative Luftfeuchtigkeit
F humidité relative

humedad del aire
E humidity
G Luftfeuchtigkeit
F humidité

humedad residual
E residual moisture
G Restfeuchte
F humidité résiduelle

humedecer
E moisten, to; wet, to; humidify, to; humidise, to
G befeuchten, anfeuchten, benetzen
F humidifier, mouiller

húmedo
E moist
G feucht
F humide

humidificación
E humidification
G Befeuchtung
F humidification

humidificador de aire
E humidifier
G Luftbefeuchter, Befeuchter
F humidificateur

identidad
E identity
G Identität
F identité

identificación
E identification
G Identifikation
F identification

identificación del impreso
E print recognition
G Druckerkennung
F identification de l'impression

identificación electrónica
E electronic identification (EID)
G elektronische Identifikation (EID)
F identification électronique

idoneidad
E suitability
G Eignung
F qualification

ignición
E ignition
G Zündung
F inflammation

English German French Spanish

ignífugo
E fire-resistant
G feuerfest
F in-inflammable

iluminación
E lighting, illumination
G Beleuchtung
F éclairage

iluminación desde atrás
E back illumination
G Beleuchtung von hinten
F éclairage par l'arrière

impacto
E impact
G Schlag, Stoß
F impact, coup

impedir
E prevent, to
G verhindern
F empêcher, éviter

impermeabilidad
E impermeability, imperviousness
G Undurchlässigkeit
F imperméabilité

impermeabilidad al aire
E air impermeability
G Luftundurchlässigkeit
F imperméabilité à l'air

impermeabilizar
E gum, to
G gummieren
F gommer

impermeable
E impermeable, impervious
G undurchlässig
F imperméable

impermeable a la humedad
E impervious to moisture
G feuchtigkeitsundurchlässig
F étanche

impermeable al agua
E water-tight, waterproof
G wasserdicht
F imperméable à l'eau

impermeable al aire
E air-tight, impermeable to air
G luftdicht, luftundurchlässig
F étanche à l'air, imperméable à l'air

impermeable al gas
E gas-tight
G gasdicht
F étanche au gaz

implantado
E implant
G Implantat
F implant

importancia
E significance
G Bedeutung
F signification

impregnar
E impregnate, to; soak, to
G imprägnieren, tränken
F imprégner

impresión
E imprint
G Aufdruck
F impression

impresión de láminas
E film printing
G Folienbedruckung
F impression de feuilles

impreso (en, sobre papel)
E printout, paper printout, hard copy
G Ausdruck, Papierausdruck, Schreiberausdruck
F imprimé, imprimé sur papier

impresora
E printer
G Drucker
F imprimante

impresora a color
E printer ink
G Druckerfarbe
F couleur d'imprimante

impresora de chorro de tinta
E ink jet printer
G Tintenstrahldrucker
F imprimante à jet d'encre

impresora de láser
E laser printer
G Laserdrucker
F imprimante à laser

imprimir
E emboss, to; imprint, to; print, to
G aufprägen, einprägen, aufdrucken, bedrucken
F imprimer, empreindre

impulso
E drive
G Antrieb
F entraînement, transmission

impureza
E impurity, contamination
G Verunreinigung
F impureté, contamination

impureza reductora
E reducing impurity
G reduzierende Verunreinigung
F pollution réductrice

impureza vestigial
E trace impurity
G Verunreinigung in Spuren
F impureté à l'état de traces

in situ
E in-situ
G in-situ
F in situ

inaccesible
E inaccessible
G unzugänglich
F inaccessible

inaccesible para niños
E child-proof
G kindersicher
F inaccessible aux enfants

inactivación
E inactivation, deactivation
G Inaktivierung
F inactivation

inactivado
E inactivated
G inaktiviert
F inactivées

inalterabilidad
E durability, resistance
G Beständigkeit
F stabilité à long terme, résistance

incandescer
E anneal, to
G glühen
F recuire

incidente
E incident, fault, failure, accident
G Vorfall, Zwischenfall, Störfall
F panne, incident

incineración
E combustion, incineration, ashing
G Verbrennung, Veraschung
F combustion, incinération

incineración de desechos
E rubbish incineration
G Müllverbrennung
F incinération des déchets

inclinación
E slope, sloping position, gradient
G Gefälle, Schräglage, Schräge, Neigung
F pente, inclinaison, position inclinée, gradient, biais

inclinado
E sloped, sloping
G geneigt, mit Gefälle, schräg
F incliné, avec une pente, oblique

incluir
E embed, to
G einbetten
F inclure

inclusión
E inclusion
G Einschluß
F inclusion

inclusión de aire
E air entrapment
G Lufteinschluß
F inclusion d'air

incoloro
E colourless
G farblos
F incolore

incompatibilidad
E incompatibility
G Inkompatibilität, Unverträglichkeit
F incompatibilité

incompatible
E incompatible
G inkompatibel
F incompatible

incompleto
E incomplete
G unvollständig
F incomplet

incorporado
E fitted
G eingebaut
F encastré

incubadora
E oven, incubator
G Wärmeschrank, Brutschrank
F incubateur

incubar
E incubate, to
G inkubieren, bebrüten
F incuber

indeleble
E indelible
G unauslöschbar
F indélébile

indemne
E undamaged
G unbeschädigt
F intact

indicación
E display
G Anzeige
F indicateur

indicador
E indicator, pointer
G Indikator, Zeiger
F indicateur, aiguille

indicador de nivel de líquido
E liquid level indicator
G Flüssigkeitsstandsanzeige
F indicateur du niveau de liquide

indicador de presión diferencial
E pressure differential indicator
G Differenzdruckanzeiger
F indicateur de pression différentielle

indicar
E display, to; indicate, to
G anzeigen
F indiquer, afficher

índice
E index, contents, list
G Verzeichnis
F répertoire, registre

índice de ácido
E acid value
G Säurezahl
F indice d'acide

índice de fusión
E melting index
G Schmelzindex
F indice de fusion

índice de iodo
E iodine number
G Iodzahl
F indice d'iode, nombre d'iode

índice de peróxido
E peroxide number, peroxide index
G Peroxydzahl
F index de peroxyde

índice de refracción
E refractive index
G Brechungsindex, Brechungszahl
F index de réfraction

índice de saponificación
E saponification value
G Verseifungszahl
F indice de saponification

índice de saturación
E saturation index
G Sättigungsindex
F indice de saturation

índice hidroxílico
E hydroxyl number
G Hydroxylzahl
F indice d'hydroxyle

inequívoco
E unambiguous, unequivocal, clear
G eindeutig
F non équivoque, clair, précis

inerte
E inert, poorly reactive
G inert, reaktionsträge
F inerte

inexactitud inherente (p. ej. de una técnica)
E inherent uncertainty (e. g. of a technique)
G inhärente Ungenauigkeit (z. B. einer Technik)
F imprécision inhérente (par ex. d'une technologie)

infeccioso
E infectious
G infektiös
F infectieux

infestación con insectos
E insect infestation
G Insektenbefall
F invasion d'insectes

inflamabilidad
E flammability
G Brennbarkeit
F combustibilité

inflamable
E flammable, ignitable
G entflammbar, entzündbar, feuergefährlich
F inflammable

fácilmente inflamable
E highly flammable
G leicht entflammbar
F facilement inflammable

influencia del medio ambiente
E environmental influence
G Umwelteinfluß
F influence de l'environnement

informar a alguien
E report to someone, to
G berichten, jemandem
F rapporter à quelqu'un

informe
E report
G Bericht
F rapport

informe anual de producción
E annual product report
G jährlicher Produktbericht
F rapport annuel de production

informe de desarrollo
E development report
G Entwicklungsbericht
F rapport de développement

informe de la situación
E status report
G Statusbericht
F rapport de situation

informe de prueba
E test report
G Prüfbericht
F rapport expérimental

informe de recepción técnica
E technical acceptance report
G Abnahmebericht
F rapport de réception technique

informe de reclamaciones
E complaint report
G Beanstandungsbericht
F compte-rendu de réclamation

informe de validación
E validation report
G Validierungsbericht
F rapport de validation

informe ecológico
E environmental report
G Umweltschutzbericht
F rapport sur l'écologie

infracción
E infringement
G Verletzung
F contrefaire un brevet

infradosificación
E sub-strength
G Unterdosierung
F hypo-dose

infusión
E infusion
G Aufguß, Infus
F infusion

ingeniería
E engineering
G Ingenieurwesen
F ingénieurie

ingeniero
E engineer
G Ingenieur
F ingénieur

ingrediente
E component, constituent, ingredient
G Bestandteil
F composant, constituant, ingrédient

inhalación
E inhalation
G Inhalation
F inhalation

inhibición
E inhibition
G Hemmung
F inhibition

inhibidor
E inhibitor
G Hemmstoff
F inhibiteur

iniciación (de una reacción)
E initiation (of a reaction)
G Initiierung (einer Reaktion)
F initiation (d'une réaction)

iniciales
E initials
G Namenszeichen
F initiales

inmunoelectroforesis
E immune electrophoresis
G Immunelektrophorese
F immunoélectrophorèse

inmunológico
E immunological
G immunologisch
F immunologique

innovador
E innovative
G innovativ
F innovant

inoculación
E inoculation
G Inokulation, Beimpfung
F inoculation

inoculación directa (para recuento microbiano)
E direct inoculation (for microbial count determination)
G Direktbeschickung (zur Keimzahlbestimmung)
F inoculation directe

inocular
E inoculate, to
G beimpfen
F ensemencer, inoculer

inodoro
E odourless
G geruchlos
F sans odeur

insaturado
E unsaturated
G ungesättigt
F insaturé

inscribir
E enter, to
G eintragen
F inscrire, enregistrer

insecticida
E insecticide
G Insektizid, insektizid
F insecticide

inseguridad
E uncertainty
G Unsicherheit
F incertitude

inseguridad analítica
E analytical uncertainty
G analytische Unsicherheit
F incertitude analytique

inserción
E reaction materials
G Ansatz
F matériaux de réaction

inserción de embalajes
E package loading
G Packguteinschub
F passage intercalé de conditionnements

inserción de la tobera
E nozzle insert
G Düseneinsatz
F garniture d'un gicleur

inserción de poliestirol
E polystyrene insert
G Polystyrol-Einsatz
F insert en polystyrène

inserción del filtro
E filter insert
G Filtereinsatz
F support de filtre

inserción del tamiz
E sieve insert
G Siebeinsatz
F segment de tamisage

insípido
E tasteless, flavourless
G geschmacklos
F insipide, fade

insoluble
E insoluble
G unlöslich
F insoluble

insonorizado
E noise-proof
G geräuschdämmend
F insonorisé

inspección
E inspection, audit, supervision
G Inspektion, Audit, Aufsicht
F inspection, audit, supervision, surveillance

inspección de un fabricante
E manufacturer audit
G Herstelleraudit
F audit d'un fabricant

English German French Spanish

English
German
French
Spanish

inspección médica periódica
E periodic health check
G regelmäßige Gesundheitsuntersuchung
F visite médicale périodique

inspección visual
E visual inspection, visual examination
G Durchsichtkontrolle, Sichtprüfung
F inspection visuelle, examen visuel

inspectoría
E inspectorate
G Inspektorat
F inspection (entité admin.)

instalación
E facility, plant, installation, mounting
G Anlage, Installation, Einrichtung, Einbau, Montage
F établissement industriel, installation (industrielle), montage

instalación para un fin determinado
E dedicated plant
G Einrichtung für einen bestimmten Zweck
F installation industrielle dédiée

instalación compacta
E compact line
G Kompaktanlage
F appareillage compact

instalación de aire comprimido
E compressed air plant
G Druckluftanlage
F installation servant à la production d'air comprimé

instalación de conducciones
E plumbing
G Verrohrung
F plomberie

instalación de pesado
E weighing facility
G Wiegeanlage
F installation de pesage

instalación de un filtro
E filter installation
G Filtereinbau
F installation d'un filtre

instalación de uso múltiple
E multi-purpose equipment
G Mehrzweckanlage
F installation technique multi-usages

instalación in situ
E on-site installation
G Installation vor Ort
F installation sur site

instalación para proceso
E processing facility, processing plant
G Prozeßanlage
F installation pour processus

instalación para uso único
E dedicated equipment
G Mono-Anlage
F équipement dédié

instalación piloto
E pilot plant
G Versuchsanlage
F usine pilote

instalado
E fitted
G eingebaut
F encastré

instalado fijamente
E permanently installed
G fest installiert
F installé de manière permanente

instalar
E apply, to; attach, to; fit, to; install, to; set up, to
G anbringen, einbauen, einrichten
F apposer, installer, poser, mettre en place

instancia
E application
G Antrag
F requête, demande

instrucción
E instruction, training
G Anweisung, Schulung
F instruction, mode d'emploi, éducation, entraînement

instrucción de embalaje
E packaging instruction
G Verpackungsanweisung
F instruction d'emballage

instrucción de fabricación
E manufacturing instructions
G Herstellungsanweisung
F instructions de fabrication

instrucción de limpieza
E cleaning procedure
G Reinigungsvorschrift
F procédure de nettoyage

instrucción de manejo
E operating instructions
G Bedienungsanleitung
F mode d'emploi, instructions opératoires

instrucción de procesado
E processing instructions
G Verarbeitungsanweisung
F instructions pour le traitement

instrucción de servicio
E operating instructions
G Bedienungsanleitung
F mode d'emploi, instructions opératoires

instrucción de trabajo
E operating procedure
G Arbeitsanweisung
F procédure opératoire

instrucción de uso
E instructions for use, operating instructions
G Gebrauchsanweisung
F instructions pour l'utilisation

instrucción estándar de trabajo
E standard operating procedure (SOP)
G Standardarbeitsanweisung
F procédures opératoires standards

instrucciones de funcionamiento
E operating manual, operating instructions
G Betriebsanleitung
F mode d'emploi, instructions de service

instrucciones de prueba
E test instructions, testing procedure
G Prüfanleitung, Prüfanweisung
F mode opératoire, instructions d'un test

instrucciones para tomar muestras
E sampling instructions
G Stichprobenanweisung
F instructions d'échantillonnage

rigor de las instrucciones para tomar muestras
E sampling criteria
G Schärfe der Stichprobenanweisung
F critères d'échantillonnage

instrumental de compresión
E compaction device, compression mould
G Preßwerkzeug
F outil de compression

instrumental de infusión
E infusion assembly
G Infusionsbesteck
F nécessaire pour infusion

English German French Spanish

instrumental de transfusión
E transfusion set
G Transfusionsbesteck
F nécessaire de transfusion

instrumental de vidrio
E glassware
G Glasgeräte
F verrerie

instrumento
E tool
G Werkzeug
F outil

instrumentos de control
E control instrumentation
G Kontrollinstrumentierung
F instruments de contrôle

instrumentos de perforación
E perforation tool
G Perforierwerkzeug
F outil de perforation

instrumentos para fabricar comprimidos
E compaction device
G Tablettierwerkzeug
F instrument de fabrication de comprimés

insuficiencia
E deficiency
G Mangel
F déficience, carence, insuffisance

intacto
E intact, sound, faultless
G intakt, einwandfrei
F intact, irréprochable

integrado en una red
E reticular
G vernetzt
F réticulaire

integridad
E integrity
G Integrität, Unversehrtheit
F intégrité

integridad de un embalaje
E package integrity
G Unversehrtheit der Verpackung
F intégrité d'un conditionnement

integridad del filtro
E filter integrity
G Filterintegrität
F intégrité d'un filtre

intensidad de cizallamiento
E shear intensity
G Scherintensität
F intensité de cisaillement

intensidad de corriente
E amperage
G Stromstärke
F ampérage

intensificación
E amplification
G Verstärkung
F amplification

intensificado
E reinforced
G verstärkt
F renforcé

interacción
E interaction
G Wechselwirkung
F interaction, action réciproque

intercambiable
E interchangeable, exchangeable, replaceable
G austauschbar, auswechselbar
F interchangeable

intercambiador de aniones
E anion exchanger
G Anionenaustauscher
F échangeur d'ions anioniques

intercambiador de calor
E heat exchanger
G Wärmetauscher
F échangeur de chaleur

intercambiador de calor de haces tubulares
E tube bundle heat exchanger
G Rohrbündelwärmetauscher
F échangeur de chaleur à faisceaux tubulaires

intercambiador de cationes
E cation exchanger
G Kationentauscher
F échangeur de cations

intercambiador de cubetas
E cell changer
G Küvettenwechsler
F échangeur de cuvette

intercambiador de iones
E ion exchanger
G Ionenaustauscher
F échangeur d'ions

intercambiador de iones de lecho mixto
E mixed bed ion exchanger
G Mischbettionenentauscher, Gemischtbett-Ionenaustauscher
F échangeur d'ions à lit mixte, échange d'ions sur lit mixte

intercambio de halógenos
E halogen exchange
G Halogenaustausch
F échange d'halogène

intercambio de iones
E ion exchange
G Ionenaustausch
F échange d'ions

interfase
E interface
G Grenzfläche
F surface de séparation, interface

interfase seriada
E serial interface
G serielle Schnittstelle
F interface série

interferencia
E interference, overlap
G Interferenz, Überschneidung
F interférence, chevauchement, recouvrement

interferencia electromagnética
E electromagnetic interference
G elektromagnetische Interferenz
F interférence électromagnétique

interlocutor
E contact person
G Ansprechpartner
F interlocuteur

interpretación
E interpretation, evaluation
G Auswertung
F interprétation, évaluation

interrupción (de una reacción)
E interruption, cessation (of a reaction)
G Unterbrechung (einer Reaktion)
F interruption (d'une réaction)

interrupción del funcionamiento
E breakdown
G Betriebsstörung
F perturbation de fonctionnement

interruptor (de desconexión)
E switch, on/off switch
G Schalter, Abschalter, Ausschalter
F interrupteur, bouton marche/arrêt

interruptor a la red
E power switch, main switch
G Netzschalter
F interrupteur de courant

interruptor de emergencia
E emergency off
G Not-Aus
F arrêt d'urgence

interruptor de encendido
E start/stop key
G An/Aus-Taste
F touche marche-arrêt

interruptor principal
E main switch, power switch
G Hauptschalter
F interrupteur principal

intervalo de calibración
E calibration interval
G Kalibrierintervall
F intervalle de calibration

intervalo de confianza
E confidence interval, confidence area
G Vertrauensintervall, Vertrauensbereich
F intervalle de confiance, plage de confiance

intervalo de destilación
E distillation range
G Destillationsbereich
F intervalle de distillation

intervalo de tolerancia
E tolerance range
G Toleranzbereich
F intervalle de tolérance

intervención
E intervention
G Eingriff
F intervention

intolerancia
E incompatibility
G Unverträglichkeit
F incompatibilité

introducción de un producto (en el mercado)
E product launch
G Produkteinführung
F lancement d'un produit

introducción en el mercado
E placing on the market, launch
G Einführung auf den Markt, Markteinführung, Inverkehrbringen
F introduction sur le marché, lancement d'un produit

inundar (con)
E flush, to (with); purge, to (with)
G durchströmen (mit)
F rincer (avec), purger

inválido
E invalid
G ungültig
F non valable

inventario
E bill of materials, list of items
G Stückliste
F liste-inventaire, liste détaillée

investigación
E investigation
G Untersuchung
F inspection

investigación clínica
E clinical research
G klinische Forschung
F recherche clinique

investigación de errores
E error (failure) investigation
G Fehleruntersuchung
F investigation des sources d'une erreur

investigación y desarrollo
E R + D (Research and Development)
G F + E (Forschung und Entwicklung)
F R + D (recherche et développement)

investigar
E investigate, to; test, to
G untersuchen, prüfen
F inspecter, tester

inyección
E injection, splashes
G Einspritzung, Spritzer
F injection, éclaboussures

inyección de muestras
E sample injection
G Probeneinspritzung
F injection d'échantillon

inyectable
E injectible
G injizierbar
F injectable

inyectables
E parenterals
G Parenteralia
F préparations injectables

inyectables de escaso volumen
E small volume parenterals (SVP)
G kleinvolumige Parenteralia
F préparations injectables de petit volume

inyectables voluminosos
E large volume parenterals (LVP)
G großvolumige Parenteralia
F préparations injectables de grand volume

inyectar
E inject, to
G injizieren
F injecter

inyector
E injection port, nozzle
G Düse, Einspritzdüse
F buse, buse d'injection, gicleur, tuyère

inyector automático
E injector, automatic
G automatischer Injektor
F injecteur automatique

inyector de implantados
E implanter
G Implantatinjektor
F injecteur d'implant

ion cargado
E charged ion
G Ion, geladenes
F ion chargé

ion complementario
E counter-ion
G Gegenion
F contre-ion, ion complémentaire

ionización
E ionisation
G Ionisierung
F ionisation

irradiación
E irradiation, radiation
G Bestrahlung
F irradiation

irradiar con
E irradiate, to (with)
G bestrahlen mit
F irradier avec

irrigar
E rinse, to
G spülen
F rincer

irrita las vías respiratorias
E irritating to respiratory system
G reizt die Atemwege
F irritant pour le système respiratoire

irrita los ojos
E irritating to eyes
G reizt die Augen
F irritant pour les yeux

irritación (química)
E irritation (chem.)
G Reizung (chemisch)
F irritation (chimique)

irritante cutáneo
E irritating to skin
G hautreizend
F irritant pour la peau

irrompible
E unbreakable, shatter-proof
G unzerbrechlich, bruchfest
F incassable

ISO certificado
E ISO-certificated
G ISO-zertifiziert
F certifié ISO

isocrático
E isocratic
G isokratisch
F isocratique

isómeros de conformación
E conformation isomers
G Konformationsisomere
F isomères de conformation

isotónico
E isotonic
G isoton
F isotonique

jarabe
E syrup
G Sirup
F sirop

jarabe antitusígeno
E cough syrup
G Hustensaft
F sirop contre la toux

jeringa
E syringe
G Spritze
F seringue

jeringa de uso único
E disposable syringe
G Einmalspritze
F seringue à usage unique

jeringa dispuesta para el uso
E prefilled syringe
G Fertigspritze
F seringue prête à l'usage

jeringa lista para el uso
E prefilled syringe
G Fertigspritze
F seringue prête à l'emploi

jeringuilla
E injection syringe
G Injektionsspritze
F seringue d'injection

juego de pesas
E set of weights
G Gewichtssatz
F série de poids

jugo (animal)
E juice
G Saft
F jus

jugo gástrico
E gastric juice, gastric fluid
G Magensaft
F suc gastrique

junta
E joint, seam, weld, seal, gasket
G Fuge, Trennfuge, Naht, Dichtung
F joint

sin juntas
E seamless
G fugenlos
F dépourvu de joint

junta de cartucho
E cartridge gasket
G Patronendichtung
F joint de cartouche

junta de construcción
E construction joint
G Arbeitsfuge
F joint de construction

junta de dilatación
E expansion joint, settlement joint
G Dehnungsfuge, Bewegungsfuge
F joint de compensation, joint dilatable, joint de dilatation

junta de goma
E rubber gasket
G Gummidichtung
F joint en caoutchouc

junta de movimiento
E settling joint
G Bewegungsfuge
F joint de dilatation

junta de una puerta
E door seal
G Türdichtung
F joint de porte

junta directiva
E board of directors, director
G Vorstand
F comité de direction

junta hinchable
E inflatable gasket
G aufblasbare Dichtung
F joint gonflable

juntas de construcción
E construction joints
G Arbeitsfugen
F joints de construction

juntura de un tubo
E crimp, seam
G Tubenfalz
F joint d'un tube

kit
E kit
G Bausatz
F kit, prêt-à-monter

lábil al calor
E heat-labile
G hitzelabil
F sensible à la chaleur

laboratorio
E laboratory, lab
G Labor
F laboratoire

laboratorio acreditado de calibración
E accredited calibration laboratory
G akkreditiertes Kalibrierlabor
F laboratoire d'étalonnage homologué

laboratorio comisionado
E contract laboratory
G Auftragslabor
F laboratoire sous-traitant

laboratorio controlado para GMP
E GMP-controlled laboratory
G GMP-Labor
F laboratoire conforme aux GMP

laboratorio de fermentación
E fermentation laboratory
G Fermentationslabor
F laboratoire de fermentation

laboratorio de seguridad biológica
E biohazard laboratory, biosafety laboratory
G Biosicherheitslabor
F laboratoire de risques biologiques

laca
E varnish, lacquer
G Lack
F vernis, laque

laca termofusible
E heat-sealing lacquer
G Heißsiegellack
F laque thermofusible

lacar
E lacquer, to
G lackieren
F laquer

lacre
E sealing wax
G Siegellack
F cire à cacheter

lactona
E lactone
G Lacton
F lactone

lactosa
E lactose
G Lactose
F lactose

ladear
E cant, to
G verkanten
F mettre sur l'arête

lado inferior
E base
G Unterseite
F face inférieure

lado superior
E upper side, top side
G Oberseite
F face supérieure, côté supérieur

lámina
E foil, film, sheet, plate, tray
G Folie, Blech
F feuille, tôle

lámina continua
E continuous foil, continuous film
G Folie, endlose
F feuille continue

lámina de estampado
E embossed film
G Prägefolie
F feuille estampée

lámina de inmersión
E immersion sword
G Tauchschwert
F lame d'immersion

lámina de plástico
E plastic film
G Plastikfolie
F film plastique

lámina divisoria para comprimidos
E tablet gate
G Tablettenablaufweichen
F déversoir pour comprimés

lámina estratificada
E laminated foil, composite foil
G Verbundfolie
F feuille stratifiée

lámina recubierta
E coated foil, coated film
G Folie, beschichtete
F feuille enduite

lámina retraíble
E shrink foil, shrink film
G Schrumpffolie
F feuille rétractable, film rétractable

lámina termoformada
E thermoforming foil, forming foil
G Tiefziehfolie, Verformfolie
F feuille thermoformée

lámina transparente
E transparent foil
G Klarsichtfolie
F feuille transparente

laminar
E coat, to; laminate, to
G beschichten
F enduire

laminilla
E lamella
G Lamelle
F lamelle

lámpara de arco de tungsteno
E tungsten arc lamp
G Wolframbogenlampe
F lampe à arc de tungstène

lámpara de señales
E control lamp
G Signallampe
F lampe de contrôle

lámpara UV
E UV lamp
G UV-Lampe
F lampe UV

lastre
E sinker
G Senkkörper
F plomb

lata
E can, tin
G Dose
F canne

lavabo
E wash basin
G Waschbecken
F évier

lavar
E rinse, to
G spülen
F rincer

lavativa
E enema
G Darmspülung, Klistier
F lavement, lavement intestinal

lecho de mortero
E mortar bed
G Mörtelbett
F lit de mortier

lecho de polvo
E powder bed
G Pulverbett
F lit de poudre

lecho filtrante
E filter bed
G Filterbett
F lit de filtre

lecho fluidificado
E fluid bed
G Wirbelschicht
F lit fluidisé

lecho mixto
E mixed bed
G Mischbett
F lit mixe

lector de anillo cromático
E colour ring code reader
G Farbringleser
F lecteur de codage de couleurs

lector electrónico de códigos
E electronic code reader
G elektronisches Codelesegerät
F déchiffreur électronique de codage

lectura de códigos
E code reading
G Codelesung
F lecture du codage

lectura de la presión
E pressure reading
G Druckablesung
F relevé de la pression

leer
E read, to; read off, to
G ablesen
F lire, relever

legible
E legible
G lesbar
F lisible

legislación
E legislation
G Gesetzgebung
F législation

lejía
E alkaline solution, lye
G Lauge
F soude

lejía madre
E mother liquor
G Mutterlauge
F eau mère, lessive-mère

lengüeta arrancable
E tear-off tab
G Aufreißlasche
F languette

lente
E lens
G Linse
F lentille

lente del objetivo
E object lens
G Objektlinse
F lentille-objet

lesión (herida)
E infringement
G Verletzung
F contrefaire un brevet

leva
E cam
G Nocke
F came

levadura
E yeast
G Hefe
F levure

levantar acta
E protocol, to; record, to; document, to
G protokollieren
F enregistrer, documenter

levigado
E eluate
G Eluat
F éluat

levógiro
E laevo-rotary
G linksdrehend
F lévogyre

ley
E law, statute
G Gesetz
F loi

Ley Alemana de Sustancias Peligrosas
E German Hazardous Substance Act
G Deutsches Gefahrstoffgesetz
F législation allemande sur les substances dangereuses

ley de protección frente a radiaciones ionizantes
E radiation protection act
G Strahlenschutzgesetz
F loi pour la protection contre les radiations

leyenda
E legend
G Zeichenerklärung
F légende

liberación
E release
G Freisetzung
F libération

liberación controlada
E controlled release
G kontrollierte Freisetzung
F libération contrôlée

liberación incompleta
E incomplete release
G unvollständige Freisetzung
F libération incomplète

liberación inmediata
E immediate release
G schnelle Freisetzung
F libération immédiate

liberación modificada
E modified release
G modifizierte Freisetzung
F libération modifiée

liberación prolongada
E sustained release
G verlängerte Freisetzung
F libération prolongée

liberación retardada
E delayed release
G verzögerte Freisetzung
F libération différée

liberación de oxígeno
E oxygen release
G Sauerstoffentwicklung
F évolution de la teneur en oxygène

liberación de un lote
E batch release
G Chargenfreigabe
F libération d'un lot

liberación de sustancia activa
E extended release of medicinal substance
G Wirkstoff-Freigabe
F libération d'un princip actif

liberación del principio activo
E release of medicinal substance, active substance release
G Arzneistoff-Freisetzung, Wirkstoff-Freigabe
F libération d'un principe actif

liberación prolongada del principio activo
E extended release
G verlängerte Wirkstoff-Freigabe
F libération prolongée d'un principe actif

liberación retardada del principio activo
E delayed release
G verzögerte Wirkstoff-Freigabe
F libération retardée d'un principe actif

liberación in vitro
E in-vitro release
G In-vitro-Freisetzung
F libération in-vitro

liberación rápida, de
E immediate release
G schnell freisetzend
F à libération immédiate

liberación temporalmente controlada
E timed release
G zeitlich gesteuerte Freigabe
F libération contrôlée

liberado
E released
G freigegeben
F libéré

liberar
E release, to
G freigeben
F libérer

liberar partículas
E shed particles, to
G Partikel abgeben
F libérer des particules

libro de entrada de mercancías
E receiving log book
G Wareneingangsbuch
F livre d'entrées de marchandises

licencia
E licence
G Lizenz
F licence

licencia de importación
E import licence
G Einfuhrerlaubnis
F license d'importation

licuar
E fluidise, to; liquify, to
G verflüssigen
F liquéfier

licuefacer
E fluidise, to; liquify, to
G verflüssigen
F liquéfier

líder de opinión
E opinion leader
G Meinungsbildner
F leader d'opinion

ligadura de superficie
E surface binding
G Oberflächenbindung
F liaison superficielle

English
German
French
Spanish

lima de ampolla
E ampoule file, ampoule cutter
G Ampullenfeile
F lime (pour ampoule)

limitación
E limitation
G Einschränkung
F limitation

límite de acción
E action limit
G Aktionsgrenze, Stopgrenze
F limite d'action

límite de alarma
E alarm limit
G Alarmlimit
F limite d'alarme

límite de alerta
E alert limit
G Warngrenze
F limite d'alerte

límite de análisis
E limit of quantitation (LOQ)
G Bestimmungsgrenze
F limite de quantitation

límite inferior de determinación
E lower limit of quantitation
G untere Bestimmungsgrenze
F limite inférieure de quantitation

límite superior de determinación
E upper limit of quantitation
G obere Bestimmungsgrenze
F limite supérieure de quantitation

límite de calidad aceptable
E acceptable quality level (AQL)
G Annehmbare Qualitätsgrenzlage (AQL)
F niveau de qualité acceptable

límite individual de calidad aceptable
E individual AQL
G Einzel-AQL
F niveau individuel de qualité acceptable

límite total de calidad aceptable
E class AQL
G Gesamt-AQL
F niveau absolu de qualité acceptable

límite de carga
E loading limit
G Belastungsgrenze
F limite de charge

límite de detección
E limit of detection (LOD)
G Nachweisgrenze
F limite de détection

límite de determinación
E limit of quantitation (LOQ)
G Bestimmungsgrenze
F limite de quantitation

límite inferior de determinación
E lower limit of quantitation
G untere Bestimmungsgrenze
F limite inférieure de quantitation

límite superior de determinación
E upper limit of quantitation
G obere Bestimmungsgrenze
F limite supérieure de quantitation

límite de error
E margin of error
G Fehlergrenze
F marge d'erreur

límite de especificación
E specification limit
G Spezifikationsgrenze
F limite de spécification

límite inferior de especificación
E lower specification limit
G untere Spezifikationsgrenze
F limite inférieure de spécification

límite superior de especificación
E upper specification limit
G obere Spezifikationsgrenze
F limite supérieure de spécification

límites estrechos de especificación
E tight specification limits
G enge Spezifikationsgrenzen
F limites étroites de spécification

límite de exclusión
E exclusion limit
G Ausschlußgrenze
F limite d'exclusion

límite de funcionamiento
E operating limit
G Betriebsgrenze
F limite de service, limite d'utilisation

límite de migración (en cromatografía)
E yield point
G Fließgrenze
F limite d'écoulement

límites de confianza
E confidence limits
G Vertrauensgrenzen
F limites de confiance

limpieza
E cleaning, purification, cleanliness
G Reinigung, Sauberkeit
F nettoyage, propreté

limpieza (de instalaciones) en sistema cerrado
E cleaning in-place (CIP)
G Reinigung (von Anlagen) im geschlossenen System
F nettoyage en place (CIP)

limpieza del producto
E product purification
G Produktreinigung
F purification d'un produit

línea de base
E baseline, zero line
G Basislinie, Nullinie
F ligne de base, ligne de zéro

línea de células de mamífero
E mammalian cell line
G Säugetierzellinie
F lignée de cellule de mammifère

línea de fractura
E rupture line, fracture line
G Bruchlinie
F ligne de rupture, ligne de fracture

línea de ruptura
E rupture line, fracture line
G Bruchlinie
F ligne de rupture, ligne de fracture

línea directriz general
E cross-functional guideline
G abteilungsübergreifende Richtlinie
F lignes directrices générales

linealidad
E linearity
G Linearität
F linéarité

Líneas directrices de la EC sobre GMP
E EC-GMP Guideline
G EG-GMP-Leitfaden
F directives GMP de la CE

linimento
E embrocation, liniment
G Einreibemittel, Liniment
F beaume, onguent, liniment

liofilización
E freeze drying, lyophilisation
G Lyophilisation, Gefriertrocknung
F lyophilisation

liofilizado
E lyophilisate, freeze-dried, lyophilised
G Lyophilisat, gefriergetrocknet
F lyophilisat, lyophilisé

liofilizador
E freeze dryer, lyophiliser
G Gefriertrockner
F lyophilisateur

lípido
E lipid
G Lipid
F lipide

lipófilo
E lipophilic
G lipophil
F lipophile

lipófobo
E lipophobic
G lipophob
F lipophobe

líquido
E liquid
G Flüssigkeit, flüssig
F liquide

líquido de cerrado hermético
E sealing liquid
G Dichtflüssigkeit
F liquide d'étanchéité

líquido de granulación
E granulating fluid
G Granulierflüssigkeit
F liquide de granulation

líquido lacrimal
E lacrimal fluid
G Tränenflüssigkeit
F liquide lacrymal

líquido refrigerante
E coolant
G Kühlflüssigkeit
F réfrigérant

líquidos biológicos
E biological fluids
G biologische Flüssigkeiten
F liquides biologiques

lisado
E lysate
G Lysat
F lysat

liso
E plane, level, smooth
G eben, glatt
F plat, lisse, poli

lista de evaluación de errores
E defect (error, failure) evaluation list
G Fehlerbewertungsliste
F registre d'évaluation d'erreurs

lista de piezas de recambio
E spare parts list
G Ersatzteilliste
F liste de pièces de rechange

lista detallada
E bill of materials, list of items
G Stückliste
F liste-inventaire, liste détaillée

listo para el uso
E ready-to-use
G gebrauchsfertig
F prêt à l'emploi

litmus
E litmus
G Lackmus
F tournesol

llama abierta
E naked flame
G offene Flamme
F flamme ouverte

llano
E plane, level
G eben
F plat

llave (de troquel)
E key (of punch)
G Paßfeder, Schlüssel (des Stempels)
F clavette, ressort d'ajustage (de poinçon)

llave en mano
E turnkey
G schlüsselfertig
F clé en main

llave hexagonal
E Allen key
G Inbusschlüssel
F clé BTR

llenado de la columna
E column packing
G Säulenfüllung
F package de colonne

llenar
E fill, to; charge, to
G einfüllen
F charger, alimenter

llenar con embudo
E funnel, to
G eintrichtern
F remplir à l'aide d'un entonnoir

lleno a rebosar
E brimful
G randvoll
F plein à ras-bord

llevar a cabo
E carry out, to; execute, to
G durchführen
F réaliser, exécuter

locales
E premises
G Räumlichkeiten
F locaux

loción
E lotion
G Lotion
F lotion

loción capilar
E medicated hair tonic
G medizinisches Haarwasser
F lotion capillaire

loción oftálmica
E eye lotion
G Augenbad
F lotion pour œil

logística
E logistics
G Logistik
F logistique

logotipo
E logo
G Logo, Firmenzeichen
F logo

longitud
E length
G Länge
F longueur

longitud de la cabeza de troquel
E punch tip length
G Stempelkopflänge
F longueur de la tête du poinçon

longitud de la columna
E column length
G Säulenlänge
F longueur de colonne

longitud de onda
E wavelength
G Wellenlänge
F longueur d'onde

longitud total
E overall length
G Gesamtlänge
F longueur totale

lote
E batch, lot
G Charge
F lot

lote de producción
E production batch
G Produktionscharge
F lot de production

lote de venta
E approved batch
G Verkaufscharge
F lot de production

lote defectuoso
E defective batch, failed batch
G Fehlcharge
F lot défectueux

English German French Spanish

lote parcial
E sub-batch, partial batch
G Teilcharge
F sous-lot, lot partiel

lote piloto
E pilot batch, trial batch
G Versuchscharge
F lot pilote

lubri(fi)cante
E lubricant
G Schmiermittel, Gleitmittel
F lubrifiant

lubri(fi)car
E grease, to; lubricate, to
G schmieren
F graisser, lubrifier

lubricación del aparato
E instrument lubrication
G Geräteschmierung
F lubrification d'un instrument

lucha antiparasitaria
E pest control
G Schädlingsbekämpfung
F lutte antiparasitaire

lugar
E location
G Ort, Lage
F endroit, lieu

lugar de almacenamiento
E storage space
G Lagerplatz
F espace de stockage

lugar de aplicación
E site of action
G Angriffspunkt
F site d'application

lugar de extracción
E point of withdrawal
G Entnahmestelle
F point de retrait

lugar de instalación
E installation location
G Aufstellungsort
F lieu d'installation

lugar de producción
E manufacturing location, manufacturing site
G Produktionsort, Produktionsstätte
F lieu de production, site de production

lugar de ruptura
E break point, breaking point
G Bruchstelle
F point de rupture

lugar de toma de muestras
E sampling location, sampling point
G Probenahmestelle
F point de prélèvement

lugar, en el
E on-site
G vor Ort
F sur site

lugares de difícil acceso
E poorly accessible points
G schwer zugängliche Stellen
F endroits difficilement accessibles

lugares inaccesibles
E inaccessible points
G unzugängliche Stellen
F endroits inaccessibles

lupa
E magnifying glass
G Lupe
F loupe

lustrado
E glossy
G glänzend
F brillant, lustré

lustre
E gloss
G Glanz
F lustre, brillance

luz difusa
E stray light
G Streulicht
F lumière diffuse

luz intermitente
E flash light
G Blinklicht
F feux clignotant

maceración
E maceration
G Mazeration
F macération

macerado
E pickled
G gebeizt
F décapé

machacar
E crush, to; grind, to; mill, to
G zerstoßen
F broyer, concasser, piler

macizo
E thick
G dick
F épais

macromolécula
E macromolecule
G Makromolekül
F macro-molécule

macroporos
E macropores
G Makroporen
F macropores

maestro
E foreman, supervisor
G Meister
F maître

magnitud
E size
G Größe
F taille

maleable
E flexible, pliable
G biegsam
F flexible, pliable

malla
E network
G Netzwerk
F réseau

mancha
E stain
G Fleck
F tache

mandíbula
E jaw (tech.)
G Backe (techn.)
F mâchoire

mandíbulas de sellado
E sealer jaws
G Siegelbacken
F mâchoires de fermeture

manejo
E handling
G Handhabung
F maniement, traitement

mango
E handle, grip
G Bügel, Griff
F prise, poignée

manguito
E socket, collar, bush, bushing (mach.)
G Buchse, Manschette, Muffe
F borne, collier, bague, anneau, manchon, collet

manguito de caldeo
E heating mantle
G Heizpilz
F manteau chauffant

manguito hermético
E sealing collar
G Dichtmanschette
F manchette d'étanchéité

manifestación de desgaste
E wear and tear
G Verschleißerscheinung
F usure

manipulación genética
E genetic engineering
G Genmanipulation
F manipulation génétique

manómetro
E manometer, pressure gauge
G Manometer, Druckmeßgerät
F manomètre, manomètre de pression

manómetro diferencial
E differential manometer
G Differenzdruckmesser
F manomètre différentiel

mantenimiento
E maintenance
G Wartung, Instandhaltung
F entretien, maintenance

mantenimiento de equipo e instalaciones
E plant maintenance
G Anlagenwartung
F maintenance d'une installation

mantenimiento del equipo
E equipment maintenance
G Wartung der Ausrüstung
F entretien de l'équipement

mantenimiento preventivo
E preventive maintenance
G vorbeugende Wartung
F entretien préventif

manual
E hand-operated, manual
G von Hand, manuell
F manuel

manual de instrucciones
E instruction manual, instrument manual
G Handbuch, Gerätehandbuch
F manuel (d'utilisation), manuel d'instructions

máquina de carga con paleta
E palletiser
G Palettiermaschine
F palettiseur

máquina de cierre
E capping machine
G Verschließmaschine
F capsuleuse

máquina de cierre de botellas
E bottle-closing machine
G Flaschenverschließmaschine
F machine d'encapsulage

máquina de cierre de cajas plegables
E folding carton sealing machine
G Faltschachtelverschließmaschine
F machine à sceller les boîtes pliantes

máquina de cierre de rosca
E screw-cap closing machine
G Schraubdeckelverschließmaschine
F machine à serrage de couvercles

máquina de comprobación de dureza
E hardness tester
G Härtetester
F machine à tester la dureté

máquina de deformación térmica
E thermoforming machine
G Thermoformmaschine
F emboutisseuse

máquina de embalaje
E bundling machine
G Bündelmaschine
F machine d'empaquetage

máquina de envasado
E filling machine
G Abfüllmaschine
F remplisseuse

máquina de fabricación de comprimidos
E tabletting machine
G Tablettiermaschine
F machine de fabrication de comprimés

máquina de lavado de tapones
E stopper washing machine
G Stopfenwaschmaschine
F machine à laver les bouchons

máquina de llenado por tubos
E tube-filling machine
G Tubenfüllmaschine
F machine de remplissage pour tubes

máquina de moldear supositorios
E suppository machine
G Zäpfchengießmaschine
F machine à mouler des suppositoires

máquina de rebordeo
E capper, crimping machine
G Bördelmaschine
F boucheuse, capsuleuse

máquina de relleno de cápsulas
E capsule filling machine
G Kapselfüllmaschine
F encapsuleuse

máquina de tambor para gragear
E pan coater
G Trommelcoater
F machine d'enrobage à tambour

máquina dosificadora de tornillo sin fin
E dosing screw conveyor
G Schneckendosiermaschine
F convoyeur à vis doseuse

máquina encapsuladora
E encapsulator
G Kapselmaschine
F encapsuleuse

máquina encartonadora
E cartoning machine
G Kartonierer
F machine à cartonner

máquina excéntrica
E eccentric machine
G Exzentermaschine
F machine excentrique

máquina para cerrar cápsulas
E capping machine
G Deckelverschließmaschine
F encapsuleur

máquina para troquelar en caliente
E blister (forming) line
G Tiefziehmaschine
F machine pour conditionnements thermoformés

máquina plegadora de cajas
E folding carton set-up machine
G Faltschachtelaufrichtmaschine
F plieuse pour boîtes pliantes

marca (de fábrica)
E trade mark
G Warenzeichen
F marque déposée

marca comercial
E brand name, registered name, trade name
G Handelsmarke
F marque de commerce

marca de graduación
E graduation mark
G Strichmarkierung, Teilstrich
F marque de graduation

marca inconstante
E marker (on leaflet)
G Flattermarke
F marque inconstante

marcado
E labelling, lettering, designation
G Beschriftung, Kennzeichnung, Bezeichnung
F étiquetage, marquage, désignation, appellation

marcado radiactivo
E radio-label
G radioaktive Markierung
F marquage isotopique

marcador
E marker, tracer
G Leitsubstanz
F marqueur, traceur

marcar
E mark, to; label, to; designate, to
G kennzeichnen, bezeichnen
F étiqueter, marquer

marcha
E run
G Lauf
F cycle, opération, expérience

marcha de ensayo
E trial run, test run
G Probelauf
F essai de fonctionnement

marchamo
E seal
G Plombe
F sceau en plomb

margen bruto
E gross margin
G Bruttomarge
F marge brute

margen de error
E margin of error
G Fehlergrenze
F marge d'erreur

márgenes
E range
G Bereich, Bandbreite
F intervalle, échelle, intervalle, gamme, zone

márgenes permitidos
E acceptable range
G zulässiger Bereich
F intervalle autorisé

márgenes de fusión
E melting range
G Schmelzbereich
F plage de fusion

márgenes de retención
E retention range
G Rückhaltebereich
F zone de rétention

marmita
E vessel, boiler
G Kessel
F chaudière, bouilloire

masa comprimible
E compression material, moulding compound
G Preßmasse
F composé comprimable, matière moulée

masa comprimida
E pellet, compressed core
G Preßling
F implant, pastille, boulette

masa para comprimidos
E tabletting mass
G Tablettiermasse
F masse de fabrication pour comprimés

masa térmica
E thermal mass
G thermische Masse
F masse thermique

máscara
E mask
G Maske
F masque

máscara contra el polvo
E dust mask
G Staubmaske
F masque contre la poussière

matar
E kill, to; destroy, to
G abtöten
F tuer, détruire

mate
E mat
G matt
F mat

materia prima
E raw material, raw product
G Rohmaterial, Rohstoff, Rohprodukt
F matière brute, produit brut

materia prima inactiva
E inactive raw material
G Rohstoff, inaktiver
F matière première inactive

material
E material
G Werkstoff
F matériau

material consumible
E consumables
G Verbrauchsmaterial
F consommables

material de cierre
E closure material, sealant
G Verschlußmaterial, Dichtungsmittel
F matériau de fermeture, matériau d'étanchéité, matériau d'obturation

material de embalaje
E packaging material
G Packmaterial, Verpackungsmaterial, Packmittel
F matériel d'emballage

material impreso de embalaje
E printed packaging material
G bedrucktes Packmaterial
F matériel d'emballage imprimé

material de envase secundario
E secondary packaging material
G Sekundärpackmittel
F matériel d'emballage secondaire

material de junta
E jointing material
G Fugenmaterial
F matériau pour joint

material de prensado
E pressing material
G Preßmaterial
F matériel de moulage, matériel de pressage

material de relleno
E contents, charge
G Füllgut
F matière de remplissage

material de relleno de la columna
E column filler
G Säulenfüllmaterial
F matériel de remplissage d'une colonne

material de sellado
E sealant
G Dichtungsmittel
F matériau d'étanchéité, matériau d'obturation

material de sutura
E suture
G Nahtmaterial
F suture

material de unión
E bonding material
G Verbindungsmaterial
F substance de liaison

material monolítico
E monolithic material
G monolithisches Material
F matériau monolithique

material muy infeccioso
E highly infectious material
G hochinfektiöses Material
F matière hautement infectieuse

material primario de envase
E primary packaging material
G Primärpackmittel
F matériel d'emballage primaire

material que desprende partículas
E particle-releasing material
G partikelabgebendes Material
F matériau libérant des particules

English German French Spanish

materiales auxilares para envasado
E packaging aids
G Packhilfsmittel
F auxiliaires de conditionnement

materiales de filtración
E filter materials
G Filtermaterialien
F matériaux de filtre

materiales de reacción
E reaction materials
G Ansatz
F matériaux de réaction

materiales rechazados
E rejected materials
G zurückgewiesene Materialien
F matériaux rejetés, matériaux refusés

materiales suministrados
E incoming goods
G angelieferte Materialien
F marchandises receptionnées

matiz del color
E colour shade, hue
G Farbton
F teinte, nuance d'une couleur

matraz
E flask
G Kolben (Glasgefäß)
F ballon, flacon

matraz cónico
E conical flask
G Spitzkolben
F ballon conique

matraz de dosificación
E dosing piston
G Dosierkolben
F piston doseur

matraz de Erlenmeyer
E Erlenmeyer flask
G Erlenmeyerkolben
F Erlenmeyer, flacon à fond plat

matraz de índice de iodo
E iodine flask
G Iodzahlkolben
F flacon d'iode

matraz de lavado
E wash bottle
G Spritzflasche
F pissette, flacon laveur

matraz esférico
E round-bottomed flask
G Rundkolben
F ballon à fond rond

matraz esmerilado
E ground-joint flask
G Schliffkolben
F ballon rodé

matraz graduado
E volumetric flask
G Meßkolben
F ballon gradué

matrices para herramientas de uso múltiple
E multi-bore die
G Matrize für Mehrfachwerkzeug
F matrice pour outil multiple

matriz (de una prensa de comprimidos)
E die (of tabletting machine)
G Matrize (an der Tabletten-presse)
F matrice (d'une presse à comprimés)

mecánico
E mechanical
G maschinell
F mécanique

mecanismo de acción
E drug mechanism
G Wirkungsmechanismus
F mécanisme d'action

mecanismo de reacción
E reaction mechanism
G Reaktionsmechanismus
F mécanisme de réaction

mecanismo de separación
E separation mechanism
G Trennungsmechanismus
F mécanisme de séparation

mechero Bunsen
E Bunsen burner
G Bunsenbrenner
F bec de Bunsen

media
E average, mean
G Durchschnitt
F moyenne

media aritmética
E arithmetic mean
G arithmetisches Mittel
F moyenne arithmétique

media caña
E recess
G Hohlkehle
F moulure creuse

medible
E measurable
G meßbar
F mesurable

medicación
E medication
G Medikation
F médication

medicación alternativa
E alternative medication
G Ausweichmedikation
F médication alternative

medicamento
E medicinal product, drug
G Arzneimittel
F médicament,
produit pharmaceutique

medicamento de uso veterinario
E veterinary medicament
G Tierarzneimittel
F médicament à usage vétérinaire

medicamento manufacturado
E finished medicinal product
G Fertigarzneimittel
F médicament fini,
produit pharmaceutique fini

medicamento para el pienso
E drugs for animal feed
G Fütterungsarzneimittel
F médicament pour nourriture animale

medicamento producido biotecnológicamente
E biopharmaceutical
G biotechnologisch hergestelltes Arzneimittel
F produit biopharmaceutique

medicamento producido mediante tecnología genética
E genetically manufactured medicinal product
G gentechnologisch hergestelltes Arzneimittel
F médicament produit par génie génétique

medición
E measurement
G Messung
F mesure

médico investigador
E trial physician, investigator
G Prüfarzt
F médecin responsable d'essais cliniques

medida
E measure, measurement, dimensions
G Maßnahme, Messung, Abmessungen, Ausmaß
F mesure, dimensions

medida de aerosol
E aerosol measurement
G Aerosolmessung
F mesure (de la dose) d'un aérosol

medida de la viscosiad
E viscometry
G Viskositätsmessung
F viscosimétrie

medida precautoria
E precaution
G Vorsichtsmaßnahme
F précaution

medida precautoria al almacenar
E storage precautions
G Vorsichtsmaßnahmen bei der Lagerung
F précautions de stockage

medidas de precaución al almacenar
E storage precautions
G Vorsichtsmaßnahmen bei der Lagerung
F précautions de stockage

medidas de seguridad
E safety precautions
G Sicherheitsmaßnahmen
F précautions de sécurité

medio
E medium
G Medium
F milieu

medio ambiente
E environment
G Umwelt
F environnement

medio de absorción
E absorbent
G Absorptionsmittel
F absorbant

medio de adsorción
E adsorbent
G Adsorptionsmittel
F adsorbant

medio de concentración
E concentration medium, enrichment medium
G Anreicherungsmedium
F médium de concentration

medio de conservación
E preservative, anti-microbial agent
G Konservierungsmittel
F conservateur

medio de contraste
E contrast medium
G Kontrastmittel
F substance de contraste

medio de contraste radiológico
E X-ray contrast medium
G Röntgenkontrastmittel
F produit de contraste aux rayons X

medio de cultivo
E culture medium, nutrient medium
G Nährmedium, Nährboden
F milieu de culture

medio de cultivo deshidratado
E dehydrated culture medium
G Trockennährmedium
F milieu déhydraté

medio de disolución
E dissolution medium
G Auflösemedium
F milieu de dissolution

medio de enriquecimiento
E concentration medium, enrichment medium
G Anreicherungsmedium
F médium de concentration

medio de envasado no impreso
E unprinted packaging material
G unbedrucktes Packmittel
F conditionnement non-imprimé

medio de envasado primario
E primary packaging material
G primäres Packmittel
F conditionnement primaire

medio de envasado secundario
E packaging material, secondary
G sekundäres Packmittel
F conditionnement secondaire

medio de lavado
E rinsing medium
G Spülmedium
F milieu de rinçage

medio de relleno
E filler
G Füllmittel
F moyen de remplissage

medio de separación
E separating medium
G Trennmittel
F milieu de séparation

medio refrigerante
E refrigerant, coolant
G Kühlmittel
F liquide de refroidissement

medio separador
E separation media
G Trennmedium
F milieu de séparation

medios de archivado
E archiving media
G Archivierungsmedien
F médium d'archivage

medios de cultivo selectivos
E selective culture medium
G Selektivnährmedien
F milieu de culture sélectif

medios de cultivo sin suero
E serum-free media
G serumfreie Nährmedien
F médium de culture exempt de sérum

medios de explotación empresarial
E utilities
G Betriebsmittel, Medien
F moyens d'exploitation

medios de producción
E utilities
G Medien, Betriebsmittel
F moyens de production

medios líquidos
E liquid media
G Flüssigmedien
F milieux liquides

medir
E measure, to; meter, to; dose, to
G messen, abmessen, dosieren
F mesurer, doser

mejora de la calidad
E quality improvement
G Qualitätsverbesserung
F amélioration de la qualité

mejorar
E improve, to
G verbessern
F améliorer

membrana
E membrane, diaphragm
G Membran
F membrane

membrana de microfiltración
E micro-filtration membrane
G Mikrofiltrationsmembran
F membrane de micro-filtration

membrana permeable
E permeable membrane
G permeable Membran
F membrane perméable

membrana semipermeable
E semi-permeable membrane
G semipermeable Membran
F membrane semi-perméable

memoria de un instrumento
E instrument memory
G Gerätespeicher
F mémoire d'un instrument

English German French Spanish

mención inicial
E sign-out log
G Ausgangsvermerk
F mention d'origine

menor calidad, de
E inferior
G minderwertig
F de mauvaise qualité

mensurable
E measurable
G meßbar
F mesurable

mercancía a granel
E bulk (material)
G Bulkware
F marchandise en vrac

mercancía devuelta
E returned goods
G zurückgegebene Ware
F marchandise retournée

merma
E impairment, damage
G Beeinträchtigung
F préjudice, dommage

mesa de abastecimiento
E feed table
G Zuführtisch
F table de chargement, table d'alimentation

mesa de laboratorio
E bench
G Labortisch
F paillasse de laboratoire

mesa de trabajo
E bench, work bench
G Arbeitstisch
F table de travail, établi

mesa para matriz
E die table
G Matrizentisch
F table d'une matrice

mesoporos
E mesopores
G Mesoporen
F mésopores

metal
E metal
G Metall
F métal

metal noble
E precious metal
G Edelmetall
F métal précieux

metal pesado
E heavy metal
G Schwermetall
F métal lourd

método
E technique, method
G Technik, Methode
F technique, méthode

método cromatográfico
E chromatographic assay
G chromatographische Methode
F méthode chromatographique

método de agitación con cesto rotatorio
E basket stirring method
G Drehkörbchenmethode
F méthode d'agitation à corbeilles

método de filtración
E filtration method
G Filtrationsmethode
F méthode de filtration

método de placas (microbiología)
E plate method (in microbiology)
G Plattengußverfahren (Mikrobiologie)
F coulage de plaques (microbiologie)

método de prueba
E test method, analytical method
G Prüfmethode
F méthode analytique, méthode de contrôle

método de separación
E separating method
G Trennmethode
F méthode de séparation

mezcla
E blend, mixture
G Mischung, Gemisch
F mixture, mélange

mezcla a agitar
E mixture to be shaken
G Schüttelmixtur
F mixture devant être agitée

mezcla a granel
E bulk mixture
G Bulkmischung
F produits en vrac

mezcla comprimible
E compactible mixture
G preßfertige Mischung
F mélange comprimable

mezcla cruzada
E cross-mix, cross-contamination
G Untermischung, Kreuzkontamination
F contamination croisée

mezcla de polvo
E powdered mixture
G Pulvermischung
F mélange de poudre

mezcla homogeneizada
E blending mixture
G Mischgut
F mélange homogénéisé

mezcla previa
E pre-mix
G Vormischung
F pré-mélange

mezclado previamente
E pre-mixed
G vorgemischt
F mélangé à l'avance

mezclador
E blender, blending apparatus
G Mischer
F mélangeur, malaxeur

mezclador cúbico
E cube mixer
G Kubusmischer
F mélangeur en cube

mezclador de circulación forzada
E forced-circulation mixer
G Zwangsmischer
F mélangeur à circulation forcée

mezclador de cizallamiento
E high-shear mixer
G Pflugscharmischer
F mélangeur à forces de cisaillement

mezclador intenso de cizallamiento
E high-shear mixer
G Mischer mit hohem Scherkraftanteil
F mélangeur avec forces de cisaillements importantes

mezclador de hélice
E propeller mixer
G Propellermischer
F mélangeur à pales

mezclador de tambor
E drum mixer
G Trommelmischer
F mélangeur à tambour

mezclador de turbulencia
E tumble blender
G Taumelmischer
F mélangeur turbulent

mezclador de volteo
E tumble blender
G Taumelmischer
F mélangeur culbuteur

mezclador planetario
E planetary mixer
G Planetenmischer
F mélangeur planétaire

mezclador por basculado
E tumbler mixer
G Freifallmischer
F mélangeur culbuteur, malaxeur à chute libre

mezclar
E blend, to; mix, to
G mischen
F mélanger

mezclar previamente
E pre-blend, to; pre-mix, to
G vormischen
F mélanger à l'avance

microbiano
E microbial
G mikrobiell
F microbien

microbiología
E microbiology
G Mikrobiologie
F microbiologie

microbiológico
E microbiological
G mikrobiologisch
F microbiologique

microcristalino
E microcrystalline
G mikrokristallin
F microcristallin

microencapsulado
E micro-encapsulated
G mikroverkapselt
F micro-encapsulé

microfiltración
E micro-filtration
G Mikrofiltration
F micro-filtration

micronización
E micronisation
G Mikronisierung
F micronisation

micronizador del chorro de aire
E air attrition mill, fluid energy mill
G Luftstrahlmühle
F microniseur à jet d'air

microonda
E microwave
G Mikrowelle
F micro-onde

microorganismos
E microorganisms
G Mikroorganismen
F micro-organismes

microorganismos apatógenos
E non-pathogenic microorganisms
G apathogene Mikroorganismen
F micro-organismes non-pathogènes

microorganismos patógenos
E pathogenic microorganisms
G pathogene Mikroorganismen
F micro-organismes pathogènes

microorganismos viables
E viable microorganisms
G lebensfähige Mikroorganismen
F micro-organismes viables

micropipetado
E micro-pipetting
G Mikropipettierung
F micro-pipettage

microplasma
E micro-plasma
G Mikroplasma
F micro-plasma

microscopio
E microscope
G Mikroskop
F microcospe

miembro de la junta directiva
E director
G Vorstandsmitglied
F directeur

migración
E migration
G Migration, Wanderung
F migration

minuciosamente
E thorough
G gründlich
F minutieusement

minuciosidad
E thoroughness
G Gründlichkeit
F minutie

minucioso
E thorough
G gründlich
F minutieusement

miscible
E miscible
G mischbar
F miscible

no miscible
E immiscible
G nicht mischbar
F non miscible

mixtura
E blend, mixture
G Mischung
F mixture, mélange

mm de presión de agua
E mm water
G mm Wassersäule
F mm de pression d'eau

modelado de sustancias
E substance modelling
G Substanzmodellierung
F modelage de substance

modelado molecular
E molecular modelling
G Molekularmodellierung
F modelage moléculaire

modelo
E stencil, template, version
G Schablone, Ausführung
F matrice, pochoir, patron, version

modernización
E re-equipping
G Umrüstung
F modernisation, réorganisation

modernizar
E upgrade, to; re-equip, to
G umrüsten, aufrüsten
F moderniser, réorganiser

modificación
E change, variation
G Änderung
F changement

modificación del procedimiento
E procedural change
G Verfahrensänderung
F modification d'un procédé

modificación química
E chemical modification
G chemische Modifikation
F modification chimique

modificado
E modified
G modifiziert
F modifié

modo a prueba de errores
E fail-safe mode
G fehlersicherer Modus
F mode indéréglable

modo de servicio
E operating mode
G Bedienungsmodus
F mode d'utilisation

módulo
E module
G Baustein
F module

moho
E fungus, mould
G Schimmel, Schimmelpilz
F moisissure, champignon

mohoso
E mouldy, mildewed
G schimmelig
F moisi

mojar
E wet, to; moisten, to
G benetzen
F humidifier, mouiller

mol
E mole
G Mol
F mole

molar
E molar
G molar
F molaire

molaridad
E molarity
G Molarität
F molarité

moldeado
E moulded
G geformt, gepreßt
F moulu

moldear supositorios
E mould, to (suppositories)
G Zäpfchen gießen
F mouler des suppositoires

moldeo por inyección
E blow moulding
G Blasverformung
F moulage par procédé pressé-soufflé

molecular
E molecular
G molekular
F moléculaire

moler
E mill, to; crush, to; grind, to
G mahlen
F broyer

molido húmedo
E wet grinding
G Naßvermahlung
F broyage humide

molienda
E grinding
G Vermahlung
F moullage

molinillo a bolas
E ball mill, pebble mill
G Kugelmühle
F broyeur à boulets

molino
E mill
G Mühle
F broyeur

molino de cilindros
E roll mill
G Walzenmühle
F broyeur à cylindres

molino de clavija
E pin mill
G Stiftmühle
F broyeur à broches

molino de pomada
E ointment mill
G Salbenmühle
F broyeur à pommade

molino triturador
E hammer mill
G Hammermühle
F broyeur à marteau

molturado
E grinding
G Vermahlung
F moullage

momento de torsión
E torque
G Drehmoment
F couple

monocromador
E monochromator
G Monochromator
F monochromateur

monocromo
E monochromatic
G monochrom
F monochromatique

monografía de farmacopea
E pharmacopoeial monograph
G Arzneibuchmonographie
F monographie de la pharmacopée

monómero
E monomer
G Monomer
F monomère

monovalente
E monovalent
G einwertig
F monovalent

montado
E fitted
G eingebaut
F encastré

montaje
E installation, mounting, assembly, set-up
G Einbau, Zusammenbau, Montage
F installation, montage, assemblage

montaje de instrumentos
E instrument set-up
G instrumenteller Aufbau
F montage des instruments

montaje previo
E pre-assembly
G Vormontage
F pré-assemblé

montar
E apply, to; attach, to; fit, to; install, to; assemble, to
G anbringen, einbauen, zusammensetzen
F apposer, installer, poser, assembler

montar (una caja plegable)
E set up, to (a folding carton)
G aufrichten (eine Faltschachtel)
F dresser, monter (un carton)

montón
E stack, pile
G Stapel
F pile

montón de reserva
E back-up stack
G Nachlegestapel
F empilement de réserve

mordaza
E jaw (tech.)
G Backe (techn.)
F mâchoire

mordaza de calefacción
E heating jaw
G Heizbacke
F mâchoire chauffante

mortero
E mortar
G Mörser, Reibschale
F mortier

mostrar
E display, to; indicate, to
G anzeigen
F indiquer, afficher

moteado
E mottled
G gesprenkelt
F madré

motor de corriente trifásica
E three-phase current motor
G Drehstrommotor
F moteur électrique triphasé

motor de propulsión
E drive motor
G Antriebsmotor
F moteur de transmission, moteur propulsif

móvil
E mobile
G fahrbar
F mobile

movimiento
E turnover, sales
G Umsatz
F chiffre d'affaires

movimiento de agitación
E shaking movement
G Schüttelbewegung
F mouvement d'agitation

movimiento de material
E material movement
G Materialbewegung
F mouvement des matériaux

mucilaginoso
E mucous
G schleimig
F muqueux

mucosa
E mucous membrane
G Schleimhaut
F muqueuse

mucosidad
E mucilage
G Schleim
F mucilage, mucus

mucoso
E mucous
G schleimig
F muqueux

muelle de retorno
E counter-spring, return spring
G Rückzugfeder
F ressort de rappel

muelle de torsión
E torsion spring
G Torsionsfeder
F ressort de torsion

muesca
E groove, notch
G Nut, Kerbe
F cannelure, sillon, rainure, fente, gorge

muesca de ruptura
E break notch, breaking notch
G Bruchkerbe, Kreuzbruchkerbe
F entaille de rupture, encoche de rupture

muestra
E sample, specimen
G Probe, Muster
F échantillon, spécimen

muestra al azar
E random sample
G Stichprobe
F échantillon prélevé au hasard

muestra al azar del abastecedor
E supplier's random sample
G Lieferantenstichprobe
F échantillon fortuit du fournisseur

muestra de dosificación
E dosing pattern
G Dosierungsschema
F schéma de dosage

muestra de prueba
E test sample
G Prüfmuster
F échantillon

muestra de referencia
E retained sample, reference sample
G Rückstellmuster
F échantillon de référence

muestra en blanco
E blank
G Blindprobe
F valeur témoin, valeur à blanc

muestra farmacéutica
E pharmaceutical sample
G Ärztemuster
F échantillon pharmaceutique

muestra gratuita
E sample
G unverkäufliches Muster
F échantillon

muestra mixta
E composite sample
G Mischprobe
F échantillon du mélange

muestra para ensayos clínicos
E clinical trial sample
G klinisches Prüfmuster
F échantillon clinique

muestra sometida a carga
E stressed sample
G beanspruchte Probe
F échantillon soumis à un effort

multicéntrico
E multicentric
G multizentrisch
F multicentrique

mutágeno
E mutagenic
G mutagen
F mutagène

muy eficaz
E highly potent, highly effective
G hochwirksam
F très efficace

muy pulido
E highly polished
G hochglanzpoliert
F poli-miroir

narcótico
E narcotic
G Rauschmittel
F narcotique

naturaleza (de una sustancia)
E nature (of a substance)
G Beschaffenheit (einer Substanz)
F nature (d'une substance)

nebulizador
E nebuliser
G Vernebler
F nébuliseur

nebulizar
E nebulise, to
G vernebeln
F nébuliser

necesidad
E requirement
G Erfordernis
F exigence

necesidades bioquímicas de oxígeno
E biochemical oxygen demand (bod) analysis
G biochemischer Sauerstoffbedarf (BSB)
F Analyse de la demande biologique d'oxygène (DBO)

necesitar
E require, to
G erfordern
F exiger, nécessiter

negocio de comisión
E manufacturing contract
G Lohnauftrag
F contrat de fabrication

neumático
E pneumatic
G pneumatisch
F pneumatique

nevera
E refrigerator
G Kühlschrank
F réfrigérateur

English German French Spanish

English
German
French
Spanish

nicho
E niche, recess
G Nische
F niche

niebla
E fog
G Nebel
F brouillard

nitrógeno
E nitrogen
G Stickstoff
F azote

nivel
E level
G Pegel, Pegelstand
F niveau

nivel de confianza
E confidence level
G Vertrauensniveau
F niveau de confiance

nivel de desarrollo
E development stage
G Entwicklungsstufe
F phase de développement

nivel de esterilidad
E clean room grade,
clean room class
G Reinraumklasse
F niveau de stérilité

nivel de líquido
E liquid level
G Flüssigkeitsstand
F niveau du liquide

nivel de llenado
E filling level
G Füllhöhe
F niveau de remplissage

nivel de pureza
E cleanliness class,
cleanliness grade
G Reinheitsklasse
F classe d'environnement

nivel de relleno
E level
G Füllstand
F niveau

nivel intermediario
E intermediate stage
G Zwischenstufe
F état intermédiaire

nivel sonoro
E noise level
G Geräuschpegel
F niveau du bruit

nivelación
E levelling
G Nivellierung
F nivellement

no acuoso
E non-aqueous
G nicht-wäßrig
F non aqueux

no combustible
E non-flammable
G nicht brennbar
F in-inflammable

no detectable
E undetectable
G nicht nachweisbar
F indétectable

no embalado
E unpacked
G unverpackt
F non emballé

no inflamable
E non-flammable
G nicht brennbar
F in-inflammable

no lineal
E non-linear
G nichtlinear
F non linéaire

no obligatorio
E without obligation
G unverbindlich
F ne comportant aucune obligation

no observancia
E non-compliance
G Nichteinhaltung
F non conformité

no polar
E non-polar
G unpolar
F non polaire

no volátil
E non-volatile
G nichtflüchtig
F non volatile

nocivo
E harmful, hazardous
G schädlich
F nocif

nombre comercial
E commercial name, brand name
G Handelsname, Markenname
F nom de commerce, nom commercial

norma
E standard
G Norm
F norme, standard

norma de trabajo
E operating procedure, instruction, working standard
G Arbeitsvorschrift, Arbeitsstandard
F procédure opératoire, instruction, norme de travail

normalidad (de una disolución)
E normality (of a solution)
G Normalität (einer Lösung)
F normalité (d'une solution)

normalización
E standardisation
G Normierung
F standardisation

normalizado
E standardised
G genormt
F standardisé

nota de llegada
E sign-in log
G Ankunftsvermerk
F mention de venue

nota inicial
E sign-out log
G Ausgangsvermerk
F mention d'origine

núcleo
E nucleus
G Kern
F noyau

núcleo del comprimido
E tablet core
G Tablettenkern
F noyau d'un comprimé

nueva formulación
E reformulation
G Umformulierung
F nouvelle formulation

número codificador inequívoco
E unequivocal code number
G eindeutige Codenummer
F code numérique non équivoque

número de aceptación
E acceptance number
G Annahmezahl
F indice d'acceptance

número de ciclos
E cycle number
G Taktzahl
F cadence

número de éster
E ester number
G Esterzahl
F nombre d'ester

número de gérmenes
E microbial count
G Keimzahl
F nombre de micro-organismes

número de gérmenes del aire
E air microbial count
G Luftkeimzahl
F nombre de micro-organismes de l'air

número de identificación del paciente
E patient identification number
G Patientennummer
F numéro d'identification d'un patient

número de lote
E batch number
G Chargennummer
F numéro de lot

número de partículas
E particle count
G Partikelzahlen
F nombre de particules

número de pedido
E order number
G Bestellnummer
F numéro de commande

número de piezas
E number of items
G Stückzahl
F nombre de pièces

número de placa
E plate number
G Bodenzahl
F nombre de plateaux

número de placas teóricas
E number of theoretical plates
G Zahl der theoretischen Böden
F nombre de plateaux théoriques

número de rechazo
E rejection number
G Rückweisezahl
F nombre de rejet

número de revoluciones
E revolutions
G Drehzahl, Umdrehungszahl
F nombre de rotations, nombre de tours

número de revoluciones del motor
E motor revolutions
G Motordrehzahl
F vitesse de rotation d'un moteur

número de serie
E serial number
G Seriennummer
F numéro de série

número de versión
E version number
G Versionsnummer
F numéro de version

número del encargo
E order number
G Auftragsnummer
F numéro de commande

número del encargo de pedido
E purchase order number
G Bestellauftragsnummer
F numéro de commande

número total de gérmenes
E total microbial count
G Gesamtkeimzahl
F nombre total de micro-organismes

nutriente
E nutrient
G Nährstoff
F aliment, produit nutritif, nutriment

oblea
E capsule, cachet
G Oblate
F capsule, cachet

oblicuidad
E slope
G Schräge
F biais

oblicuo
E sloping
G schräg
F incliné, oblique

obligación (contabilidad)
E liability (financial)
G Verbindlichkeit (finanz.)
F passif (finance)

obligatorio
E binding, compulsory
G verbindlich, obligatorisch, verpflichtend
F obligatoire

obra de malla
E network
G Netzwerk
F réseau

observación especial
E observation, special
G Beobachtung, besondere
F observation particulière

observancia
E compliance
G Einhaltung
F conformité

obsoleto
E obsolete, out-dated
G überholt, veraltet
F obsolète, périmé, suranné, vieillot

obstruido
E clogged, blocked
G verstopft
F obstrué, bouché

obtención
E production, extraction
G Gewinnung
F production

obturar por vitrificación (ampollas)
E flame-seal, to (ampoules)
G zuschmelzen (Ampullen)
F obturer par vitrification (ampoules)

ocular
E ocular
G Okular
F occulaire

oficina de patentes
E patent office
G Patentamt
F office des brevets

ojal
E eye, eyelet
G Öse
F œillet

ojal de inoculación
E inoculating loop
G Impföse
F œillet d'inoculation

oleaginoso
E oily
G ölig
F huileux

oleoso
E oily
G ölig
F huileux

oligoelementos
E trace elements
G Spurenelemente
F oligoélément

oligómero
E oligomers
G Oligomere
F oligomères

olor
E fragrance, odour
G Duft, Geruch
F odeur

omisión
E omission
G Auslassung
F omission

opaco
E opaque
G undurchsichtig, lichtundurchlässig
F opaque

opalescencia
E opalescence
G Opaleszenz
F opalescence

opciones del aparato
E instrument options
G Geräteoptionen
F options d'un équipement

operación en etapa única
E single step operation
G in einem Arbeitsgang
F opération en une seule étape

operador
E operator
G Durchführender
F exécutant, opérateur

optim(iz)ación
E optimisation
G Optimierung
F optimisation

oral
E oral
G oral
F oral

orden de magnitud
E order of magnitude
G Größenordnung
F ordre de magnitude

ordenar
E classify, to
G sichten, klassieren
F classifier

organigrama
E organisation chart, organogram
G Organigramm
F organigramme

organismos modificados genéticamente
E genetically modified organisms (GMO)
G genetisch veränderte Organismen
F organismes génétiquement modifiés (OGM)

organismos oficiales
E authorities
G Behörde
F autorité réglementaire

Organización Mundial de la Salud (OMS)
E World Health Organisation (WHO)
G Weltgesundheitsorganisation
F organisation mondiale de la santé (OMS)

orientar
E align, to
G ausrichten
F aligner, ajuster, centrer

orificio
E orifice
G Mündung
F orifice

orificio (válvula) de seguridad (antideflagrante)
E ex-duct, explosion vent
G Ex-Kanal
F canal de purge anti-déflagrant, orifice de purge anti-déflagrant

orificio de descarga
E sink
G Ausguß
F évier

orificio de descompresión
E pressure relief opening
G Druckentlastungsöffnung
F ouverture de décompression

orificio de entrada de líquido
E inlet
G Einfluß
F orifice d'entrée de liquide

orificio de matriz
E pitch die
G Matrizenbohrung
F forure d'une matrice

orificio de salida de una columna
E column outlet
G Auslaßöffnung einer Säule
F sortie d'une colonne

orificio de salida del aire
E air outlet
G Luftaustrittsöffnung
F sortie d'air

orificio de ventilación
E vent
G Belüftungsloch
F orifice de ventilation, orifice de purge

orín
E rust
G Rost
F rouille

sin orín
E rust-free
G rostfrei
F dépourvu de rouille

oscilación
E oscillation, vibration
G Schwingung, Vibration
F oscillation, vibration

oscurecimiento
E darken
G Verdunkelung
F obscurcissement

osmolalidad
E osmolality
G Osmolalität
F osmolalité

osmómetro
E osmometer
G Osmometer
F osmomètre

ósmosis
E osmosis
G Osmose
F osmose

ósmosis inversa
E reverse osmosis (RO)
G Umkehrosmose
F osmose inverse

ovalidad
E ovality
G Ovalität
F forme ovale

oxidable
E oxidisable
G oxydierbar
F oxydable

oxidación
E oxidation
G Oxydierung
F oxydation

oxidado electrolíticamente
E anodised
G eloxiert
F oxydé (électrolytiquement)

oxidante
E oxidising agent
G Oxydationsmittel
F oxydant

oxidarse
E rust, to
G rosten
F rouiller

óxido de aluminio
E alumina, aluminium oxide
G Aluminiumoxid
F oxyde d'aluminium

oxigenación
E oxygenation
G Oxigenierung
F oxygénation

English German French Spanish

oxígeno
E oxygen
G Sauerstoff
F oxygène

oxígeno disuelto
E dissolved oxygen (DO)
G gelöster Sauerstoff
F oxygène dissous

oximación
E oximation
G Oximierung, Oximbildung
F oximation

ozon(iz)ación
E ozonisation
G Ozonisierung
F ozonisation, ozonation

ozono
E ozone
G Ozon
F ozone

paciente
E patient
G Patient
F patient

País Miembro (UE) de Referencia (para registro de medicamentos)
E Reference Member State (EU) (RMS)
G Erstzulassender (EU) Mitgliedsstaat
F pays rapporteur (UE)

pala
E blade
G Schaufel
F pale, pelle

pala de agitación
E paddle stirrer
G Blattrührerapparatur
F pale d'agitation

palanca
E lever
G Hebel
F levier

paleta
E pallet
G Palette
F palette

paleta de aluminio
E aluminium pallet
G Alupalette
F alupalette, palette en aluminium

paleta de madera
E wooden pallet
G Holzpalette
F palette en bois

paleta de plástico
E plastic pallet
G Kunststoffpalette
F palette en plastique

panel de mandos
E operating panel
G Bedienungsfeld
F tableau d'utilisation

paño de limpieza
E cleaning cloth, cleaning tissue
G Reinigungstuch
F chiffon, serpillière

pantalla
E display, screen
G Anzeige, Bildschirm
F indicateur, écran

pantalla análoga
E analogue display
G Analoganzeige
F affichage numérique

pantalla de aviso de avería
E fault (failure) display
G Störanzeige
F affichage d'une erreur

pantalla de cristal líquido
E liquid crystal display (LCD)
G Flüssigkristallanzeige
F affichage à cristaux liquides

pantalla electroluminiscente
E LED readout
G LED-Anzeige
F affichage électroluminescent

pantalla integrada
E integrated display
G integrierte Anzeige
F indicateur intégré

pantalla óptica
E visual display
G optische Anzeige
F indicateur optique

pantalla protectora
E protective screen, partition
G Schutzschirm, Stellwand
F écran de protection, mur de partage

pantalla protectora de vidrio de seguridad
E safety glass screen
G Schutzschirm aus Sicherheitsglas
F écran de protection constitué de verre de sécurité

papel de filtro
E filter paper
G Filtrierpapier
F papier filtre

papel de tornasol
E litmus paper
G Lackmuspapier
F papier de tournesol

par
E torque
G Drehmoment
F couple

par motor
E torque
G Drehmoment
F couple

parado
E at rest
G im Ruhezustand
F à l'arrêt, immobilisé

parámetro crítico
E critical parameter
G kritischer Parameter
F paramètre critique

parámetro de prueba
E testing parameter
G Prüfparameter
F paramètre d'analyse

parámetro de servicio
E operational parameter
G Betriebsparameter
F paramètre de service

parar
E lock, to
G arretieren
F fermer à clef

pared
E wall
G Wandung
F paroi

pared celular
E cell wall
G Zellwand
F membrane cellulaire

pared de matriz
E die wall
G Matrizenwand
F paroi d'une matrice

pared de un recipiente
E vessel wall
G Gefäßwand
F paroi d'un récipient

pared revocada
E plastered wall
G verputzte Wand
F mur revêtu d'un crépi

párpado
E eye lid
G Augenlid
F paupière

parte
E part, moiety
G Teil
F partie, portion

participación
E participation, involvement
G Beteiligung
F participation

partícula
E particle, particulate matter
G Partikel, Teilchen
F particule

sin partículas
E particle-free
G partikelfrei
F libre de particules

partícula de polvo
E dust particles
G Staubpartikel
F particules de poussière

partícula de vidrio
E glass particle
G Glaspartikel
F particule de verre

partícula fina
E fine particle
G Feinkorn
F particule fine

partículas de vidrio sinterizado
E fused glass particles
G Sinterglasteilchen
F particules de verre fritté

partículas procedentes del aire
E airborne particles
G aus der Luft stammende Partikel
F particules aéroportées

partículas viables
E viable particles
G lebensfähige Partikel
F particules viables

pasamuros
E wall opening, duct
G Wanddurchführung
F ouverture dans le mur, conduite

pasante
E trainee
G Praktikant
F stagiaire

pasivación (p. ej. de acero)
E passivation (e. g. of steel)
G Passivierung (z. B. von Stahl)
F passivation (par ex. de l'acier inoxydable)

pasivado
E passivated
G passiviert
F passivé

pasivo (contabilidad)
E liability (financial)
G Verbindlichkeit (finanz.)
F passif (finance)

paso
E passage
G Durchlauf
F passage

paso (de un líquido)
E flow
G Durchfluß
F débit

paso a paso
E stepwise
G schrittweise
F étape par étape

paso de tamiz
E fines (sieve)
G Durchgang beim Sieben, Siebdurchgang
F passant (tamisage)

paso derecho, de
E right-handed
G rechtsgängig
F droit

paso izquierdo, de
E left-hand
G linksgängig
F à pas gauche

paso seguro, de
E non-crushing, hard-wearing
G trittsicher
F sûr à la marche

pasta
E paste
G Paste
F pâte

pasta cutánea
E cutaneous paste
G Paste zur Anwendung auf der Haut
F pâte pour utilisation cutanée

pasta oral
E oral paste
G Paste zum Einnehmen
F pâte pour utilisation orale

paste(u)rización
E pasteurisation
G Pasteurisierung
F pasteurisation

pastilla
E pastille
G Pastille
F pastille

pastoso
E pasty, paste-like, doughy
G pastenartig, pastös, teigartig
F pâteux

patentado
E patented
G patentiert
F breveté

patente
E patent
G Patent
F brevet

aprobación de patente
E patent approval
G Erteilung eines Patentes
F approbation de brevet

violación de patente
E infringement of a patent
G Verletzung eines Patentes
F violation de brevet

patógeno
E pathogen, pathogenic
G Krankheitserreger, pathogen
F pathogène, pathogénique

patológico
E pathological
G pathologisch
F pathologique

patrón
E scale, standard, stencil, template
G Maßstab, Schablone
F échelle, standard, matrice, pochoir, patron

patrón de conducción de aire
E air flow pattern
G Luftführung
F modèle d'écoulement d'air

pavimento
E flooring, floor covering
G Fußbodenbelag
F revêtement de sol

pavimento compensador
E screed, floor leveller
G Ausgleichsestrich
F chape de compensation

pavimento de resina sintética
E synthetic resin screed
G Kunstharzestrich
F couche de résine synthétique

pavimento inclinado
E sloping flooring, screed
G Gefälleestrich
F chape inclinée

pedido
E order
G Bestellung
F commande

pegajoso
E sticky, tacky
G klebrig
F collant, gluant

pegar
E glue, to
G leimen, kleben
F coller

película acuosa de revestimiento
E aqueous film coating
G wäßrige Filmbeschichtung
F film aqueux,
couche aqueuse pelliculaire

película adhesiva
E adhesive film
G Klebefolie
F film adhésif

película de revestimiento
E coating
G Filmüberzug
F film de revêtement

película transparente
E transparent foil
G Klarsichtfolie
F feuille transparente

película tubular
E tubular film, film tube
G Schlauchfolie
F feuille en gaine

peligro biológico
E biohazard
G Biogefahr, Gefahr durch
biologische Agenzien
F danger biologique,
risque biologique

peligro de explosión
E explosion hazard
G Explosionsgefahr
F danger d'explosion

peligro de incendio
E fire hazard
G Feuergefahr
F risque d'incendie

peligroso
E hazardous, dangerous
G gefährlich
F dangereux

pellet
E pellet
G Pellet
F pellet

pender sobre
E project, to; protrude, to
G überhängen, überstehen
F saillir, faire saillir

pendiente
E gradient, slope
G Gefälle, Neigung
F pente, inclinaison, gradient

pendiente, con
E sloped
G geneigt, mit Gefälle
F incliné, avec une pente

penetración
E penetration, permeation
G Penetration, Durchdringung
F pénétration

penetrar
E penetrate, to
G eindringen
F pénétrer

peptona
E peptone
G Pepton
F peptone

percolación
E percolation
G Perkolation
F percolation

percolar
E percolate, to
G perkolieren
F extrahir par percolation

pérdida
E loss
G Verlust
F perte

pérdida calórica
E heat loss, waste heat
G Wärmeverlust, Abwärme
F déperdition de chaleur, chaleur perdue

pérdida de calidad
E loss of quality
G Güteminderung
F perte de qualité, baisse de qualité

pérdida de evaporación
E evaporative loss
G Verdunstungsverlust
F perte due à l'évaporisation

pérdida de peso (al desecar)
E weight loss (on drying)
G Gewichtsverlust (bei der Trocknung)
F perte de poids (lors de la dessication)

pérdida de producción
E production downtime
G Produktionsausfall
F période d'immobilisation en production

pérdidas por desecación
E loss on drying
G Trocknungsverlust
F pertes dues au séchage

perfeccionado
E reviewed
G überarbeitet
F révisé

perfeccionar
E review, to
G überarbeiten
F réviser, remanier

perfil de comprimido
E tablet profile
G Tablettenprofil
F profil du comprimé

perfil de contaminación (de un producto)
E contamination profile (of a product)
G Kontaminationsprofil (eines Produktes)
F profil de contamination (d'un produit)

perfil de impurezas
E impurity profile
G Verunreinigungsprofil
F profil d'impuretés

perfil de liberación
E release profile
G Freisetzungsprofil
F profil de libération

perfil químico
E chemical profile
G chemisches Profil
F profil chimique

perforación
E perforation, bore
G Perforierung, Bohrung
F perforation, forage, percement

perforaciones de aguja
E pin holes
G Nadellöcher
F perforations d'aiguille

perforado
E perforated
G gelocht
F perforé

perforadora
E punching station
G Lochstanze
F poinçonneuse

English German French Spanish

perforar
E die-cut, to; punch, to; stamp, to; pierce, to; perforate, to
G ausstanzen, durchstechen, perforieren
F découper à l'emporte-pièce, poinçonner, transpercer, perforer

perímetro
E circumference
G Umfang
F circonférence, périmètre, étendue

período de funcionamiento
E standing time
G Standzeit
F période d'utilisation

período de incubación
E period of incubation
G Inkubationsdauer
F période d'incubation

período de uso (de filtros)
E period of use (of filters)
G Standzeit (von Filtern)
F période d'utilisation (de filtres)

período de validez
E period of validity
G Gültigkeitsdauer
F durée de validité

peritaje
E expert opinion
G Begutachtung
F opinion d'expert

perito
E qualified person, expert, assessor
G Sachkundiger, Sachverständiger, Begutachter
F personne compétente, expert

perjudicado
E defective, damaged
G beschädigt
F défectueux, endommagé

perjudicial
E harmful
G gesundheitsschädlich
F dangereux

perjudicial para la salud si entra en contacto con la piel
E harmful in contact with skin
G gesundheitsschädlich bei Hautkontakt
F dangereux pour la santé lors d'un contact cutané

perjudicial para la salud si se ingiere
E harmful if swallowed
G gesundheitsschädlich beim Verschlucken
F dangereux pour la santé si ingéré

perjudicial para la salud si se inhala
E harmful by inhalation
G gesundheitsschädlich bei Inhalation
F dangereux pour la santé si inhalé

perjuicio
E impairment, damage
G Beeinträchtigung, Beschädigung
F préjudice, dommage, dégâts

perjuicio para la salud
E damage to health
G Gesundheitsschaden
F préjudice à la santé

permanencia en el estómago
E gastric duration, gastric residence
G Aufenthalt im Magen
F durée de résidence gastrique

permeabilidad
E transmittance, permeability, leak, leakage
G Durchlässigkeit, Permeabilität, Undichtigkeit
F perméabilité, fuite

permeabilidad al aire
E air permeability
G Luftdurchlässigkeit
F perméabilité à l'air

permeabilidad al vapor de agua
E water vapour permeability
G Wasserdampfdurchlässigkeit
F perméabilité à la vapeur d'eau

permeable
E permeable, leaky
G durchlässig, permeabel, undicht
F perméable, non étanche

permeable al aire
E permeable to air
G luftdurchlässig
F perméable à l'air

permiso de fabricación
E manufacturing authorisation
G Herstellerlaubnis
F autorisation de fabrication

permiso de producción
E production licence
G Produktionsgenehmigung
F autorisation de production

permitido
E permissible
G zulässig
F permis

perno
E bolt, pin
G Bolzen, Stift (technisch)
F boulon, cheville, broche, pointeau, goupille

peróxido de hidrógeno
E hydrogen peroxide
G Wasserstoffperoxid
F eau oxygénée, peroxide d'hydrogène

persona autorizada
E authorised person, authorised individual
G befugte Person, autorisierte Person
F personne autorisée

persona cualificada
E qualified person
G sachkundige Person
F personne qualifiée

personal de servicio
E operating personnel
G Bedienungspersonal
F personnel de service

personal en posición clave
E key personnel
G Personal in Schlüsselstellung
F personnel occupant un poste à responsabilités

pesar
E weigh in, to
G einwiegen
F peser

peso
E weight
G Gewicht
F poids

peso al envasar
E filling weight, shot weight
G Füllgewicht
F poids de remplissage

peso del comprimido
E tablet weight
G Tablettengewicht
F poids d'un comprimé

peso en vacío
E dead weight, net weight, tare
G Leergewicht
F poids à vide

peso específico
E specific gravity
G spezifisches Gewicht
F poids spécifique

peso individual
E individual weight
G Einzelgewicht
F poids individuel

peso inicial
E initial weight
G Einwaage
F poids initial

English German French Spanish

peso máximo
E maximum weight
G Höchstgewicht
F poids maximum

peso molecular
E molecular weight
G Molekulargewicht
F poids moléculaire

peso seco
E dry weight
G Trockengewicht
F poids sec, extrait sec

pesticida
E pesticide
G Pestizid, Schädlingsvertilgungsmittel
F pesticide

pH
E pH
G pH-Wert
F pH

pH metro
E pH meter
G pH-Meter
F pH-mètre

picaporte
E latch, door handle
G Klinke, Türklinke
F loquet, poignée de porte

picnómetro
E pycnometer, specific gravity meter
G Pyknometer
F pycnomètre

pico
E peak
G Peak
F pic

pico doble
E double peak
G Doppelpeak
F pic double

pico extraño
E extraneous peak
G nicht zugehöriger Peak
F pic étranger

pico fantasma
E ghost peak
G Geisterpeak
F pic fantôme

pie
E base
G Untergestell
F socle

piedra de construcción
E module
G Baustein
F module

piedra de ebullición
E boiling chip
G Siedestein
F pierre facilitant l'ébullition

pieza bruta
E blank
G Rohling
F ébauche, pièce brute

pieza de empalme
E extension
G Ansatzstück
F rallonge

pieza de montaje
E attachment, module
G Anbauteil
F accessoire, dispositif adaptable, module

pieza de recambio
E spare part, replacement part
G Ersatzteil, Austauschteil
F pièce de rechange

pieza de unión
E connector
G Verbindungsstück
F raccord

pieza desgastable
E part subject to wear
G Verschleißteil
F pièce sujette à l'usure

pieza insertable
E extension
G Ansatzstück
F rallonge

piezas móviles
E movable parts
G bewegliche Teile
F pièces mobiles

pigmento
E dye, stain, pigment
G Farbe, Pigment
F colorant, teinture, pigment

pigmento vegetal
E vegetable dye
G Pflanzenfarbstoff
F pigment végétal

pila
E stack, pile
G Stapel
F pile

pila termoeléctrica
E thermocouple
G Thermoelement
F thermocouple

píldora
E pill
G Pille
F pilule

piñón
E pinion
G Ritzel
F pignon

pinza
E terminal, tongs
G Klemme, Zange
F pince, borne, tenailles

pinza de crisol
E tongs
G Tiegelzange
F pince à creuset

pinzas
E tweezers, clamp
G Pinzette, Klammer
F brucelles, pinces

pipeta
E pipette
G Pipette
F pipette

pipeta (de toma de muestras)
E powder sampler, sampling device, sampling pipette
G Stechheber
F dispositif d'échantillonnage, pipette de prélèvement

pipeta calibrada
E calibrated pipette
G Vollpipette
F pipette calibrée

pipetear
E pipette off, to
G abpipettieren
F pipetter

pirogenicidad
E pyrogenicity
G Pyrogenität
F pyrogénicité

pirógenos
E pyrogens
G Pyrogene, fiebererzeugende Substanzen
F pyrogènes

sin pirógenos
E pyrogen-free
G pyrogenfrei
F dépourvu de pyrogènes

pirólisis
E pyrolysis
G Pyrolyse
F pyrolyse

piso de servicio técnico
E technical floor
G Technikgeschoß
F étage du service technique

piso intermedio
E mezzanine
G Zwischengeschoß
F étage intermédiaire

pistilo
E pestle
G Pistill
F pilon

pistola de llama
E flame gun
G Flammpistole
F pistolet chalumeau

pistón
E piston
G Kolben (technisch)
F piston

pivote
E pin
G Stift (technisch)
F broche, pointeau, goupille

píxel
E pixel
G Pixel
F pixel

placa de contacto
E contact plate
G Abklatschplatte
F plaque de contact

placa de desviación
E baffle
G Ablenkplatte
F plaque déflectrice, chicane

placa de Petri
E Petri dish
G Petrischale
F boîte de Petri

placa de sedimentación
E settling plate
G Sedimentationsplatte
F plaque de sédimentation

placa del suelo
E bottom plate
G Bodenplatte
F dalle (de sol)

placa giratoria
E revolving plate feeder, turntable
G Aufgabedrehteller
F plateau tournant

placa para cromatografía en capa fina (CCF)
E TLC plate (thin layer chromatography)
G DC-Platte (Dünnschichtchromatographie)
F plaque de CCM (chromatographie en couche mince)

placebo
E placebo
G Placebo
F placebo

plan de almacenamiento
E stacking plan (in warehouse)
G Stapelplan (im Lager)
F plan de stockage (entrepôt)

plan de limpieza
E cleaning schedule
G Reinigungsplan
F programme de nettoyage

plan de producción
E production schedule
G Produktionsplan
F schéma de production

plan de prueba
E testing schedule
G Prüfplan
F protocole opératoire

plan de toma de muestras
E sampling plan
G Probenahmeplan
F programme d'échantillonnage

plan de validación
E validation protocol
G Validierungsplan
F protocole de validation

plan del edificio
E building (facility) floor plan
G Gebäudeplan
F plan de l'édifice

plan escalonado
E graduated plan
G Stufenplan
F plan échelonné

plan graduado
E graduated plan
G Stufenplan
F plan échelonné

plan higiénico
E sanitation programme
G Hygieneplan
F programme sanitaire

plan para decidir problemas
E problem decision plan
G Problementscheidungsplan
F plan de solutionnement d'un problème

plancha
E sheet, plate, tray
G Blech
F tôle

planificación de necesidades
E requirements planning
G Bedarfsplanung
F planification des besoins

plano
E plan, plane, level
G Grundriß, eben
F plan (horizontal), plat

plano de los pisos
E floor plan
G Stockwerksplan
F plan d'étage

plano del lugar
E site plan, layout
G Lageplan
F schéma, plans du site

plano inclinado
E inclined plane
G schiefe Ebene
F plan incliné

planta química
E chemical plant
G Chemiebetrieb
F usine chimique

plantas empresariales
E plant, factory, facility
G Betriebsstätte
F usine, installations, site de fabrication

planteamiento
E reaction materials
G Ansatz
F matériaux de réaction

plantilla
E stencil, template
G Schablone
F matrice, pochoir, patron

plasticidad
E plasticity
G Plastizität
F plasticité

plástico
E plastic, plastic material
G Kunststoff, plastisch
F plastique

plastificante
E softening agent, plasticiser
G Weichmacher
F plastifiant

plataforma de control
E operating platform
G Bedienungsbühne
F plate-forme de commande

plataforma elevadora
E lifting platform
G Hebebühne
F plate-forme de levage

platillo de balanza
E weighing pan, weighing scale
G Waagschale
F plateau de balance

platino
E circuit board
G Platine
F platine

plato giratorio
E turntable
G Drehteller
F plateau tournant

plazo
E time limit, deadline
G Frist
F délai, terme

plegable
E flexible, pliable, foldable, tiltable
G biegsam, abklappbar
F flexible, pliable, rabattable

plegadora
E folding machine
G Falzmaschine
F plieuse

plegamiento espacial (p. ej. de una proteína)
E spatial folding (e. g. of protein)
G räumliche Faltung (z. B. eines Proteins)
F pliage spatial (par ex. des protéines)

plegar
E fold, to; crimp, to; seam, to
G falzen
F plier

plexiglás
E Plexiglas, acrylic glass
G Plexiglas
F plexiglas

pliego de datos de seguridad
E safety data sheet, material safety data sheet (MSDS)
G Sicherheitsdatenblatt
F feuillet de données sur la sécurité, feuille de données de sécurité

pliegue
E fold
G Falte
F pli

plomo
E sinker
G Senkkörper
F plomb

población celular
E cell population
G Zellpopulation
F population de cellules

pocillo del blíster
E well, cup (of blister)
G Napf (beim Blister)
F blister, emballage à bulles

poder colorante
E dyeing power
G Färbkraft
F pouvoir colorant

polar
E polar
G polar
F polaire

polaridad
E polarity
G Polarität
F polarité

polarímetro
E polarimeter
G Polarimeter
F polarimètre

polarizador
E polariser
G Polarisator
F polariseur

polea
E casters
G Laufrollen, Lenkrollen
F rouleau porteur, galet de guidage, poulie de guidage

poleas de guía
E guide rollers
G Führungsrollen
F rouleaux de guidage

policíclico
E polycyclic
G polycyclisch
F polycyclique

poliesterol expandido
E expanded polystyrene (EPS)
G expandiertes Polystyrol (EPS)
F polystyrène expansé

polímero
E polymer
G polymer
F polymère

polímero acuoso
E aqueous polymer
G wäßriges Polymer
F polymère aqueux

polivalente
E multivalent
G mehrwertig
F polyvalent

polución de aguas residuales
E waste water pollution
G Abwasserverschmutzung
F pollution des eaux résiduelles

polucionante
E polluting, harmful
G umweltverschmutzend
F polluant

polvo
E powder
G Pulver, Puder
F poudre

polvo oral
E oral powder
G Pulver zum Einnehmen
F poudre à utilisation orale

polvo suelto
E loose powder
G loses Pulver
F poudre en vrac

polvo vulnerario
E dusting powder
G Streupulver
F poudrage

pomada
E ointment
G Salbe
F pommade

pomada auricular
E ear ointment
G Ohrensalbe
F pommade auriculaire

pomada con elevado contenido en grasa
E fatty ointment
G Fettsalbe
F pommade

pomada evanescente
E water-soluble cream
G abwaschbare Salbe
F crème évanescente

pomada nasal
E nasal ointment
G Nasensalbe
F pommade nasale

pomada oftálmica
E eye ointment
G Augensalbe
F pommade pour les yeux

pomada rectal
E rectal ointment
G Rektalsalbe
F pommade rectale

English German French Spanish

pomada vaginal
E vaginal ointment
G Vaginalsalbe
F pommade vaginale

ponente
E person responsible, clerk
G Sachbearbeiter
F responsable

poner en funcionamiento
E put into operation, to
G in Betrieb setzen
F mettre en fonctionnement

poner en marcha
E start, to; start-up, to
G anfahren
F démarrer

poner en peligro (la calidad)
E endanger, to (quality)
G gefährden (Qualität)
F mettre en danger, compromettre (la qualité)

porciones insaponificables
E unsaponifiable matter
G unverseifbare Anteile
F portions insaponifiables

poros, sin
E pore-free
G porenfrei
F dépourvu de pores

porosidad
E porosity
G Porosität
F porosité

poroso
E porous
G porös
F poreux

portacubetas
E cell mount, cell holder
G Küvettenhalter
F support de cuvette

portaobjetos (microscopio)
E slide
G Objektträger
F porte-objet

portátil
E mobile
G fahrbar
F mobile

portavoz
E chairman, spokesman
G Obmann, Vorsitzender
F porte-parole

posibilidad de lavar las manos
E hand wash facility
G Handwaschgelegenheit
F possibilité de lavage des mains

posición
E location
G Ort, Lage
F endroit, lieu

posición cero
E zero adjustment
G Nulleinstellung
F mise à zéro

posición de desecho
E reject position
G Ausschußposition
F position de rejet

posición de la válvula
E valve setting
G Ventilstellung
F position d'une vanne

posicionador de válvulas
E flap positioner
G Klappensteller
F positionneur de clapet

posología
E dosage
G Dosierung
F posologie

postigo
E hatch, slippage
G Durchreiche, Durchschlupf
F porte coupée, décalage

potenciación
E potentation
G Potenzierung
F potentialisation

potencial de riesgos
E hazard potential
G Gefahrenpotential
F potentiel de danger

potencial redox
E redox potential
G Redoxpotential
F potentiel redox

potenciómetro
E potentiometer
G Potentiometer
F potentiomètre

pozo
E duct
G Schacht
F conduite, bouche

pozo de evacuación de aire
E exhaust air shaft, exhaust air flue
G Abluftschacht
F puits d'évacuation d'air

practicable
E accessible, walk-in
G begehbar
F accessible

practicante
E trainee
G Praktikant
F stagiaire

Prácticas Clínicas Correctas (GCP)
E Good Clinical Practice (GCP)
G Gute Klinische Praxis
F bonnes pratiques cliniques (GCP)

Prácticas Correctas de Fabricación (GMP)
E Good Manufacturing Practice (GMP)
G Gute Herstellungspraxis (GMP)
F bonnes pratiques de fabrication (GMP)

Prácticas Correctas de Laboratorio (GLP)
E Good Laboratory Practice (GLP)
G Gute Laborpraxis (GLP)
F bonnes pratiques de laboratoire (GLP)

preamplificación
E pre-amplification
G Vorverstärkung
F préamplification

precintado
E sealed
G verplombt
F fermé hermétiquement

precintado de un frasco
E tamper-proof seal
G Entnahmesicherung
F sécurité de prélèvement

precintar
E seal, to
G siegeln
F sceller, clore

precinto
E band, banderole, tape, seal
G Banderole, Plombe
F banderole, sceau en plomb

precio de compra
E purchase cost
G Kaufpreis
F prix d'achat

precipitación (química)
E precipitation, precipitate
G Ausfällung, Fällung
F précipitation, précipité

precipitado
E precipitation, precipitate
G Ausfällung, Fällung, Niederschlag
F précipitation, précipité

precipitador
E separator
G Abscheider
F séparateur

precipitar
E precipitate, to; separate, to
G ausfällen, abscheiden
F précipiter, séparer, sécréter

precisión
E precision
G Präzision
F précision

preciso
E precise
G präzise
F précis

predecesor
E predecessor
G Vorgänger
F prédécesseur

preformulación
E pre-formulation
G Präformulierung
F préformulation

preimpreso
E pre-printed
G vorbedruckt
F imprimé à l'avance

preinserción
E pre-insertion
G Voreinschub
F pré-insertion

prensa de alta velocidad
E high-speed tabletting press
G Hochgeschwindigkeitstablettenpresse
F presse à comprimés haute vitesse

prensa de comprimidos
E tablet press
G Tablettenpresse
F presse à comprimés, pastilleuse

prensa automática de comprimidos
E automated tablet press
G instrumentierte Tablettenpresse
F presse à comprimés avec instruments

prensa de palanca
E lever press
G Hebelpresse
F presse à bascule

prensa excéntrica
E eccentric tablet press
G Exzenterpresse
F presse excentrique à comprimés

prensa extrusora
E extruder
G Strangpresse
F extrudeuse

prensa manual
E hand press
G Handpresse
F presse manuelle

prensa rápida
E high-speed press
G Hochleistungspresse
F presse rapide

prensa rotatoria
E rotary press
G Rundläuferpresse
F presse rotative

prensa rotatoria doble
E double rotary press
G Doppelrundläuferpresse
F presse rotative double

prensar
E express, to
G auspressen
F presser

preparación
E preparation, formulation
G Zubereitung
F préparation, formulation

preparación de medio de cultivo
E culture media preparation
G Nährmedienherstellung
F préparation des milieux de culture

preparación de muestras
E sample preparation
G Probenvorbereitung
F préparation d'un échantillon

preparación de turba
E mud pack preparation
G Moorzubereitung
F préparation de tourbe

preparación de una solución
E preparation of solution
G Lösungsherstellung
F préparation d'une solution

preparación del trabajo
E work scheduling
G Arbeitsvorbereitung
F planification du travail

preparación estéril
E sterile form
G sterile Zubereitung
F forme stérile

preparación para ensayo ciego
E blinding
G Verblindung
F préparation pour essai en aveugle

preparado de prueba
E test preparation
G Prüfpräparat
F préparation pour test

preparado de referencia
E reference medication (preparation)
G Referenzpräparat
F préparation de référence

preparado para funcionar
E ready for operation
G betriebsbereit
F prêt au service, prêt à l'utilisation, prêt à l'emploi

preparado retard
E depot drug
G Depotpräparat
F médicament retard

preparar (columna)
E bake off, to (column)
G verbacken (Säule)
F agglutiner (colonne)

preparar grageas (con cubierta de azúcar)
E pan-coat, to
G dragieren
F dragéifier

prerrecubrir (grageas)
E precoat, to (tablets)
G andecken (beim Dragieren)
F pré-enrober

prerreglaje
E pre-setting
G Voreinstellung
F pré-réglage

prescripción
E instruction, specification, regulation, prescription
G Vorschrift, Verordnung (rechtlich), Verschreibung
F instruction, spécification, décret, ordonnance

conforme a las prescripciones
E complying with specification
G vorschriftsmäßig
F en conformité avec les spécifications

prescripción de prueba
E test instructions
G Prüfvorschrift
F instructions d'un test

English German French Spanish

English German French Spanish

prescripción de vestuario
E gowning procedure
G Bekleidungsvorschrift
F règles vestimentaires, instructions vestimentaires

prescripción estándar
E standard specification
G Normvorschrift
F spécification standard

prescripción médica
E medical prescription
G ärztliche Verordnung
F ordonnance, prescription

prescripciones de eliminación
E disposal regulations
G Entsorgungsvorschriften
F régulations concernant les rejets

prescripciones de fabricación
E master formula, manufacturing instructions
G Herstellungsvorschrift
F instructions de fabrication

prescripciones sobre desechos
E waste regulations
G Abfallbestimmungen
F dispositions (légales) concernant les déchets

preselección
E pre-selection
G Vorauswahl
F pré-sélection

presencia
E presence
G Anwesenheit
F présence

presentación (de una solicitud de autorización)
E submission (of an application for marketing approval)
G Einreichung (eines Zulassungsantrags)
F déposition (d'une demande d'autorisation de mise sur le marché)

presentar (una solicitud de autorización)
E submit, to (application for marketing approval)
G einreichen (Zulassungsantrag)
F soumettre (une demande d'autorisation de mise sur le marché)

presidente
E chairman, spokesman
G Obmann, Vorsitzender
F porte-parole

presión
E pressure
G Druck
F pression

sobrepresión
E positive pressure
G Überdruck
F surpression

presión atmosférica
E atmospheric pressure
G Atmosphärendruck
F pression atmosphérique

presión atmosférica baja
E sub-atmospheric pressure
G Atmosphärenunterdruck
F dépression atmosphérique

presión baja
E negative pressure
G Unterdruck
F souspression

presión de aire
E air pressure
G Luftdruck
F pression d'air

presión de prensado
E moulding pressure
G Preßdruck
F pression de pressage, pression de moulage

presión de rotura
E bursting pressure
G Berstdruck
F pression d'éclatement

presión de sellado
E sealing pressure
G Siegeldruck
F pression de scellage, pression de fermeture

presión de soporte
E support pressure
G Stützdruck
F pression de soutien

presión de trabajo
E working pressure
G Arbeitsdruck, Betriebsdruck
F pression de travail

presión de vapor
E vapour pressure, steam pressure
G Dampfdruck
F pression de vapeur

presión diferencial
E pressure differential
G Differenzdruck
F pression différentielle

presión empresarial
E working pressure
G Betriebsdruck
F pression de travail

presión interna
E internal pressure
G Innendruck
F pression interne

presión osmótica
E osmotic pressure
G osmotischer Druck
F pression osmotique

presión parcial
E partial pressure
G Partialdruck
F pression partielle

presupuestos uniformes
E uniform preconditions
G einheitliche Voraussetzungen
F conditions préalables uniformes

pretratamiento
E pre-treatment
G Vorbehandlung
F traitement préalable

pretratamiento de muestras
E sample pre-treatment
G Probenvorbehandlung
F prétraitement d'échantillons

primeros auxilios
E first aid
G Erste Hilfe
F secours d'urgence, premiers secours

principio activo (medicamento)
E active substance, active pharmaceutical ingredient (API)
G Wirkstoff (im Arzneimittel)
F principe actif (d'un médicament)

principio de unidades de montaje
E modular design
G Baukastenprinzip
F design modulaire

prión bovino
E bovine prion
G Rinderprion
F prion bovin

prión celular (prpc)
E cellular prion (prpc)
G zelluläres Prion
F prion cellulaire (prpc)

priones específicos de la encefalopatía espongiforme ovina
E scrapie-specific prions (prpsc)
G Scrapie-spezifische Proteine (prpsc)
F prions spécifiques à la scrapie (prpsc)

probar
E test, to
G prüfen
F tester

probeta
E test tube, beaker
G Reagenzglas, Becherglas
F tube à essais, bécher, gobelet

probeta graduada
E graduated measuring cylinder
G graduierter Meßzylinder
F éprouvette graduée

procedencia del producto
E product origin
G Produktherkunft
F origine du produit

procedimiento
E procedure
G Verfahren
F procédé

procedimiento administrativo
E method of administration
G Verwaltungsverfahren
F méthode d'administration

procedimiento de cubierta simple
E single coating process
G Einschichtverfahren
F procédé monocouche

procedimiento de desinfección
E disinfecting procedure
G Desinfektionsverfahren
F procédé de désinfection

procedimiento de fabricación
E manufacturing procedure
G Herstellungsverfahren
F procédure de fabrication

procedimiento de granulación
E granulating process
G Granulierverfahren
F procédé de granulation

procedimiento de inmersión, en
E by immersion
G im Tauchverfahren
F procédé par immersion

procedimiento de lecho fluidificado
E fluidisation
G Wirbelschichtverfahren
F fluidisation

procedimiento de prueba
E analytical procedure, testing procedure
G Prüfverfahren
F procédure de test

procedimiento de purga gaseosa
E gas flow-through process
G Gasdurchströmungsverfahren
F procédé de circulation des gaz

Procedimiento de Reconocimiento Mutuo en la UE
E Mutual Recognition Procedure (MRP)
G Gegenseitiges Anerkennungsverfahren bei der Zulassung von Arzneimitteln in der EU
F procédure de reconnaissance mutuelle

procesable
E processable
G verarbeitungsfähig
F traitable

procesar
E process, to; reprocess, to
G aufarbeiten
F traiter

proceso
E operation, processing, reprocessing
G Aufarbeitung, Bearbeitung, Verarbeitung, Vorgang
F fabrication, mise en forme, processus, traitement

proceso automático
E machine processing
G maschinelle Verarbeitung
F traitement automatique

proceso manual
E manual processing
G manuelle Verarbeitung
F traitement manuel

proceso no observado
E unattended operation
G nicht unter Beobachtung stehender Vorgang
F processus non soumis à un contrôle

proceso de autorización
E release procedure
G Freigabeverfahren
F processus de libération

proceso de destilación
E distillation process
G Destillationsprozeß
F processus de distillation

proceso electrónico de datos
E EDP (Electronic Data Processing)
G EDV (Elektronische Datenverarbeitung)
F traitement électronique des données, informatique

procesos de trabajo en área estéril
E clean room operations
G Arbeitsvorgänge im Reinraum
F opérations en zone d'atmosphère contrôlée

producción
E production, manufacture, generation (of), extraction
G Produktion, Gewinnung, Erzeugung
F production, engendrement

producción a escala piloto
E pilot scale production
G Produktion im Versuchsmaßstab
F production à l'échelle pilote

producción de partículas
E particle generation
G Partikelerzeugung
F génération de particules

producción de polvo
E dust production
G Staubentwicklung
F production de poussière

producción de ruido
E noise development
G Geräuschentwicklung
F émissions sonores

producción de vapor
E steam generation
G Dampferzeugung
F production de vapeur

producción por contrata
E contract manufacturing
G Auftragsherstellung
F production par un sous-traitant

producción por encargo
E contract manufacturing
G Auftragsproduktion
F production par un sous-traitant

producir
E compile, to
G erstellen
F compiler, produire

producto acabado
E finished product
G Fertigprodukt
F produit fini

producto bruto
E raw product, crude product
G Rohprodukt
F produit brut

producto colateral
E by-product
G Nebenprodukt
F sous-produit, produit secondaire

producto comercial
E commercial product
G Handelsware
F produit commercial

producto de degradación
E degradation product, decomposition product
G Abbauprodukt, Zersetzungsprodukt
F produit de dégradation, produit de décomposition

producto de desecho
E waste material
G Abfallprodukt
F déchets

producto de desintegración
E degradation product
G Zerfallsprodukt
F produit de dégradation

producto de limpieza
E cleansing agent, detergent
G Reinigungsmittel
F agent de nettoyage

producto de plasma sanguíneo
E blood plasma product, blood plasma derivative
G Blutplasmaderivat
F produit d'origine plasmatique

producto de venta libre
E over-the-counter (OTC) product
G frei verkäufliches Produkt, OTC-Produkt
F produit sans ordonnance, produit en vente libre

producto desechado
E rejected product
G verworfenes Produkt
F produit rejeté

producto estéril
E sterile product
G Sterilprodukt
F produit stérile

producto intermediario
E intermediate product
G Zwischenprodukt
F produit intermédiaire

producto médico
E medical device
G Medizinprodukt
F produit à usage médical

producto natural
E natural product
G Naturprodukt
F produit naturel

producto para automedicación
E over-the-counter (OTC) medicament
G Selbstmedikationsprodukt
F produit sans ordonnance

producto para pulir
E polish
G Poliermittel
F produit de polissage

producto reciclado
E reprocessed product
G wiederaufbereitetes Produkt
F produit recyclé

producto sanguíneo
E blood product
G Blutprodukt
F produit sanguin

producto secundario
E by-product
G Nebenprodukt
F sous-produit, produit secondaire

producto semiacabado
E semi-manufactured product
G Halbfertigware
F produit intermédiaire

producto semiterminado
E semi-finished product
G Vorprodukt
F produit semi-fini

productor de esporas
E spore former
G Sporenbildner
F producteur de spores

productos colaterales microbianos
E microbial by-products
G mikrobielle Nebenprodukte
F produits secondaires microbiens

productos éticos
E ethical products
G ethische Produkte
F produits éthiques

productos homeopáticos
E homeopathic products
G homöopathische Erzeugnisse
F produits homéopathiques

productos inocuos
E harmless products
G unschädliche Mittel
F produits inoffensifs

productos inyectables de gran volumen
E large volume parenterals (LVP)
G großvolumige Parenteralia
F produits injectables de grand volume

productos inyectables de poco volumen
E small volume parenterals (SVP)
G kleinvolumige Parenteralia
F produits injectables de petit volume

productos manufacturados
E manufactured goods, finished goods
G Fertigwaren
F produits manufacturés

productos oftálmicos
E ophthalmic products
G Ophthalmica
F produits ophtalmiques

productos para la salud
E health care products
G Gesundheitsprodukte
F produits d'hygiène grand public

productos químicos
E chemicals
G Chemikalien
F produits chimiques

productos radiofarmacéuticos
E radio-pharmaceuticals
G Radiopharmazeutika
F produits radiopharmaceutiques

productos secundarios
E secondary products
G Sekundärprodukte
F produits secondaires

profiláctico
E prophylactic
G prophylaktisch
F prophylactique

profilaxia
E prophylaxis
G Prophylaxe
F prophylaxe

profundidad de inmersión
E immersion depth
G Eintauchtiefe
F profondeur d'immersion

profundidad de penetración
E penetration depth
G Eindringtiefe
F profondeur de pénétration

programa sanitario
E sanitation programme
G Hygieneplan
F programme sanitaire

programable
E programmable
G programmierbar
F programmable

programación
E programming
G Programmierung
F programmation

programación de la longitud de onda
E wavelength programming
G Wellenlängenprogrammierung
F programmation de la longueur d'onde

programador
E programmer
G Programmierer
F programmeur

proliferación celular
E cell proliferation
G Zellvermehrung
F prolifération de cellules

prolongación de un plazo
E deadline extension
G Fristverlängerung
F prolongation d'un délai

prolongación del plazo de patente
E patent prolongation
G Patentfristerneuerung
F prorogation d'un brevet

prolongar
E extend, to; prolong, to
G verlängern
F prolonger, rallonger

promedio
E average, mean
G Durchschnitt
F moyenne

promoción de un producto
E product promotion
G Produktförderung
F mesures propres à favoriser un produit

promover
E convey, to
G fördern
F transporter

propagación
E spreading
G Spreizung
F propagation

propelente
E propellant (gas)
G Treibgas
F gaz propulseur

propiedad
E property
G Eigenschaft
F propriété, caractéristique

propiedad deslizante
E slip property
G Gleiteigenschaft
F propriété lubrifiante

propiedad física
E physical characteristic
G physikalische Eigenschaft
F caractéristique physique

propiedad fluida
E flow property
G Fließeigenschaft
F propriété d'écoulement

propiedad intelectual
E intellectual property
G intellektuelles Eigentum
F propriété intellectuelle

propiedades físicas
E physical characteristics
G physikalische Eigenschaften
F caractéristiques physiques

propiedades fisicoquímicas
E physical-chemical characteristics
G physikalisch-chemische Eigenschaften
F caractéristiques physico-chimiques

proporción
E ratio
G Verhältnis
F rapport, taux

proporción de mezcla
E blending ratio
G Mischungsverhältnis
F proportions de mélange, titration

proporción de polvo
E dust concentration
G Staubanteil
F concentration en poussière

propulsión
E drive
G Antrieb
F entraînement, transmission

propulsión por cadena
E chain drive
G Kettenantrieb
F entraînement par chaînes

propulsión por correa
E belt drive
G Riemenantrieb
F entraînement par courroie

propulsión por correa trapezoidal
E belt drive
G Keilriemenantrieb
F entraînement par courroie trapézoïdale

propulsión por émbolo
E piston drive
G Kolbenantrieb
F entraînement par piston

prospectivo
E prospective
G prospektiv
F prospective

prospecto acompañante (del medicamento)
E package leaflet, package insert
G Beipackzettel
F notice (d'un emballage)

prospecto informativo del medicamento
E package insert, package leaflet
G Packungsbeilage
F notice explicative

prospecto informativo del medicamento previamente plegado
E pre-folded package insert
G vorgefaltete Packungsbeilage
F notice explicative dépliante

proteasa
E protease
G Protease
F protéase

protección
E screening
G Abschirmung
F screening, tri, dépistage

protección (eléctrica)
E fuse
G Schütz
F protection

protección antioxidante
E rust protection
G Rostschutz
F protection contre la rouille

protección auricular
E ear protector, ear defender
G Gehörschutz
F protection auriculaire

protección bucal
E face mask
G Mundschutz
F masque de protection facial

protección contra el polvo
E dust guard
G Staubschutz
F protection contre les poussières

protección de patentes
E patent protection
G Patentschutz
F protection d'un brevet

protección facial
E face protection
G Gesichtsschutz
F protection faciale

protección frente a la colisión
E impact protection
G Stoßschutz
F protection anti-chocs

protección frente al fuego (de un aparato)
E flame protector (of instrument)
G Brandschutz (eines Gerätes)
F ignifugation, ignifugeage (d'un instrument)

protección frente al goteo
E drop protection
G Tropfschutz
F protection anti-gouttes

protección frente al salpicado
E spray protection
G Spritzschutz
F couvercle anti-éclaboussures

protección ocular
E eye protection
G Augenschutz
F protection oculaire

protección respiratoria
E respiratory protection
G Atemschutz
F masque respiratoire de protection

protector cónico
E conical screener
G konischer Abschirmer
F protection cônique

protegido contra explosión
E explosion-protected
G explosionsgeschützt
F protégé contre une explosion

protegido frente a explosión
E explosion-protected
G Ex-geschützt
F protégé contre les explosions

protegido frente al fuego
E fire-proof
G feuergeschützt
F ignifugé, à l'épreuve du feu

protegido frente al polvo
E dustproof
G staubgeschützt
F imperméable à la poussière

proteína priónica (prp)
E prion proteins (prp)
G Prionproteine
F protéines-prions (prp)

protocolar
E protocol, to; record, to; document, to
G protokollieren
F enregistrer, documenter

protocolo
E record
G Protokoll
F enregistrement, référence

protocolo de deficiencias
E deficiency protocol
G Mängelprotokoll
F procès-verbal des défauts

protocolo de embalaje
E batch packaging record
G Verpackungsprotokoll
F compte rendu de conditionnement

protocolo de fabricación
E batch processing record
G Herstellungsprotokoll
F protocole de fabrication

protocolo de lotes
E batch record
G Chargenprotokoll
F relevé d'un lot, enregistrement d'un lot, compte rendu d'un lot

protocolo de prueba
E test protocol
G Prüfprotokoll
F procès-verbal d'un test

protocolo del ensayo
E testing schedule
G Prüfplan
F protocole opératoire

prototipo
E prototype
G Erstausführung
F prototype

protozoos
E protozoa
G Protozoen
F protozoaires

proveedor
E supplier, vendor
G Lieferant
F fournisseur

proveer
E supply, to
G liefern, versorgen mit
F fournir, livrer

provisional
E temporary
G vorläufig
F temporaire

provocar
E cause, to
G verursachen
F provoquer

proyecto
E draft
G Entwurf
F ébauche

proyecto de ley
E draft bill
G Gesetzesentwurf
F projet de loi

prueba
E trial, experiment, analysis, control test, detection, evidence, proof
G Versuch, Prüfung, Nachweis, Beweis
F essai, expérience, analyse, test de contrôle, détection, preuve

prueba (test) de integridad
E integrity test
G Integritätstest
F test d'intégrité

prueba biológica
E biological testing
G biologische Prüfung
F examens biologiques

prueba de accidentes, a
E accident-proof
G unfallsicher
F protégé contre les accidents

prueba de aceptación (p. ej. de software)
E acceptance test (e. g. for software)
G Akzeptanztest (z. B. für Software)
F test d'acceptance (par ex. pour logiciel)

prueba de aptitud
E suitability test
G Eignungsprüfung
F test de qualification

prueba de baño con colorante azul
E blue dye bath test
G Blaubadtest
F test au bain bleu

prueba de carga
E challenge test
G Belastungstest
F test de stimulation

prueba de contacto directo
E direct contact test
G Abklatschtest
F test de contact direct

prueba de eficacia antimicrobiana
E anti-microbial effectiveness test
G Konservierungsmittelbelastungstest
F test d'efficacité anti-microbien

prueba de escape
E leak test
G Lecktest
F essai d'étanchéité

prueba de estabilidad
E stability test
G Haltbarkeitsuntersuchung
F test de stabilité

English German French Spanish

prueba de estanqueidad
E leak test
G Dichtigkeitsprüfung
F essai d'étanchéité, essai de fuite, essai de perte

prueba de estanqueidad del blíster
E blister tightness test
G Blisterdichtigkeitstest
F test d'étanchéité du blister

prueba de estimulación con bacterias
E microbial challenge test
G Bakterienbelastungstest
F test de stimulation microbien

prueba de explosión, a
E explosion-proof
G explosionssicher
F anti-déflagrant

prueba de identidad
E identity test
G Identitätsprüfung
F test d'identité

prueba de integridad
E integrity testing
G Integritätsprüfung
F test d'intégrité

prueba de integridad del filtro
E filter integrity test
G Filterintegritätstest
F test d'intégrité de filtre

prueba de límites
E limit test
G Grenzprüfung
F test de limites

prueba de mantenimiento del vacío
E vacuum test
G Vakuumhaltetest
F test de maintien du vide

prueba de penetración térmica
E heat penetration test
G Hitzedurchdringungstest
F essai de pénétration thermique

prueba de prelavado con torunda de algodón
E wipe test, swab test
G Wischtest
F essai de prélèvement par tampon d'ouate

prueba de presión de vejiga
E bubble point test
G Blasendrucktest
F essai de point de bulle

prueba de pureza
E purity test
G Reinheitsprüfung
F test de pureté

prueba de referencia
E reference sample
G Bezugsmuster
F échantillon de référence

prueba de retención de la presión
E pressure test
G Druckhaltetest
F test de pression de retenue

prueba estéril
E sterility test
G Steriltest
F test de stérilité

prueba fisiológica
E physiological testing
G physiologische Prüfung
F examen physiologique

prueba organoléptica
E organoleptic testing
G Sinnesprüfung
F test organoleptique

prueba toxicológica
E toxicological testing
G toxikologische Prüfung
F étude toxicologique

publicación
E publication
G Veröffentlichung
F publication

puente de hidrógeno
E hydrogen bond
G Wasserstoffbrückenbindung
F liaison hydrogène

puerta corrediza
E sliding door
G Schiebetür
F porte coulissante

puerta de protección contra incendios
E fire protection door
G Brandschutzklappe
F porte de protection anti-incendie

puerta falsa
E slippage
G Durchschlupf
F décalage

puesta a cero
E zero adjustment
G Nulleinstellung
F mise à zéro

puesta en marcha
E start-up
G Inbetriebnahme
F mise en service

puesta en servicio
E start-up
G Inbetriebnahme
F mise en service

puesto de trabajo
E place of work, employment, job
G Arbeitsplatz, Arbeitsstelle
F poste de travail, emploi

pulido
E smooth, ground
G glatt, geschliffen
F lisse, poli, moulu

pulido del vidrio
E ground glass
G Glasschliff
F polissage de verre

pulido eléctricamente
E electro-polished
G elektropoliert
F électro-poli

pulir
E polish, to; smooth, to
G polieren, glätten
F polir

pulverizador
E atomiser
G Zerstäuber
F atomiseur, pulvérisateur

pulverizar
E pulverise, to; powder, to; grind, to; crush, to; grind, to; mill, to; spray, to; atomise, to; vaporise, to
G pulverisieren, zerstoßen, aufsprühen, zerstäuben
F pulvériser, broyer, concasser, piler, atomiser

pulverulento
E powdery
G pudrig
F poudreux

punta
E spike
G Spike
F pointe, ajout

punta de jeringa
E injection tip
G Injektionsspitze
F pointe d'injection

punta de pipeta
E pipette tip
G Pipettenspitze
F pointe de pipette

punto cero (en diagrama)
E zero (in diagram)
G Nullpunkt (beim Diagramm)
F point zéro

punto de congelación
E freezing point
G Gefrierpunkt, Eispunkt
F point de congélation

punto de descarga de la cadena de envasado
E line clearance (at a packaging line)
G Linienabnahme (an der Verpackungslinie)
F ligne de dégagement (d'une chaîne de conditionnement)

punto de descongelación
E dewpoint
G Taupunkt
F point de rosée

punto de ebullición
E boiling point
G Siedepunkt
F point d'ébullition

punto de fusión
E melting point
G Schmelzpunkt
F point de fusion

punto de fusión (de ampollas)
E fusion point (of ampoules)
G Abschmelzhöhe (von Ampullen)
F point de fusion (d'ampoules)

punto de fusión inmediata
E instant melting point
G Sofortschmelzpunkt
F point de fusion instantané

punto de fusión instantánea
E instant melting point
G Sofortschmelzpunkt
F point de fusion instantané

punto de goteo
E dropping point
G Tropfpunkt
F point de goutte, température de liquéfaction

punto de ignición
E flash point
G Flammpunkt
F point d'inflammation

punto de medida
E measuring point
G Meßpunkt
F point de mesure

punto de medida de presión
E pressure-measuring point
G Druckmeßdose
F point de mesure de la pression

punto de reblandecimiento
E softening point
G Erweichungspunkt
F point de ramollissement

punto de referencia
E reference point
G Bezugspunkt
F point de référence

punto de ruptura (de una ampolla)
E cutting point (of an ampoule)
G Brechpunkt (einer Ampulle)
F point de rupture (d'une ampoule)

punto de solidificación
E solidification point
G Erstarrungspunkt
F point de solidification

punto eutéctico
E eutectic point
G Eutektikum
F point d'eutexie

punto más frío (en autoclave)
E coldest spot (autoclave)
G kältester Punkt (beim Autoklav)
F point le plus froid

punzonadora
E punch, punching station
G Stanze, Lochstanze
F poinçon, poinçonneuse

punzonar
E die-cut, to; punch, to; stamp, to; emboss, to
G ausstanzen, stanzen
F découper à l'emporte-pièce, poinçonner, estamper

pupitre de mando
E operator console, panel
G Bedienpult
F pupitre de commande, tableau de commande

pureza
E purity
G Reinheit
F pureté

pureza del pico
E peak purity
G Peakreinheit
F pureté de pic

pureza enantiómera
E enantiomeric purity
G enantiomere Reinheit
F pureté énantiomère

pureza óptica
E optical purity
G optische Reinheit
F pureté optique

pureza química
E chemical purity
G chemische Reinheit
F pureté chimique

pureza quiral
E chiral purity
G chirale Reinheit
F pureté chirale

purga con gases inertes
E inert gas purging
G Inertbegasung
F purge au gaz rare

purgar (con)
E flush, to (with); purge, to (with)
G durchströmen (mit), begasen
F rincer (avec), purger

purificación (química)
E purification
G Aufreinigung
F purification

purificación de agua
E water purification
G Wasseraufbereitung
F traitement des eaux usées

purificación de muestras
E sample clean-up
G Probenaufreinigung
F nettoyage d'échantillons

purificado
E purified
G gereinigt
F purifié

putrefacción
E putrefaction
G Fäulnis
F putréfaction

quebradizo
E brittle
G brüchig, spröde
F cassant, fragile

quebrado (vidrio)
E cracked (glass)
G gesprungen (Glas)
F fêlé

quebrar
E bend, to; buckle, to
G knicken
F casser, couder

química analítica
E analytical chemistry
G analytische Chemie
F chimie analytique

química húmeda
E wet chemistry
G Naßchemie
F chimie humide

químicamente húmedo
E wet chemical
G naßchemisch
F chimique humide

químicamente puro
E chemically pure
G chemisch rein
F chimiquement pur

quimioluminiscencia
E chemiluminescence
G Chemilumineszenz
F chimiluminescence, chimioluminescence

quiralidad
E chirality
G Chiralität
F chiralité

R & S (riesgo y seguridad)
E R & S (risk and safety)
G R & S (Risiko und Sicherheit)
F R & S (risque et sécurité)

frases de R & S
E R & S phrases
G R & S-Sätze
F phrases de R & S

racemado
E racemate
G Razemat
F racémate

racémico
E racemic
G razemisch
F racémique

radiación
E radiation
G Strahlung
F radiation

radiación infrarroja
E infrared radiation
G Infrarotstrahlung
F rayonnement infrarouge

radiación térmica
E convective heat
G Wärmestrahlung
F rayonnement thermique

radiador
E reflux condenser
G Rückflußkühler
F radiateur à reflux

raer
E scrape, to; scrape off, to
G schaben, abkratzen
F racler

raíz cuadrada
E square root
G Quadratwurzel
F racine carrée

raja
E slit
G Schlitz
F fente, fissure, rainure

rama
E division
G Sparte
F département, section

ramificación
E branching
G Verzweigung
F ramification

rancio
E rancid
G ranzig
F rance

randomizado
E randomised
G randomisiert
F randomisé

ranura
E corrugation, groove
G Riffelung, Rille, Nut
F cannelure, striage, rainure, sillon

ranura de ruptura
E break notch, break score
G Bruchrille
F encoche de rupture, entaille de rupture

rascador
E scraper
G Schaber, Abstreifer
F racloir

rascar
E scrape, to; scrape off, to
G schaben, abkratzen
F racler

raspador
E scraper
G Schaber, Abstreifer
F racloir

raspar
E scrape, to; scrape off, to
G schaben, abkratzen
F racler

rastrillo del agitador
E stirrer rake
G Rührwerksrechen
F râteau d'agitateur

rayo de referencia
E reference beam
G Referenzstrahl
F faisceau de référence

rayo doble
E double beam
G Doppelstrahl
F double faisceau

rayos gamma
E gamma rays
G Gammastrahlen
F rayons gamma

razonamiento
E rationale, reasoning
G Begründung
F exposé des motifs, explication

reacción cinética
E kinetic reaction
G kinetische Reaktion
F réaction cinétique

reacción colateral
E side reaction
G Nebenreaktion
F réaction secondaire

reacción de apertura de anillo
E ring-opening reaction
G Ringöffnungsreaktion
F réaction ouvrant un anneau

reacción de primer orden
E first-order reaction
G Reaktion 1. Ordnung
F réaction de premier ordre

reacción de segundo orden
E second-order reaction
G Reaktion 2. Ordnung
F réaction de second ordre

reacción de sustitución
E substitution reaction
G Substitutionsreaktion
F réaction de substitution

reacción endotérmica
E endothermic reaction
G endothermische Reaktion
F réaction endothermique

reacción espontánea
E spontaneous reaction
G Spontanreaktion
F réaction spontanée

reacción exotérmica
E exothermic reaction
G exothermische Reaktion
F réaction exothermique

reacción indeseable
E adverse reaction
G unerwünschte Reaktion
F réaction indésirable, effet adverse

reacción inflamatoria
E inflammatory reaction
G Entzündungsreaktion
F réaction inflammatoire

reacción térmica
E thermal reaction
G thermische Reaktion
F réaction thermique

reactivo
E reagent
G Reagenz
F réactif

reactivo de componente único
E single-component reagent
G Einkomponenten-Reagenz
F réactif à composant unique

reactivo de doble componente
E dual-component reagent
G Zweikomponenten-Reagenz
F réactifs à deux composants

reactivo de Karl Fischer
E Karl Fischer reagent
G Karl-Fischer-Lösung
F réactif de Karl Fischer

reactivo listo para el uso
E ready-to-use reagent
G gebrauchsfertiges Reagenz
F réactif prêt à l'emploi

reactor
E reactor
G Reaktor
F réacteur

realización
E fulfilment, realisation, version
G Erfüllung, Ausführung
F réalisation, version

realizar
E carry out, to; execute, to; implement, to
G durchführen, implementieren
F réaliser, exécuter, implémenter, établir

reblandecedor del agua
E water-softener
G Wasserenthärter
F adoucisseur d'eau

reblandecer
E soften, to
G erweichen
F ramollir

reblandecimiento del agua
E water softening
G Wasserenthärtung
F adoucissage de l'eau

rebordear
E flange, to; bead, to; border, to
G umbördeln
F sertir

rebordear cantos
E crimp, to; cap, to
G verbördeln
F capsuler

rebosadero
E overflow
G Überlauf
F débordement

recepción central de mercancías
E central receiving
G zentrale Warenannahme
F réception de marchandises

recepción técnica (de una máquina)
E final acceptance (of a machine)
G Abnahme (einer Maschine)
F réception technique (d'une machine)

receptor
E receptor
G Rezeptor
F récepteur

receta
E prescription
G Verordnung, Verschreibung, Rezept
F ordonnance

con receta médica
E prescription only
G rezeptpflichtig
F disponible seulement sur ordonnance

de receta obligatoria
E prescription
G verschreibungspflichtig
F vendu sur ordonnance

rechazar
E reject, to
G zurückweisen
F rejeter

rechazo
E rejection
G Zurückweisung
F rejet

rechazo (p. ej. de una patente)
E rejection (e. g. of a patent)
G Ablehnung (z. B. eines Patentes)
F refus (par ex. d'un brevet)

reciclaje
E re-cycling
G Wiederverwertung
F recyclage

recipiente
E bin, container, vessel
G Behälter, Behältnis, Gefäß
F bac, container, cuve, récipient

recipiente a presión
E pressure vessel
G Druckgefäß
F récipient sous pression

recipiente colector
E collection vessel
G Auffanggefäß
F cuve de collecte, récipient de collecte

recipiente de cuello ancho
E jar, wide-necked vessel
G Weithalsgefäß
F fiole, jarre

recipiente de depósito
E reservoir
G Vorratsgefäß
F réservoir

recipiente de desbordamiento
E overflow vessel
G Überlaufgefäß
F récipient de débordement

recipiente de desechos
E waste disposal vessel
G Abfallbehälter
F récipient d'élimination des déchets, poubelle

recipiente de dosis múltiple
E multi-dose container, multiple-dose container
G Mehrdosenbehältnis
F récipient multi-doses, conditionnement multi-doses

recipiente de dosis única
E single dose container, single unit dose container
G Einzeldosisbehältnis
F récipient à dose unique, récipient monodose

recipiente de inactivación
E inactivation vessel
G Inaktivierungsgefäß
F récipient servant à l'inactivation

recipiente de vidrio con cierre de rosca
E screw cap glass container
G Schraubglas
F pot fileté

recipiente final
E final container
G Endbehältnis
F récipient final

recipiente flexible
E squeeze bottle
G Quetschflasche
F flacon souple doseur

recipiente para muestras
E sample vessel
G Probengefäß
F récipient pour échantillon

recipiente portátil
E mobile vessel
G fahrbarer Behälter
F cuve mobile, cuve sur roues

recipiente presurizado
E pressurised container
G Druckbehälter
F récipient pressurisé, récipient soumis à la pression

reclamación
E complaint
G Reklamation, Beanstandung
F réclamation

reclamación de patente
E patent claim
G Patentanspruch
F droits liés à un brevet

reclamación por vicios
E deficiency report
G Mängelrüge
F compte-rendu des insuffisances

reclamado
E required
G gefordert
F exigé

recoger
E collect, to; entrap, to
G auffangen
F capter, recueillir

recolección de células
E cell harvesting
G Zellernte
F récolte de cellules

recombinante
E recombinant
G rekombinant
F recombinant

recomendación
E recommendation
G Empfehlung
F notes explicatives

reconocimiento de la zona de adherencia
E splice recognition
G Klebestellenerkennung
F identification de l'aire de collage

reconstitución
E reconstitution
G Wiederherstellung
F rétablissement, reconstitution

recorrido
E run
G Lauf
F cycle, opération, expérience

recorrido de visita
E visitor tour
G Besuchergang
F circuit de visite

recristalización
E recrystallisation
G Umkristallisation
F recristallisation

recta (línea)
E straight, straight line
G Gerade
F ligne droite

rectangular
E rectangular
G rechtwinkelig
F rectangulaire

rectificación
E correction
G Berichtigung
F correction

rectificado
E rectified
G rektifiziert
F rectifié

rectificador de corriente
E rectifier
G Stromgleichrichter
F redresseur de courant

recualificación
E requalification
G Requalifizierung
F requalification

recubierto
E covered
G verkleidet
F revêtu, recouvert

recubierto (comprimidos)
E coated (tablets)
G überzogen (Tabletten)
F enduit (comprimés)

recubrimiento
E coating
G Beschichtung, Belag
F couche, enduction, revêtement

recubrimiento (de conducciones)
E cladding (of piping)
G Verkleidung (von Rohrleitungen)
F revêtement (de tuyauteries)

recubrimiento de la pared
E deposit
G Wandbelag
F dépôt

recubrir
E coat, to; laminate, to
G beschichten
F enduire

recubrir (comprimidos)
E coat, to; cap, to (tablets)
G deckeln, überziehen (Tabletten)
F capsuler, enrober (comprimés)

recuento de etiquetas
E label count
G Etikettenzählung
F comptage d'étiquettes

recuento de gérmenes
E microbial count determination
G Keimzahlbestimmung
F détermination du nombre de micro-organismes

recuento de partículas viables
E viable particle count
G Zählung lebensfähiger Partikel
F comptage de particules viables

recuperación
E recovery
G Rückgewinnung, Wiedergewinnung
F récupération, rendement

recuperación de calor
E heat recovery
G Wärmerückgewinnung
F récupération de la chaleur

recuperación de solventes
E solvent recovery
G Lösungsmittelrückgewinnung
F récupération des solvants

recuperar
E recover, to
G wiedergewinnen
F récupérer

red
E net, grid
G Netz
F grille

red anular
E main ring
G Ringleitung
F boucle de recirculation

red de alambre
E mesh wire
G Drahtnetz
F tamis métallique

red de canales
E duct network, ducting
G Kanalnetz
F système de canalisation

redacción (de documentos)
E compilation (of documents)
G Erstellung (von Dokumenten)
F compilation des documents

redactar
E compile, to
G erstellen
F compiler, produire

redondeado a la cifra inferior
E rounded off
G abgerundet
F arrondi, arrondi au chiffre inférieur

redondear
E flange, to; bead, to; border, to
G umbördeln
F sertir

redondear a la cifra inferior
E round off, to
G abrunden
F arrondir

reducción
E deconcentration
G Abreicherung
F élimination

reducción de gérmenes
E microbial reduction
G Keimreduktion
F réduction microbienne

reducción del punto de congelación
E depression of freezing point
G Gefrierpunktserniedrigung
F abaissement du point de congélation

reducir
E diminish, to; reduce, to; lower, to
G vermindern, reduzieren, senken
F diminuer, réduire, abaisser, baisser

reducirse
E shrink, to
G schrumpfen
F rétrécir

reductor
E reducer
G Reduzierstück
F réducteur

reembalaje
E re-packaging
G Wiederverpackung
F action de réemballer

reemplazar
E replace, to
G ersetzen
F remplacer

reensamblaje
E re-assembly
G Wiederzusammenbau
F réassemblage

referencia
E cross reference
G Querverweis
F référence

referencia a
E reference to
G Verweis auf
F référence à

referir a
E refer to, to
G verweisen auf
F faire référence à

reflujo
E reflux, back flow
G Rückfluß
F reflux

reformulación
E reformulation
G Umformulierung
F nouvelle formulation

reforzado
E reinforced
G verstärkt
F renforcé

refractómetro
E refractometer
G Refraktometer
F réfractomètre

refrigeración
E refrigeration
G Kälteerzeugung
F réfrigération

refrigerador
E cooler, condenser
G Kühler
F réfrigérant

refrigerador a bolas
E bulb cooler
G Kugelkühler
F réfrigérant à boules

refrigerador de reflujo
E reflux condenser
G Rückflußkühler
F radiateur à reflux

refringencia
E refringence
G Brechungsvermögen
F réfringence

refuerzo
E amplification
G Verstärkung
F amplification

regeneración
E regeneration
G Regenerierung
F régénération

registrador de temperatura
E temperature recorder
G Temperaturschreiber
F enregistreur de température

registrador de valores medidos
E transducer
G Meßwertaufnehmer
F capteur, transducteur

registrador gráfico
E chart recorder
G Diagrammschreiber
F enregistreur graphique

registradora
E recorder, chart recorder
G Schreiber
F enregistreur

registradora de canales múltiples
E multi-channel recorder
G Mehrkanalschreiber
F enregistreur à canaux multiples

registradora de línea de puntos
E dotted-line recorder
G Punktschreiber
F enregistreur par ligne pointillée

registrar (datos)
E log, to; record, to; register, to; enter, to (data)
G aufzeichnen, eintragen, erfassen (Daten)
F enregistrer, inscrire (des données)

registro
E record, log, registration, recording, manhole
G Aufzeichnung, Registrierung, Aufnahme, Mannloch
F enregistrement, trou d'homme

registro de datos
E data recording
G Datenaufnahme
F enregistrement de données

registro de diagramas
E recorder chart
G Schreiberstreifen
F bande de papier d'enregistreur

reglamento de seguridad
E safety regulation
G Sicherheitsvorschriften
F règlement de sécurité

reglas concernientes a riesgos y peligros
E risk and safety phrases
G Risiko- und Gefahrensätze
F règles concernant les risques et la sécurité

reglas de etiquetado
E labelling rules
G Etikettierungsregeln
F règles d'étiquetage

reguera
E gutter
G Rinne
F gouttière

regulable
E controllable, adjustable
G regulierbar, einstellbar, regelbar
F ajustable

regulación
E adjustment, setting
G Einstellung, Regulierung
F ajustement, réglage

regulación del flujo
E flow regulation
G Durchflußregulierung
F régulation du débit

regulación fina
E fine adjustment
G Feinregulierung
F réglage fin

regulador
E controller, control valve
G Regler
F régulateur

regulador de fuelle cruzado
E cross-bellows controller
G Kreuzbalgregler
F régleur pneumatique

regulador de presión
E pressure regulator, reducing valve
G Druckregler
F régulateur de pression

regulador de temperatura
E temperature controller
G Temperaturregler
F régulateur de température

regulador de tensión
E voltage regulator
G Spannungsregler
F régulateur de tension

regulador variable de flujo
E flowmeter, variable
G variabler Volumenstromregler
F régulateur de flux

regular
E adjust, to
G einstellen
F ajuster, régler

regusto
E after-taste
G Nachgeschmack
F arrière-goût

reintroducir
E reintroduce, to
G wiedereinschleusen
F réintroduire

relé
E relay
G Relais
F relais

relevador
E relay
G Relais
F relais

relevante
E relevant, pertinent
G relevant
F pertinent, approprié

rellenado de una ampolla
E ampoule filling
G Ampullenabfüllung
F remplissage d'une ampoule

rellenante de una fisura
E crack-filling
G rißüberbrückend
F colmatant (une fissure)

relleno con medio de cultivo
E culture medium filling, media fill
G Nährmedienabfüllung
F remplissage des milieux de culture

relleno uniforme
E uniform filling
G gleichmäßige Füllung
F remplissage uniforme

remache
E rivet
G Niete
F rivet

remache avellanado
E countersunk rivet
G Senkniete
F rivet conique

remodelación
E reworking
G Umarbeitung
F retraitement

remuneración
E remuneration
G Vergütung
F rémunération

rendimiento
E yield, throughput, capacity, performance
G Ausbeute, Ertrag, Durchsatz, Leistung
F rendement, capacité, débit, performance

rendimiento bruto
E raw yield
G Rohausbeute
F rendement brut

rendimiento de aire
E air throughput
G Luftdurchsatz
F débit d'écoulement d'air

rendimiento de granulación
E granulation performance
G Granulationsleistung
F rendement de transformation en granulé

rendimiento de la máquina de comprimidos
E tablet output
G Tablettierausstoß
F débit de production de comprimés

rendimiento de producción
E production output
G Produktionsleistung
F rendement d'une production

rendimiento de un motor
E motor performance
G Motorleistung
F performance d'un moteur

rendimiento en comprimidos
E tablet output
G Tablettenausstoß
F débit de production de comprimés

rendimiento en muestras
E sample throughput
G Probendurchsatz
F capacité d'analyse d'échantillons

rendimiento en producto
E product yield
G Produktausbeute
F taux de récupération d'un produit

rendimiento final
E final yield
G Endausbeute
F rendement final

rendimiento horario
E output per hour
G Stundenleistung
F rendement horaire, débit horaire

rendimiento real
E actual yield
G Ausbeute, tatsächliche
F rendement réel

rendimiento secundario
E secondary yield
G Sekundärausbeute
F rendement secondaire

rendimiento separador
E separation performance
G Trennungsleistung
F performance de séparation

rendimiento separador de la columna
E column performance
G Trennleistung der Säule
F performance d'une colonne

rendimiento teórico
E theoretical yield
G theoretische Ausbeute
F rendement théorique

rendimiento total
E total yield
G Gesamtausbeute
F rendement total

renovación del aire
E air exchange
G Luftwechsel
F renouvellement d'air

renovar
E upgrade, to
G aufrüsten
F moderniser

reología
E rheology
G Rheologie
F rhéologie

reorganización
E re-equipping
G Umrüstung
F modernisation, réorganisation

reorganizar
E re-equip, to
G umrüsten
F moderniser, réorganiser

reparación
E repair
G Reparatur, Instandsetzung
F réparation

repelente de la humedad
E moisture-repelling
G feuchtigkeitsabweisend
F qui répulse l'humidité

repetición
E repetition
G Wiederholung
F répétition

repetitividad
E repeatability
G Wiederholbarkeit
F répétitivité

repetitividad de la precisión
E precision repeatability
G Wiederholbarkeit der Präzision
F répétitivité de la précision

repleción
E overfill(ing)
G Überfüllung
F quantité en excès

representación gráfica
E graph
G grafische Darstellung
F graphe

reprocesado
E reprocessing
G Nacharbeitung, Wiederaufbereitung
F traitement complémentaire, retraitement, retouche

reproducible
E reproducible
G reproduzierbar
F reproductible

reproductibilidad
E reproducibility
G Reproduzierbarkeit
F reproductibilité

requerimiento
E requirement
G Anforderung, Erfordernis
F exigence

requerimiento legal
E legal requirement
G gesetzliche Anforderung
F exigence légale

requerimientos del usuario
E user requirements, user specifications
G Lastenheft
F cahier des charges, spécifications de l'usager

requerir
E require, to
G erfordern
F exiger, nécessiter

requisito de seguridad
E safety requirements
G Sicherheitsanforderungen
F consignes de sécurité

resaltar
E project, to; protrude, to
G überhängen
F saillir, faire saillir

resbaladizo
E smooth
G glatt
F lisse, poli

resbalar
E slip, to
G gleiten
F couler, glisser

reservado
E retentive
G zurückhaltend
F réservé, effacé, réticent

residuo
E residue
G Rückstand, Rest
F résidu

residuo de destilación
E distillation residue
G Destillationsrückstand
F résidu de distillation

residuo de evaporación
E residue on evaporating
G Verdampfungsrückstand
F résidus de vaporisation

residuo de filtración
E filter residue
G Filterrückstand
F résidu de filtration

residuo de ignición
E residue on ignition
G Glührückstand
F résidu d'ignition

residuo de prensado
E residue
G Preßrückstand
F résidu de pressage

residuo de tamizado
E overs, residue
G Siebrückstand
F résidu de tamisage

residuo de un producto
E product residue
G Produktrückstand
F résidu d'un produit

residuo seco
E residue on drying
G Trockenrückstand
F résidu de séchage

residuo visible
E visible residue
G sichtbarer Rückstand
F résidu visible

residuos
E rubbish, waste
G Müll
F déchets, résidus

residuos radiactivos
E radioactive waste
G radioaktiver Abfall
F résidu radioactif

resina
E resin
G Harz
F résine

resina acrílica
E acrylic resin
G Acrylharz
F résine acrylique

resina de intercambio iónico
E ion exchange resin
G Austauscherharz
F résine échangeuse d'ions

resina sintética
E synthetic resin
G Kunstharz
F résine synthétique

resistencia
E toughness
G Zähigkeit
F viscosité

resistencia a la abrasión
E frictional resistance
G Abriebfestigkeit
F résistance à la friction

resistencia a la filtración
E filtration resistance
G Filtrationswiderstand
F résistance au filtrage

resistencia a la flexión
E flexural strength, flexional strength
G Beugungsfestigkeit, Biegefestigkeit
F résistance à la flexion, résistance au pliage, résistance au fléchissement

resistencia a la fricción
E frictional resistance
G Reibungswiderstand
F résistance à la friction, résistance au frottement

resistencia a la luz
E light-fastness
G Lichtbeständigkeit
F résistance à la lumière

resistencia a la presión
E pressure resistance
G Druckfestigkeit
F résistance à la pression

resistencia a la rotura
E breaking strength, breaking resistance
G Bruchfestigkeit
F résistance à la rupture

resistencia a la tracción y a la presión
E traction-compression resistance
G Zug- und Druckfestigekit
F résistance à la traction et à la compression

resistencia a los choques
E impact resistance
G Schlagfestigkeit
F résistance au choc

resistencia al desgarro
E resistance to tearing, tear strength, tensile strength
G Reißfestigkeit, Zerreißfestigkeit
F résistance au déchirement

resistencia al desgaste
E resistance to wear
G Verschleißwiderstand
F résistance à l'usure

resistencia al estallido
E bursting strength
G Berstdruckfestigkeit
F résistance à l'éclatement

resistencia al pandeo
E resistance to bending
G Knickechtheit
F résistance à la plicature

resistencia al plegado
E flexing resistance
G Falzechtheit
F résistance au pliage

resistencia del filtro
E filter resistance
G Filterwiderstand
F résistance du filtre

resistencia eléctrica
E resistance, electrical
G elektrischer Widerstand
F résistance électrique

resistencia específica
E specific resistance
G spezifischer Widerstand
F résistance spécifique

resistente
E resistant, tough
G widerstandsfähig, resistent, zäh
F résistant, visqueux, épais

resistente a la abrasión
E non-abrasive, resistant to abrasion
G abriebfest
F résistant à l'abrasion

resistente a la agitación
E shock-resistant
G erschütterungsbeständig
F résistant aux chocs

resistente a la corrosión
E resistant to corrosion
G korrosionsbeständig
F résistant à la corrosion

resistente a la decoloración
E resistant to fading
G lichtecht
F résistant à la décoloration

resistente a la fricción
E resistance to abrasion
G Reibeechtheit
F résistance à l'abrasion

resistente a la humedad
E moisture-resistant
G feuchtigkeitsbeständig
F résistant à l'humidité

resistente a la luz
E light-fast
G lichtbeständig
F résistant à la lumière

resistente a la presión
E pressure-resistant
G druckfest
F résistant à la pression

resistente a los ácidos
E acid-resistant
G säurebeständig
F résistant aux acides

resistente a los golpes
E impact-resistant
G stoßfest
F résistant aux chocs

resistente a solventes
E solvent-resistant
G lösungsmittelbeständig
F résistant aux solvants

resistente al calor
E heat-resistant
G hitzebeständig
F résistant à la chaleur

resistente al envejecimiento
E age-resistant
G alterungsbeständig
F résistant au vieillissement

resistente al fuego
E fire-resistant
G feuerfest
F in-inflammable

resistente al jugo gástrico
E gastro-resistant
G magensaftresistent
F résistant au suc gastrique

resorción
E resorption
G Resorption
F résorption

English German French Spanish

resorte
E spring
G Feder (Sprung-)
F ressort

responsabilidad
E responsibility
G Verantwortlichkeit
F responsabilité

responsabilidad (jurídica)
E liability (legal)
G Haftung (rechtlich)
F responsabilité (juridique)

responsable
E responsible person
G Verantwortlicher
F personne responsable

responsable de farmacovigilancia
E pharmaco-vigilance manager, drug safety manager
G Stufenplanbeauftragter
F personne responsable de la pharmaco-vigilance

restablecimiento
E reconstitution
G Wiederherstellung
F rétablissement, reconstitution

restitución
E reimbursement
G Erstattung
F remboursement

resto
E residue
G Rückstand
F résidu

restos
E debris
G Bruch
F débris

restricción
E limitation
G Einschränkung
F limitation

resultado
E result
G Ergebnis
F résultats

resultados esperados
E expected results
G erwartete Ergebnisse
F résultats escomptés

resultado de la prueba
E analytical result
G Testergebnis
F résultat d'analyse

resumen de características del producto
E summary of product characteristics (SPC)
G Zusammenfassung der Produktmerkmale
F résumé des caractéristiques du produit

retardado
E delayed
G verzögert
F retardé

retardo
E delay
G Verzögerung
F retard

retención
E retention
G Retention
F rétention

retener
E lock, to
G arretieren
F fermer à clef

retícula
E grating
G Gitter, Gitterrost
F grille

reticular
E reticular, net-like
G netzförmig, vernetzt
F réticulaire

retículo
E network, crosswires
G Netzwerk, Fadenkreuz
F réseau, réticule

retículo cristalino
E lattice
G Kristallgitter
F réseau cristallin

retirada
E recall
G Rückruf
F rappel

retirada de un producto
E product recall
G Produktrückruf
F rappel d'un produit

retocado
E reprocessing
G Nacharbeitung
F traitement complémentaire, retouche

retorno
E return, reverse flow
G Retoure, Rücklauf
F renvoi, rappel, retour

retorta
E flask
G Kolben (Glasgefäß)
F ballon, flacon

retraerse
E shrink, to
G schrumpfen
F rétrécir

retrasado
E delayed
G verzögert
F retardé

retraso
E delay, time lag
G Verzögerung, Zeitverzögerung
F retard

retraso de la ebullición
E boiling retardation
G Siedeverzug
F retardement de l'ébullition

retromarcado
E traceability
G Rückverfolgbarkeit, Rückführbarkeit
F traçabilité

reutilizable
E returnable, re-usable
G Mehrweg-, wiederverwendbar
F réutilisable

reutilización
E re-use
G Wiederverwendung
F réutilisation

revalidación
E revalidation
G Revalidierung
F revalidation

reventar
E burst, to
G bersten
F éclater

revestido
E covered
G verkleidet
F revêtu, recouvert

revestido de plástico
E plastic-coated
G kunststoffbeschichtet
F revêtu de plastique

revestimiento
E coat, film, cover, coating, jacket, mantle
G Überzug, Verkleidung, Belag, Ummantelung
F couche, pellicule, revêtement, gaine, enveloppe

revestimiento (de recipientes)
E lining (of containers)
G Auskleidung (von Behältern)
F garnissage (de récipients)

revestimiento coloreado
E colour coating
G Farbüberzug
F revêtement de couleur

revestimiento de superficies
E surface coating
G Oberflächenbeschichtung
F revêtement de surface

revestimiento del suelo
E flooring, floor covering, floor finishing
G Bodenbelag, Fußbodenbelag
F revêtement de sol

revestimiento plástico
E plastic coating
G Kunststoffbeschichtung
F revêtement plastique

revisado
E reviewed
G überarbeitet
F révisé

revisar
E revise, to; review, to
G revidieren, überarbeiten
F réviser, remanier

revocado
E plastered
G verputzt
F crépi

revoluciones (por minuto)
E revolutions (per minute)
G Umdrehungen (pro Minute)
F rotations (par minute)

riesgo de lesión
E risk of injury
G Verletzungsgefahr
F risque de blessures

riesgo para la salud
E health risk
G Gesundheitsrisiko
F risque pour la santé

riesgo para la seguridad
E safety risk
G Sicherheitsrisiko
F danger

rígido
E rigid
G starr, steif
F rigide

robustez
E robustness
G Robustheit
F robustesse

robustez del proceso
E process robustness
G Robustheit des Prozesses
F robustesse d'un procédé

robusto (p. ej. instrumento, método)
E rugged (e. g. instrument, method)
G robust (z. B. Gerät, Methode)
F robuste (par ex. instrument, méthode)

rociado
E splashes
G Spritzer
F éclaboussures

rociado con agua caliente
E hot water spraying
G Heißwasserberieselung
F aspersion d'eau chaude

rociar
E wet, to; moisten, to
G benetzen
F humidifier, mouiller

rodamiento a bolas
E ball bearing
G Kugellager
F roulement à billes

rodapié en forma de garganta
E fluted skirting
G Hohlkehlsockel
F plinthe à gorge arrondie

rodeado de
E encased
G eingeschlossen, umgeben von
F enchâssé

rodillo
E roller, drum
G Walze
F rouleau, cylindre, tambour

rodillo de imprenta
E printing roller
G Druckwalze
F cylindre à imprimer

roedor
E rodent
G Nagetier
F rongeur

roldana
E casters
G Laufrollen, Lenkrollen
F rouleau porteur, galet de guidage, poulie de guidage

rollo (p. ej. de una lámina)
E sheet (e. g. of foil)
G Bahn (z. B. Folien-)
F bande (d'étoffe)

rollo de grabado
E engraving roll
G Gravurrolle
F rouleau de gravure

rollo de prensado previo (comprimidos)
E pre-pressing roller
G Vordruckrolle (Tablettenpresse)
F rouleau presseur

rollo principal de prensa
E main compression roll
G Hauptdruckrolle
F rouleau presseur principal

romper por el cuello (ampolla)
E snap, to (an ampoule)
G abknicken (eine Ampulle)
F casser (une ampoule)

romper una ampolla
E break an ampoule, to
G Ampulle aufbrechen
F casser une ampoule

ropa de calle
E street clothing
G Straßenkleidung
F vêtements de ville

ropa de seguridad
E safety clothing
G Sicherheitskleidung
F vêtement de sécurité

ropa de trabajo
E working clothing
G Arbeitskleidung
F vêtement de travail

cesto para ropa de trabajo
E clothing receptacle
G Kleidungsaufnahmebehälter
F corbeille pour vêtements de travail

ropa de uso único
E disposable jump-suit
G Einmalanzug
F combinaison à usage unique

ropa para área estéril
E clean room clothing
G Reinraumkleidung
F vêtement protecteur pour zone d'atmosphère contrôlée

ropa protectora
E protective clothing
G Schutzkleidung
F vêtement de protection

ropa sin pelusa
E lint-free clothes
G fusselfreie Kleidung
F vêtement qui ne peluche pas

rosca
E thread
G Gewinde
F filetage

de paso derecho
E right-handed
G rechtsgängig
F à droite

de paso izquierdo
E left-handed
G linksgängig
F à gauche

rosca de tornillo
E screw thread
G Schraubgewinde
F filetage

rosca de tubo
E tube thread
G Tubengewinde
F filets du tube

rotación
E recirculation
G Umlauf
F recirculation

rotación específica
E specific rotation
G spezifische Drehung
F rotation spécifique

rotación óptica
E optical rotation
G optische Drehung
F rotation optique

rotor
E rotor
G Rotor
F rotor

rotulación
E designation
G Bezeichnung
F désignation, appellation

rotulado
E labelling, lettering
G Beschriftung, Kennzeichnung
F étiquetage, marquage

rotular
E label, to; designate, to
G bezeichnen
F étiqueter

rueda de aletas
E rotor, impeller, fan wheel, blade, vane
G Laufrad, Flügelrad
F ailette

rueda de dosificación
E dosing wheel
G Dosierrad, Dosierstern
F roue de dosage

rueda de paletas
E fan wheel, blade, vane
G Flügelrad
F ailette

rueda de ventilador
E fan wheel
G Gebläserad
F roue de ventilateur

rueda portante
E rotor, impeller
G Laufrad, Flügelrad
F ailette

rugosidad de superficie
E surface rawness
G Oberflächenrauhigkeit
F rugosité de la surface

ruido
E noise
G Lärmbelastung
F pollution par le bruit

ruido (de fondo)
E noise
G Rauschen
F bruit

ruido (de fondo) en la línea de base
E baseline noise
G Basislinienrauschen
F bruit de fond d'une ligne de base

ruptura de hilo
E thread rupture
G Fadenbruch
F rupture de fil

ruptura de vidrio
E breakage of glassware
G Glasbruch
F débris de verre

ruptura del tamiz
E sieve rupture
G Siebbruch
F rupture de trémie

saco filtrante
E sack filter
G Sackfilter
F sac filtrant

sacudir
E shake, to; shake out, to; vibrate, to
G rütteln, ausschütteln
F secouer

sala de máquinas
E machine room
G Maschinenraum
F salle des machines

sala de preparación de medios de cultivo
E culture media preparation room
G Nährmedienküche
F salle de préparation des milieux de culture

salida
E outlet, discharge outlet, orifice, drain
G Auslauf, Auslaß, Ablauf, Austritt
F sortie, orifice, sortie de vidange, sortie de purge

salida de presión
E pressure release outlet
G Druckablaß
F sortie de régulation de pression

salida del detector
E detector outlet
G Detektorauslaß
F sortie de détecteur

salificación
E salt formation
G Salzbildung
F formation de sels

salinidad
E salinity
G Salzigkeit, Salinität
F salinité

salirse
E run off, to
G auslaufen
F couler, s'écouler

salpicado
E mottled
G gesprenkelt
F madré

salpicadura
E splashes
G Spritzer
F éclaboussures

saneamiento
E reorganisation, restructuring
G Sanierung
F assainissement

sanguijuela
E leech
G Blutegel
F sangsue

saponificación
E saponification
G Verseifung
F saponification

saponificar
E saponify, to
G verseifen
F saponifier

English German French Spanish

saturación
E saturation
G Sättigung
F saturation

saturado
E saturated
G gesättigt
F saturé

secado al aire
E air-dried
G luftgetrocknet
F séché à l'air

secado al vacío
E vacuum drying
G Vakuumtrocknung
F dessication sous vide

secado en bandeja
E tray drying
G Hordentrocknung
F dessication sur claies

secado final
E final drying
G Nachtrocknen
F séchage final

secador
E drying oven
G Trockenschrank
F séchoir

secador de cilindros
E drum dryer
G Walzentrockner
F séchoir à cylindres

secador de circulación de aire
E circulatory dryer
G Umlufttrockner
F séchoir à circulation d'air

secador de lecho fluidificado
E fluid bed dryer
G Wirbelschichttrockner
F sécheur en lit fluidisé

secar
E dry, to; desiccate, to
G trocknen, eintrocknen
F sécher, dessiquer

secar atomizando
E spray-dry, to
G sprühtrocknen
F séchage par atomisation

sección de llenado
E filling section
G Abfüllstrecke
F chemin de remplissage

sección transversal
E cross-section
G Querschnitt
F section transversale, coupe transversale

secreto empresarial
E company secret
G Betriebsgeheimnis
F secret d'entreprise

sector
E division
G Sparte
F département, section

sector farmacéutico
E pharmaceutical division
G Pharma-Sparte
F division pharmaceutique

secuencia
E sequence
G Reihenfolge
F séquence

secuencia (de un proceso)
E sequence of operation
G Ablauf (eines Prozesses)
F déroulement d'un procédé

secuencia de ciclos
E cycle sequence
G Zyklussequenz
F séquence de cycles

secuenciación
E sequencing
G Sequenzierung
F séquençage

secuestración
E complex formation
G Komplexbildung
F formation de complexes

sedante
E sedative
G Beruhigungsmittel
F sédatif, calmant

sedimentar
E sediment, to
G sedimentieren
F sédimenter

sedimento
E sediment
G Ablagerung, Bodensatz
F dépôt, sédiment

segregación
E segregation, separation
G Abtrennung
F séparation, ségrégation

seguimiento de un lote
E batch traceability
G Chargenrückverfolgbarkeit
F traçabilité d'un lot

seguridad
E safety, security
G Sicherheit, Unbedenklichkeit
F sécurité

seguridad biológica
E biosafety
G biologische Sicherheit
F bio-sécurité

seguridad de datos
E data security
G Datensicherheit
F sécurité des données

seguridad de dosificación
E dosage security
G Dosierungssicherheit
F sécurité de dosage

seguridad de un producto
E product safety
G Produktsicherheit
F sécurité d'un produit

seguridad del personal
E personnel safety, personnel protection
G Personenschutz
F sécurité du personnel

seguridad en el trabajo
E safety at work
G Arbeitssicherheit
F sécurité du travail

seguridad informática
E computer security
G Computersicherheit
F sécurité informatique

selección
E selection
G Auswahl, Auslese
F sélection

selectividad
E selectivity
G Selektivität
F sélectivité

sellado
E seal
G Versiegelung
F joint, fermeture

sellar
E seal, to
G siegeln, versiegeln
F sceller, clore, fermer hermétiquement

sellar (ampollas)
E tip seal, to (ampoules)
G abschmelzen (Ampullen)
F obturer (des ampoules)

sellar al calor
E heat seal, to
G heißsiegeln
F thermosceller

sembrar
E inoculate, to
G beimpfen
F ensemencer, inoculer

sembrar (colonias microbiológicas)
E smear, to (microbiological colonies)
G ausstreichen (mikrobiol. Kolonien)
F ensemencer (colonies microbiol.)

semiconductor
E semiconductor
G Halbleiter
F semi-conducteur

semisólido
E semi-solid
G halbfest
F semi-solide

señal acústica
E acoustic signal
G akustisches Signal
F signal acoustique

señal de alarma
E alarm
G Warnsignal
F alarme

señal óptica
E visual signal, display
G optisches Signal, optische Anzeige
F signal optique, indication visuelle

sensibilidad
E sensitivity
G Empfindlichkeit
F sensibilité

sensibilidad de detección
E detection sensitivity
G Detektionsempfindlichkeit
F sensibilité de détection

sensible
E sensitive
G empfindlich
F sensible

sensible a la corrosión
E corrodible, sensitive to corrosion
G korrosionsempfindlich
F sensible à la corrosion

sensible a la humedad
E moisture-sensitive
G feuchtigkeitsempfindlich
F sensible à l'humidité

sensible al calor
E heat-sensitive
G hitzeempfindlich
F sensible à la chaleur

sensor
E sensor
G Fühler
F capteur

sensor de conductividad
E conductivity sensor
G Leitfähigkeitsmesser
F capteur de conductivité

sensor de luminiscencia
E luminescence scanner
G Lumineszenztaster
F scanner à luminescence

sensor de nivel
E level sensor
G Pegelmesser
F détecteur de niveau

sensor de presión atmosférica
E air pressure sensor
G Luftdruckfühler
F détecteur de pression atmosphérique

sensor de temperatura
E temperature sensor
G Temperatursensor, Temperaturfühler
F sonde de température, sonde thermique

sensor del contenido
E product scanner
G Füllguttaster
F palpeur de remplissage

sensor térmico
E temperature sensor
G Wärmefühler
F sonde thermique

sentido antihorario
E anticlockwise
G gegen Uhrzeigersinn
F contre le sens des aiguilles d'une montre

sentido de la rotación
E direction of rotation
G Drehrichtung
F direction de rotation

sentido horario
E clockwise
G im Uhrzeigersinn
F dans le sens des aiguilles d'une montre

separación
E segregation, separation, demixing
G Abtrennung, Trennung, Entmischung
F séparation, ségrégation, démixtion

separación de gotitas
E drop-collection
G Tröpfchenabscheidung
F collecte de gouttelettes

separación de solventes
E solvent separation
G Lösungsmittelabscheidung
F séparation des solvants

separación espacial
E physical segregation
G räumliche Trennung
F ségrégation physique

separación magnética de células
E magnetic cell separation
G magnetische Zelltrennung
F clivage cellulaire magnétique

separación por centrifugación
E cyclone separation
G Zyklonabscheidung
F séparateur à cyclone

separado
E separated, segregated
G abgetrennt
F séparé, détaché, isolé

separador
E separator
G Abscheider
F séparateur

separador de aceite
E oil separator, oil trap
G Ölabscheider
F siphon de dépôt d'huile, séparateur d'huile, déshuileur

separador de agua
E water separator
G Wasserabscheider
F séparateur d'eau

separador de formas
E parting agent
G Formentrennmittel
F séparateur de formes

separador de vapor
E steam separator
G Dampfabscheider
F séparateur de vapeur

separar
E separate, to
G abscheiden
F séparer, sécréter

septo
E septum
G Septum
F septum

serie
E series
G Serie, Baureihe
F série

English German French Spanish

serie de dilución
E dilution series
G Verdünnungsreihe
F séries de dilution

serie de ensayos
E screening
G Reihenuntersuchung
F screening, série d'analyses

serie de perforaciones
E row of perforations
G Lochreihe
F série de perforations

serpentín de calefacción
E heating coil
G Heizschlange
F serpentin chauffant

serpentín de calefacción sumergido
E immersed heating coil
G untergetauchte Heizschlange
F serpentin chauffant immergé

serpentín de calentamiento
E heating coil
G Aufheizspirale
F serpentin chauffant

serpentín para el agua de refrigeración
E cooling water loop
G Kühlwasserschleife
F boucle d'eau de refroidissement

serpentín refrigerador
E cooling coil
G Schlangenkühler
F serpentin de refroidissement

servicio de donantes de sangre
E blood donor service
G Blutspendewesen
F banque du sang

servicio externo de ventas
E field force, sales force
G Außendienst
F force de vente

siembra
E inoculation
G Beimpfung
F inoculation

significado
E significance
G Bedeutung
F signification

silenciador
E silencer, attenuator
G Schalldämpfer
F silencieux, amortisseur de son

silicato
E silicate
G Silikat
F silicate

siliconización
E siliconisation
G Silikonisierung
F siliconisation

símbolo CE
E CE symbol
G CE-Zeichen
F symbole CE

símbolo de peligro
E hazard symbol
G Gefahrensymbol
F symbole de danger

simultáneamente
E simultaneous
G gleichzeitig
F simultanément

simultáneo
E simultaneous
G gleichzeitig
F simultanément

sincronizador del tiempo
E timer
G Zeitgeber
F minuterie

sinéresis
E synaresis
G Synärese
F synérèse

sínter de vidrio
E glass sinter
G Glassinter
F fritte de verre

sinterizar
E sinter, to
G sintern
F fritter

síntesis
E synthesis
G Synthese
F synthèse

sistema colector
E collection system
G Sammelsystem
F système de collecte

sistema de acoplamiento
E docking system
G Andocksystem
F système d'amarrage, système de fixation

sistema de alarma
E alarm system
G Alarmsystem
F système d'alarme

sistema de alimentación
E feed system
G Eintragsvorrichtung
F système d'alimentation

sistema de aspiración
E aspiration system, evacuation system
G Absaugvorrichtung
F système d'aspiration, système d'évacuation

sistema de aspiración de polvo
E dust exhausting device, dust extraction
G Staubabsauganlage
F système d'aspiration de la poussière

sistema de ayuda para pipetear
E pipetting aid
G Pipettierhilfe
F système d'aide au pipettage

sistema de canalización
E piping system
G Rohrleitungssystem
F système de canalisation

sistema de conducciones
E ducting system
G Schachtsystem
F système de canalisation

sistema de control
E control system
G Leitsystem
F système de contrôle

sistema de eliminación
E disposal system
G Entsorgungssystem
F système d'élimination

sistema de evacuación
E aspiration system, evacuation system
G Absaugvorrichtung
F système d'aspiration, système d'évacuation

sistema de expertos
E expert system
G Expertensystem
F système expert

sistema de fijación
E docking system
G Andocksystem
F système d'amarrage, système de fixation

sistema de gestión de datos de laboratorio (LIMS)
E laboratory information management system (LIMS)
G Laborinformations- und -management-System (LIMS)
F système de gestion des données de laboratoire (LIMS)

sistema de gestión de un proceso
E process control system
G Prozeßleitsystem
F système de gestion d'un procédé

sistema de lavado
E trickle installation, trickle plant
G Berieselungsanlage
F système de ruissellement

sistema de medida del nivel de relleno
E level-measuring device
G Füllstandsmesser
F dispositif de mesure d'un niveau

sistema de pipeteo
E pipetting system, pipettor
G Pipettiersystem
F système de pipettage

sistema de pipeteo con canales múltiples
E multi-channel pipetting system
G Vielfachkanalpipettiersystem
F système de pipettage à canaux multiples

sistema de presurización
E pressurisation system
G Drucksystem
F système de pressurisation

sistema de prueba (para calibrar)
E calibrating equipment
G Prüfmittel (zur Kalibrierung)
F équipement de calibration

sistema de pulverización
E spraying system
G Sprühsystem
F système de pulvérisation

sistema de retromarcado
E tracing system
G Rückverfolgungssystem
F système de suivi, système d'observation

sistema de servicio
E operating system
G Bedienungssystem
F système d'exploitation

sistema de tratamiento de agua
E water treatment system
G Wasseraufbereitungsanlage
F système de traitement de l'eau

sistema de ventilación
E ventilation system
G Belüftungsanlage, Lüftungsanlage, Belüftungssystem, raumlufttechnische Anlage
F système de ventilation

sistema de vigilancia
E monitoring system
G Überwachungssystem
F système de contrôle, système de surveillance

sistema de vigilancia de comprimidos
E tablet monitoring system
G Tablettenüberwachungssystem
F système de surveillance des comprimés

sistema empresarial de propuestas
E employee suggestion scheme
G betriebliches Vorschlagswesen
F schéma interne de suggestions pour employés

sistema lógico de aplicación
E application software
G Anwendungssoftware
F logiciel d'application

sistema robot
E robotic system
G Robotersystem
F analyseur robot

sistema sanitario
E health care
G Gesundheitswesen
F système de santé

sistema terapéutico transdérmico
E transdermal delivery system
G Transdermales Therapeutisches System
F système thérapeutique transdermique

sistemas logísticos
E logistic systems
G logistische Systeme
F systèmes logistiques

situación
E location
G Lage, Ort
F endroit, lieu

sobrante
E excess
G Überschuß
F excès

sobre
E bag
G Beutel
F poche, sac, sachet

empaquetar en sobres
E package in bags, to
G in Beutel verpacken
F empaqueter, emballer

sobre (como forma de administración)
E sachet
G Beutel
F sachet

sobre de pared doble
E bag in bag
G Beutel in Außenbeutel
F sac à double paroi

sobrecarga
E overload, overloading
G Überlastung
F surcharge

sobrecarga de columna
E column overloading
G Säulenüberladung
F surcharge de la colonne

sobredosificación
E overdose
G Überdosierung
F surdosage, surdose

sobredosificado
E overdosed
G überdosiert
F surdosé, surdosage

sobreinoculación
E transfer inoculation
G Überimpfung
F repiquage

sobrenadante
E supernatant
G Überstand
F surnageant

sobrepresión
E positive pressure, excess pressure
G Überdruck
F surpression

sobrepresión atmosférica
E excess atmospheric pressure
G Atmosphärenüberdruck
F surpression atmosphérique

sobresalir
E project, to; protrude, to
G überhängen, überstehen
F saillir, faire saillir

sobresaturación
E supersaturation
G Übersättigung
F sursaturation

sociedad
E company
G Gesellschaft
F société, compagnie

English German French Spanish

sociedad anónima
E public liability company
G Aktiengesellschaft
F société anonyme

sociedad matriz
E parent company
G Mutterfirma
F société mère

software configurable
E configurable software
G konfigurierbare Software
F logiciel configurable

software de aplicación
E application software
G Anwendungssoftware
F logiciel d'application

soldado
E welded
G verschweißt
F soudé

soldado orbitalmente
E orbitally welded
G orbital geschweißt
F soudé par soudure orbitale

soldadura
E joint, weld, welding seam
G Naht, 'Schweißnaht
F joint, soudure

soldadura del encaje
E lock seam
G Falznaht
F couture de pliage

soldadura orbital
E orbital fusion welding
G Orbitalschweißen
F soudure orbitale

soldar
E weld, to; seam weld, to
G schweißen, nahtschweißen
F souder

soldar a tope
E butt-weld, to
G stumpfschweißen
F souder par rapprochement

soldar por puntos
E spot-weld, to
G punktschweißen
F souder par points

solicitud
E application
G Antrag
F requête, demande

solicitud a la FDA (EE.UU.) para investigar clínicamente un nuevo medicamento
E Investigational New Drug Application (IND)
G Antrag an die FDA auf klinische Prüfung eines Arzneimittels
F demande d'autorisation d'étude clinique d'un nouveau médicament (IND) auprès de la FDA

solicitud de aprobación de un producto por la FDA
E New Drug Application (NDA)
G Antrag auf Produktzulassung bei der FDA
F demande d'autorisation d'un médicament auprès de la FDA

solicitud de autorización
E application for marketing authorisation
G Zulassungsantrag
F demande d'autorisation de mise sur le marché

solicitud de autorización de un producto (para la venta)
E application for marketing authorisation
G Produktzulassungsantrag
F demande d'autorisation de mise sur le marché

solicitud de autorización de venta de medicamentos en la UE
E Medicines Marketing Authorisation Application (MAA)
G Antrag auf Zulassung zum Inverkehrbringen von Arzneimitteln in der EU
F demande d'autorisation de mise sur le marché (AMM)

solicitud de cambio
E change request
G Änderungsantrag
F demande de modification

solicitud de patente
E patent filing, patent application
G Patentanmeldung, Patentbeantragung, Patenteinreichung
F demande de brevet, dépôt de demande de brevet

solicitud de permiso a la FDA (EE.UU.) para poner a la venta un medicamento
E Product License Application (PLA), application for marketing approval
G Antrag auf Vertriebsgenehmigung eines Arzneimittels bei der FDA
F demande d'autorisation de mise sur le marché (AMM)

solidez
E firmness, solidity
G Festigkeit
F solidité

solidificar
E solidify, to
G erstarren
F solidifier

sólido
E solid
G fest
F solide

solubilidad
E solubility
G Löslichkeit
F solubilité

solubilizante
E solubiliser
G Lösungsvermittler
F solubilisant

soluble
E soluble
G löslich
F soluble

difícilmente soluble
E sparingly soluble
G schwer löslich
F difficilement soluble

fácilmente soluble
E readily soluble
G leicht löslich
F facilement soluble

insoluble
E insoluble
G unlöslich
F insoluble

muy difícilmente soluble
E very slightly soluble
G sehr schwer löslich
F très difficilement soluble

muy fácilmente soluble
E very soluble
G sehr leicht löslich
F très soluble

poco soluble
E slightly soluble
G wenig löslich
F peu soluble

prácticamente insoluble
E practically insoluble
G praktisch unlöslich
F pratiquement insoluble

soluble en el intestino delgado
E entero-soluble
G dünndarmlöslich
F entéro-soluble

English German French Spanish

English German French Spanish

solución
E solution
G Lösung
F solution

solución insaturada
E unsaturated solution
G ungesättigte Lösung
F solution non-saturée

solución saturada
E saturated solution
G gesättigte Lösung
F solution saturée

solución sobresaturada
E supersaturated solution
G übersättigte Lösung
F solution sursaturée

solución colorante
E staining liquid
G Färbelösung
F solution de teinture

solución colorimétrica
E colorimetric solution
G Farbvergleichslösung
F solution colorimétrique

solución de cultivo
E culture broth
G Nährlösung
F bouillon de culture

solución de enjuague bucal
E mouthwash
G Mundspüllösung
F solution pour bain de bouche

solución de hemofiltración
E solution for haemofiltration
G Hämofiltrationslösung
F solution d'hémofiltration

solución de infusión
E infusion solution
G Infusionslösung
F solution de perfusion

solución de lavado
E rinsing solution
G Spüllösung
F solution de rinçage

solución de lavado auricular
E ear wash
G Ohrenspüllösung
F solution de lavage auriculaire

solución de referencia
E reference solution
G Vergleichslösung
F solution de référence

solución de tamponamiento
E buffer solution
G Pufferlösung
F solution tampon

solución fijadora
E fixing solution
G Fixierlösung
F solution de fixation

solución inyectable
E injection solution
G Injektionslösung
F solution injectable

solución madre
E stock solution
G Stammlösung
F solution mère

solución nutritiva
E culture broth
G Nährlösung
F bouillon de culture

solución para gargarismos
E gargle
G Gurgellösung
F solution pour gargarisme

solución reactiva
E reagent solution
G Reagenzlösung
F solution réactive

solución salina
E saline solution
G Kochsalzlösung
F solution saline

solución salina fisiológica
E physiological saline
G physiologische Kochsalzlösung
F solution saline physiologique

solución volumétrica
E volumetric solution
G Maßlösung
F solution volumétrique

solvente
E solvent
G Lösungsmittel
F solvant

solvente inorgánico
E inorganic solvent
G anorganisches Lösungsmittel
F solvant inorganique

solvente orgánico
E organic solvent
G organisches Lösungsmittel
F solvant organique

solvente viscoso
E viscous solvent
G viskoses Lösungsmittel
F solvant visqueux

sombrerete
E cover, hood
G Haube, Abdeckung
F couvercle, capuchon

sombrero
E head covering, headgear
G Kopfbedeckung
F bonnet

sonda
E probe
G Sonde
F sonde

sonda de toma (de muestras)
E removal probe, sampling probe
G Entnahmesonde
F sonde d'échantillonnage

sonda térmica
E thermocouple, heat sensor
G Thermofühler
F sonde thermique

sondeo
E bearing
G Peilung
F sondage, coussinet

soporte
E support brace, stand, frame, bearing (mach.), base, mount, support
G Stütze, Gestell, Lager (Maschinenteil), Untergestell, Halterung, Stativ
F support, cadre, assise, socle, trépied

soporte del casquete
E cover fitting
G Haubenhalterung
F garniture de couvercle

soporte del filtro
E filter stand
G Filtergestell
F support de filtre

soporte del troquel
E punch holder
G Stempelhalter
F support de poinçon

sosa alcalina
E sodium hydroxide solution
G Natronlauge
F soude

spray sublingual
E sub-lingual spray
G Sublingualspray
F aérosol sublingual

status de autorización
E release status
G Freigabestatus
F statut de libération

status de desarrollo
E development status
G Entwicklungsstatus
F état de développement

status de seguridad
E safety status
G Sicherheitsstatus
F statut de sécurité

stocks
E inventory, stock
G Lagerbestand
F inventaire, stock

subcultivo
E sub-culture
G Subkultur
F culture repiquée

subcutáneo
E subcutaneous
G subkutan
F sous-cutanée

sublimación
E sublimation
G Sublimierung
F sublimation

sublote
E partial batch, sub-batch
G Teilcharge
F sous-lot

succionar
E aspirate, to
G ansaugen
F aspirer

suelo
E floor, soil
G Boden
F sol, plancher

suelo de cemento
E cement flooring
G Zementestrich
F chape de ciment

suelo del tamiz
E sieve screen
G Siebboden
F tamis

suelo perforado
E perforated base
G Lochboden
F base perforée

suero
E serum
G Serum
F sérum

suero fetal bovino
E foetal calf serum
G fötales Kälberserum
F sérum fœtal de veau

sueros de origen animal
E animal sera
G tierische Seren
F sérums d'origine animale

sumergir(se)
E immerse, to; dip, to; submerge, to
G eintauchen, untertauchen
F immerger

sumidero
E floor drain
G Bodenabfluß, Fußbodenabfluß, Gulli
F égoût, bouche d'égout

suministrar
E supply, to
G liefern, versorgen mit
F fournir, livrer

suministro
E supply, feed
G Versorgung, Zufuhr
F alimentation, charge

suministro de agua
E water supply
G Wasserversorgung
F alimentation en eau

suministro de prospectos
E leaflet feed
G Prospektzuführung
F approvisionnement en dépliants

suministro de un producto
E product feed
G Produktzufuhr
F alimentation en produit

suministro de vapor externo
E external steam
G externe Dampfzufuhr
F vapeur externe

suministro eléctrico
E power supply
G Stromversorgung
F alimentation en courant

suministro por cinta
E conveyor
G Bandzufuhr
F convoyeur

superficie
E surface, area
G Oberfläche, Fläche
F surface, superficie, aire

superficie de cultivo
E seed layer, culture surface
G Kulturrasen
F surface de culture

superficie de la membrana
E membrane area
G Membranfläche
F surface de membrane

superficie de trabajo
E working surface
G Arbeitsoberfläche
F surface de travail

superficie del comprimido
E tablet surface
G Tablettenoberfläche
F surface d'un comprimé

superficie del filtro
E filter surface
G Filterfläche, Filteroberfläche
F surface d'un filtre,
superficie d'un filtre

superficie del pico
E peak area
G Peakfläche
F surface de pic

superficie en contacto con el producto
E product contact surface
G produktberührende Oberfläche
F surface au contact d'un produit

superficie específica
E specific surface area
G spezifische Oberfläche
F aire spécifique

superficie limitante
E interface
G Grenzfläche
F surface de séparation, interface

superficie lisa
E smooth surface
G glatte Oberfläche
F surface polie, surface lisse

superficie plana
E flat surface
G ebene Fläche
F surface plane

superficie rugosa
E rough surface
G rauhe Oberfläche
F surface rugueuse

superficie total
E total area
G Gesamtfläche
F surface totale, aire totale

English German French Spanish

supervisar
E monitor, to; supervise, to
G überwachen
F contrôler, surveiller

supervisión
E supervision, monitoring
G Aufsicht, Überwachung
F supervision, surveillance, contrôle

suplemento
E addition, supplementation, supplement, overage
G Zugabe, Ergänzung, Aufschlag
F adjonction, complément, supplément, majoration

suplencia
E deputisation
G Stellvertretung
F suppléance

suplente
E deputy
G Stellvertreter
F suppléant, remplaçant

supositorio vaginal
E vaginal suppository, pessary
G Vaginalzäpfchen
F suppositoire vaginal

supositorios
E suppositories
G Suppositorien
F suppositoires

surco
E gutter
G Rinne
F gouttière

surco de ruptura
E break notch, break score
G Bruchrille
F encoche de rupture, entaille de rupture

surtido
E product range
G Sortiment
F sortiment

susceptible a la corrosión
E susceptible to corrosion
G korrosionsanfällig
F susceptible à la corrosion

suspender
E suspend, to
G suspendieren
F suspenser

suspensibilidad
E suspendibility
G Suspendierbarkeit
F suspensif

suspensión
E suspension, suspension device
G Suspension, Aufhängung, Suspendierung
F suspension

suspensión de lacado
E lacquering fluid
G Lackiersuspension
F suspension de laquage

suspensión mediante resorte
E spring suspension
G Federaufhängung
F suspension à ressort

sustancia a analizar
E analyte
G Analyt
F analyte, substance à analyser

sustancia activa (materia prima)
E bulk pharmaceutical chemical (BPC)
G Wirkstoff (als Rohstoff)
F matière première en vrac

sustancia adhesiva
E adhesive, glue
G Kleber
F colle

sustancia amarga
E bitter component
G Bitterstoff
F composant amer, substance amère

sustancia aromática
E aromatic substance
G Aromastoff
F substance aromatique

sustancia auxiliar
E excipient, adjuvant
G Hilfsstoff
F excipient, adjuvant

sustancia de partida
E starting material, raw material
G Ausgangsstoff
F matériel de départ, matière première

sustancia de referencia estándar
E standard reference material
G Standardreferenzsubstanz
F substance de référence standard

sustancia emparentada
E related substance
G verwandte Substanz
F substance apparentée

sustancia extraíble
E extractable substance
G extrahierbare Substanz
F substance extractible

sustancia inicial
E starting material, raw material
G Ausgangsstoff
F matériel de départ, matière première

sustancia irritante
E irritating substance
G reizende Substanz
F substance irritante

sustancia medicamentosa
E medicinal substance, active substance, drug
G Arzneistoff
F principe actif

sustancia medicamentosa ópticamente activa
E chiral medicinal substance
G chiraler Arzneistoff
F médicament optiquement actif

sustancia narcótica
E narcotic substance
G Betäubungsmittel
F substance narcotique

sustancia neutralizante (para inactivar desinfectantes)
E neutralising substance, inactivating substance (for disinfectant)
G Enthemmer (zur Inaktivierung von Desinfektionsmitteln)
F substance neutralisante

sustancia nutricia
E nutrient
G Nährstoff
F aliment, produit nutritif, nutriment

sustancia peligrosa
E hazardous material, dangerous material
G Gefahrstoff
F matériel dangereux

sustancia sólida
E solid
G Feststoff
F solide

sustancia tensioactiva
E surfactant
G grenzflächenaktiver Stoff
F tensioactif

sustancia venenosa
E toxin, poison
G Giftstoff
F toxine

sustancias activas naturales
E natural active substances
G natürlich vorkommende Wirkstoffe
F principes actifs naturels

sustancias contaminantes
E contaminants
G kontaminierende Stoffe
F contaminants

English German French Spanish

sustancias petroquímicas
E petrochemicals
G petrochemische Substanzen
F substances pétrochimiques

sustitución
E substitution, deputisation
G Substitution, Stellvertretung
F substitution, suppléance

sustitución nucleófila
E nucleophilic substitution
G nukleophile Substitution
F substitution nucléophilique

sustituir
E replace, to
G ersetzen
F remplacer

sustituto
E deputy
G Stellvertreter
F suppléant, remplaçant

sustrato
E substrate
G Substrat
F substrat

sutura
E joint, weld
G Naht
F joint

sin sutura
E seamless
G nahtlos
F dépourvu de joint

tabajador cualificado
E skilled worker
G Facharbeiter
F ouvrier qualifié

tabique (de separación)
E partition (wall), baffle
G Trennwand, Zwischenwand
F mur de séparation

tabla
E table
G Tabelle
F tableau, table

tablero de control
E operator console, panel
G Bedienpult
F pupitre de commande, tableau de commande

tablero de instrumentos
E panel, instrument panel
G Armaturentafel, Instrumententafel
F tableau de bord, tableau d'instruments

tallado
E ground
G geschliffen
F moulu, poli

taller
E workshop
G Werkstatt
F atelier

talón de entrega
E delivery note
G Lieferschein
F bordereau de livraison

tamaño
E format, size
G Format, Größe
F format, taille

tamaño de las partículas
E particle size
G Partikelgröße, Teilchengröße
F taille des particules

tamaño de un lote
E batch size
G Losgröße, Chargengröße
F taille d'un lot

tamaño de una cápsula
E capsule size
G Kapselgröße
F taille d'une capsule

tamaño del envase
E package size
G Packungsgröße
F taille de l'emballage

tamaño del grano
E particle size
G Korngröße
F taille des particules

tamaño del orificio de la malla
E mesh size
G Maschenweite
F ouverture de maille

tamaño del poro
E pore size
G Porengröße
F taille d'un pore

tamaño molecular
E molecular size
G Molekülgröße
F taille moléculaire

tamaño nominal
E nominal size
G Nenngröße
F taille nominale

tamaño uniforme de las partículas
E uniform particle size
G Gleichkorn
F taille des particules uniforme

tambor
E drum
G Trommel
F tambour

tambor de fibras
E fibre drum
G Fibertrommel
F tambour à fibres

tamiz
E sieve
G Sieb
F tamis

tamiz agitador
E sieve shaker
G Siebschüttler
F tamis secoueur

tamiz base
E bottom screen
G Bodensieb
F tamis bas, crible bas

tamiz de alambre
E wire sieve
G Drahtsieb
F tamis en toile métallique

tamiz de malla gruesa
E coarse sieve
G Grobsieb
F tamis grossier

tamiz fino
E fine sieve
G Feinsieb
F tamis fin

tamiz vibrante
E vibrating sieve, vibrating screen
G Rüttelsieb
F tamis vibrant

tamizado
E fines (sieve)
G Durchgang (beim Sieben), Siebdurchgang
F passant (tamisage)

tamizado del aire
E air sieving
G Luftstrahlsiebung
F tamisage d'air

tamizado húmedo
E wet sieving
G Naßsiebung
F tamisage humide

tamizar
E sieve, to; sift, to
G sieben
F tamiser

tampón
E tampon, buffer
G Tampon, Puffer
F tampon

tampón vaginal
E medicated vaginal tampon
G Vaginaltampon
F tampon vaginal

tangente
E tangent
G Tangente
F tangente

tanino
E tanning agent
G Gerbstoff
F tannin

tanque de conservación
E storage tank
G Aufbewahrungstank
F récipient de stockage

tanque (de) depósito
E storage vessel, holding tank reservoir
G Lagertank, Vorratstank
F récipient de stockage, cuve de stockage

tapa
E lid, cover, flap
G Deckel, Klappe
F couvercle, clapet, volet

tapa de botella
E bottle cap
G Flaschenverschluß
F capsule à bouteilles

tapa de cierre de golpe
E snap cap, snap lid
G Schnappdeckel
F couvercle à enclenchement

tapa de rosca (p. ej. de autoclave)
E swivel lid (e. g. of autoclave)
G Drehdeckel (z. B. eines Autoklaven)
F couvercle pivotant (par ex. d'un autoclave)

tapadera
E lid, cover
G Deckel, Abdeckhaube
F couvercle

tapón
E plug, stopper
G Stopfen
F bouchon, tampon

tapón cuentagotas
E drop closure, dropper insert
G Tropfverschluß, Tropfeinsatz
F obturateur doseur, bouchon à compte-gouttes

tapón de caucho butílico
E butyl rubber stoppers
G Stopfen aus Butylgummi
F bouchon en caoutchouc butyle

tapón de goma
E rubber stopper
G Gummistopfen
F bouchon en caoutchouc

tapón esmerilado
E ground stopper
G Schliffstopfen
F bouchon rodé

taquímetro
E revolution counter, tachymeter, tachometer, velocimeter
G Drehzahlmesser, Geschwindigkeitsmesser, Umdrehungszähler
F compte-tours, tachymètre

tara
E dead weight, net weight, tare
G Leergewicht, Tara
F poids à vide, tare

tarar
E tare, to
G tarieren, austarieren
F tarer

tasa de disolución
E dissolution rate
G Auflösungsrate
F vitesse de dissolution

tasa de errores
E failure rate
G Fehlerrate
F taux d'erreur

tasa de extinción
E mortality rate
G Absterberate
F taux de mortalité

tasa de liberación
E release rate
G Freisetzungsrate
F vitesse de libération

tasa de liberación in vitro
E in-vitro release rate
G In-vitro-Freisetzungsrate
F vitesse de libération in-vitro

tasa de mortalidad
E mortality rate
G Absterberate
F taux de mortalité

tasa de pulverización
E spray rate
G Sprührate
F vitesse de pulvérisation

tasa de recuperación
E recovery rate
G Wiederfindungsrate
F taux de récupération, taux de rendement

tasa de renovación de aire
E air exchange rate
G Luftwechselrate
F taux de renouvellement d'air

tasa de separación de partículas
E particle separation rate
G Partikelabscheiderate
F taux de retenue des particules

techo
E ceiling
G Decke
F plafond

techo de hormigón
E concrete ceiling
G Betondecke
F plafond en béton

techo falso
E false ceiling
G eingezogene Decke
F faux plafond

techo intermedio
E intermediate ceiling, suspended ceiling
G Zwischendecke
F faux plafond

techo suspendido
E suspended ceiling
G abgehängte Decke
F faux plafond

tecla
E key
G Taste
F touche

teclado
E key board
G Tastatur(feld)
F clavier

teclado de membrana plástica
E membrane key pad
G Folientastatur
F clavier à effleurement

técnica
E technique, method
G Technik, Methode
F technique, méthode

English
German
French
Spanish

English German French Spanish

técnica de encartonar
E cartoning technology
G Kartoniertechnik
F technique d'encartonnage

técnica de medición, regulación y control
E measuring and control technology
G Meß-Steuer-Regel (MSR) -Technik
F techniques de mesure, de réglage et de contrôle

técnica de proceso aséptico
E aseptic process, aseptic technology
G aseptische Prozeßtechnik
F procédé aseptique, technique aseptique

técnica del procedimiento
E process technology
G Verfahrenstechnik
F technique des procédés

técnica para el área estéril
E clean room engineering
G Reinraumtechnik
F ingénierie des zones d'atmosphère contrôlée

técnico de servicio
E service technician
G Servicetechniker
F technicien

tecnología genética
E gene technology
G Gentechnologie
F génie génétique

tejido
E tissue
G Gewebe
F tissu

tejido fino
E fine tissue
G Feingewebe
F tissu fragile

tejido mucoso
E mucosal tissue
G Schleimhautgewebe
F tissu d'une muqueuse

tejido sintético
E synthetic tissue
G Kunststoffgewebe
F tissu synthétique, tissu en plastique

tela metálica
E wire mesh
G Drahtgewebe
F toile métallique

telemando
E remote control, remote operation
G Fernbedienung
F télécommande

temperatura
E temperature
G Temperatur
F température

temperatura adiabática
E adiabatic temperature
G adiabatische Temperatur
F température adiabatique

temperatura ambiente (ambiental)
E room temperature, ambient temperature
G Raumtemperatur, Umgebungstemperatur
F température ambiante

temperatura de entrada
E inlet temperature
G Eingangstemperatur, Einlaßtemperatur
F température d'entrée, température d'admission

temperatura de esterilización
E sterilisation temperature
G Sterilisationstemperatur
F température de stérilisation

temperatura de salida
E outlet temperature
G Auslaßtemperatur
F température de sortie

temperatura de solidificación
E solidification temperature
G Erstarrungstemperatur
F température de solidification

temperatura de un proceso
E process temperature
G Prozeßtemperatur
F température d'un procédé

temporal
E temporary
G vorläufig
F temporaire

tenacidad
E toughness
G Zähigkeit
F viscosité

tenaz
E resistant, tough
G widerstandsfähig, zäh
F résistant, visqueux, épais

tenazas para cerrar tubos
E crimping tongs
G Falzzange
F pincettes, pinces, tenailles

teñidor
E stainer
G Färbegerät
F appareil à teindre

teñir
E stain, to
G färben
F colorer, teinter, teindre

tensión
E tension, stress, strain
G Spannung, Zug, Beanspruchung
F tension, traction, soumission à un effort

tensión (eléctrica)
E voltage
G Spannung
F tension

tensión de cizallamiento
E shear stress
G Scherspannung
F contrainte de cisaillement

tensión de empuje
E shear stress
G Schubspannung
F contrainte de poussée

tensión de flexión
E flexional strain, flexural stress
G Biegespannung, Biegebeanspruchung
F tension de pliage, tension de fléchissement, sollicitation à la flexion

tensión de la red
E line voltage
G Netzspannung
F tension du secteur

tensión estática
E static stress
G statische Beanspruchung
F stress statique

tensión sobre el material
E material stress
G Materialbeanspruchung
F sollicitation du matériel

tensión superficial
E surface tension
G Oberflächenspannung
F tension superficielle

teoría del genoma
E genomics
G Genomlehre
F génomique

terapéutico
E therapeutic
G therapeutisch
F thérapeutique

terapia a largo plazo
E long-term therapy
G Langzeittherapie
F thérapie à long terme

teratógeno
E teratogenic
G teratogen
F tératogène

terminación
E completion
G Beendigung
F achèvement

terminal
E terminal
G Klemme
F pince, borne

terminal de cable
E cable terminal, cable lug
G Kabelklemme, Kabelschuh
F serre-fils, cosse de câble

terminal de control
E control panel
G Bedienterminal
F terminal de contrôle

termodilatación
E thermal expansion
G Wärmeausdehnung
F thermodilatation

termoelástico
E thermo-elastic
G thermoelastisch
F thermo-élastique

termoplástico
E thermo-plastic
G thermoplastisch
F thermoplastique

termostato
E thermostat
G Thermostat
F thermostat

ternario
E ternary
G ternär
F ternaire

test
E analysis, control test
G Prüfung
F analyse, test de contrôle

test de aceptación en fábrica
E factory acceptance test (FAT)
G Werksabnahme
F réception en usine

testigo
E blank
G Blindprobe
F valeur témoin, valeur à blanc

tiempo de calentamiento
E heat-up time
G Aufheizzeit
F temps de réchauffement

tiempo de contacto
E contact time
G Kontaktzeit
F temps de contact

tiempo de desecación
E drying time
G Trocknungszeit
F temps de séchage

tiempo de desintegración
E disintegration time
G Zerfallszeit
F temps de désintégration

tiempo de detención (por avería)
E downtime
G Stillstandzeit (wegen Reparatur)
F temps d'immobilisation

tiempo de enfriamiento
E cool-down time
G Abkühlzeit
F temps de refroidissement

tiempo de esterilización
E sterilisation time, duration of sterilisation
G Sterilisationszeit
F temps de stérilisation, durée de stérilisation

tiempo de eyección
E ejection time
G Ausstoßzeit
F temps d'éjection

tiempo de funcionamiento
E running time
G Laufzeit
F durée d'opération, durée d'un cycle

tiempo de generación
E doubling time
G Generationszeit
F temps de doublement

tiempo de incubación
E incubation time
G Bebrütungszeit
F temps d'incubation

tiempo de inmersión
E immersion period
G Eintauchzeit
F période d'immersion

tiempo de paso
E processing time
G Durchlaufzeit
F temps de traitement

tiempo de pérdida de producción
E production down time
G Produktionsausfallzeit
F période d'immobilisation en production

tiempo de permanencia
E residence time
G Verweilzeit
F temps de résidence

tiempo promedio de permanencia
E mean residence time (MRT)
G mittlere Verweilzeit
F temps de résidence moyen

tiempo de recuperación (en área estéril)
E recovery time (in clean room)
G Erholzeit (im Reinraum)
F temps de récupération

tiempo de reequipamiento
E re-equipping time
G Umrüstzeit
F temps de réorganisation

tiempo de respuesta
E response time
G Ansprechzeit
F temps de réponse

tiempo de retención
E retention time
G Retentionszeit
F temps de rétention

tiempo de retraso
E delay time
G Verzögerungszeit
F retard

tiempo de solidificación
E solidification time, setting time
G Erstarrungszeit, Abbindezeit
F temps de solidification

tiempo de vida media
E half-life
G Halbwertszeit
F demi-vie

tiempo invertido
E time required
G Zeitaufwand
F temps requis

tiempo muerto
E dead time
G Totzeit
F temps mort

tinción de Gram
E Gram staining
G Gramfärbung
F méthode de coloration de Gram

tindalización
E fractional sterilisation
G Tyndallisation
F tyndallisation

tinta
E ink
G Tinte
F encre

tintura
E dye, stain, pigment, tincture
G Farbe, Färbemittel, Tinktur
F colorant, teinture, pigment

tintura madre
E tincture standard
G Urtinktur
F teinture standard

tipo de aglutinante
E binding agent type
G Bindemitteltyp
F type de liant

tipo de construcción
E design
G Bauart
F design

tipo de membrana
E membrane type
G Membrantyp
F type de membrane

tipo de troquel
E punch type
G Stempeltyp
F type de poinçon

tipo de vidrio
E glass type
G Glasart
F type de verre

tira (p. ej. de una lámina)
E sheet (e. g. of foil)
G Bahn (z. B. Folien-)
F bande (d'étoffe)

titulación
E titration
G Titration
F titration, dosage

titulación inversa
E back titration
G Rücktitration
F dosage en retour

titulación retrógrada
E back titration
G Rücktitration
F dosage en retour

título
E titre
G Titer
F titre

título estándar
E volumetric standard
G Urtiter
F substance standard de titrimétrie

toallas de uso único
E disposable towels
G Einmalhandtücher
F serviette à usage unique

tobera
E nozzle
G Düse
F buse, gicleur, tuyère

tobogán
E chute
G Rutsche
F toboggan

tobogán de carga
E charge chute
G Befüllrutsche
F toboggan de charge, toboggan d'alimentation, glissoir de charge

tolerancia
E tolerance
G Toleranz
F tolérance

fuera de la tolerancia
E out of tolerance
G außer Toleranz
F hors des limites de tolérance

tolerancias prefijadas
E specified tolerances
G festgelegte Toleranzen
F tolérances spécifiques

tolva
E funnel, hopper
G Trichter, Schütttrichter
F entonnoir, trémie, trémie d'alimentation, entonnoir d'alimentation

toma
E recording, withdrawal
G Aufnahme, Entnahme
F enregistrement, retrait

toma de muestra
E sampling
G Probenahme, Musterziehung
F échantillonnage, prélèvement d'un échantillon

toma de tierra
E ground, earth, earthing
G Ableitung, Erdung
F mise à la terre, prise de terre

tonel
E barrel
G Faß
F tonneau

tonel de acero inoxidable
E stainless steel drum
G Edelstahlfaß
F tonneau en acier inoxydable

tonel de plástico
E plastic barrel
G Kunststoffaß
F tonneau en plastique

tonicidad
E tonicity
G Tonizität
F tonicité

tópico
E topical
G topisch
F topique

tornasol
E litmus
G Lackmus
F tournesol

tornillo avellanado
E countersunk screw
G Senkschraube
F vis conique

tornillo con tuerca
E screw with nut
G Schraube mit Mutter
F vis avec écrou

tornillo de ajuste
E adjusting screw
G Justierschraube
F vis de mise au point

tornillo de aletas
E wing screw
G Flügelschraube
F vis à oreilles

tornillo dosificante
E dosing screw, feed screw
G Dosierschnecke
F vis de dosage

tornillo hexagonal
E Allen screw
G Inbusschraube
F vis à six pans creux femelle

tornillo micrométrico
E fine adjusting screw, micrometer screw
G Mikrometerschraube
F micromètre, vis micromètre

tornillo moleteado
E knurled screw
G Rändelschraube
F vis moletée

English German French Spanish

tornillo sin fin
E worm gear, worm screw
G Schnecke, Förderschnecke
F vis sans fin, vis d'Archimède

tornillo sin fin dosificador de polvo
E powder feeder
G Pulverdosierschnecke
F vis doseuse pour poudre

tornillo transportador
E worm gear, worm screw
G Förderschnecke
F vis sans fin, vis d'Archimède

torre de lavado
E washing tower, spray tower
G Rieselturm
F tour d'arrosage

torre de refrigeración
E cooling tower
G Kühlturm
F tour de refroidissement

torre de tamizado
E sieve tower
G Siebturm
F tour de tamisage

torsión
E torsion
G Verdrillung
F torsion

torunda
E swab, gauze, pad
G Tupfer
F tampon d'ouate, gaze

torunda de algodón
E cotton plug
G Wattebausch
F tampon d'ouate

toxicidad
E toxicity
G Toxizität, Giftigkeit
F toxicité

tóxico
E poison, toxin, toxic, poisonous
G Gift, toxisch, giftig
F poison, toxique

tóxico para la piel
E toxic in contact with skin
G giftig bei Hautkontakt
F toxique au contact de la peau

tóxico si entra en contacto con la piel
E toxic in contact with skin
G giftig bei Hautkontakt
F toxique au contact de la peau

tóxico si se ingiere
E toxic if swallowed
G giftig beim Verschlucken
F toxique si ingéré

tóxico si se inhala
E toxic by inhalation
G giftig beim Einatmen
F toxique si inhalé

toxicología
E toxicology
G Toxikologie
F toxicologie

toxina
E toxin, poison
G Toxin, Giftstoff
F toxine

trabajador manual
E workman, tradesman
G Handwerker
F ouvrier, artisan

tracción
E tension, drive
G Spannung, Zug, Antrieb
F tension, traction, entraînement, transmission

traje impermeable al agua
E waterproof jump-suit
G wasserdichter Anzug
F combinaison imperméable à l'eau

trama
E raster, screen
G Raster
F trame

trampa de insectos
E insect trap
G Insektenfalle
F piège à insectes

tranquilizante
E sedative
G Beruhigungsmittel
F sédatif, calmant

transcripción
E transcription
G Transkription
F transcription

transcripción de datos
E data transcription
G Datentranskription
F transcription de données

transcurso de la reacción
E course of a reaction
G Reaktionsverlauf
F déroulement d'une réaction

transductor
E transducer
G Meßwertaufnehmer
F capteur, transducteur

transferencia
E transfer
G Übertragung
F transfert

transferencia de muestras
E sample transfer
G Probenübertragung
F transfert d'échantillons

transferencia tecnológica
E technology transfer
G Technologietransfer
F transfers de technologie

transferencia térmica
E heat transfer
G Wärmeübertragung
F transfert de chaleur

transferir
E transfer, to; relocate, to
G übertragen, verlagern
F transférer, déplacer

transformación
E processing, reworking
G Verarbeitung, Bearbeitung, Umarbeitung
F fabrication, mise en forme, traitement, retraitement

transformación automática
E machine processing
G maschinelle Verarbeitung
F traitement automatique

transformación manual
E manual processing
G manuelle Verarbeitung
F traitement manuel

transformador
E converter
G Umwandler
F convertisseur

transformar en pellets
E pelletise, to
G pelletieren
F pastiller, transformer en pastilles

transición de fase
E phase transition
G Phasenübergang
F transition de phase

transición térmica uniforme
E uniform heat transfer
G gleichmäßiger Wärmeübergang
F transition thermique uniforme

transitorio
E temporary
G vorläufig
F temporaire

translúcido
E translucent
G lichtdurchlässig
F translucide

transmisión
E transmission, drive, gear ratio
G Getriebe, Übersetzung (im Getriebe)
F transmission, engrenage

transmisión UV
E UV transmittance
G UV-Transmission
F transmission UV

transmisor de presión
E pressure transmitter
G Druckaufnehmer
F transmetteur de pression

transparencia
E transparency
G Durchsichtigkeit
F transparence

transparencia para la luz
E light transmittance
G Lichtdurchlässigkeit
F transparence

transparente
E clear, transparent
G klar, durchsichtig
F transparent

transpiración
E effluvium
G Ausdünstung
F effluent, efflux

transportador
E conveyor-
G Förder-
F convoyeur

transportador de cinta
E conveyor belt
G Bandförderer
F convoyeur

transportador de tornillo sin fin
E worm drive
G Schneckenförderer
F vis d'Archimède

transportador de tubos
E tube carriage
G Schlauchwagen
F chariot dévidoir

transporte
E carryover
G Übertrag
F report, somme intermédiaire

transvasar
E refill, to
G umfüllen
F transvaser

trasegar
E refill, to
G umfüllen
F transvaser

trasladar
E transfer, to; relocate, to
G verlagern
F transférer, déplacer

tratado con chorro de arena
E sand-blasted
G sandgestrahlt
F traité au jet de sable

tratamiento
E handling
G Handhabung
F maniement, traitement

tratamiento alcalino
E alkaline treatment
G alkalische Behandlung
F traitement alcalin

tratamiento biológico
E biological treatment
G biologische Behandlung
F traitement biologique

tratamiento de superficies
E surface treatment
G Oberflächenbehandlung
F traitement de surface

tratamiento subsiguiente
E secondary treatment
G Nachbehandlung
F traitement secondaire

tratamiento térmico
E heat treatment
G Wärmebehandlung
F traitement thermique

trato (con)
E handling (of)
G Umgang (mit)
F maniement, traitement

traza
E trace
G Spur
F trace

traza determinable, de
E traceable
G rückverfolgbar
F traçable

trazabilidad
E traceability
G Rückverfolgbarkeit, Rückführbarkeit
F traçabilité

traza-testigo de la auditoría
E audit trail
G Auditweg
F trace-témoin de l'audit

trepidación
E vibration
G Erschütterung
F vibration

trepidar
E shake, to; vibrate, to
G rütteln
F secouer

trinquete
E latch, door handle
G Klinke
F loquet, poignée de porte

trípode
E stand
G Stativ
F trépied

trituración
E trituration
G Trituration
F trituration

trituradora
E homogeniser, shredder
G Zerkleinerer
F hachoir

triturar
E crush, to; grind, to; mill, to; homogenise, to; shred, to
G zerstoßen, zerkleinern
F broyer, concasser, piler, hacher

troceadora
E chopper
G Zerhacker
F hachoir, couperet

tronco de cono
E truncated cone
G Kegelstumpf
F troncature d'un cône

troquel
E hob, punch, punching station
G Stempel (zum Tablettieren), Prägestempel, Lochstanze
F poinçon, poinçonneuse

troquel inferior
E lower punch
G Unterstempel
F poinçon inférieur

troquel superior
E upper punch, top punch
G Oberstempel
F poinçon supérieur

troquel para comprimidos
E tabletting punch
G Tablettierstempel
F poinçon de fabrication de comprimés

troquelado
E embossment, embossed
G Prägung, geprägt
F estampage, estampé

troqueladora
E punch
G Stanze
F poinçon

troquelar
E stamp, to; emboss, to; punch, to; mark, to
G prägen, stanzen, einstanzen, stempeln
F poinçonner, estamper

tubería (gas, agua)
E piping (gas, water)
G Leitung (Gas, Wasser)
F conduite (de gaz, d'eau)

tubería de acero inoxidable
E stainless steel piping
G Edelstahlrohrleitung
F tuyauterie en inox

tubería de alimentación
E feed
G Zuleitung
F tuyauterie d'alimentation

tubería flexible
E tubing
G Schlauchleitung
F tuyauterie

tubo
E tube, duct, channel
G Rohrbogen, Kanal, Schlauch, Tube
F tube, tuyau

tubo (de ensayo) de vidrio
E glass tube
G Glasröhrchen
F tube de verre

tubo acodado
E pipe bend
G Knierohr
F tuyau coudé

tubo aerosol
E aerosol can
G Aerosoldose
F bidon d'aérosol, bombe aérosol

tubo ascensional
E dip tube
G Steigrohr
F colonne d'ascension

tubo de congelación
E cryotube
G Gefrierröhrchen
F tube de congélation

tubo de empalme
E extension pipe
G Ansatzrohr
F tuyau de rallonge

tubo de ensayo
E test tube
G Reagenzglas
F tube à essais

tubo de ensayo Eppendorf
E Eppendorf reaction vessel
G Eppendorf-Reaktionsgefäß
F fiole Eppendorf

tubo de envasado
E filling tube
G Abfüllschlauch
F tuyau de remplissage

tubo de evacuación de aire
E exhaust pipe
G Abluftrohr
F conduite d'évacuation d'air

tubo de goma
E rubber tube
G Gummischlauch
F tube en caoutchouc

tubo de humo
E smoke tube
G Rauchröhrchen
F tube de fumée

tubo de inmersión
E dip tube
G Tauchrohr, Eintauchrohr
F colonne d'immersion, tube plongeur

tubo de llenado
E feed tube
G Füllrohr
F tube de remplissage

tubo de presión
E pressure tubing
G Druckschlauch
F tuyauterie apte à la pression

tubo de relleno
E filling tube, charging tube
G Einfüllrohr
F conduite d'alimentation

tubo de silicona
E silicone tubing
G Silikonschlauch
F tube de silicone

tubo en Y
E Y-duct
G Hosenrohr
F tube en Y

tubo montante
E dip tube
G Steigrohr
F colonne d'ascension

tubuladura
E support
G Stutzen
F support, embout

tubuladura de acceso
E access port
G Eintrittsstutzen
F tubulure d'accès

tubuladura de alimentación
E charge port, nipple
G Befüllstutzen
F orifice de charge, orifice d'alimentation

tubuladura de carga
E charge port, nipple
G Befüllstutzen
F orifice de charge, orifice d'alimentation

tubuladura de toma de muestra
E sampling port
G Probeentnahmestutzen
F tubulure de prélèvement d'échantillon

tuerca
E nut
G Mutter, Schraubenmutter
F écrou

tuerca moleteada
E knurled nut
G Rändelmutter
F écrou moleté

túnel de esterilización
E tunnel steriliser
G Hitzetunnel
F tunnel de stérilisation

túnel de retracción
E shrinking tunnel
G Schrumpftunnel
F tunnel de rétraction

turbidez
E turbidity
G Trübung
F turbidité

turbio
E turbid, cloudy
G trüb
F turbide, trouble

turbulencia
E turbulence
G Turbulenz
F turbulence

turbulencia del aire
E air turbulence
G Luftverwirbelung
F turbulence d'air

turno de trabajo
E operation, shift (working)
G Arbeitsgang, Arbeitsschicht
F opération, travail en trois-huit, équipe (de travail)

ubicación
E site, location
G Standort
F emplacement

ultrafiltración
E ultrafiltration
G Ultrafiltration
F ultrafiltration

ultrasonido
E ultrasound
G Ultraschall
F ultra-son

ultravioleta
E ultraviolet
G ultraviolett
F ultraviolet

ungüento
E ointment
G Salbe
F pommade

unidad
E unit
G Einheit
F unité

unidad (de un ordenador)
E disk drive (computer)
G Laufwerk (Computer)
F minuterie, lecteur (d'un ordinateur)

unidad de destilación a etapas múltiples
E multi-stage distillation unit
G Mehrstufendestillationsanlage
F unité de distillation à plusieurs étages

unidad de dosificación
E dosage unit
G Dosiereinheit, Dosierungseinheit
F unité de dosage, dose unitaire

unidad de envío
E dispatch unit
G Versandeinheit
F unité d'expédition

unidad de medición
E unit of measurement
G Meßgröße
F unité de mesure

unidad de medida
E unit of measurement
G Maßeinheit
F unité de mesure

unidad de secuenciación
E sequencing unit
G Sequenzierungseinheit
F unité de séquençage

unidad formadora de colonias
E colony-forming unit (CFU)
G koloniebildende Einheit (KBE)
F unité formant colonie

unidad propulsora
E drive unit
G Antriebseinheit
F unité de transmission

unidades defectuosas
E defective units
G fehlerhafte Einheiten
F unités défectueuses

uniforme
E uniform
G einheitlich, gleichmäßig
F uniforme

uniformidad
E uniformity, consistency
G Einheitlichkeit, Gleichförmigkeit
F uniformité, consistance

uniformidad cromática
E colour uniformity
G Farbuniformität
F uniformité de couleur

uniformidad de la dosificación
E dose uniformity
G Einheitlichkeit der Dosierung
F uniformité d'une dose

uniformidad del contenido
E content uniformity (CU)
G Einheitlichkeit des Gehaltes
F uniformité du contenu

uniformidad del peso
E uniformity of weight
G Gewichtseinheitlichkeit
F uniformité du poids

unión esférica
E ball + socket joint
G Kugelgelenk
F rotule, joint à rotule

unívoco
E unambiguous, clear
G eindeutig
F clair, précis

untabilidad
E spreadability
G Streichfähigkeit
F aptitude à être étendu

untar
E apply, to
G auftragen
F appliquer, étendre

untar con cepillo
E brush coat, to
G einstreichen (mit einer Bürste)
F enduire à la brosse

uso bucal
E oromucosal use
G Anwendung in der Mundhöhle
F usage bucco-mucosal

uso cutáneo
E cutaneous use
G Anwendung auf der Haut
F pour usage cutané

uso dental
E dental use
G dentale Anwendung
F usage dental

uso duradero
E sustained use
G Dauergebrauch
F utilisation permamente (d'un instrument)

uso endocervical
E endocervical use
G endozervikale Anwendung
F usage endo-cervical

uso endosinusal
E endosinusial use
G Anwendung in den Nebenhöhlen
F pour usage sinusien

uso epidural
E epidural use
G epidurale Anwendung
F usage épidural

uso gingival
E gingival use
G Anwendung am Zahnfleisch
F pour usage gingival

uso oftálmico
E ocular use, ophthalmic use
G Anwendung am Auge
F pour usage ophtalmique

uso oral, para
E for oral use
G Einnehmen, zum
F pour administration orale

uso otológico
E auricular use
G Anwendung am Ohr
F pour usage auriculaire

uso por inadvertencia
E inadvertent use
G versehentlicher Gebrauch
F utilisation par inadvertance

uso único, de
E disposable
G Einweg-
F jetable, à usage unique

usuario
E user
G Benutzer
F utilisateur

utensilios para elaborar comprimidos
E tablet tooling
G Tablettenwerkzeug
F presse-outil pour comprimés

vaciado
E drain
G Abguß
F conduit d'écoulement, drain

vaciamiento de un recipiente
E vessel emptying
G Gefäßentleerung
F action de vider un flacon, action de vider un récipient

vaciar
E empty, to; evacuate, to
G entleeren
F vider, évacuer

vacío
E vacuum, recess
G Vakuum, Aussparung
F vide, évidure, échancrure

vacío de membrana
E membrane vacuum
G Membranvakuum
F vide à diaphragme

vacuna
E vaccine
G Impfstoff
F vaccin

vacuna viral
E viral vaccine
G Virusimpfstoff
F vaccin viral

vacuna viva
E live vaccine
G Lebendimpfstoff
F vaccin vivant

valencia
E valency
G Wertigkeit
F valence

validable
E validatable
G validierbar
F validable

validación
E validation
G Validierung
F validation

validación acompañante
E concurrent validation
G begleitende Validierung
F validation concurrente

validación analítica
E analytical validation
G analytische Validierung
F validation analytique

validación concomitante a la producción
E concurrent validation
G produktionsbegleitende Validierung
F validation concurrente

validación de la limpieza
E cleaning validation
G Reinigungsvalidierung
F validation du nettoyage

validación de un proceso
E process validation
G Prozeßvalidierung
F validation d'un procédé

validación informática
E computer validation
G Computervalidierung
F validation d'ordinateur, validation informatique

validación retrospectiva
E retrospective validation
G retrospektive Validierung
F validation retrospective

validez
E validity
G Gültigkeit
F validité

válido a partir de
E valid from
G gültig ab
F valide à partir de

valor de concentración máxima de trabajo
E MAC value
G MAK-Wert
F taux de concentration maximal de travail

valor en blanco
E blank value
G Leerwert, Blindwert
F valeur à blanc, valeur témoin

valor límite
E limit
G Grenzwert
F limite

valor nominal
E nominal value, required value
G Nennwert, Sollwert
F valeur nominale

valor real
E actual value
G Istwert
F valeur actuelle

valor testigo
E blank value
G Blindwert
F valeur témoin, valeur à blanc

válvula
E valve, flap
G Ventil, Klappe
F vanne, clapet, volet

válvula activada por reflujo
E throttle check valve, throttle non-return valve
G Drosselrückschlagventil
F soupape de retenue

válvula antideflagrante
E explosion panel
G Ex-Klappen
F clapet anti-déflagrant

válvula con tres vías
E three-way valve
G Dreiwegeventil
F vanne trois voies

válvula de aspiración
E aspiration valve
G Ansaugventil
F vanne d'aspiration

válvula de bloqueo
E blocking valve
G Sperrventil
F vanne de verrouillage

válvula de bomba
E pump valve
G Pumpenventil
F vanne de pompe

válvula de cierre
E shut-off flap, on/off valve, lid flap
G Absperrklappe, Absperrventil, Verschlußklappe
F clapet de fermeture, valve d'arrêt, clapet de fermeture

válvula de descompresión
E pressure relief valve
G Druckentlastungsklappe
F soupape de sûreté (pour la pression)

válvula de entrada
E inlet valve
G Einlaßventil
F vanne d'entrée

English German French Spanish

válvula de entrada de aire
E air inlet cover
G Zuluftklappe
F couvercle d'entrée d'air

válvula de evacuación de aire
E exhaust valve
G Abluftregelklappe
F clapet d'évacuation d'air

válvula de hedor
E stench trap, siphon
G Geruchsverschluß
F siphon

válvula de inyección
E injection valve
G Einspritzventil
F vanne d'injection

válvula de mariposa
E butterfly valve
G Drosselventil
F vanne papillon

válvula de membrana
E diaphragm valve
G Membranventil
F vanne à membrane

válvula de relleno
E filling valve, filling nozzle, charging valve
G Füllventil, Einfüllklappe
F vanne d'alimentation, buse de remplissage

válvula de retención
E flap trap, non-return valve, check valve, back flow preventer, back flow flap
G Rückschlagklappe, Rückschlagventil, Rückstauklappe
F clapet anti-retour, vanne anti-retour, clapet antirefouleur

válvula de salida
E drain valve, outlet valve
G Ablaßventil, Auslaßventil
F vanne de purge, vanne de sortie

válvula de seguridad
E safety valve
G Sicherheitsventil
F vanne de sécurité

válvula de vaciamiento
E emptying valve
G Entleerventil
F valve de vidange

válvula de vapor
E steam valve
G Dampfventil
F soupape de vapeur

válvula de ventilación
E ventilation valve, vent flap
G Belüftungsventil, Entlüftungsklappe
F valve de ventilation, clapet de ventilation, volet de ventilation

válvula electromagnética
E solenoid valve
G elektromagnetisches Ventil
F vanne solénoïde

válvula esférica
E ball valve
G Kugelventil
F clapet à billes, soupape à billes, vanne à billes

válvula estranguladora de retención
E throttle check valve, throttle non-return valve
G Drosselrückschlagventil
F soupape de retenue

válvula magnética
E solenoid valve
G Magnetventil
F vanne magnétique

válvula reductora
E reducing valve
G Reduzierventil
F vanne de détente

válvula reguladora
E regulating valve, control flap, control valve
G Regelventil, Regelklappe
F vanne de régulation, clapet de réglage

válvula rotativa
E rotary valve
G Drehschieber
F valve rotatoire

vapor
E steam, vapour
G Dampf
F vapeur d'eau

vapor de agua saturado
E saturated steam
G gesättigter Wasserdampf
F vapeur d'eau saturée

vapor de agua sobrecalentado
E super-heated steam
G gespannter Wasserdampf
F vapeur surchauffée

vapor de una planta
E plant steam
G Betriebsdampf
F vapeur d'une installation

vapor primario
E primary steam
G Primärdampf
F vapeur primaire

vapor purificado
E purified steam
G gereinigter Dampf
F vapeur purifiée

vapor puro
E clean steam, pure steam
G Reindampf, Reinstdampf
F vapeur pure

vapor saturado
E saturated steam
G Sattdampf
F vapeur saturée

vapor sobrecalentado
E super-heated steam
G gespannter Wasserdampf
F vapeur surchauffée

vaporización
E vaporisation
G Verdampfung, Verdunstung
F vaporisation

variabilidad
E variability
G Variabilität
F variabilité des résultats

variabilidad de un proceso
E process variability
G Prozeßvariabilität
F variabilité du processus

variación
E change, variation
G Änderung
F changement

variación de la tensión
E voltage variation
G Spannungsänderung
F variation de tension

variar
E vary, to; fluctuate, to
G schwanken
F fluctuer

vaselina
E vaseline
G Vaselin
F vaseline

vasija
E ladle, scoop
G Schöpfkelle
F louche

vaso graduado
E graduated beaker
G Meßbecher
F coupe, gobelet

vegetal
E plant, plant-based, phyto-
G pflanzlich
F végétal

vejación
E baffle
G Schikane
F chicane

vejiga
E bubble, blister
G Blase
F bulle

vellocino
E fleece
G Vlies
F toison

velocidad de absorción
E absorption rate
G Absorptionsgeschwindigkeit
F vitesse d'absorption

velocidad de agitación
E stirring speed, agitating speed
G Rührgeschwindigkeit
F vitesse d'agitation

velocidad de cinta
E belt speed
G Bandgeschwindigkeit
F vitesse du tapis

velocidad de compresión
E compression speed
G Preßgeschwindigkeit
F vitesse de compression

velocidad de difusión
E diffusion speed
G Diffusionsgeschwindigkeit
F vitesse de diffusion

velocidad de disolución
E dissolution rate, dissolution speed, speed of solubility
G Auflösegeschwindigkeit, Lösungsgeschwindigkeit
F vitesse de dissolution, vitesse de solubilisation

velocidad de enfriamiento
E cooling rate
G Abkühlungsgeschwindigkeit
F vitesse de refroidissement

velocidad de flujo
E flow rate
G Fließgeschwindigkeit, Durchflußgeschwindigkeit
F débit

velocidad de la mesa para matriz
E die plate speed
G Matrizentischgeschwindigkeit
F vitesse de la table d'une matrice

velocidad de propulsión
E drive speed, impeller speed
G Antriebsgeschwindigkeit, Laufradgeschwindigkeit
F vitesse de roulement, vitesse de transmission

velocidad de reacción
E reaction velocity, reaction speed
G Reaktionsgeschwindigkeit
F vitesse de réaction

velocidad de revolución
E impeller speed, drive speed
G Laufradgeschwindigkeit
F vitesse de roulement, vitesse de transmission

velocidad de rodamiento
E drive speed, impeller speed
G Antriebsgeschwindigkeit
F vitesse de transmission, vitesse de roulement

velocidad de separación
E separation rate
G Abscheiderate
F vitesse de séparation

velocidad de troceo
E chopper speed
G Zerhackergeschwindigkeit
F vitesse de hachoir

velocidad de una máquina
E machine speed
G Maschinengeschwindigkeit
F vitesse de machine

velocidad del aire
E air velocity
G Luftgeschwindigkeit
F vitesse de l'air

velocidad del flujo
E flow rate
G Strömungsgeschwindigkeit
F débit

velocidad del troquel
E punch speed, punch velocity
G Stempelgeschwindigkeit
F vitesse d'un poinçon

velocidad inicial
E start speed, initial speed
G Anfangsgeschwindigkeit
F vitesse initiale

velocidad máxima
E maximum speed
G Höchstgeschwindigkeit
F vitesse maximale

velocidad media
E average speed
G durchschnittliche Geschwindigkeit
F vitesse moyenne

venda de gasa
E gauze bandage
G Mullbinde
F bande de gaze

vendaje
E bandage
G Verband
F pansement, bandage

vendaje de una herida
E wound dressing
G Wundauflage
F pansement

vendaje oclusivo
E occlusive dressing
G Okklusivverband
F bandage d'occlusion

veneno
E poison, toxin
G Gift, Giftstoff, Toxin
F poison, toxine

venenoso
E poisonous, toxic
G giftig
F toxique

venta
E sales
G Vertrieb
F ventes

venta libre, de
E non-prescription
G nicht verschreibungspflichtig
F vendu sans ordonnance

venta sólo en farmacias, de
E for sale in pharmacies only
G apothekenpflichtig
F en vente seulement en pharmacie

ventana de observación
E observation window,
observation port
G Beobachtungsfenster, Schauglas
F fenêtre d'observation

ventana visual
E observation window
G Sichtfenster
F fenêtre de visée

ventas (volumen de)
E sales
G Absatz, Verkauf
F ventes

ventilación
E ventilation
G Belüftung
F ventilation

ventilación del tanque
E tank aspiration
G Tankbelüftung
F aération du réservoir

ventilador
E ventilator, fan
G Ventilator, Gebläse
F ventilateur

ventilador centrífugo
E centrifugal fan
G Zentrifugalventilator
F ventilateur centrifuge

ventilar
E deaerate, to; ventilate, to; vent, to
G entlüften, belüften
F désaérer, aérer, ventiler

verificación
E verification
G Verifizierung
F vérification

versión
E edition, version, issue
G Ausgabe, Version, Ausführung
F édition, version

versión básica
E standard construction
G Grundausführung
F fabrication standard

versión especial
E special version
G Sonderausführung
F version spéciale

verter
E decant, to; spill, to; tilt, to
G abgießen, verschütten, kippen
F décanter, transvaser, renverser, répandre, basculer

vestigio
E trace
G Spur
F trace

vestuario
E gowning room, locker room, changing room
G Ankleideraum, Spindraum, Umkleide
F vestiaire

vestuario estéril
E sterile gowns, sterile clothing
G Sterilraumkleidung
F vêtement pour zone stérile

veterinario
E doctor of veterinary medicine, vet
G Tierarzt
F vétérinaire

vía de administración
E application route
G Applikationsweg
F voie d'application

vía de degradación
E degradation path, metabolic path
G Abbauweg
F chemin de dégradation

vía de desarrollo
E development route
G Entwicklungsweg
F route de développement

vía de síntesis
E synthesis route
G Syntheseweg
F voie de synthèse

vía evolutiva
E development route
G Entwicklungsweg
F route de développement

viabilidad
E viability
G Lebensfähigkeit
F viabilité

viable
E accessible, walk-in, viable
G begehbar, lebensfähig
F accessible, viable

vial
E vial
G Fläschchen, Gläschen
F flacon, récipient, fiole

vial de inyección
E injection vial
G Injektionsflasche
F flacon d'injection

vial de muestras
E sample vial
G Probenfläschchen
F flacon d'échantillon

vial de vidrio
E glass vial
G Glasfläschchen
F flacon en verre, fiole en verre

vibración
E vibration
G Vibration, Schwingung, Erschütterung
F vibration

sin vibración
E vibration-free
G erschütterungsfrei
F exempt de vibration

vibrador
E vibrator, shaker
G Rüttler
F secoueuse, secoueur, vibreur

vidrio de silicato bórico
E borosilicate glass
G Borosilikatglas
F verre de borosilicate

vidrio laminado
E laminated glass
G laminiertes Glas
F verre stratifié

vidrio sinterizado
E fused glass
G Sinterglas
F verre fritté

vigilancia
E monitoring
G Überwachung
F contrôle, surveillance

vigilancia continua
E continuous monitoring
G ständige Überwachung
F contrôle continu

vigilar
E monitor, to; supervise, to
G überwachen
F contrôler, surveiller

virología
E virology
G Virologie
F virologie

virus
E virus, viruses
G Virus, Viren
F virus

viscosidad
E viscosity, toughness
G Viskosität, Zähigkeit
F viscosité

viscosímetro de esfera descendiente
E falling sphere viscosimeter
G Kugelfallviskosimeter
F viscosimètre à sphère descendante

viscoso
E viscous
G viskos, dickflüssig, zähflüssig
F visqueux

visita del lugar
E on-site visit
G Ortsbesichtigung
F visite sur site

visualizar
E visualise, to
G sichtbarmachen
F visualiser

volátil
E volatile
G flüchtig
F volatile

componentes volátiles
E volatile components
G flüchtige Bestandteile
F composants volatiles

no volátil
E non-volatile
G nicht flüchtig
F non-volatile

volatilización
E volatilisation
G Verflüchtigung
F volatilisation

volatilizar(se)
E volatilise, to; strip, to; evaporate, to
G sich verflüchtigen, ausdampfen, abdampfen
F volatiliser, passer à la vapeur, évaporer, faire évaporer, faire s'évaporer

volcar
E tilt, to
G kippen
F basculer

voltaje de funcionamiento
E operating voltage
G Betriebsspannung
F voltage, tension de régime

voltímetro
E voltmeter
G Spannungsmesser
F voltmètre

volumen de bucle
E loop volume
G Schleifenvolumen
F volume de la boucle

volumen de carrera del émbolo
E stroke volume
G Hubvolumen
F volume de course

volumen de distribución
E dispensing volume
G Verteilungsvolumen
F volume de délivrance

volumen de inyección
E injection volume
G Einspritzvolumen
F volume d'injection

volumen de negocios
E turnover, sales
G Umsatz
F chiffre d'affaires

volumen de producción
E output
G Ausstoß (Menge)
F niveau de production, niveau de rendement

volumen de relleno
E filling volume
G Füllvolumen
F volume de charge

volumen del poro
E pore volume
G Porenvolumen
F volume d'un pore

volumen efectivo
E effective volume
G Nutzungsvolumen
F volume effectif

volumen muerto
E dead volume
G Totvolumen
F volume mort

volumen nominal
E nominal volume
G Nennvolumen
F volume nominal

volumen residual
E residual volume
G Restvolumen
F volume résiduel

volumetría
E volumetry
G Volumetrie
F volumétrie

volumetría de precipitación
E precipitation titration
G Fällungstitration
F titrage de précipitation, dosage de précipitation

volumétrico
E volumetric
G volumetrisch
F volumétrique

voluminoso
E voluminous
G voluminös
F volumineux

voluntario
E volunteer
G Proband
F volontaire

voluntario sano
E healthy volunteer
G gesunder Freiwilliger
F volontaire sain

vulnerabilidad
E vulnerability
G Anfälligkeit
F vulnérabilité

zócalo
E base, socket
G Sockel
F socle

zócalo de la pared
E wall skirting
G Wandsockel
F bordure d'un mur

zócalo triangular
E triangular skirting
G Dreikantsockel
F bordure triangulaire

zona
E range
G Bereich
F intervalle

zona permitida
E acceptable range
G zulässiger Bereich
F intervalle autorisé

zona de acceso controlado
E controlled access area
G kontrollierter Zugangsbereich
F zone d'accès contrôlé

zona de acceso limitado
E limited access area
G Bereich mit eingeschränktem Zugang
F zone d'accès limité

zona de adherencia
E splice point
G Klebestelle
F aire de collage

zona de atmósfera controlada
E climate-controlled area
G Bereich mit kontrolliertem Klima
F zone d'atmosphère contrôlée

zona de detección
E detection range
G Detektionsbereich
F zone de détection

zona de expulsión
E reject position
G Auswurfstelle
F emplacement de l'éjection

zona de medición
E measuring range
G Meßbereich
F gamme de mesure

zona de relleno
E filling section
G Füllbereich
F zone de remplissage

zueco distribuidor
E feed shoe
G Füllschuh
F sabot distributeur

zumo (vegetal)
E juice
G Saft
F jus